DISEASES OF THE PITUITARY

CONTEMPORARY ENDOCRINOLOGY

P. Michael Conn, SERIES EDITOR

6. ***G Protein-Coupled Receptors and Disease,*** edited by *ALLEN M. SPIEGEL,* 1997
5. ***Natriuretic Peptides in Health and Disease,*** edited by *WILLIS K. SAMSON AND ELLIS R. LEVIN,* 1997
4. ***Endocrinology of Critical Disease,*** edited by *K. PATRICK OBER,* 1997
3. ***Diseases of the Pituitary:*** *Diagnosis and Treatment,* edited by *MARGARET E. WIERMAN*, 1997
2. ***Diseases of the Thyroid,*** edited by*LEWIS E. BRAVERMAN,* 1997
1. ***Endocrinology of the Vasculature,*** edited by *JAMES R. SOWERS*, 1996

Diseases of the Pituitary

Diagnosis and Treatment

Edited by

Margaret E. Wierman, MD

University of Colorado Health Sciences Center and Veterans Affairs Medical Center, Denver, CO

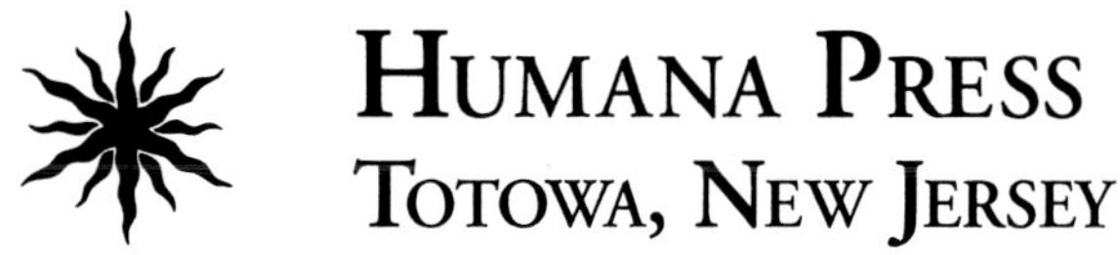

Humana Press
Totowa, New Jersey

999 Riverview Drive, Suite 208
Totowa, New Jersey 07512

For additional copies, pricing for bulk purchases, and/or information about other Humana titles, contact Humana at the above address or at any of the following numbers: Tel: 201-256-1699; Fax: 201-256-8341; E-mail: humana@mindspring.com or visit our website at http://www.humanapress.com

This publication is printed on acid-free paper. ∞
ANSI Z39.48-1984 (American National Standards Institute)
Permanence of Paper for Printed Library Materials.

Printed in the United States of America. 10 9 8 7 6 5 4 3 2 1

Library of Congress Cataloging in Publication Data

Diseases of the Pituitary/edited by Margaret E. Wierman.
p. cm.—(Contemporary endocrinology; 3)
Includes index.
ISBN 0-89603-364-3 (alk. paper)
1. Pituitary gland—Diseases. I. Wierman, Margaret E. II. Series: Contemporary endocrinology (Totowa, NJ) 3. [DNLM: 1. Pituitary Diseases—diagnosis. 2. Pituitary Diseases—therapy. WK 550 D611 1997]
RC658.D55 1997
616.4'7—dc21
DNLM/DLC
for Library of Congress

97-16899
CIP

PREFACE

The goal of *Pituitary Disease: Diagnosis and Treatment* is to provide a comprehensive overview of the normal function of the pituitary and the diagnosis and treatment of pituitary disorders. The past decade has brought a wealth of new information concerning the physiology of hypothalamic–pituitary target-organ function, as well as a better understanding of disease states. New advances in the fields of developmental biology and molecular and structural biology have advanced our ability to diagnose and treat disorders of the pituitary gland.

In this volume, advances in basic science are reviewed as they apply to our conceptualization of the normal hypothalamic–pituitary interactions and processes that disrupt that function. As an important background, Cheryl Pickett and Arthur Gutierrez-Hartmann review the latest information concerning the mechanisms controlling pituitary differentiation, which has shed new light on the underlying defects in congenital hypopituitarism. Mary Lee Vance then reviews the approach to deficiency states that result in a lack of all anterior pituitary hormones. Next, Virginia Sarapura outlines the latest information concerning prolactin biology, followed by a strategy for the evaluation of patients with hyperprolactinemia by Janet Schlecte. Ian Chapman and Michael Thorner update the current advances in our understanding of the control of growth hormone production, while Mary Hunter and Ron Rosenfeld review the approach to deficiency states and Ilan Shimon and Shlomo Melmed review the diagnosis and therapy of acromegaly. The newest information on the normal physiology of ACTH is reviewed by Lawrence Crapo and Richard Dorin and the evaluation and treatment options in glucocorticoid states is outlined by Maria Magiakou, George Mastorakos, and George Chrousos. The latest data on the normal function of the hypothalamic–pituitary–gonadal axis is presented by François Pralong and William Crowley and the approach to deficiency states by Corrine Welt and Janet Hall. A discussion of the newest approach to the diagnosis and treatment of glycoprotein pituitary tumors is presented in chapters on alpha-subunit tumors by Tamis Bright and E. Chester Ridgway, LH and FSH tumors by Eun Jig Lee and Larry Jameson, and TSH tumors by Mary Samuels. The update on normal TSH function is provided by Joshua Safer and Fred Wondisford. In addition to tumors, infiltrative diseases of the pituitary provide a challenge to the clinician and are reviewed by Mike McDermott. Importantly, a review of new advances in pituitary imaging is provided by John Stears. An approach to the appropriate surgical intervention in pituitary disorders is reviewed by Kevin Lillehei, and the invaluable aid of careful immunohistochemical analysis of surgical specimens in the appropriate diagnosis and treatment of pituitary disease is discussed by Bette DeMasters.

By presenting the newest information on the normal physiology of pituitary hormones, coupled with discussions by acknowledged experts on the approach to the diagnosis and treatment of pituitary disorders, we hope to broaden the reader's fund of knowledge in a concise single text. This work will serve as a reference for students and fellows in training, as well as an update for both basic scientists and clinicians interested in pituitary disease.

We thank the many contributors to this volume, without whose major efforts this book would not be possible.

Margaret E. Wierman, MD

CONTENTS

CONTRIBUTORS

TAMIS M. BRIGHT, MD, *Division of Endocrinology, Texas Tech University, El Paso, TX*
IAN M. CHAPMAN, MD, *Department of Medicine, University of Virginia Health Sciences Center, Charlottesville, VA*
GEORGE P. CHROUSOS, MD, *Division of Developmental Endocrinology, NIH, Bethesda, MD*
LAWRENCE M. CRAPO, MD, PHD, *Department of Medicine, Santa Clara Valley Medical Center, San Jose, CA*
WILLIAM F. CROWLEY, MD, *Division of Reproductive Endocrinology, Massachusetts General Hospital, Reproductive Endocrinology Sciences Center, Boston, MA*
RICHARD DORIN, MD, *Division of Endocrinology, VAMC, Albuquerque, NM*
JANET E. HALL, MD, *Department of Medicine, National Center for Infertility Research, Massachusetts General Hospital, Boston, MA*
ARTHUR GUTIERREZ-HARTMANN, MD, *Division of Endocrinology, University of Colorado Health Sciences Center, Denver, CO*
MAYA K. HUNTER, MD, *Division of Endocrinology, Oregon Health Sciences University, Portland, OR*
J. LARRY JAMESON, MD, *Division of Endocrinology and Molecular Medicine, Northwestern University Medical School, Chicago, IL*
B. K. KLEINSCHMIDT-DEMASTERS, MD, *Department of Pathology, University of Colorado Health Sciences Center, Denver, CO*
EUN JIG LEE, MD, *Department of Medicine, Northwestern University Medical School, Chicago, IL*
KEVIN O. LILLEHEI, MD, *Department of Neurosurgery, University of Colorado Health Sciences Center, Denver, CO*
MARIA ALEXANDRA MAGIAKOU, MD, *Division of Pediatric Endocrinology, NICHD, NIH, Bethesda, MD*
GEORGE MASTORAKOS, MD, *Division of Pediatric Endocrinology, NICHD, NIH, Bethesda, MD*
MICHAEL T. MCDERMOTT, MD, *Department of Medicine, University of Colorado Health Sciences Center, Denver, CO*
SHLOMO MELMED, MD, *Department of Medicine, Cedars-Sinai Medical Center, Los Angeles, CA*
CHERYL A. PICKETT, MD, *Department of Medicine, University of Colorado Health Sciences Center, Denver, CO*
FRANCOIS P. PRALONG, MD, *Division of Endocrinology, Massachusetts General Hospital, Reproductive Endocrinology Science Center, Boston, MA*
E. CHESTER RIDGWAY, MD, *Department of Medicine, University of Colorado Health Sciences Center, Denver, CO*
RON G. ROSENFELD, MD, *Department of Pediatrics, Oregon Health Sciences University, Portland, OR*
JOSHUA D. SAFER, MD, *Department of Medicine, Beth Israel Hospital, Boston, MA*
MARY H. SAMUELS, MD, *Department of Medicine, Oregon Health Sciences University, Portland, OR*

VIRGINIA D. SARAPURA, MD, *Department of Medicine, University of Colorado Health Sciences Center, Denver, CO*
JANET A. SCHLECHTE, MD, *Department of Internal Medicine, University of Iowa, Iowa City, IA*
ILAN SHIMON, MD, *Department of Medicine, Cedars-Sinai Medical Center, Los Angeles, CA*
JOHN STEARS, MD, *Department of Radiology, University of Colorado Health Sciences Center, Denver, CO*
MICHAEL O. THORNER, MD, *Department of Medicine, University of Virginia Health Sciences Center, Charlottesville, VA*
MARY LEE VANCE, MD, *Department of Medicine, Division of Endocrinology, University of Virginia Health Sciences Center, Charlottesville, VA*
CORRINE K. WELT, MD, *Department of Medicine, National Center for Infertility Research, Massachusetts General Hospital, Boston, MA*
FREDRIC E. WONDISFORD, MD, *Thyroid Unit, Department of Medicine, Harvard Medical School, Beth Israel Hospital, Boston, MA*

1 Molecular and Cellular Ontogeny of Distinct Pituitary Cell Types

Cheryl A. Pickett, MD, PHD,
and Arthur Gutierrez-Hartmann, MD

CONTENTS

INTRODUCTION

The development of the anterior pituitary gland has been studied extensively over several decades. With its five distinct cell types, the anterior pituitary provides a model system for investigations of the mechanisms involved in cellular commitment and tissue-specific gene expression. In recent years these studies have begun to yield fascinating information that will be valuable to our general understanding of the molecular interactions that take place during differentiation. In this chapter, we will review the current state of knowledge concerning the role of trophic/growth factors and hormones, the nuclear transcription factors, and the genetic elements required for normal development of the five distinct cell types of the anterior pituitary. We will also discuss the molecular basis of abnormal differentiation/development of the human pituitary and the potential role that aberrancy of these mechanisms may play in certain pituitary disorders. This is a broad topic, and we cannot do justice to all the many invaluable studies that have contributed to our understanding of pituitary development; instead we will concentrate on those areas in which our knowledge is most complete.

From: *Contemporary Endocrinology, Vol. 3: Diseases of the Pituitary: Diagnosis and Treatment*
Edited by M. E. Wierman Humana Press Inc., Totowa, NJ

Pituitary ontogeny has been most extensively examined in the mouse and rat. Much less is known about the timing of events during human pituitary development, although in general, the appearance of anatomical structures, hormones, and regulatory factors appears to follow relatively similar temporal patterns. We will be presenting data primarily derived from studies in the mouse and rat but, where possible, will include information on human pituitary development. Interpretation of ontological studies is significantly complicated by disparate criteria for gestational age, as well as by the multiple approaches and methods utilized. Hence, we will attempt to point out where various studies differ and analyze potential explanations for these discrepancies. Much has been accomplished in identifying crucial factors involved in development of the anterior pituitary. However, a clear understanding of the temporal appearance of these factors and the interplay between them during differentiation of the phenotypically distinct cells of the pituitary remains to be elucidated.

ANATOMICAL AND CYTOLOGICAL DEVELOPMENT

Anatomical Development of the Anterior Pituitary

The adult pituitary gland is made up of an anterior lobe (adenohypophysis) and a posterior lobe (neurohypophysis). The anterior lobe has three components: the pars distalis, pars intermedia, and pars tuberalis. In adults, the pars distalis is the main source of anterior pituitary hormone secretion. The posterior lobe consists primarily of the pars nervosa and the pituitary stalk or infundibulum. The anterior pituitary gland arises from a structure known as Rathke's pouch, which first appears as an invagination in the oral ectoderm (stomadeal epithelium), anterior to the roof of the primitive mouth on embryonic d 8.5 in the mouse (E_m 8.5) *(1–3)* or d 12 in the rat (E_r 12) *(4)* (Fig. 1). By E_m 12 and E_r 14, Rathke's pouch detaches from the oral epithelium, becomes an independent structure, and shows signs of cellular proliferation. The ventral epithelium of Rathke's pouch gives rise to the pars distalis, whereas the dorsal epithelium gives rise to the pars intermedia. The two structures can be clearly identified by E_m 14 (E_r 16 in the rat) *(1–4)*. The posterior lobe of the pituitary arises as an outpouching from the floor of the third ventricle and hence is an anatomic extension of the central nervous system. Direct contact between the developing Rathke's pouch and the floor of the diencephalon can be observed by E_m 10. Outpouching of the floor of the third ventricle commences over the next several days, forming the infundibular recess. The lumen of this diverticulum narrows and begins to be obliterated by E_m 15.5 *(1–3)*.

In the human, Rathke's pouch begins to form around the fourth and fifth fetal weeks and the anterior wall of the pituitary primordium begins to contact the diencephalon *(5)*. At the sixth fetal week, formation of the diencephalon diverticulum commences and continuity between Rathke's pouch and the primitive oral cavity is lost. Pituitary development is essentially complete by the 14th week of gestation. One significant difference between human pituitary development and that of the rodent is that the major events of differentiation appear to be accomplished during the first trimester in the human, whereas in the rodent differentiation of the pituitary begins at approximately midgestation and are not completed until after birth.

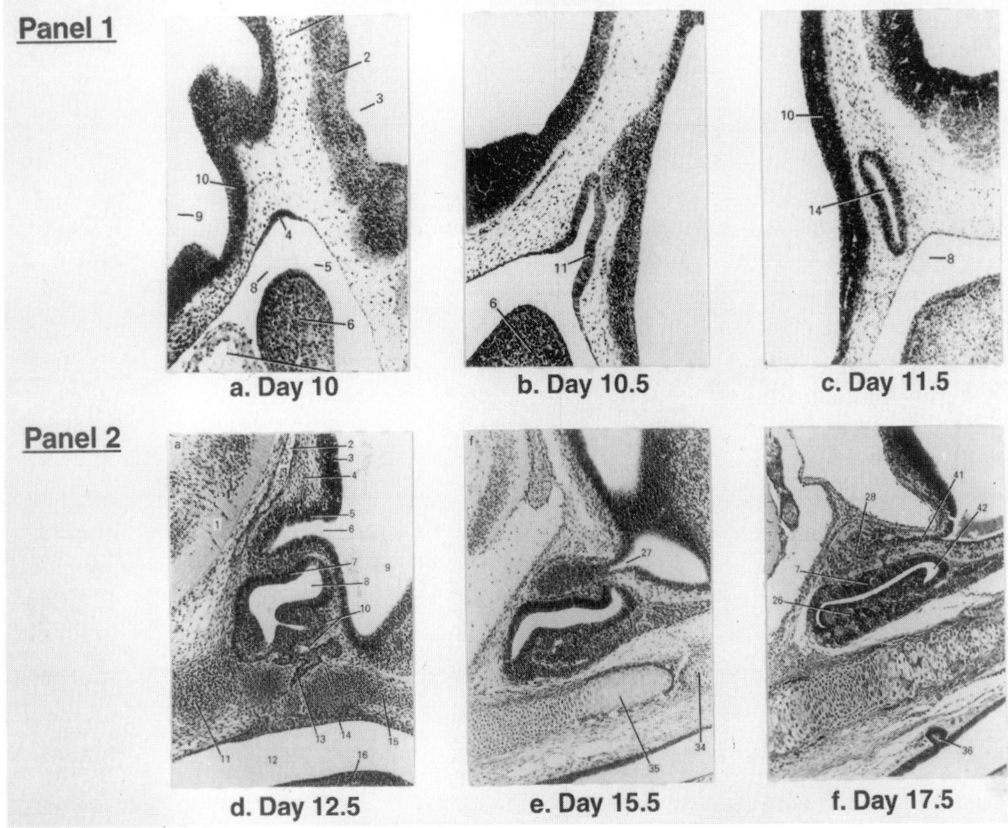

Fig. 1. Pituitary Development in the Fetal Mouse.

Panel 1 **(a-c)**

1. Cephalic mesenchyme.
2. Neuroepithelial cells forming the wall of the hindbrain.
3. Fourth ventricle.
4. Peripheral boundary of entrance to Rathke's pouch.
5. Rostral part of pharyngeal region of foregut.
6. Mandibular component of first branchial arch.
8. Oropharynx.
9. Third ventricle.
10. Neuroepithelial cells forming the wall of the diencephalon.
11. Ectodermal cells lining Rathke's pouch.
14. Lumen of Rathke's pouch.

Panel 2 **(d-f).**

2. Basilar artery.
3. Wall of diencephalon (hypothalamus).
4. Cephalic mesenchyme tissue.
5. Wall of infundibular recess of third ventricle.
6. Entrance to infundibular recess.
7. Pars intermedia.
8. Ectodermally lined lumen of Rathke's pouch.
9. Third ventricle.
10. Early evidence of vascular differentiation.
11. Mesenchymal condensation.
12. Oropharynx.
13. Remnant of connecting stalk between roof of oropharynx and Rathke's pouch.
14. Endodermal lining of roof of pharyngeal region of oropharynx.
15. Mesenchymal condensation.
16. Dorsal surface of tongue.
26. Pars anterior.
27. Entrance to infundibular recess reduced to narrow slit.
28. Pars nervosa—lumen now obliterated.
34. Cartilage primordium of presphenoid bone.
35. Cartilage primordium of postphenoid bone.
36. "Pharngeal" pituitary.
41. Stalk of pituitary.
42. Narrow cleft representing remnant of lumen of Rathke's pouch.

(Reproduced with permission from Kaufman, MH. *The Atlas of Mouse Development,* Academic Press, London, 1992.)

Vascular Development

Development of the vascular supply to the anterior pituitary is of particular interest in that many hypothalamic trophic factors and circulating hormones are known to affect anterior pituitary hormone synthesis and secretion in the adult state and hence, may be crucial in the development of the anterior pituitary. The adult hypothalamo-hypophysial vascular system is comprised of a network of capillaries lying on the surface of the median eminence (ME), from which superficial and deep capillary loops arise. This plexus is supplied by several arteries: the superior hypophysial arteries from the internal carotid arteries, the posterior infundibular arteries, and a branch from the posterior communicating artery. The blood supply to the pars distalis consists of several long portal vessels that arise from the capillary plexus of the ME and multiple short portal vessels from the posterior pituitary. In the adult, the pars distalis receives no major direct arterial blood supply. Rather, the pars distalis receives venous blood directly via this capillary plexus from the hypothalamus (70%) or from the posterior pituitary (30%). Development of the vascular supply of the pituitary has been studied extensively in both the mouse and rat. Immature blood vessels are detectable at E_r 14 on the surface of the ME and pars distalis *(1,6)*. However, vascularization of the interior of the pars distalis is not evident until E_m 16–18 and the portal vessels do not begin to develop until E_m 17–18. Deep capillary loops do not reach the internal layer of the ME until postnatal (p.n.) days 1–2 *(1)*. Whereas the adult hypothalamo-hypophysial portal system is not achieved until 2–3 wk postnatally, these studies suggest that during the early stages of pituitary development, a vascular link between the infundibular process and the pars distalis may exist across the surface of the developing pituitary *(1,6)*. Since the first axonal terminals from the hypothalamus reach the ME at E_m 16, such a superficial capillary link could, potentially, provide the anatomical basis for a hypothalamic humoral controlling mechanism as early as E_m 17. Finally, the studies of Dearden and others *(1)* suggest that early in development (E_m 16) there is a direct arterial supply from the internal carotids to the developing pars distalis, which would provide an avenue for circulating hormones to reach the pituitary. Whereas these vascular connections are established relatively early, at least some of the crucial events in pituitary cell differentiation would appear to precede them, and hence may occur independently of hypothalamic growth factors or circulating hormones.

Distinct Cell Types of the Anterior Pituitary— Temporal Appearance

Immunohistochemical studies indicate that five phenotypically distinct hormone secreting cell types appear during anterior pituitary ontogeny (for earlier reviews, *see* refs. *7–10*). These cell types are believed to arise from one common lineage. They include, in order of initial appearance (in the rat and mouse): corticotrophs, producing POMC; thyrotrophs, producing the β-subunit (β-SU) of TSH (TSHβ); gonadotrophs, producing the β-SU of FSH (FSHβ) and of LH (LHβ); somatotrophs, producing GH; and lactotrophs, producing PRL. The hormones TSH, LH, and FSH are comprised of a common α-glycoprotein subunit (α-GSU) and distinct β-subunits. Of note, a subset of cells, referred to as somatolactotrophs, appear to maintain the ability to produce both

GH and PRL into adult life. A sixth, nonhormone secreting population of cells is also found within the adult anterior pituitary. These "folliculo-stellate" cells are thought to be of neuroectoderm origin due to their morphology and immunostaining with glial markers *(11)*.

In the rat, the first hormonal evidence of pituitary organ commitment appears to be the appearance of the α-GSU of the glycoprotein hormones (TSH, LH, and FSH). mRNA transcripts for the α-GSU can be detected on E_r 11.5 *(12)*. Transcripts for pro-opiomelanocortin (POMC) are detected at E_r 13–14, TSHβ at E_r 14.5, LHβ at E_r 16.5, and FSHβ at E_r 17.5 *(12)* (Table 1). The GH transcripts are detectable at 17.5–18.5 d and PRL at 18.5 d. Immunohistochemical studies by Watanabe in the rat *(4)*, suggest a close correlation between appearance of mRNA and detectable levels of immunoreactive hormone (on or within 1d of mRNA detectability). Histological and electron microscopy studies in the mouse indicate that the appearance of hormone immunoreactivity correlates well with granulation of cells and with active secretory function (except in the case of somatotrophs, in which secretory activity lagged several weeks behind appearance of immunoreactivity) *(1)*.

The differentiation of specific cell types has also been studied in the human fetal pituitary. The *in situ* immunohistochemical studies of Ikeda et al. *(5)* and of Asa et al. *(13)*, indicate that ACTH can be detected at 8–9 wk gestation; GH at 8–13 wk; α-GSU at 9 wk; and TSHβ and FSHβ staining can be detected at 12–13 wk. The two groups differed considerably on the timing of appearance of LHβ and PRL. Asa et al. *(13)* observed both hormones at 12 wk gestation, whereas Ikeda et al. *(5)* were unable to detect LHβ or PRL until 21 wk. Recent studies by Asa et al. *(14)* of secretion of fetal pituitaries in primary culture, correlated well with this laboratory's *in situ* data. Studies examining the appearance of mRNA by *in situ* hybridization in the human fetus have not yet been reported. When compared to data in the fetal rodent, GH and PRL expression in the human would appear to be present considerably earlier in gestation, relative to the gonadotrophins and TSH. Especially interesting is the appearance of GH immunoreactivity at a stage just shortly after the appearance of ACTH and considerably before the appearance of the gonadotrophins. Further investigation will be necessary to substantiate this difference and to establish its significance.

Distinct Cell Types—Topological Development

There appears to be a definite topological development of the specific pituitary cell phenotypes as demonstrated in several studies *(4,12)*. These studies are intriguing in that they potentially provide clues as to the role of local and circulating factors in initial pituitary differentiation. The nearby mesoderm and neuroectoderm may well provide paracrine factors that function as initial signals for pituitary differentiation. Some of these paracrine factors will be discussed in more detail in the next section. In addition, this adherence to a specific topological pattern of development could relate to exposure to circulating factors or to substances secreted by the differentiating pituitary cells themselves. Clearly, further investigation in these areas is needed to establish the mechanisms dictating the topological development of specific cell types.

Table 1
Development of the Rat Anterior Pituitary

Embryonic day	*8*	*9*	*12*	*13*	*14*	*15*	*16*	*17*	*18*	*20*	*Postnatal*
Anatomy	Rathke's pouch appears		Rathke's pouch detaches		Separate pars distalis and pars intermedia		First HTH axons appear in ME				
Vascular development					Superficial immature vessels—pars distalis		Arterial connection to internal cartoid artery	Deep vessels—pars distalis	Portal vessels appear		Deep capillar loops tc ME 1–2d
Anterior pituitary hormones			α-GSU (E 11.5)		POMC	TSHβ		LHβ	GH FSHβ PRL		
HTH hormone receptors						CRHR[a]		GRHR[a]	GnRHR[a]		
Growth factors, hormones and receptors			FGF[a]			GR	ER[a,b]		GRH[a]	CRH[a]	
Transacting factors	Oct-1[b]	P-LIM[b]		SF-1[a,b]	Pit-1[c] TEF	—	Pit-1[c]				

[a]Data are from the fetal mouse.
[b]Appearance of immunoreactive protein (all other data indicates mRNA).
[c]*See text*. There is some controversy concerning the timing of appearance of Pit-1 mRNA transcripts.

THE ROLE OF GROWTH FACTORS AND HORMONES IN PITUITARY DIFFERENTIATION

The hypothalamic trophic factors, growth hormone releasing hormone (GRH), corticotroph releasing hormone (CRH), gonadotrophin releasing hormone (GnRH), and thyrotrophin releasing hormone (TRH), are known to stimulate the synthesis and secretion of hormones from their respective target cells in the adult pituitary. These trophic factors also promote expansion of populations of their target cells and in some cases act as mitogens. In addition to the hypothalamic trophic factors, several other hormones, neurotransmitters, and growth factors have been implicated in pituitary development. These include, but perhaps are not limited to dopamine, somatostatin, vasopressin, estrogen, thyroid hormone, inhibins and activins, glucocorticoids, retinoic acid, insulin and the insulin-like growth factors (IGFs), nerve growth factor (NGF), epidermal growth factor (EGF), the transforming growth factors (TGFs), and the basic fibroblast growth factors (bFGFs).

The Hypothalamic Trophic Factors

Considerable information as to the role of the hypothalamic trophic hormones in regulation of pituitary hormone gene expression and expansion of specific committed cell types has been obtained in recent years using molecular genetic approaches. In the case of somatotrophs, GRH has clearly been shown to mediate activation of GH gene expression *(15,16)*, although an understanding of the exact mechanism involved has been hampered by the lack of GRH receptors (GRHR) in established pituitary cell lines *(17)*. Evidence obtained utilizing a transgenic mouse model overexpressing GRHR (*see* Table 2) has demonstrated that GRH also acts to expand populations of both somatolactotrophs and somatotrophs *(18–21)*. It is, however, the discovery and characterization of several spontaneously occurring dwarf mouse phenotypes with abnormalities in expression of the GRHR that has been particularly valuable in defining the role of GRH in the differentiation of somatolactotrophs. (These and several other mouse gene mutations affecting pituitary development are summarized in Table 2.) Homozygous *little* (lit/lit), Snell (dw/dw), and Ames (df/df) mice all appear normal in size, at birth, but demonstrate severe dwarfism within several months after birth. The *little* mouse, which is approximately two-thirds the size of normal mice and exhibits somatotroph hypoplasia with a profound decrease in pituitary GH mRNA and protein, results from a mutation in the GRHR gene *(22,23)*. In addition, a decrease in PRL synthesis has been observed in these mice. The Snell and Ames mice exhibit a more severe dwarfism and hypocellularity of the anterior pituitary *(22,24–26)*. Somatotrophs, lactotrophs, and thyrotrophs are all significantly diminished, and in addition to their dwarf phenotype, these mice are hypothyroid and infertile. The Snell dwarf appears to result from a mutation in the gene for Pit-1/GHF-1 transcription factor. Although the underlying gene defect in the Ames mouse remains unclear, Pit-1/GHF-1 is also deficient in these animals *(22,24,27)*. As discussed in detail in the section entitled the POU Domain Gene Family, Pit-1/GHF-1 appears to be necessary for expression of the GRHR gene *(28,29)*. In both the Snell and Ames dwarf phenotypes, mice fail to respond to GRH and fail to express the GRHR *(22,24,27,29)*. Hence, the GRHR is necessary for optimal development of the GH, PRL, and TSH cell types of the anterior pituitary *(22,23,27)*.

Table 2
Mouse Gene Mutations Affecting Pituitary Development/Hormone Expression

Mutant designation	*Gene/ domain*	*Chromosome/ mutation*	*Functional defect*	*Phenotype/ hormonal deficit*	*Anatomic defect*	*Inheritance*	*Reference*
Little mouse (lit/lit)	GRHR (N-term extra cellular domain)	Chromosome 6 D60G	GRHR not expressed or incompetent binding	Dwarf (2/3 normal) ↓ GH ↓ PRL ↓ # GH cells	Hypoplasia	Autorecessive	Lin *(23)* Cheng *(22)*
Snell mouse (dw/dw)	Pit-1	Chromosome 16 W261C	Pit-1 low to absent ↓ GRHR	Dwarf (1/3 normal) Infertile, hypothyroid ↓ GH, PRL, and TSH ↓ # GH, PRL, and TSH cells	Hypoplasia	Autorecessive	O'Hara *(25)* Camper *(28)* Cheng *(22)*
Ames mouse (df/df)		Chromosome 11 Deletion exons IV and V. Missing POU spec.- and homeodomains of Pit-1	Pit-1 absent ↓ GRHR	Dwarf (1/3 normal) Infertile, hypothyroid ↓ GH, PRL, and TSH ↓ # GH, PRL, and TSH cells	Hypoplasia	Autorecessive	Buckwalter *(24)* Gage *(27)* Cheng *(22)*
Jackson mouse	Pit-1	Chromosome 16 Genomic rearrangement	Truncated Pit-1 No DNA binding	Dwarf		Autorecessive	Camper *(28)* Li *(30)*

rdw mouse				Dwarf Hypothyroid ↓ GH and PRL ↑ TSHβ mRNA	Hypoplasia	Autorecessive	Koto *(174)* Shibayama *(179)* Ono *(178)*
Others:							
Spontaneous dwarf (dr)				Dwarf			Okuma *(177)*
Pygmy mouse (pg)				Dwarf			King *(173)*
Transgenic—hGRH mouse	hGRH	Metallothionein/hGRH fusion gene	hGRH overexpression	↑ growth - ↑ wt organomegaly ↑ GH secretion ↑ # GH cells	Hyperplasia and adenomas	Autodominant	Hammer *(172)* Mayo *(19)* Lloyd *(20)*
Toxic fusion construct—GH mouse		GH promoter—diphtheria toxin	GH promoter activation produces diphtheria toxin	Dwarf No GH cells ↑ # PRL cells			Behringer *(171)*
Oncogene, construct—Pit-1		Pit-1 promoter—SV 40 T antigen	Pit-1 promoter activation produces SV 40 T antigen	Pituitary tumors No GH, PRL, or TSHβ. No αGSU	Pituitary tumors		Lew *(175)*
Transgenic—CREB	CREB		Nonphosphorylatable CREB	Dwarf ↓ GH			Struthers *(97)*

The observation that these GRHR deficient mice are not completely devoid of somatotrophs suggests that some somatotrophs may arise via a GRH/GRHR-independent mechanism *(27,30)*. Indeed, Lin et al. *(23)* have demonstrated that somatotrophs arise in a GRHR-independent manner in the Snell mouse, suggesting that GRH is not required for initial stem cell differentiation, but becomes crucial later in development for continued replication or for cell survival. Another line of evidence to support this contention is provided by studies in human fetal pituitary cell primary cultures by Asa et al. *(14)*. Secretion of GH from pituitary cells in culture was detectable at 8–9 wk of gestation, but at this stage there was no significant response to GRH. At 12–13 wk, GH was clearly stimulated by the addition of GRH, suggesting that the somatotroph commitment precedes GRH responsiveness.

Corticotrophs also increase in number after exposure to CRH both in vivo and in culture *(31–33)*, and there is evidence that CRH increases their mitotic activity *(32)*. The studies of Asa et al. *(14)* in cultured human fetal pituitary cells suggest that, like GRH, CRH responsiveness lags behind the actual secretion of ACTH (by 5–6 wk). However, Hotta et al. *(34)*, have described coincident basal and CRH-stimulated secretion of POMC products (β-endorphin) in the fetal rat pituitary beginning at E_r 15 (the earliest day examined). The CRH immunoreactivity itself was not detected in the fetal pituitary until E_r 19.5 suggesting that the ability of the corticotrophs to respond to CRH was present prior to significant delivery of this factor to the anterior pituitary *(34)*.

The regulation of gonadotrophin gene expression by GnRH has proven difficult to define; however, it would appear that specific pulse frequencies of GnRH can selectively stimulate α-GSU, LHβ, or FSHβ transcription *(35,36)*. Chronic GnRH stimulation inhibits FSHβ and LHβ transcription *(36)*. The temporal pattern of pulsatile GnRH release to the developing pituitary and gonadotrophin response to this has not been well defined. TRH has been found to stimulate expression of both the α-GSU and TSHβ genes in thyrotrophs *(37,38)*. In somatolactotrophs, TRH stimulates PRL gene transcription while inhibiting expression of GH *(39)*. TRH appears to have complex effects upon somatolactotrophs, acting either to promote or to inhibit proliferation depending upon the concentration of TRH administered *(40)*. Little data are available as to the role of TRH during differentiation of thyrotrophs, lactotrophs, or somatotrophs. As with GH and ACTH synthesis, the studies of Asa et al. *(14)* suggest that in human fetal pituitary cells in culture, α-GSU, LHβ, and TSHβ immunoreactivity appear prior to the onset of responsiveness to their respective hypothalamic hormones.

Other hypothalamic and pituitary factors may play a role in differentiation of the pituitary cell subtypes. These include vasopressin, which has been implicated in control of ACTH, β-endorphin, and PRL, and two inhibitory factors, dopamine and somatostatin, with important functions in regulating pituitary gene expression and/or secretion. Dopamine, the predominant inhibitor of PRL secretion, is in fact present in high concentration in the human fetal hypothalamus by 15 wk of gestation *(41)*; however, its role, if any, in regulating differentiation is unknown. Messenger RNA for all five receptor subtypes of somatostatin (SRIH), a potent inhibiter of GH and PRL secretion *(42,43)*, has been identified in the pituitary *(44,45)*; however, only receptor types and II and V are expressed to any significant extent. In normal adult anterior pituitary cells, somatostatin receptors can be found only on somatotrophs and thyrotrophs; however, gonadotrophin and α-GSU producing pituitary adenomas have been described that express somatostatin receptors *(46–48)*. It is presently unclear whether negative regulation by dopamine or somatostatin is involved in maintaining normal development of the pituitary.

Paracrine/Autocrine Growth Factors

The role of growth factors, encountered from direct contact with mesenchymal tissue or from endogenous secretion, in regulating cell-specific differentiation in the pituitary has not been extensively studied. However, potential roles for nerve growth factor (NGF), epidermal growth factor (EGF), the fibroblast growth factors (FGFs), and the transforming growth factors (TGFs), including activin and inhibin, have been suggested.

Activins and inhibins are members of the transforming growth factor-β (TGF-β) family that has powerful effects on growth and differentiation *(49)*. These proteins appear to modulate activity of gonadotrophs and somatotrophs. Within the pituitary gland, both α- and β-subunits of these growth factors are synthesized by the gonadotrophs, hence, these factors have autocrine effects on gonadotrophs. Activin A stimulates growth and differentiation of gonadotroph cells, and particularly of FSH secretion *(50)*. Inhibins compete for the same classes of activin binding sites and in general antagonize the effects of activin. Activin also has paracrine effects on somatotrophs. It inhibits GRH-stimulated cAMP synthesis, GH synthesis and secretion, and somatotroph proliferation in vitro *(51,52)*. TGF-β1, a mesenchymal growth factor, is also produced in anterior pituitary tissues *(53)*. In primary cultures of lactotrophs, TGF-β1 has been shown to exert a potent inhibitory action on basal and estrogen-induced secretion of PRL *(53)*, on basal PRL mRNA levels *(54)*, and on estrogen-induced proliferation of lactotrophs *(53)*. Taken together, these findings suggest that TGF-β is a negative regulator of lactotroph activity. Secretion of other pituitary hormones (LH, FSH, GH) is not affected by TGF-β1 *(53)*. These data suggest a possible role for TGF-β in differentiation of the lactotroph phenotype. TGF-α mRNA and protein have also been described in the normal pituitary *(55)* and in pituitary tumors *(56)*, where it appears to be localized in lactotrophs and somatotrophs *(57)*. This factor is structurally and functionally related to epidermal growth factor (EGF) and appears to act through the EGF receptor *(58)*. Although these data suggest that the TGF family of growth factors may be important in pituitary differentiation, the temporal appearance of these factors and of cellular response to them has not been studied.

Low levels of NGF mRNA have been detected in the pituitary and NGF-like immunoreactivity has been found within the gland. Furthermore, both somatolactotroph and lactotroph cells express receptors for NGF *(59–61)*. NGF has been shown to increase the number and rate at which mature lactotrophs appear in primary cultures of neonatal rat pituitary cells *(61)*. Overexpression of NGF in lactotrophs of transgenic mice resulted in massive lactotroph hyperplasia and late tumorogenesis *(62)*. Taken together, these data implicate NGF as a regulator of lactotroph proliferation and differentiation, however, its precise role in vivo is yet to be determined.

EGF has also been implicated in pituitary differentiation. EGF receptors have been documented to be present on all subtypes of pituitary cells *(63)*. Furthermore, mRNA for EGF is present in both somatotrophs and gonadotrophs *(63)*, suggesting that EGF may have both autocrine and paracrine functions. In the GH4/GH3 somatolactotroph cell lines, EGF appears to induce a phenotypic switch, manifested by alterations in morphology, a decrease in growth rate, and an alteration of the relative transcription of the GH and PRL genes, resulting in a significant increase in and predominance of PRL expression *(64–66)*. Several recent studies utilizing primary cell cultures, enriched in corticotrophs, suggest that EGF may act as a mitogen to corticotrophs *(31,33)* and EGF also appears to increase expression of POMC mRNA as well as ACTH secretion from these cells *(67)*. Little is known about the effects of EGF on other cell types of the anterior pituitary. Whereas these studies suggest that EGF may play a significant role in differentiation of pituitary cells during fetal development, further investigation is needed in this area.

Basic fibroblast growth factor (bFGF), a potent angiogenic factor *(68)*, is found in high concentration in the adult anterior pituitary, and has been implicated in pituitary differentiation *(69)*. The ontogeny of bFGF has been examined recently by Schechter et al. *(6)*. FGF immunostaining was demonstrated not only in perihypophyseal connective tissue (by E_r 15), but also within a subpopulation of gonadotrophs (by E_r 16), particularly those abutting developing capillaries. Thus, the temporal and spatial appearance of FGF in the developing pituitary would allow for a role in terminal differentiation events.

Circulating Hormones and Growth Factors

The temporal appearance of other hormones such as estrogen, thyroid hormone, and glucocorticoids and of their receptors in the developing pituitary is poorly characterized. These hormones will be discussed in more detail below in relation to their function as activators of specific receptor transcription factors.

TRANSCRIPTION FACTORS IN PITUITARY ONTOGENY

Several classes of transcription factors have been implicated in differentiation events. Examples that will be discussed here include the homeodomain transcription factors, of which the POU domain and LIM domain factors are a subset; and the bZIP; helix loop helix; and Zinc finger families of transcription factors. These transcription factors often exhibit tissue-specific and/or temporally restricted distribution which would appear to allow for the activation of a unique combination of target genes, resulting in a given stem cell entering a specific morphogenic pathway. The mechanisms underlying regulation of target gene expression are complicated and still poorly understood. Regulation may include both competition and cooperation between transcription factors for binding to recognition elements, posttranslational modifications affecting DNA binding or transactivation properties, and variation in the temporal pattern of expression of the transcription factors and their modifiers.

Homeodomain Transcription Factors in Pituitary Differentiation

Homeodomain transcription factors appear to be critical in specifying distinct cell fates. Pit-1/GHF-1 was the first homeobox protein shown to bind to specific DNA sequences and to activate specific genes. As a tissue-specific transcription factor whose expression is confined to the pituitary, it was the first example of a mammalian homeodomain factor regulating ontogeny of a discrete cellular phenotype.

The POU Domain Gene Family

The POU homeodomain transcription factors include Pit-1, Oct-1, Oct-2, and Unc-86. These factors share a novel motif, the POU-specific domain, upstream of the homeodomain. The discovery that specific POU domain genes are expressed selectively during the course of mammalian development suggests functions in early differentiation (for review, *see* ref. *70*).

Pit-1/GHF-1. Pit-1/GHF-1 was cloned *(71,72)* based on knowledge of the sequence of critical regulatory regions of both the GH and PRL genes *(73,74)*. Pit-1 is expressed exclusively in the anterior pituitary in GH, PRL, and TSH producing cells. The exact timing of appearance of Pit-1 transcripts is somewhat controversial. Simmons et al. *(12)* reported that Pit-1 transcripts were undetectable on E_r 13.5 but were present at E_r 15.5 in the rat embryo, whereas Dolle et al. *(75)* were able to detect transcripts at E_r 13.5 with a marked increase at E_r 14 and 15. Both groups reported that Pit-1 protein could not be detected until E_r 15. The relative expression of Pit-1 mRNA appeared to increase progressively through postnatal d 10 *(12)*. Initiation of Pit-1 expression correlated both spatially and temporally with activation of its distal target genes; hence, Pit-1 appears to be selectively activated in the caudomedial part of the developing gland, preceding activation of PRL, GH, and TSHβ genes in this region *(12,75)*. The exception to this spatial correlation was the appearance of TSHβ transcripts in the rostral tip of the developing pituitary in the apparent absence of significant Pit-1 expression *(12)*, hence raising some question about the role or Pit-1 in specifying TSHβ cell ontogeny *(30,76)*. Transcripts for Pit-1 can also be detected in corticotrophs and gonadotrophs, but apparently these cells fail to express the Pit-1/GHF-1 protein *(12)*.

Several isoforms of Pit-1 have been described that result from alternative mRNA splicing. These include Pit-1β (also referred to as Pit-1a or GHF-2) *(77–79)*, and Pit-1T *(80)*. The biological significance of these various isoforms remains unclear; however, Pit-1β appears to selectively stimulate the GH promoter *(77,78)*, whereas Pit-1T selectively stimulates the TSHβ promoter *(80,81)*. Furthermore, Pit-1 and Pit-1T have synergistic effects on the TSHβ promoter *(81)*. These findings suggest that distinct isoforms may provide specificity of function within the cells in which Pit-1 is expressed.

The mechanisms involved in activation of the Pit-1 gene are of considerable interest because they may give insights into early steps in cell differentiation. Interestingly, the 5′ flanking sequence of the Pit-1 gene contains an enhancer in which five Pit-1 binding sites are located, and the proximal promoter itself contains two Pit-1 binding sites *(82)*. At least three of the Pit-1 sites within the enhancer have been shown to be important for activation of the gene, suggesting that Pit-1 positively autoregulates its own expression. In addition, binding elements for retinoic acid receptor, vitamin D3 receptor, CREB (three sites), and a cell-specific factor have been identified in the enhancer sequence. These elements may be important in initial activation of the Pit-1 gene. The Pit-1 gene is activated at the same time during gestation in dw/dw (Snell) mice as in the wild-type mouse, and Pit-1 expression was detectable in a subgroup of cells in the Snell mice until postnatal d 0 *(76)*. Since the Snell mice lack functional Pit-1 protein, these data suggest that Pit-1 autoregulation is not critical for initial activation or early maintenance events and that Pit-1-independent mechanisms must be sufficient to dictate the temporally and spatially specific patterns of expression of this transcription factor. Autoregulation by Pit-1/GHF-1 may be required later to maintain significant Pit-1 gene activation and thus the lack of the positive autoregulatory function may account for the later loss of Pit-1 gene activation in the Snell dwarf *(76)*. It has been suggested that Pit-1/GHF-1 autoregulation serves a memory function to maintain the lactotroph, thyrotroph, and somatotroph cell phenotypes *(76)*.

Pit-1 appears to play multiple roles in specifying cell phenotype and function. Pit-1 clearly has the ability to activate the PRL, GH, and TSHβ genes in vitro systems. The lack of expression of the PRL, GH, TSHβ, and GRHR genes in Pit-1 defective mice and humans suggests that Pit-1 is required for full expression of these genes in vivo. The failure of proliferation of thyrotroph, somatotroph, and lactotroph cell types in the Snell dwarf indicates that Pit-1 is also critical for proliferation and/or survival of these three cell types. Furthermore, addition of antisense oligonucleotides for Pit-1, thus decreasing Pit-1 expression, reduces the proliferation rate of rat pituitary GC cells *(83)*. The mechanisms by which Pit-1 functions as a morphogen remain to be clearly elucidated. One mechanism by which Pit-1 regulates cell proliferation is illustrated by the Snell mouse, wherein Pit-1 deficiency results in failure to express the GRHR, with the resulting phenotype demonstrating hypoplasia of GH, PRL, and TSH secreting cells. It is possible that Pit-1 regulates other genes encoding trophic factors and/or their receptors that are required for proliferation of lactotrophs, somatotrophs, and thyrotrophs. Functional interactions between Pit-1 and other morphogenic signals such as the retinoic acid receptor may also occur *(82)*.

Finally, Pit-1 clearly functions in mediating regulation of the GH, PRL, and TSHβ genes by hormones and other growth factors. Several studies have shown that the Pit-1-binding sites in the PRL gene regulatory region are required for control of PRL gene transcription by TRH, calcium, dopamine, Ras, cAMP, and phorbol esters. Similarly, Pit-1 binding sites in the TSHβ and GH genes can mediate TRH and activin responsiveness, respectively. Functional interactions between Pit-1 and other transcription factors such as the ER on the PRL promoter *(84)*, and the TR on the GH promoter *(85)*, probably contribute to restriction of certain signals to a given cell type.

Oct-1. Oct-1, another member of the POU-domain transcription factor family, appears to be expressed in a wide variety of cell types, including the anterior pituitary. In the developing mouse it is expressed much earlier that Pit-1, on E_m 8 *(86)*. Oct-1 can bind to the proximal Pit-1 binding element on the PRL promoter *(87)* as well as to similar Pit-1 binding sites in other pituitary-specific genes such as the Pit-1 gene itself *(88)*. Furthermore, Pit-1 and Oct-1 can associate, in the absence of DNA, via their POU domains. Coexpression of Pit-1 and Oct-1 results in synergistic transcriptional effects on genes under control of the native PRL promoter or of a single Pit-1 response element *(89)*. These data provide the possibility that a combinatorial pattern of heterodimeric and homodimeric interactions between these two different members of the POU-domain gene family coexpressed in the developing pituitary, could regulate differential gene activation.

LIM Homeodomain Factors

The LIM homeodomain factors include Lin 11, Isl 1, and Mec 3. This family of transcription factors appear to mediate crucial events in organogenesis and terminal differentiation. Recently, P-LIM was identified as a LIM homeobox protein that is selectively expressed in the pituitary *(90)*. P-LIM was observed in all stratified regions in which each of the five pituitary cell types initially appear. This factor appears to be expressed throughout mammalian pituitary development, but is highest at the early stage of development of Rathke's pouch, where it can be detected as early as E_r 9, and declines with time. It continues to be expressed specifically in the anterior and intermediate lobes of the pituitary in the adult mouse. It is present prior to discernible signal for α-GSU, Pit-1, and RXRγ *(90)*. P-LIM binds to and activates the promoter of the α-GSU gene *(90)*. In addition, it appears to synergize with Pit-1 in transcriptional activation of genes encoding terminal pituitary differentiation markers (Pit-1, TSHβ, and PRL) *(90)*. Although further functional analysis will be required, it is possible that this factor may exert actions during early pituitary cell commitment, either directly or by interaction with Pit-1.

bZIP Transcription Factors in Pituitary Differentiation

The bZIP family of transcription factors is characterized by a conserved DNA-binding domain, containing clusters of basic amino acids, immediately adjacent to a conserved dimerization domain. This dimerization domain contains a leucine residue at every seventh position: the leucine zipper motif. These factors can form homodimers and heterodimers with other members of the bZIP family, depending upon the compatibility of the leucine zipper domain. Included in this family of transcription factors are: the Fos-Jun transcription factors, cAMP response element binding-activating transcription factor (CREB-ATF), the CCAAT/enhancer-binding protein (C/EBP), and the thyrotroph embryonic factor (TEF)/albumin D box-binding proteins (DBP) (for review, *see* ref. *91*).

TEF

TEF was cloned based on its ability to bind to the proximal Pit-1 binding element of the PRL promoter, but may in fact be functionally more important in regulating TSHβ expression. *In situ* hybridization studies have demonstrated that TEF transcripts first appear in the rostral part of the anterior pituitary gland on E_r 14. This pattern of gene expression corresponds temporally as well as spatially to the pattern of TSHβ gene expression. This restricted pattern of TEF gene expression was maintained through E_r 16, whereas in the juvenile and adult rat, TEF transcripts were observed in several tissues. Drolet et al. *(92)* have demonstrated three independent binding domains for TEF within the proximal TSHβ promoter and TEF was able to transactivate a reporter gene under the transcriptional control of the TSHβ promoter. A TEF binding domain was also identified within the proximal PRL promoter and in the GH promoter. Although TEF was able to produce an increase in transcription of PRL and GH promoter-reporter constructs, this was to a much lesser extent than with the TSHβ promoter, suggesting that TEF may not exert substantial transcriptional effects on PRL or GH promoters in vivo *(92)*. Because of the spatial and temporal pattern of TEF expression, and its relatively selective activation of the TSHβ gene expression, it is possible that TEF functions alone or in concert with other factors to specifically establish the TSH cell, in the developing anterior pituitary gland.

CREB

Cyclic AMP (cAMP), specific CRE (cAMP response element) binding sites, and factors that bind to these sites, have been implicated in the regulation of many genes. In the human anterior pituitary, α-GSU transcription appears to be regulated by cAMP through two tandem CREs *(93)*. Of note, there is no evidence for this region conferring cAMP responsiveness in the rodent (*see* ref. *36*). Pit-1/GHF-1 gene transcription is also regulated at least in part by two CRE sites within the promoter region *(10,94)*. Since the GRHR is a G_s-linked cell surface receptor *(95,96)*, it has been hypothesized that the Pit-1/GHF-1 gene functions as the link between GRHR and increased GH gene transcription via CREB activation of Pit-1 expression. Although this has not been demonstrated directly, studies with transgenic mice, overexpressing a dominant-negative (nonphosphorylatable) variant of CREB, indicate that the loss of functional CREB results in dwarfism and somatotroph hypoplasia *(10,97)*. Interestingly, targeting of the inactive CREB transgene to lactotrophs had no effect on the expansion of this cell population. Basal CREB activity was shown to be elevated by enhanced phosphorylation in GH-secreting pituitary adenomas, some of which harbor an oncogenic Gαs mutation *(98)*. Whereas the ubiquitous nature of CRE makes it unlikely that these mechanisms control differentiation, several studies have suggested that other transcription factors may bind within the CRE region of the human α-GSU *(93,99,100)*. Hence, the CRE-binding proteins may act in concert with other transcription factors to confer tissue specificity to these CRE-regulated genes.

Helix-Loop-Helix Transcription Factors

The basic-helix-loop-helix (bHLH) class of transcriptional activators contain a conserved domain rich in basic amino acids, preceding an amphipathic α-helix, followed by a loop region, and then by a second conserved α-helix. The basic region is necessary for DNA binding, whereas the HLH domain is required for dimerization. Since bHLH proteins bind to DNA as dimers, the intact bHLH motif is required for transcriptional activation. Members of this transcription factor family bind to DNA elements containing the loose consensus sequence referred to as an E-box motif and are able to heterodimerize readily. This ability to heterodimerize is an elegant mechanism for regulating DNA binding activity, by providing both a mechanism for activation and for inhibition of transcription. Hence, other members of the bHLH family can act as inhibitors of a given factor by forming nonfunctional heterodimers. The bHLH family of transcription factors have been implicated in the establishment of a wide variety of highly differentiated cell lineages.

CUTE

Recently, Therrien and Drouin *(101)* have described an element of the proopiomelanocortin (POMC) promoter containing an E-box motif typical of binding sites for bHLH transcription factors. They were also able to identify a cell-specific E-box binding protein in nuclear extracts from a POMC expressing corticotroph tumor cell line, AtT-20 cells. This protein was named CUTE, for corticotroph upstream transcription element binding protein. The CUTE proteins appear to be specific to POMC expressing cells in that they were not found in multiple other cell lines tested, including the GH3 pituitary somatolactotroph. The temporal pattern of appearance of CUTE during pituitary development has not been examined, but it is tempting to speculate that this factor may be important in specifying differentiation of the corticotroph cell. There is also recent evidence to suggest that CUTE may synergize with a novel homeobox containing factor, Ptx 1, which appears to be restricted to POMC expressing cells during certain stages of embryogenesis *(102)*.

Id

Id, another member of the bHLH group of transcription factors, contains the HLH domain, but lacks the basic region, and thus is unable to bind to DNA on its own. It is able to heterodimerize with other bHLH proteins, inhibiting their ability to bind to DNA. In general, expression of Id-like proteins is highest during early development and decreases as tissues become more fully differentiated. Jackson et al. *(103)*, have found several factors in pituitary cell extracts that bind to a bHLH consensus sequence. These extracts were also found to contain several factors that interact with Id protein. Messenger RNA for Id was present in pituitary tumor cell lines but absent in normal adult pituitary tissue, suggesting that Id is decreased in the more differentiated pituitary cells and, hence, implying a possible role for Id-like proteins during pituitary cell differentiation *(103)*. Using Id as a functional probe, the bHLH protein, "upstream stimulating factor" (USF), which appears to be important in regulating α-GSU promoter function, was identified *(104)*.

Zinc Finger Transcription Factors

Zn-15

Recent studies of the proximal GH promoter have identified an unusually well conserved sequence between the proximal and distal Pit-1 binding sites (referred to as the GH-Z box), which, when mutated, resulted in markedly impaired GH expression *(105)*. A systematic search for factors binding this region in pituitary cells identified Zn-15, a novel transcription factor possessing an unusual DNA binding domain consisting of three Cys/His zinc fingers in the context of 12 other potential zinc fingers. Studies with GC pituitary cell nuclear extracts suggest that endogenous Zn-15 does complex with this region of the GH promoter in the GC cell. In transient transfection studies, Zn-15 expression stimulated activation of the GH promoter, whereas Pit-1 had little effect. Expression of both Zn-15 and Pit-1 simultaneously resulted in synergistic activation as compared to Zn-15 alone. These data suggest that functional interactions between Pit-1 and Zn-15 may be an important component in the regulation of GH gene expression.

Nuclear Hormone Receptors and Pituitary Gene Regulation

Nuclear hormone receptors represent one of the largest transcription factor families known (for review, *see* refs. *106,107*). They mediate the signals of a broad variety of hormones including the steroid hormones, thyroid hormones and retinoids, which will be discussed here.

SF-1. Horn et al. *(108)* have described a conserved element of the α-GSU gene, termed the gonadotropin-specific element (GSE), that interacts with a gonadotroph-specific protein. More recent data by Ingraham et al. *(109)* suggests that this factor is identical to steroidogenic factor 1 (SF-1) or adrenal 4-binding protein, a member of the nuclear hormone receptor superfamily, initially discovered in the adrenal gland *(110,111)*. In studies of mice with homozygous disruption of the Ftz-F1 gene, which encodes both SF-1 and a related isoform, immunohistochemical analysis of pituitary sections failed to detect LH, FSH, or the GnRH receptor *(109)*. In contrast, TSH, GH, PRL, ACTH, and Pit-1 protein expression were comparable to that in normal mice. Further an analysis revealed normal levels of POMC transcripts and low levels of α-GSU transcripts, whereas LHβ and FSHβ transcripts were absent in the Ftz-F1 disrupted animals. SF-1 transcripts are found specifically in the gonadotrophin-derived cell line, the αT3-1 cell, and not in cell lines derived from the hypothalamus or in other pituitary-derived cell lines. Finally, in normal pituitary cells, the patterns of expression of SF-1 and gonadotroph-specific markers (α-GSU, LHβ, FSHβ) colocalize *(109)*.

During embryogenesis, SF-1 transcripts are initially detectable at E_m 13.5 and increase to much higher levels by E_m 17.5 *(109)*. This would place the appearance of SF-1 after the onset of α-GSU expression (E 12.5), and prior to the onset of LHβ and FSHβ (E 16.5) *(12,112)*. The studies of Horn et al. *(108)* suggest that SF-1 may interact with the GSE to regulate α-GSU expression in gonadotrophs. Recently, Shupnik et al. *(133)* have demonstrated that SF-1 can bind to a specific region of the LHβ gene with sequence homology to the GSE. Taken together these data are consistent with the hypothesis that SF-1 may regulate the expression of α-GSU, LHβ, and possibly FSHβ during ontogenesis of the gonadotroph phenotype.

ER. Estrogen clearly has significant effects on the expression of gonadotrophins and prolactin and may play a role in cellular commitment. Some of the effects of estrogen on pituitary hormone expression appear to be indirectly mediated through the hypothalamus. However, several studies have demonstrated direct enhancement of βLH gene transcription in response to estradiol *(114–116)*, and the PRL gene distal enhancer requires the ligand-activated estrogen receptor in combination with Pit-1 for full activation *(12,84)*.

ER expression is detectable in all cells of the normal adult pituitary and in pituitary tumors, but is highest in gonadotrophs and lactotrophs *(117,118)*. Interestingly, ER expression was absent in GH tumors, but present in both PRL and GH/PRL producing tumors, suggesting that divergence of somatotrophs and lactotrophs might involve regulation of the ER gene. Studies of ER expression during pituitary development are limited. In mice, functional ERs are detectable in neonates; increasing in number and responsivity over the first several weeks of life *(25)*. Human fetal lactotrophs show a functional response to estrogen at 12 wk gestation *(14)*. Immunocytochemistry or *in situ* hybridization studies on fetal pituitary are needed to establish the timing of ER appearance during gestation.

GR. Glucocorticoid hormones modulate expression of many genes *(119)*. Both glucocorticoid-inducible and glucocorticoid-repressible genes have been described. In the pituitary, the most thoroughly studied effect of glucocorticoids is the repression of the POMC gene. A glucocorticoid-dependent response element mediating GR repression of POMC gene transcription has been characterized *(120)*. The region of the promoter containing this GRE also contains binding sites for several nuclear transactivating factors that appear to act synergistically in regulating POMC gene expression. Hence, the GRE most likely functions as a means to control/repress POMC gene transactivating factors. Glucocorticoids also negatively regulate α-GSU gene expression in human placental cells via interaction with a site overlapping a CRE *(100)*. In the GH3, somatolactotroph cell line, glucocorticoids have been shown to decrease PRL mRNA expression while increasing GH mRNA *(10,121)*.

The available evidence suggests that GR mRNA and immunoreactivity are present in developing fetal rat pituitary glands as early as E_r 15 (the earliest time examined) *(122)*. In the fetus, GR ligand binding properties are similar to those in the adult; however, the biological activity of the GR at this stage of development has been questioned *(123)*. Whether the GR plays a significant role in morphogenesis and initial cell commitment is unclear.

Thyroid Hormone Receptor. In the rat, the ligand-activated thyroid hormone receptor (TR) appears to be an important negative regulator of both α- and TSHβ gene transcription *(124–127)*. Like the ER and the GR, TR appears to exert its effect through interaction with other *trans*-activating factors binding in the region of a specific TR element (TRE). In contrast to TSH, GH gene expression is activated by the TR, and a specific TRE has been identified in the GH promoter *(128,129)*. Although the precise role of the TR during cellular differentiation remains to be characterized, it is possible that complex interactions between this and other transcription factors serves to define precise patterns of development.

Retinoic Acid Receptor. A retinoic acid response element (RARE) has been identified within the mouse Pit-1 gene that appears to be involved in synergistic activation of Pit-1 expression by Pit-1 and a retinoic acid receptor (RAR) *(82)*. Indeed, the RARE in the Pit-1 gene appears to be absolutely dependent upon Pit-1 for retinoic receptor function. As retinoic acid has also been implicated in control of critical aspects of organogenesis *(107,130)*, these findings have led to the suggestion that the combined action of Pit-1 and retinoic acid are required for sustained activation of the Pit-1 gene *(82)*.

The Ets Family of Transcription Factors

The Ets superfamily is a novel structural class of transactivating phosphoproteins that have important roles in the control of growth and development *(131,132)*. Recent data utilizing transient transfection in cultured pituitary and heterologous systems has suggested a synergistic interaction between Ets-1 and Pit-1 in mediating PRL promoter activity and has mapped this response to a composite element consisting of an Ets-1 binding domain and the distal Pit 1 domain on the proximal rat PRL (rPRL) promoter *(133)*. When studied in nonpituitary cells, coexpression of Pit-1 and Ets-1 resulted in marked synergistic activation of the rPRL promoter *(134)*.

Specific expression of Ets transcription factors in the anterior pituitary during embryogenesis has not been examined. However, *in situ* hybridization studies of the expression of Ets-1 and Ets-2 in the mouse suggest both tissue-specific and temporally specific patterns of expression of both these genes beginning as early as E_m 8 *(135)*. Specific studies to determine the temporal pattern of expression of Ets transcription factors and their relation to expression of Pit-1 are clearly needed.

HUMAN SYNDROMES ASSOCIATED WITH ABERRANT DEVELOPMENT OF THE ANTERIOR PITUITARY

Pituitary Deficiency Syndromes

A number of syndromes have been described in humans that are associated with abnormal pituitary function. Many of these include other neuro-opthalmological abnormalities such as septo-optic dysplasia, anencephaly, and midline craniofacial defects.

Abnormalities that are limited primarily to the pituitary have also been described, and although still somewhat poorly understood, include congenital hypopituitarism, congenital pituitary agenesis, idiopathic hypopituitarism, pituitary dwarfism, combined pituitary hormone deficiency, Kallman's syndrome, and isolated central hypothyroidism. As one may infer from the names of these disorders, considerable overlap appears to exist between these syndromes and stringent criteria for their classification have not been established.

Idiopathic and Congenital Hypopituitarism

The terms idiopathic pituitary dwarfism or idiopathic hypopituitarism have generally been used to describe patients presenting in childhood or adulthood (as opposed to infancy) with pituitary hormone deficiencies and a history of perinatal trauma or asphyxia *(136–139)*. Magnetic resonance imaging studies of these individuals have disclosed a common abnormality consisting of: an adenopophysis and sella turcica of abnormal volume and/or configuration, attenuation or transection of the pituitary stalk, and an "ectopic" neurohypophysis *(136–139)*. However, interestingly, a similar MRI image has also been described in congenital hypopituitarism, which typically presents in infancy with hypoglycemia, microgenitalia, and evidence of multiple anterior pituitary hormone deficiencies, but with the absence of a history of birth trauma *(140)*. Pituitary abnormalities in the idiopathic syndromes suggest a primary hypothalamic lesion (or a stalk lesion) as opposed to a primary pituitary lesion. In congenital hypopituitarism the response to stimulation with hypothalamic factors is more variable; some patients demonstrating a response suggestive of hypothalamic disease, whereas others respond in a manner consistent with a primary pituitary disorder. Taken together, these findings suggest the possibility that these disorders may represent a spectrum of severity, dependent both upon the degree of compromise between hypothalamic and pituitary communication and the timing of the defect in development.

Pit-1 Deficiency

Several patients with combined pituitary hormone deficiency who harbor specific mutations in the Pit-1 gene have now been described (Table 3). These growth-impaired patients manifest varying degrees of hypothyroidism with deficiencies of GH, PRL, and TSH *(140–143)*. The Pit-1 mutations range from absence of Pit-1 expression to point mutations in either the homeodomain or the POU-specific domains. Most of the Pit-1 proteins harboring point mutations have the ability to bind DNA, but are unable to transactivate GH or PRL gene expression. The ability to transactivate the TSHβ gene, and hence the expression of TSH, is more variable than that of the other Pit-1-dependent genes. These findings account for the severe deficiency of measurable GH and PRL, with variable levels of TSH in these patients. Both sporadic and familial forms of Pit- 1 gene mutations have been reported, with sporadic forms being somewhat more common *(142)*. Interestingly, considerable variability in the degree of hypoplasia of the anterior pituitary, by MRI, was observed in these patients. These latter findings remain to be explained, but have been postulated to relate to differential effects of a specific Pit-1 mutation on morphogenesis vs hormone expression *(142)*.

Table 3
Human Gene Mutations Affecting Pituitary Development/Hormone Expression

Gene Product Domain	*Mutation*	*Functional Defect*	*Phenotype Hormonal Deficit*	*Anatomic Defect/MRI*	*Inheritance*	*Reference*
Pit-1 POU homeo domain	R271W	Unable to transactivate	↓ GH ↓ PRL, Basal TSH normal, Abnormal TRH stim.	Normal or hypoplastic	Sporadic and familial auto recessive	Radovick *(143)* Cohen *(141)* Ohta *(176)*
Pit-1 POU-specific domain	Nonsense mutation R172→ Stop codon	Absent Pit 1	↓ GH ↓ PRL ↓ TSH		Familial autorecessive	Tatsumi *(180)*
Pit-1 POU-specific domain	A158P	Unable to transactivate	↓ GH ↓ PRL ↓ TSH	Normal or hypoplastic	Familial autorecessive and comp hetero with Pit-1deletion	Pfaffle *(142)*
Pit 1 POU-specific domain	R143Q					Ohta *(176)*
Pit 1 Activation domain	P24L	Unable to transactivate	↓ GH, ↓ PRL TSH low normal		Familial autorecessive	Ohta *(176)*
βTSH	G29R	βSU unable to complex with αGSU	↓ TSH (1/5 with ↓ GH)	Normal	Familial autorecessive	Hayashizaki *(145,146)*

Isolated TSH Deficiency

Familial inherited TSH deficiency is an autosomally recessive disease causing typical symptoms of cretinism, with mental and growth retardation and defects in pubertal development *(144–149)*. In individuals studied, TSH was undetectable in the blood, yet normal levels of other glycoprotein hormones (LH and FSH) were found *(148)*. TRH administration produced a dramatic increase in α-GSU, but not in TSH or the free βSU, indicating that these patients do not produce active β-subunits *(148)*. These investigators have now demonstrated that patients from several families with inherited TSH deficiency carry a single base mutation in the TSHβ gene in a highly conserved region of the βSU. This mutation apparently produces a conformationally abnormal βSU that cannot associate with the αGSU *(145,148)*

Kallman's Syndrome

The syndrome described by Kallman et al. *(150)*, includes hypogonadotropic hypogonadism coupled with varying degrees of anosmia. The primary defect is a failure of GnRH neurons to migrate to their appropriate position in the hypothalamus, hence the cells of the anterior pituitary are not exposed to GnRH via the portal system (for review, *see* refs. *151,152*). Despite this lack of GnRH input into the pituitary throughout development, it is possible to produce LH and FSH secretion and normalize the pituitary-gonadal axis in patients with this syndrome via repeated pulsatile iv injections of GnRH *(151,152)*.

Pituitary Adenomas and Hyperplasia

Pituitary Hyperplasia

It has been known for some time that in humans, chronic stimulation by several of the hypothalamic trophic factors can produce hyperplasia of specific pituitary cell subtypes. This can in some cases produce radiographic changes suggestive of a pituitary adenoma. For instance, Nelson's syndrome, a condition of hyperplasia of corticotrophs of the anterior pituitary is a frequent result of long-standing adrenal insufficiency arising as a result of loss of negative feedback on CRH secretion. In long-standing severe primary hypothyroidism, elevated secretion of TRH produces hyperplasia of both thyrotrophs and lactotrophs. Hyperplasia of GH and ACTH producing cells has also been described in syndromes of ectopic production of GRH and CRH. Other hormones can also contribute to hyperplasia of the pituitary. For instance, lactotroph hyperplasia frequently occurs during pregnancy, presumably owing to high levels of circulating estrogens. These conditions most likely represent expansion of previously committed cells, however, it remains unclear whether stem cells within the adult pituitary can be induced into differentiating into a specific subtype.

Pituitary Adenomas

Recent studies using molecular genetic techniques have demonstrated the clonal nature of human pituitary tumors *(153)*. Although one or more somatic mutations must underlie pituitary tumor development, currently no single common mutation has been identified that contributes to the pathogenesis of all pituitary tumor phenotypes. Obviously, many of the factors discussed above are potential candidates for promoting tumor growth. One well described mutation in the Gsα-subunit of adenylyl cylase has been shown to be requisite for the development of approximately 40% of somatotroph adenomas *(154,155)*. However, these mutations appear to be restricted to pituitary tumors of somatotroph lineage and do not appear to contribute to tumor formation in other pituitary cell types. Examples of other abnormalities identified in human pituitary tumors include increased frequency of the *hst* oncogene (a member of the fibroblast growth family) *(156)*, amplification of the v-*fos* gene *(157)*, decreased numbers of EGF-Rs *(158)*, and increased protein kinase C activity *(159)*. Ras (a protein with crucial roles in signal transduction of a number of hormones) mutations appear to be rare in pituitary adenomas, having been described in only one invasive lactotroph adenoma *(160–162)*. Deletion mutations in chromosome 11 have been found in 16 of 80 pituitary macroadenomas, but these mutations were not in the same region of the chromosome *(163)*. Hence, no causal relationship between any growth factor or oncogene and the adenoma that expresses them has yet been demonstrated.

Another interesting aspect of pituitary adenomas is that many are plurihormonal. In addition to GH, most pituitary adenomas of acromegalic patients produce PRL and occasionally they also produce α-GSU and TSH *(164,165)*. TSH secreting adenomas produce excessive amounts of α-GSU relative to TSH, and in addition, frequently elaborate GH *(166,167)*. Less commonly these tumors secrete PRL or FSH (*see* ref. *168*). Adenomas that produce both ACTH and α-GSU have also been described *(169)*. Finally, many clinically nonfunctioning adenomas produce significant amounts of the free α-GSU *(170)*. These observations suggest that pituitary adenomas arise via dedifferentiation to multipotential progenitor cells. It is anticipated that further investigation into the mechanisms that result in pituitary tumorigenesis will give important insights into normal pituitary differentiation and may also provide the basis for targeted treatment of these tumors.

ACKNOWLEDGMENTS

This work was supported in part by National Institutes of Health grants to A.G. H. (DK 37667) and to C.A.P. (K8 DK02408 and F32 DK08974), and by the Lucille P. Markey Charitable Trust.

REFERENCES

1. Dearden NM, Holmes RL. Cyto-differentiation and portal vascular development in the mouse adenohypophysis. J Anat 1976; 121:551–569.
2. Kaufman MH. The Atlas of Mouse Development. Academic, London, 1992.
3. Rugh R. The Mouse: Its Reproduction and Development. Burgess Publishing, Minneapolis, MN, 1968.
4. Watanabe YG, Daikoku S. An immunohistochemical study on the cytogenesis of adenohypophysial cells in fetal rats. Dev Biol 1979; 68:557–567.
5. Ikeda H, Suzuki J, Sasano N, Niizuma H. The development and morphogenesis of the human pituitary gland. Anat Embryol 1988; 178:327–336.
6. Schechter JE, Pattison A, Pattison T. Development of the vasculature of the anterior pituitary: ontogeny of basic fibroblast growth factor. Developmental Dynamics 1993; 197:81–93.
7. Borrelli E. Pitfalls during development: controlling differentiation of the pituitary gland. Trends Genetics 1994; 10:222–224.
8. Karin M, Castrillo J-L, Theill LE. Growth hormone gene regulation: a paradigm for cell type-specific gene activation. Trends Genetics 1990; 6:92–96.
9. Voss JW, Rosenfeld MG. Anterior pituitary development: short tales from dwarf mice. Cell 1990; 70:527–530.

10. Theill LE, Karin M. Transcriptional control of GH expression and anterior pituitary development. Endocrine Rev 1993; 14:670–689.
11. Coates PJ, Doniach I. Development of folliculo-stellate cells in the human pituitary. Acta Endocrinologica 1988; 119:16–20.
12. Simmons DM, Voss JW, Ingraham HA, Holloway JM, Broide RS, Rosenfeld MG, Swanson LW. Pituitary cell phenotypes involve cell-specific Pit-1 mRNA translation and synergistic interactions with other classes of transcription factors. Genes Dev 1990; 4:695–711.
13. Asa SL, Kovacs K, Lazlo FA, Domokos I, Ezrin C. Human fetal adenohypophysis: histologic and immunocytochemical analysis. Neuroendocrinology 1986; 43:308–316.
14. Asa SL, Kovacs K, Singer W. Human fetal adenohypophysis: morphologic and functional analysis in vitro. Neuroendocrinology 1991; 53:562–572.
15. Barinaga M, Yamnamoto G. Rivier C, Vale W, Evans R, Rosenfeld MG. Transcriptional regulation of growth hormone gene expression by growth hormone-releasing factor. Nature 1983; 306:84–85.
16. Gick GG, Zeytin F, Brazeau P, Ling NC, Esch F, Bancroft FC. Growth hormone releasing factor regulates growth hormone mRNA in primary cultures of rat pituitary cells. Proc Natl Acad Sci USA 1984; 81:1553–1555.
17. Zeytin FN, Gick GG, Brazeau P, Ling N, McLaughlin M, Bancroft C. Growth hormone (GH)-releasing factor does not regulate GH release or GH mRNA levels in GH3 cells. Endocrinology 1984; 114:2054–2059.
18. Asa SL, Kovacs K, Stefaneanu L, Horvath E, Billestrup N, Gonzales-Manchon C, Vale W. Pituitary mammosomatotroph adenomas develop in old mice transgenic for growth hormone releasing hormone. Proc Soc Exp Biol Med 1990; 193:232–235.
19. Lloyd RV, Jin L, Chang A, Kulig E, Camper SA, Ross BD, Downs TR, Frohman LA. Morphologic effects of hGRH gene expression on the pituitary, liver, and pancreas of MT-hGRH transgenic mice. Amer J Pathol 1992; 141:895–906.
20. Mayo KE, Hammer RE, Swanson LW, Brinster RL, Rosenfeld MG, Evans RM. Dramatic pituitary hyperplasia in transgenic mice expressing a human growth hormone-releasing factor gene. Mol Endocrinol 1988; 2:606–612.
21. Stefaneanu L, Kovacs K, Horvath E, Asa SL, Losinski NE, Billestrup N. Price J. Vale W. Adenohypophysial changes in mice transgenic for human growth hormone-releasing factor (hGRF): A histological, immunocytochenlical and electron microscopic investigation. Endocrinology 1989; 125:2710–2718.
22. Cheng TC, Beamer WG, Phillips JA, Bartke A, Mallonee RL, Dowling C. Etiology of growth hormone deficiency in Little, Ames and Snell dwarf mice. Endocrinology 1983; 113:1669–1678.
23. Lin S-C, Lin CR, Gukovsky I, Lusis AJ, Sawchenko PE, Rosenfeld MG. Molecular basis of the little mouse phenotype and implications for cell type-specific growth. Nature 1993; 364:208–213.
24. Buckwalter MS, Katz RW, Camper SA. Localization of the panhypopituitary dwarf mutation (df) on mouse chromosome 11 in intersubspecific backcross. Genomics 1991; 10:515–526.
25. Slabaugh MB, Lieberman ME, Rutledge JJ, Gorski J. Ontogeny of growth hormone and prolactin gene expression in mice. Endocrinology 1982; 110:1489-1497.
26. O'Hara BF, Bendotti D, Reeves RH, Oster-Granite MI, Coyle JT, Gearhart JD. Genetic mapping and analysis of somatostatin expression in Snell dwarf mice. Mol Brain Res 1988; 4:283–292.
27. Gage PJ, Lossie AC, Scarlett LM, Lloyd RV, Camper SA. Ames dwarf mice exhibit somatotrope commitment but lack growth hormone-releasing factor response. Endocrinology 1995; 136:1161–1167.
28. Lin C, Lin S-C, Chang C-P, Rosenfeld MG. Pit-1-dependent expression of the receptor for growth hormone releasing factor mediates pituitary cell growth. Nature 1992; 360:765–768.
29. Camper SA, Saunders TL, Katz RW, Reeves RH. The Pit-l transcription factor gene is a candidate for the Snell dwarf mutation. Genomics 1990; 8:586–590.
30. Li S, Crenshaw EB, Rawson EJ, Simmons DM, Swanson LW, Rosenfeld MG. Dwarf locus mutants lacking three pituitary cell types result from mutations in the POU domain gene pit-1. Nature 1990; 347:528–533.
31. Gertz BJ, Contreras LH, McComb KI, Kivacs JB, Tyrrel JB, Dallman MG. Chronic administration of corticotropin-releasing factor increases pituitary corticotroph number. Endocrinology 1987; 120:381–388.
32. Childs GV, Rougeau D, Unabia G. Corticotropin-releasing hormone and epidermal growth factor: Mitogens for anterior pituitary corticotropes. Endocrinology 1995; 136:1595–1602.

33. Asa SL, Kovacs K, Hammer GD, Liu B, Roow BA, Low MJ. Pituitary corticotroph hyperplasia in rats implanted with a medullary thyroid carcinoma cell line transfected with a corticotropin-releasing hormone complementary deoxyribonucleic acid expression vector. Endocrinology 1992; 131:715–720.
34. Hotta M, Shibasaki T, Masuda A, Imaki T, Demura H, Olmo H, Daikoku S, Benoit R, Ling N, Shizume K. Ontogeny of pituitary responsiveness to corticotropin-releasing hormone in rat. Regulatory Peptides 1988; 21:245–252.
35. Dalkin AC, Haisenleder DJ, Ortolano GA, Ellis TR, Marshall JC. The frequency of gonadotropin-releasing-hormone stimulation differentially regulates gonadotropin subunit messenger ribonucleic acid expression. Endocrinology 1989; 125:917–922.
36. Gharib SD, Wierman ME, Shupnik MA, Chin WW. Molecular biology of the pituitary gonadotropins. Endocrine Reviews 1990; 11:177–199.
37. Murakami M, Muri M, Kato Y. Kobayashi I. Hypothalamic thyrotropin-releasing hormone regulates pituitary beta- and alpha-subunit mRNA levels in the rat. Neuroendocrinology 1991; 53:276–280.
38. Shupnik MA, Greenspan SL, Ridgway EC. Transcriptional regulation of thyrotropin subunit genes by thyrotropin-releasing hormone and dopamine in pituitary cell culture. J Biol Chem. 1986; 261:12,675–12,679.
39. Tashjian AH, Jr., Barowsky NJ, Jensen DK. Thyroptropin-releasing hormone: Direct evidence for stimulation of prolactin production by pituitary cells in culture. Biochem Biohys Res Commun 1971; 43:516–523.
40. Ramsdell JS. Thyrotropin-releasing hormone inhibits GH4 pituitary cell proliferation by blocking entry into S phase. Endocrinology 1990; 126:472–479.
41. Hyyppa M. Hypothalamic monamines in human fetuses. Neuroendocrinology 1972; 9:257–266.
42. Patel YC, Srikant CB. Somatostatin mediation of adenohypophysial secretion. Annual Rev Physiol 1986; 48:551–567.
43. Lamberts S, Krening E, Reubi J-C. The role of somatostatin and its analogs in the diagnosis and treatment of tumors. Endocrine Rev. 1991; 12:450–482.
44. Bruno J-F, Xu Y, Song J, Berelowitz M. Tissue distribution of somatostatin receptor subtype messenger ribonucleic acid in the rat. Endocrinology 1993; 133:2561–2567.
45. Wulfsen I, Meyerhorf W, Fehr S, Richter D. Expression patterns of rat somatostatin receptor genes in pre- and postnatal brain and pituitary. J Neurochem 1993; 61:1549–1552.
46. Srkalovic G, Cai R-Z, Schally AV. Evaluation of receptors for somatostatin in various tumour tissues using different analogues. J Clin Endocrinol Metab 1990; 70:661–669.
47. Reubi JC, Heitz PU, Landolt AM. Visualization of somatostatin receptors and correlation with immunoreactive growth hormone and prolactin in human pituitary adenomas. Evidence for different tumour subclasses. J Clin Endocrinol Metab 1987, 65:65–73.
48. Katznelson L, Oppenheim DS, Coughlin JF, Kliman B. Scheinfeld DA, Klibanski A. Chronic somatostatin analogue administration in patients with α-subunit secreting pituitary tumors. J Clin Endocrinol Metab 1992; 75:1318–1325.
49. Massague J. The TGF-beta family of growth and differentiation factors. Cell 1987; 49:437–438.
50. Katayama T, Shioto K, Takahashi M. Activin A increases the number of follicle stimulating hormone cells in anterior pituitary cultures. Mol Cell Endo 1990; 69:179–185.
51. Billestrup N, Gonzalez, Manchon C, Potter E, Vale W. Inhibition of somatotroph growth and growth hormone biosynthesis by activin in vitro. Mol Endocrinol 1990; 4:356–362.
52. Bilezikjian LM, Corrigan AZ, Vale W. Activin-A modulate growth hormone secretion from cultures of rat anterior pituitary cells. Endocrinology 1990; 126:2369–2376.
53. Sarkar DK, Kim KH, Minami S. Transforming growth factor-β1 messenger RNA and protein expression in the pituitary gland: its action on prolactin secretion and lactotropic growth. Mol Endo 6:1825–1833.
54. Delidow BC, Billis WM, Agarwal P. White. Inhibition of prolactin gene transcription by transforming growth factor-β in GH3 cells. Mol Endo 1991; 5:1716–1722.
55. Samsoondar J. Kobrin MS, Kudlow JE. α-Transforming growth factor secreted by untransformed bovine anterior pituitary cells in culture. J Biol Chem 1986; 261: 14408–14413.
56. Finley EL, Ramsdell JS. A transforming growth factor-α pathway is expressed in GH4C1 rat pituitary tumors and appears necessary for tumor formation. Endocrinology 1994; 135:416–422.

57. Kobrin MS, Asa SL, Samsoondar J, Kudlow JE. α-Transforming growth factor in the bovine anterior pituitary gland: secretion by dispersed cells and immunohistochemical localization. Endocrinology 1987; 121:1412–1416.
58. Marquardt H, Hunkapiller MW, Hoodk L.E., Todaro GJ. Rat transforming growth factor type 1: structure and relation to epidermal growth factor. Science 1984; 223:1079–1082.
59. Patterson JC, Childs GV. Nerve growth factor in the anterior pituitary: regulation of secretion. Endocrinology 1994; 135:1697–1704.
60. Patterson JC, Childs GV. Nerve growth factor and its receptor in the anterior pituitary. Endocrinology 1994; 135:1689–1696.
61. Missale C, Boroni F, Frassine M, Caruso A, Spano P. Nerve growth factor promotes the differentiation of pituitary mammotroph cells in vitro. Endocrinology 1995; 136:1205–1213.
62. Borelli E, Sawchenko PE, Evans RM. Pituitary hyperplasia induced by ectopic expression of nerve growth factor. Proc Natl Acad Sci USA 1992; 89:2764–2768.
63. Fan X, Childs GV. Epidermal growth factor and transforming growth factor-α messenger ribonucleic acids and their receptors in the rat anterior pituitary: localization and regulation. Endocrinology 1995; 136:2284–2293.
64. Murdoch GH, Potter E, Nicolaisen AK, Evans RM, Rosenfeld MG. Epidermal growth factor rapidly stimulates prolactin gene transcription. Nature 1982; 300 192–194.
65. Schonbrunn A, Krasnoff M, Westendorf J, Tashjian AJ. Epidermal growth factor and thyrotropin—releasing hormone act similarly on a clonal pituitary cell strain. J Cell Biol 1980; 85:786–797.
66. Johnson L, Baxter J, Vlodavsky I, Gospodrowicz D. Epidermal growth factor and expression of specific genes: effects on cultured rat pituitary cells are dissociable from the mitogenic response. Proc Natl Acad Sci USA 1980; 77:394–398.
67. Childs GV. Epidermal growth factor enhances ACTH secretion and expression of POMC mRNA by corticotropes in mixed and enriched cultures. Mol Cell Neurosci 1991; 2:235–241.
68. Gospodarowicz D, Ferrara N, Schweigerer L, Neufeld G. Structural characterization and biological functions of fibroblast growth factors. Endocrine Rev 1987; 8:95–114.
69. Gospodarowicz D, Ferrara N. Fibroblast growth factor and the control of pituitary and gonad development and function. Steroid Biochem. 1989; 32:183–191.
70. Rosenfeld MG. POU-domain transcription factors: powerful developmental regulators. Genes Dev 1991; 5:897–907.
71. Bodner M, Castrillo JL, Theill LE, Derrinck T, Ellisman M, Karin M. The pituitary specific transcription factor GHF-1 is a homeobox-containing protein. Cell 1988; 55:505–518.
72. Ingraham HA, Chen RP, Mangalam HP, Elsholtz HP, Flynn SE, Lin CR, Simmons DM, Swanson L, Rosenfeld MG. A tissue-specific transcription factor containing a homeodomain specifies a pituitary phenotype. Cell 1988; 55:519–529.
73. Crenshaw EB, III, Kalla K, Simmons DM, Swanson LW, Rosenfeld MG. Cell-specific expression of the prolactin gene in transgenic mice is controlled by synergistic interactions between Pit-1 recognition elements. Genes Dev 1989; 3:959–972.
74. Lira SA, Crenshaw EB, III, Glass CK, Swanson LW, Rosenfeld MG. Identification of rat growth hormone genomic sequence targeting pituitary expression in transgenic mice. Proc Natl Acad Sci USA 1989; 85:4755–4759.
75. Dolle P, Castrillo J-L, Theill LE, Deerinck T, Ellisman M, Karin M. Expression of GHF-1 protein in mouse pituitaries correlates both temporally and spatially with the onset of growth hormone gene activity. Cell 1990; 60:809–820.
76. Lin S-C, Li S, Drolet DW, Rosenfeld MG. Pituitary ontogeny of the Snell dwarf mouse reveals Pit-1-independent and Pit-1-dependent origins of the thyrotrope. Development 1994; 120:515.
77. Theill LE, Hattori K, Lazzaro D, Castrillo J-L, Karin M. Differential splicing of the GHF-1 primary transcript gives rise to two functionally distinct homeodomain proteins. EMBO J 1992; 11:2261–2269.
78. Morris AE, Kloss B, McChesney RE, Bancroft C, Chasin LA. An alternatively spliced Pit-1 isoform altered in its ability to trans-activate. Nucleic Acids Res 1992; 20:1355–1361.
79. Konzak KE, Moore DD. Functional isoforms of Pit-l generated by alternative mRNA splicing. Mol Endocrinol 6:241–247.
80. Haugen BR, Wood WM, Gordon DF, Ridgway EC. A thyrotrope-specific variant of Pit-1 transactivates the thyrotropin β promoter. J Biol Chem 1993; 268:20,818–20,824.

81. Haugen BR, Gordon DF, Nelson AR, Wood WM, Ridgway EC. The combination of Pit-l and Pit-1T have a synergistic stimulatory effect on the thyrotropin β-subunit promoter but not the growth hormone or prolactin promoters. Mol Endocrinol 1994; 8:1574–1582.
82. Rhodes SJ, Chen R, DiMattia GE, Scully KM, Kalla KA, Lin S-C, Yu VC, Rosenfeld MG. A tissue-specific enhancer confers Pit-1-dependent morphogen inducibility and autoregulation on the pit-1 gene. Genes Dev 1993; 7:913–932.
83. Castrillo JL, Theill LE, Karin M. Function of the homeodomain protein GHF1 in pituitary cell proliferation. Science 1991; 253:197–199.
84. Day RN, Koikw A, Sakai M, Muramatsu M, Maurer RA. Both Pit-1 and the estrogen receptor are required for estrogen responsiveness of the rat prolactin gene. Mol Endocrin 1990; 4:1964–1971.
85. Schaufele F, West BL, Baxter JD. Synergistic activation of the rat growth hormone promoter by Pit-1 and the thyroid hormone receptor. Mol Endocrinol 1992; 6:656–665.
86. He X, Treacy MM, Simmons DM, Ingraham HA, Swanson LW, Rosenfeld MG. Expression of a large family of POU-domain regulatory genes in mammalian brain development. Nature 1989; 340:35–42.
87. Elsholtz HP, Albert VR, Treacy MN, Rosenfeld MG. A two-base change in a POU factor-binding site switches pituitary-specific to lymphoid-specific gene expression. Genes Dev 1990; 4:43–51.
88. Chen C, Ingraham HA, Treacy MN, Albert VA, Wilson L, Rosenfeld MG. The pituitary POU-domain protein Pit-1 can positively and negatively regulate transcription of its own promoter. Nature 1990; 346:583–586.
89. Voss JW, Wilson L, Rosenfeld MG. POU-domain proteins Pit-1 and Oct-1 interact to form a heteromeric complex and can cooperate to induce expression of the prolactin promoter. Genes Dev 1991; 5: 1309–1320.
90. Bach I, Rhodes SJ, Pearse RV, Heinzel T, Gloss B, Scully KM, Sawchenko PE, Rosenfeld MG. P-Lim, a LIM homeodomain factor, is expressed during pituitary organ and cell commitment and synergizes with Pit-1. Proc Natl Acad Sci 1995; 92:2720–2724.
91. Busch SJ, Sassone-Corsi P. Dimers, leucine zippers and DNA-binding domains. Trends Genet 1990; 6:36–40.
92. Drolet DW, Scully KM, Simmons DM, Wegner M, Chu K, Swanson LW, Rosenfeld MG. TEF, a transcription factor expressed specifically in the anterior pituitary during embryogenesis, defines a new class of leucine zipper proteins. Genes Dev 1991; 5:1739–1753.
93. Delegeane AM, Ferland LH, Mellon PL. Tissue specific enhancer of the human glycoprotein hormone α subunit gene: dependence on cAMP inducible elements. Mol Cell Biol 1987; 7:3994–4002.
94. McCormick A, Brady H. Theill LE, Karin M. Regulation of the pituitary-specific homeobox gene GHF-1 by cell-autonomous and environmental cues. Nature 1990; 345:829–832.
95. Bilezikjian LM, Erlichman J, Fleischer N. Vale W. Differential activation of type I and type II 3′, 5′-cyclic adenosine monophosphate -dependent protein kinases by growth hormone releasing factor. Mol Endocrinology 1987; 1:137–146.
96. Bilezikjian LM, Vale W. Stimulation of adenosine 3′,5′ -monophosphate production by growth hormone-releasing factor and its inhibition by somatostatin in anterior pituitary cells in vitro. Endocrinology 1983; 113:1726–1731.
97. Struthers RS, Vale WW, Arias C, Sawchenko PE, Montminy MR. Somatotroph hypoplasia and dwarfism in transgenic mice expressing a non-phosphorylatable CREB mutant. 1991; Nature 350:622–624.
98. Bertherat J. Chanson P, Montminy M. The cyclic ,adenosine 3′,5′-monophosphate responsive factor CREB is constitutively activated in human somatotroph adenomas. Mol Endocrinol 1995; 9:777–783.
99. Schoderbek WE, Kim KE, Ridgway EC, Mellon PL, Maurer RA. Analysis of DNA sequences required for pituitary-specific expression of the glycoprotein hormone α-subunit gene. Mol Endocrinol 1992; 6:893–903.
100. Akerblom IE, Slater EP, Becto M, Baxter JD, Mellon PL. Negative regulation by glucocorticoids through interference with a cAMP responsive enhancer. Science 1988; 241:350–353.
101. Therrien M, Drouin J. Cell-specific helix-loop-helix factor required for pituitary expression of the proopiomelanocortin gene. Mol Cell Biol 1993; 13:2342–2353.
102. Tremblay J, Lamonerie T, Lanctot C, Therrien M, Drouin J. A novel homeobox transcription factor is expressed in early pituitary development and is a major determinant for cell-specific transcription of the proopiomelanocortin gene. Endocr Soc Meeting Abstr 1995; OR18–2.

103. Jackson SM, Barnhart KM, Mellon PL, Gutierrez-Hartmann A, Hoeffler JP. Helix-loop-helix proteins are present and differentially expressed in different cell lines from the anterior pituitary. Mol Cell Endocrinology 1993; 96:167–176.
104. Jackson SM, Gutierrez-Hartmann A, Hoeffler JP. Upstream stimulatory factor, a basic helix loop helix zipper protein, regulates the activity of the alpha-glycoprotein hormone subunit gene in pituitary cells. Mol Endocrinol 1995; 9:278–291.
105. Lipkin SM, Naar AM, Kalla KA, Sack RA, Rosenfeld MG. Identification of a novel zinc finger protein binding a conserved element critical for Pit-1-dependent growth hormone gene expression. Genes Dev 1993; 7:1674–1687.
106. Mangelsdorf DJ, Thummel C, Beato M, Herrlich P, Schutz G, Umesono K, Blumberg B, Kastner P, Mark M, Chambon P, Evans RM. The nuclear receptor superfamily: The second decade. Cell 1995; 83:835–839.
107. Green S, Chambon P. Nuclear receptors enhance our understanding of transcription regulation. Trends Genetics 1988; 4:309–314.
108. Horn F, Windle JJ, Barnhart KM, Mellon PL. Tissue-specific gene expression in the pituitary: The glycoprotein hormone α-subunit gene is regulated by a gonadotrope-specific protein. Mol Cell Biol 1992; 12:2143–2153.
109. Ingraham HA, Lala DS, Ikeda Y, Luo X, Shen W-H, Nachtigal MW, Abbud R, Nilson JH, Parker KL. The nuclear receptor steroidogenic factor L acts at multiple levels of the reproductive axis. Genes Dev 1994; 8:2302–2312.
110. Honda S-I, Morohashi K-I, Nomura M, Takeya H. Kitajima M, Omura T. Ad4BP regulating steriodogenic P-450 gene is a member of steroid hormone receptor superfamily. J Biol Chem 1993; 268:7494–7502.
111. Lala DS, Rice DA, Parker KL. Steriodogenic factor 1, a key regulator of steroidogenic enzyme expression, is the mouse homolog of fushi tarazu-factor 1. Mol Endocrinol 1993; 6:1249–1258.
112. Japon MG, Rubenstein M, Low MJ. In situ hybridization analysis of anterior pituitary homone gene expression during fetal mouse development. J Histochem Cytochem 1994; 42:1117–1125.
113. Shupnik MA, Fallest PC. Steriodogenic factor-1 binds to a region of the rat LHβ gene which confers a synergistic response to cyclic amp and protein kinase C activation. Endocr Soc Meeting Abst 1995; P1–521.
114. Shupnik MA, Gharib SD, Chin WW. Divergent effects of estradiol on gonadotropin gene transcription in pituitary fragments. Mol Endo 1989; 3:474–480.
115. Shupnik MA, Weinmann CM, Notides AC, Chin WW. An upstream region of the rat luteinizing hormone β gene binds estrogen receptor and confers estrogen responsiveness. J Biol Chem 1989; 264:80–86.
116. Shupnik MA, Rosenzweig BA. Identification of an estrogen-responsive element in the rat LHα gene. J Biol Chem 1991; 266:17084–17091.
117. Friend KE, Chiou YK, Lopes MBS, Laws ER, Jr., Hughes KM, Shupnik MA. Estrogen receptor expression in human pituitary: correlation with immunohistochemistry in normal tissue, and immunohistochemistry and morphology in macroadenomas. J Clin Endo Metab 1994; 78: 1497–1504.
118. Stefaneanu L, Kovacs K, Horvath E, Lloyd RV, Buchfelder M, Fahlbusch R. Smyth H. In situ hybridization study of estrogen receptor messenger ribonucleic acid in human adenohypophysial cells and pituitary adenomas. J Clin Endo Metab 1994; 78:83–88.
119. Beato M, Herrlich P, Schutz G. Steroid hormone receptors: many actors in search of a plot. Cell 1995; 83:851–857.
120. Drouin J, Trifiro MA, Plante RK, Nemer M, Eriksson P, Wrange O. Glucocorticoid receptor binding to a specific DNA sequence is required for hormone-dependent repression of pro-opiomelanocortin gene transcription. Mol Cell Biol 1989; 9:5303–5314.
121. Elsholtz HP. Molecular biology of prolactin: Cell-specific and endocrine regulators of the prolactin gene. Seminars of Reprod Endocrinol 1992; 10:183–195.
122. Cintra A, Solfrini V, Bunnemann B, Okret S, Bortolotti F. Gustafsson J-A, Fuxe K. Prenatal development of glucocorticoid receptor gene expression and immunoreactivity in the rat brain and pituitary gland: a combined in situ hybridization and immunocytochemical analysis. Neuroendocrinology 1993; 57:1133–1147.
123. Meaney MJ, Sapolsky RM, McEwen BS. The development of the glucocorticoid receptor system in the rat limbic brain, I. Ontogeny and autoregulation. Dev Brain Res 1985; 18:159–164.
124. Wondisford FE, Farr EA, Radovick S, Steinfelder HJ, Moates JM, McClaskey JH, Weintraub BD. Thyroid hormone inhibition of human thyrotropin β-subunit gene expression is mdiated by a cis-acting element located in the first exon. J Biol Chem 1989; 264:14601–14604.

125. Chatterjee VKK, Lee J-K, Rentoumis A, Jameson JL. Negative regulation of the thyroid-stimulating hormone α gene by thyroid hormone: receptor interaction adjacent to the TATA box. Proc Natl Acad Sci USA 1989; 86:9114–9118.
126. Carr FE, Burnside J, Chin WW. Thyroid hormones regulate rat thyrotropin S gene promoter activity expressed in GH3 cells. Mol Endo 1989; 3:709–716.
127. Burnside J, Darling DS, Carr FE, Chin WW. Thyroid hormone regulation of the rat glycoprotein hormone α-subunit gene promoter activity. J Biol Chem 1989; 264:6886–6891.
128. Brent GA, Harney JW, Chen Y, Warne RG, Moore DD, Larsen PR. Mutations of the rat growth hormone promoter which increase and decrease response to thyroid hormone define a consensus thyroid hormone response element. Mol Endocrinol 1989; 3:1996–2007.
129. Glass CK, Franco R, Weinberger C, Albert VR, Evans RM, Rosenfeld MG. A c-erbA binding site in rat growth hormone gene mediates trans-activation by thyroid hormone. Nature 1987; 329:738–741.
130. Sporn MB, Roberts AB. Role of retinoids in differentiation and carcinogenesis. Cancer Res. 1983; 43:3034–3040.
131. Macleod K, Leprince D, Stehelin D. The ets gene family. Trends Biochem Sci 1992; 17:251–256.
132. Wasylyk B. Hahn SH, Giovane A. The Ets family of transcription factors. Eur J Biochem 1993; 211:7–18.
133. Bradford AP, Conrad KE, Wasylyk C, Wasylyk B, Gutierrez-Hartmann A. Functional interaction of c-Ets-1 and GHF-1/Pit-1 mediates Ras activation of pituitary-specific gene expression: Mapping of the essential c-Ets-1 domain. Mol Cell Biol 1995; 15:2849–2857.
134. Bradford AP unpublished results.
135. Maroulakou IG, Papas TS, Green JE. Differential expression of ets-1 and ets-2 protooncogenes during murine embryogenesis 1994; 1551–1565.
136. Abrahams JJ, Trefelner E, Boulware SD. Idiopathic growth hormone deficiency: MR findings in 35 patients. American J Neurorad 1991; 12:155–160.
137. Kuroiwa T, Yasufumi O, Hasuo K, Yasumori K, Mizushima A, Masuda K. MR imaging of pituitary dwarfism. American J Neurorad 1991; 12:161–164.
138. Root AW. Magnetic resonance imaging in hypopituitarism. J Clin Endocrinol Metab 1991; 72:10,11.
139. Proto G, Mazzolini A, Grimaldi F. Bertolissi F, Pozzi-Mucelli RS, Magnaldi S. Idiopathic anterior hypopituitarism: magnetic resonance imaging and clinical correlation. J Endocrinol Invest 1992; 15:283–287.
140. Brown RS, Bhatia V, Hayes E. An apparent cluster of congenital hypopituitarism in central Massachusetts: magnetic resonance imaging and hormonal studies. J Clin Endocrinol Metab 1991; 72:12–18.
141. Radovick S, Nations M, Du Y, Berg LA, Weintraub BD, Wondisford FE. A mutation in the POU-homeodomain of Pit-1 responsible for combined pituitary hormone deficiency. Science 1992; 257:1115–1118.
142. Cohen LE, Wondisford FE, Salvatoni A, Maghnie M, Brucker-Davis F, Weintraub BD, Radovick S. A "hot spot" in the Pit-1 gene responsible for combined pituitary hormone deficiency: Clinical and molecular correlates. J Clin Endocrin Metab 1995; 80:679–684.
143. Pfaffle RW, DiMattia GE, Parks JS, Brown MR, Wit JM, Jansen M, Van der Nat H, Van den Brande JL, Rosenfeld MG, Ingraham HA. Mutation of the POU-specific domain of Pit-1 and hypopituitarism without pituitary hypoplasia. Science 1992; 257:1118–1121.
144. Labbe A, Dubray C, Gaillard G, Besse G, Assali P, Malpucch G. Familial growth retardation with isolated thyroid-stimulating hormone deficiency. Clin Pediatr 1984; 23:675–678.
145. Hayashizaki Y, Hiraoka Y, Tatsumi K, Hashimoto T, Furuyama J-I, Miyai K, Nishijo K, Matsuura M, Kohno H. Labbe E, Matsubara K. Deoxyribonucleic acid analyses of five families with familial inherited thyroid stimulating hormone deficiency. J Clin Endocrinol Metab 1990; 71:792–796.
146. Hayashizaki Y, Miyai K, Onishi T, Kumahara Y, Effects of corticotrophin releasing factor and growth hormone releasing factor on pituitary hormone secretion in patients with congenital thyrotropin (TSH) deficiency. Horm Metab Res 1986; 18:842–846.
147. Miyai K, Azukizawa M, Kumahara Y. Familial isolated thyrotropin deficiency with cretinism. N Engl J Med 1971; 285:1043–1048.
148. Hayashizaki Y, Hiraoka Y, Endo Y, Matsubara K. Thyroid-stimulating hormone (TSH) deficiency caused by a single base substitution in the CAGYC region of the β-subunit. EMBO J 1989; 8:2291–2296.
149. Dacou-Voutekais C, Feltquate DM, Drakopoulou M, Kourides IA, Dracopoli NC. Familial hypothyroidism caused by a nonsense mutation in the thyroid-stimulating hormone β-subunit gene. Am J Human Genet 1990; 46:988–993.

150. Kallman FJ, Schenfeld WA, Barrera SE. The genetic aspects of primary eunuchoidism. Am J Ment Defic 1944; 48:203–236.
151. Crowley WF, Jameson JL. Gonadotlopin-releasing hormone deficiency: perspectives from clinical investigation. Endocr Rev 1992; 13:635–640.
152. Schwanzel-Fukuda M, Jorgenson KL, Bergen HT, Weesner GD, Pfaff DW. Biology of normal luteinizing hormone-releasing hormone neurons during and after their migration from olfactory placode. Endocr Rev 1992; 13:623–634.
153. Alexander JM, Biller BM, Bikkal H, Zervas NT, Arnold A, Klibanski A. Clinically nonfunctioning pituitary tumors are monoclonal in origin. J Clin Invest 1990; 86:336–340.
154. Vallar L, Spada A, Giannattasio G. Altered Gsα adenylate cyclase activity in human GH secreting adenomas. Nature 1987; 330:566–568.
155. Spada A, Arosis M, Bassetti M, Vallar L, Clementi E, Bazzoni N. Mutations in the alpha subunit of the stimulatory regulatory protein of adenylyl cyclase (Gs) in human GH-secreting pituitary adenomas. Biochemical, clinical and morphological aspects. Pathol Res Pract 187:567–570.
156. Gonsky R, Herman V, Melmed S, Fagin J. Transforming DNA sequences present in human prolactin-secreting pituitary tumors. Mol Endocrinol 1991; 5:1587–1695.
157. U HS, Kelley P, Lee WH. Abnormalities of the human growth hormone gene and protooncogenes in some human pituitary adenomas. Mol Endocrinol 1988; 2:85–89.
158. Birman P, Michard M, Li JY, Peillon F, Bression D. Epidermal growth factor-binding sites, present in normal human and rat pituitaries, are absent in human pituitary adenomas. J Clin Endocrinol Metab 1987; 65:275–281.
159. Alvaro V, Levy L, Dubray C. Invasive human pituitary tumors express a point-mutated α-protein kinase-C. J Clin Endocrinol Metab 1993; 77:1125–1129.
160. Karga HJ, Alexander JM, Hedley-Whyte ET, Klibanski A, Jameson JL. Ras mutations in human pituitary tumors. J Clin Endocrinol Metab 1992; 75:914–919.
161. Cai WY, Alexander JM, Hedley-Whyte ET, Scheithauer BW, Jameson JL, Zervas NT, Klibanski A. Ras mutations in human prolactinomas and pituitary carcinomas. J Clin Endocrinol Metab 1994; 78:89–93.
162. Pei L, Melmed S. Scheithauer B. Kovacs K, Prager D . H-Ras mutations in human pituitary carcinoma metastases. J Clin Endocrinol Metab 1994; 78:847–854.
163. Boggild MD, Jenkinson S. Pistorello M. Molecular genetic studies of sporadic pituitary tumors. J Clin Endocrinol Metab 1994; 78:387–392.
164. Kontogeorgos G. Kovacs K, Scheithauer BW, Rologis D, Orphanidis G. α-subunit immunoreactivity in plurihormonal pituitary adenomas of patients with acromegaly. Mod Pathol 1991; 4:191–195.
165. Furuhata S. Kameya T. Otani M, Toya S. Prolactin presents in all pituitary adenomas of acromegalic patients. Hum Pathol 1993; 24:10–15.
166. Kourides IA, Ridgway EC, Weintraub BD, Bigos ST, Gershengorn MC, Maloof R. Thyrotropin induced hyperthyroidism: use of alpha and beta subunit levels to identify patients with pituitary tumors. J Clin Endocrinol Metab 1977; 45:534–543.
167. Lamberg BA, Pelkonen R. Gordin A. Hyperthyroidism and acromegaly caused by pituitary TSH- and GH-secreting tumors. Acta Endocrinol 1983; 103:7–14.
168. Kuzuya N, Inque K, Ishibashi M, Murayama Y, Koide Y, Ito K, Yamaji T, Yamashita K. Endocrine and immunohistochemical studies on thyrotropin (TSH)-secreting pituitary adenomas: Responses of TSH, α-subunit, and growth hormone to hypothalamic releasing hormones and their distribution in adenoma cells. J Clin Endocrin Metab 1990; 71:1103–1111.
169. Berg KK, Scheithauer BW, Felix I, Kovacs K, Horvath E, Klee GG, Laws ER. Pituitary adenomas that produce adrenocorticotropic hormone and α-subunit: clinicopathological, immunohistochemical, ultrastructural, and immunoelectron microscopic studies in nine cases. Neurosurg 1990; 26:397–403.
170. Oppenheim DS, Kana AR, Sangha JS, Klibanski A. Prevalence of α-subunit hypersecretion in patients with pituitary tumors: Clinically nonfunctioning and somatotroph adenomas. J Clin Endocrinol Metab 1990; 70:859–864.
171. King JWB. Pygmy, a dwarfing gene in the house mouse. J Heredity 1950; 41:249–252.
172. Koto M, Sato T. Okamoto M, Adachi J. Rdw rats, a new hereditary dwarf model in the rat. Experimental Animals 1988; 37:21–30.
173. Shibayama K, Ohyama Y. Ono M, Furudate S. Expression of mRNA coding for pituitary hormone and pituitary-specific transcription factor in the pituitary gland of the rdw rat with hereditary dwarfism. J Endocrin 1993; 138:301–313.

174. Ono M, Harigai T. Furudate S. Pituitary-specific transcription factor Pit-1 in the rdw rat with growth hormone- and prolactin-deficient dwarfism. J Endocrin 1994; 143:479–487.
175. Okuma S. Kawashima S. Spontaneous dwarf rat. Exp Anim 1980; 29:301–304.
176. Ohta K, Nobukuni Y, Mitsubchi H, Fujimoto S, Matsuo N, Inagaki H, Endo F, Matsuda I. Mutations in the Pit-l gene in children with combined pituitary hormone deficiency. Biochem Biophys Res Commun 1992; 189:851–855.
177. Tatsumi K, Miyai K, Notomi T. Kaibe K, Amino N. Mizuno Y. Kohno H. Cretinism with combined hormone deficiency caused by a mutation in the PIT1 gene. Nature Genet 1992; 1:56–58.
178. Hammer RE, Brinster RL, Rosenfeld MC;, Evans RM, Mayo KE. Expression of human growth hormone-releasing factor in transgenic mice results in increased somatic growth. Nature 1985; 315:413–416.
179. Behringer RR, Mathews LS, Palmiter RD, Brinster RL. Dwarf mice produced by genetic ablation of growth hormone-expressing cells. Genes Dev 1988; 2:453–461.
180. Lew D, Brady H, Klausing K, Yaginuma K, Theill LE, Stauber C, Karin M, Mellon PL. GHF-1-promoter-targeted immortalization of a somatotropic progenitor cell results in dwarfism in transgenic mice. Genes Dev 1993; 7:683–693.

2 Hypopituitarism

Differential Diagnosis and Treatment

Mary Lee Vance, MD

CONTENTS

INTRODUCTION

Hypopituitarism refers to the congenital absence or acquired loss of pituitary hormone secretion, which may be an isolated deficiency or multiple hormone deficiencies. The diagnosis of pituitary hormone deficiency can usually be made in the outpatient setting with a combination of the clinical assessment and hormone measurements. Hypopituitarism is most commonly acquired, and occurs most often with pituitary disease, usually a benign adenoma. Pituitary failure may also result from treatment of the adenoma (surgery, radiation). Causes of pituitary hormone deficiency are listed in Table 1 *(1–23)*. The loss of pituitary function has numerous effects, depending on which hormone or hormones is/are deficient. Table 2 lists the hypothalamic and pituitary hormones and target organs. It is apparent from this list that some deficiencies can be life threatening, i.e., adrenocorticotropin (ACTH) deficiency results in adrenal insufficiency, thyrotropin (TSH) deficiency results in hypothyroidism. Loss of the gonadotropins, luteinizing hormone (LH), and follicle-stimulating hormone (FSH) produce hypogonadism and infertility. If the posterior pituitary is compromised, diabetes insipidus (DI) results in polyuria and polydipsia; if the patient does not ingest adequate fluid, the resultant volume depletion and hypernatremia can be severe.

Growth hormone deficiency during childhood results in retardation of linear growth. More recently GH deficiency in adults has become recognized as being associated with alterations in body composition and, possibly, with the risk of premature mortality *(24)*. Growth hormone-deficient adults have an increased amount of body fat, particularly intrabdominal adipose tissue, and decreased muscle mass. In addition to physical

From: *Contemporary Endocrinology, Vol. 3: Diseases of the Pituitary: Diagnosis and Treatment*
Edited by M. E. Wierman Humana Press Inc., Totowa, NJ

Table 1
Causes of Hypopituitarism

Hypothalamic Releasing Hormone Deficiency
- Tumor, hamartoma, chordoma, third ventricle cyst, meningioma
- Metastatic disease: breast, lung, prostate, colon, lymphoma, plasmacytoma
- Infiltrative disease: giant cell granuloma, sarcoidosis, eosinophilic granuloma, Wegener's granulomatosis
- Radiation: cranial, pituitary, nasopharyngeal
- Postoperative
- Congenital

Pituitary Hormone Deficiency
- Pituitary adenoma: prolactinoma, GH secreting, ACTH, gonadotrope (LH, FSH, FSH), TSH, null cell, nonsecretory, astrocytoma (posterior lobe)
- Intrasellar tumor: craniopharyngioma, Rathke's cleft cyst, dermoid cyst, gangliocytoma, paraganglioma, esthesioneuroblastoma, sarcoma, lipoma, hemangiopericytoma, germ cell tumor
- Infiltrative disease: hemochromatosis, lymphocytic hypophysitis, sarcoidosis
- Infection: tuberculosis, brucellosis, mycosis, syphilis, abscess
- Internal carotid artery aneurysm, cavernous angioma
- Empty sella
- Trauma
- Parasellar meningioma
- Pituitary apoplexy: hemorrhage into a pituitary tumor, postpartum pituitary hemorrhage (Sheehan's syndrome)
- Postoperative

Table 2
Hypothalamic and Pituitary Hormones and Target Tissues

Hypothalamic hormone	*Pituitary hormone*	*Target organ*	*Pituitary hormone function*
CRH	ACTH	Adrenal cortex	Stimulates cortisol synthesis
TRH	TSH	Thyroid gland	Stimulates T_4, T_3 synthesis
GnRH	LH	Ovaries, testes	Stimulates estrogen, testosterone synthesis
GnRH	FSH	Ovaries, testes	Stimulates ovulation, spermatogenesis
Dopamine	Prolactin	Breast	Stimulates breast milk production
GHRH	GH	All tissues	Stimulates liner growth, anabolism
Somatostatin	GH	All tissues	—
TRH, GnRH	α-subunit	Unknown	Binds to β-subunit: LH, FSH, TSEH
Vasopressin (ADH)	—	Kidney	Stimulates free water absorption
Oxytocin	—	Uterus, breast	Stimulates uterine contraction, milk ejection

CRH, corticotropin releasing hormone; TRH, thyrotropin releasing hormone; GnRH, gonadotropin releasing hormone; GHRH, growth hormone releasing hormone; ADH, antidiuretic hormone.

Table 3
Suggested Screening Hormone Studies in Suspected Pituitary Disease

Deficiency
Morning cortisol (8:00–9:00 AM)
Thyroxine (T4), T3 resin uptake, TSH
LH, FSH, testosterone (men), estradiol (women)
IGF-1[a]
Serum, urine osmolality, serum sodium
Pituitary Hormone Hypersecretion
Prolactin
IGF-1[a]
α-subunit[a]
24h urine free cortisol

[a]IGF-1 and α-subunit, must be interpreted according to age- and sex-matched normal subjects.

changes, adults with GH deficiency may experience diminished exercise tolerance, easy fatiguability, and a general sense of ill health *(25)*.

Pituitary hormone deficiency must not only be recognized promptly, but the etiology must be sought and treatment instituted. Treatment consists of correcting the cause and replacement of the deficient target organ hormone in as physiologic manner as possible.

DIAGNOSIS OF HYPOPITUITARISM

Clinical and Biochemical

The symptoms and signs of hypopituitarism are those of the target gland deficiency; the challenge is to determine the etiology of hormone deficiency. Suggested screening studies are listed in Table 3. Since hypopituitarism is most often caused by a pituitary adenoma, the evaluation should also seek to determine the cause of pituitary failure; suggested screening studies for pituitary tumor hypersecretion are also listed in Table 3. The most common pituitary hormone deficiencies are those of growth hormone and the gonadotropins (LH, FSH). Since adults have completed linear growth, there are no obvious signs of the loss of this hormone. Changes in body composition are gradual and subtle (increased adipose mass, diminished muscle mass) and are frequently attributed to aging. Measurement of the serum IGF-1 (insulin-like growth factor-1) concentration provides an indication of overall GH secretion. This value must be interpreted according to age- and sex-matched normal values, and not all commercial laboratories provide information on values in normal subjects according to age and sex. Childhood pituitary hormone deficiency is most commonly that of isolated GH deficiency with resultant retardation of linear growth. Definitive diagnosis of GH deficiency in adults and children usually involves a stimulation test such as insulin-induced hypoglycemia, administration of growth hormone releasing hormone (GHRH), clonidine, or L-dopa.

The diagnosis of secondary hypogonadism is most easily made in premenopausal women who have a change in menstrual function (oligomenorrhea, amenorrhea) or who seek medical consultation for infertility. Postmenopausal women and men usually come to diagnosis because of the mass effect of a pituitary lesion (headache, visual loss). Many men report loss of libido or erectile function only with *specific* questioning (men do not often volunteer this information or assume their sexual dysfunction is caused by aging). Hot flashes and development of gynecomastia are also consequences of subnormal testosterone concentrations. Men with secondary hypogonadism usually have normal male hair distribution and beard growth and normal testicular size (it may take years for these to change). The hypothalamic/pituitary etiology of hypogonadism is established by measuring serum gonadotropins (LH, FSH), which are usually low or inappropriately normal in women with secondary amenorrhea, in postmenopausal women, or in men with a low serum testosterone concentration. Administration of gonadotropin releasing hormone (GnRH) with measurement of serum LH and FSH responses may be misleading; in the circumstance of longstanding gonadotropin deficiency, LH and FSH may not increase with a single injection of GnRH, but may do so after repeated administration. Thus, this test is of limited utility.

Symptoms of hypothyroidism include fatigue, weight gain or difficulty losing weight, constipation, cold intolerance, loss of mental acuity, and a general sense of ill health. Physical examination may reveal periorbital puffiness, dry or sallow skin, normal thyroid size, and delayed or deliberate relaxation of peripheral reflexes. Loss of the lateral portion of the eyebrows usually occurs with longstanding hypothyroidism. Hormone measurements should include both TSH and thyroxine (T4) levels. A low serum T4 in conjunction with a normal serum TSH indicates that the cause of hypothyroidism is lack of central stimulation, either a hypothalamic thyrotropin releasing hormone (TRH) or a pituitary TSH deficiency. A common error is to measure only serum TSH as a screening test for hypothyroidism and assume that a normal TSH excludes thyroid gland failure.

Adrenal insufficiency poses the greatest threat to the patient's health and well being. Since adrenal aldosterone secretion is not primarily dependent upon ACTH stimulation, patients may not have the severe volume depletion and characteristic hyponatremia and hyperkalemia that occurs with primary adrenal insufficiency. Symptoms of adrenal insufficiency are nonspecific and include generalized fatigue, headache, loss of appetite, and weight loss; orthostatic symptoms may also occur. Physical findings include a decline in blood pressure on standing and lack of hyperpigmentation as occurs with primary adrenal failure. The best screening test is measurement of a morning serum cortisol concentration; simultaneous measurement of serum ACTH is helpful if the cortisol is very low and the ACTH is inappropriately in the normal range. Definitive diagnosis of secondary adrenal insufficiency may require a stimulation test, preferably one that tests the entire hypothalamic-pituitary adrenal axis such as insulin-induced hypoglycemia or the metyrapone test.

Diabetes insipidus (DI) is characterized by polyuria, including frequent nocturia, and polydipsia. When DI is complete, the patient may report hourly urination and excessive thirst, with a preference for cold water to relieve the thirst. Simultaneous serum and urine osmolality and serum sodium measurements are indicated; if the patient is ingesting adequate fluid, the serum osmolality and sodium will be normal but the urine osmolality will be very low. A water deprivation test is the definitive study to diagnose DI and should only be performed in a hospitalized patient who is under close supervision with hourly monitoring of weight, blood pressure, and urine volume. Diabetes insipidus more commonly occurs in the setting of a craniopharyngioma, Rathke's cleft cyst, or a metastatic lesion; these types of lesions have a predilection for involving the hypothalamus, the site of vasopressin synthesis.

Deficiency of prolactin is not clinically evident except in the postpartum women who are unable to nurse. The more common occurrence in a patient with a pituitary adenoma is hyperprolactinemia, either from a prolactin or a prolactin and GH secreting tumor or as a result of impaired dopamine inhibition of prolactin (secondary hyperprolactinemia) by a large mass.

The diagnosis of pituitary hormone deficiency can usually be made in the outpatient setting by clinical assessment and by measuring the target glad hormone and its regulatory pituitary hormone and assessing the relationship between the two hormone values.

Anatomic Diagnosis

The most common cause of hypopituitarism is a pituitary adenoma. Therefore, it is imperative to image the pituitary gland and surrounding structures (hypothalamus, optic chiasm, cavernous sinus). The best study is a magnetic resonance imaging (MRI) scan, before and after gadolinium administration. The MRI scan images all of these structures and provides valuable information on the anatomic relationships among them, which is particularly important if pituitary surgery is indicated. Since 10% of normal subjects have a small hypodense area in the pituitary (consistent with a microadenoma), the imaging findings must be correlated with endocrine function *(26)*. If the patient is unable to undergo an MRI study (ferrous metal in the body, claustrophobia, obesity), a properly performed head CT scan can provide reliable information on pituitary size and the presence of a mass. The CT scan should be performed with thin sections (1.5 mm) through the gland and in the coronal plane, before and after contrast administration. Although the optic chiasm is not visualized, the detection of a pituitary microadenoma (as small as 3–4 mm) is possible if the study is performed correctly *(27)*.

Ophthalmologic Diagnosis

If a patient has a large pituitary mass (>10 mm), a complete ophthalmologic examination, including visual fields, is indicated. The evaluation should include assessment of visual acuity and ocular motility and as well as visual fields. Visual field examination is best done with an automated instrument such as the Goldmaml, Octopus, or Humphries. Bitemporal visual loss is the classical finding in patients with a large pituitary mass compressing the optic chiasm. However, some tumors extend more anteriorly and may involve only one optic nerve, producing a unilateral deficit. Similarly, if the tumor extends laterally and invades the cavernous sinus, ocular paresis may result. The most common motility disorder is a third nerve palsy which results in ptosis and inability to adduct the eye. Optic atrophy occurs if there has been longstanding compression of the optic chiasm or an optic nerve; the time required for this to occur is not known If a patient is found to have an abnormal visual examination, this needs to be followed closely after treatment.

TREATMENT OF HYPOPITUITARISM

Hormone replacement is necessary once the deficiency is identified. In patients with a large pituitary adenoma, resection of the tumor or treatment of a prolactin secreting adenoma with a dopamine agonist drug may result in spontaneous recovery of the deficient pituitary hormone or hormones. Conversely, surgery and/or radiation may produce deficiency *(28–39)*. Thus, the patient should be assessed for the need for hormone replacement both before and after treatment. The most important replacements are glucocorticoid and thyroid hormone to prevent significant morbidity and potential mortality. The need for glucocorticoid replacement should be established before beginning thyroid hormone therapy because administration of thyroxine in the setting of unrecognized and untreated adrenal insufficiency can precipitate an adrenal crisis with hypotension and shock.

Glucocorticoid Replacement

Glucocorticoid replacement should aim to mimic the normal circadian secretion of cortisol secretion. The most physiologic method of accomplishing this is to use hydrocortisone, which is short acting and does not require metabolism by the liver. The minimum hydrocortisone dose that restores adequate energy and vitality should be given since over-replacement causes excessive bone loss and increases the risk for development of osteoporosis *(40)*. Other side-effects of an excessive glucocorticoid dose include weight gain, edema, an increase in blood pressure, and glucose intolerance. A suggested starting hydrocortisone dose is 15 mg on awakening and 5 mg at 6:00 PM, for a total daily dose of 20 mg; the total daily dose should not exceed 30 mg. Some patients have difficulty taking a medication twice a day; in this circumstance a trial of prednisone, 5 mg on awakening, is reasonable. The long half-life of dexamethasone and risk for developing side-effects makes this preparation a less attractive choice. There is no reliable laboratory test to assess the appropriateness of the glucocorticoid replacement regimen. Careful questioning of the patient regarding symptoms of under- or over-replacement is necessary, and close monitoring of weight and blood pressure (supine and standing) is helpful. Regardless of the type of glucocorticoid used, the patient should be educated about the need to increase the dose (usually double the daily dose) during times of intercurrent illness. The patient should also wear an identifying engraved necklace or bracelet to indicate that he or she has adrenal insufficiency and requires steroid replacement.

Thyroid Hormone Replacement

Thyroid hormone replacement is most effectively administered as thyroxine (T4) once daily. The beginning dose should be selected according to the patient's baseline T4 level, his or her age, and the coexistence of other diseases, particularly coronary artery disease. It is prudent to begin replacement in older adults with a low dose (0.025 mg/d) and gradually increase the dose over several weeks to minimize the risk of precipitating angina. Thyroid hormone increases both the metabolic rate and cardiac oxygen consumption. Assessment of the suitability of the thyroxine dose is made on the basis of clinical symptoms and measurement of the serum T4 concentration. Since the etiology of thyroid failure is TSH deficiency, measurement of TSH is not reliable and may provide misleading information. The patient's symptoms, weight, blood pressure, and pulse rate should be followed and the prescribed dose should be taken for at least a month before increasing the dose.

Gonadal Steroid Replacement

Both men and women should receive gonadal steroid replacement for its medical benefits, even if the patient is not interested in restoration of sexual function. Hypogonadism produces accelerated bone loss in both women and men and increases the risk of developing osteoporosis *(41,42)*. Other consequences of hypogonadism include an increased risk of premature development of coronary artery disease in women *(43)* and loss of muscle mass in men. Men with hypogonadism should be given testosterone unless there is a contraindication such as prostate cancer. The use of oral testosterone preparations should be avoided; the only oral testosterone preparations available in the United States are hepatotoxic. The conventional method of testosterone replacement has been a long acting testosterone ester, either testosterone enanthate or testosterone cipionate. These preparations are usually administered by im injection every 2 or 3 wk and are effective in restoring sexual function. However, this method of replacement cannot be considered physiologic; serum testosterone concentrations are usually above the normal range for 1–2 d after the injection and decline to lower than normal values a few days before the next injection. More recently, two transdermal preparations have become available in the United States *(44–47)*. A patch applied to the shaved scrotum (Testoderm), and a patch that can be applied to the arms, abdomen, thigh, or back (Androderm), are more physiologic methods of replacing testosterone. These transdermal patches are applied each day, continuous dermal absorption results in stable serum testosterone levels throughout 24 h. The scrotal patch (Testoderm) is a little more difficult to use, requiring shaving of the scrotum, and adherence may be a problem with sweating or showering. Replacement with the Androderm patch usually requires application of 2 patches/d but does not require shaving or avoidance of exercise or showering. Both transdermal preparations are considerably more expensive than the long acting im preparations. Regardless of the preparation selected, the patient should have a prostate examination and measurement of the serum prostate specific antigen (PSA) level before beginning therapy. Monitoring of serum lipid concentrations, particularly LDL and HDL cholesterol, is also advisable.

There are several estrogen and progesterone preparations available for gonadal steroid replacement in women. The most convenient method to replace gonadal steroids is with an oral contraceptive preparation. Alternatively, conjugated estrogens plus progesterone (usually medroxyprogesterone) can be administered cyclically or continuously. With continuous estrogen and progesterone administration withdrawal bleeding is avoided, and this may be more acceptable to some women. Addition of progesterone is necessary in women who have a uterus and may provide some benefit for breast tissue. A transdermal estrogen preparation is also available for replacement therapy. Women should have regular breast and pelvic examinations, including a pap smear; yearly mammography is recommended in all women over 40 yr and in those with a family history of breast cancer.

Vasopressin (ADH) Replacement

An arginine vasopressin analog, desmopressin acetate (dDAVP), is the preferred method of treating patients with DI. Desmopressin acetate is now available in two delivery systems—the intranasal preparation (nasal spray or rhinal tube) and a oral form (tablets). The dose and frequency of administration of the nasal preparation must be adjusted according to the patient's symptoms; some patients can be treated with a once daily intranasal dose, others require the medication twice daily. If the patient is using dDAVP tablets, the recommended starting regimen is twice daily. Return of symptoms of polyuria and polydipsia indicates the need for another dose. Periodic monitoring of the serum sodium is helpful to detect over-replacement, excessive treatment is apparent if hyponatremia develops.

Growth Hormone Replacement

In the United States, growth hormone replacement is approved only for children. Treatment of childhood GH deficiency with GH results in acceleration of the linear growth velocity as well as changes in body composition (reduced fat mass, increased muscle mass). Whereas several European countries have approved GH replacement for GH-deficient adults, it is not yet approved in the United States. Several studies of GH administration to GH-deficient adults have demonstrated a beneficial effect on body composition, some studies also report improvement of exercise endurance and muscle strength with GH therapy *(48–52)*. As with other hormone replacement therapies, over-replacement is to be avoided. Consequences of excessive GH administration include edema, increased blood pressure, carpal tunnel syndrome, and glucose intolerance. The optimal GH dose in adults has not yet been determined, but the lowest effective dose should be used to reduce the risks of developing symptoms and signs of acromegaly.

SUMMARY

Loss of pituitary function is relatively easy to diagnose and treat with the available hormone assays and medications *(53)*. Perhaps the most difficult aspect of this disorder is consideration of the diagnosis in the setting of nonspecific symptomatology. The patient with hypopituitarism or a history of a pituitary tumor requires regular and lifelong medical care to monitor hormone replacement therapy and to detect tumor recurrence. With adequate replacement, the patient can expect to lead a productive and active life.

REFERENCES

1. Percy AK, Elveback LR, Okazaki H, Kurland LT. Neoplasms of the central nervous system: epidemiologic considerations. Neurology 1972; 22:40–48.
2. Kurland LT. The frequency of intracranial and intraspinal neoplasms in the resident population of Rochester, Minnesota. J Neurosurg 1958; 15:627–641.
3. Sandler LM, Richards NT, Carr DH, Mashiter K, Joplin GF. Long term follow-up of patients with Cushing's disease treated by interstitial irradiation. J Clin Endocrinol Metab 1987; 65:441–447.
4. Lam KSL, Tse VKC, Wang C, Yeung RTT, Ma JTC, Ho JHC. Early effects of cranial irradiation on hypothalamic-pituitary function. J Clin Endocrinol Metab 1987; 64:418–424.
5. Samaan NA, Vieto R. Schultz PN, et al. Hypothalamic, pituitary and thyroid dysfunction after radiotherapy to the head and neck. J Rad Onc Biol Phys 1982; 8: 1857–1867.
6. Wakai S. Fukushima T. Teramoto A, Sano K. Pituitary apoplexy: its incidence and clinical significance. J Neurosurg 1981; 55: 187–193.

7. Cardoso ER, Peterson EW. Pituitary apoplexy: a review. Neurosurgery 1984; 14:363–373.
8. Veldhuis JD, Hammond JM. Endocrine function after spontaneous infarction of the human pituitary: report, review, and reappraisal. Endocr Rev 1980; 1:100–107.
9. Barkan AL. Case report: pituitary atrophy in patients with Sheehan's syndrome. Am J Med Sci 1989; 1:38–40.
10. Sherif IH, Vanderley CM, Beshayah S, Bosairi S. Sella size and contents in Sheehan's syndrome. Clin Endocrinol 1989; 30:613–618.
11. Ishikawa SE, Furuse M, Saito T, Okada K, Kuzuya T. Empty sella in control subjects and patients with hypopituitarism. Endocrinol Japon 1988; 35:665–674.
12. Nakagawa YK, Matsumoto TF, Takase K. Exploration of the pituitary stalk and gland by high-resolution computed tomography: comparative study of normal subjects and cases with microadenoma. Neuroradiology 1984; 26:473–478.
13. Pocecco M, de Campo C, Marinoni S. et al. High frequency of empty sella syndrome in children with growth hormone deficiency. H'elv Paediat Acta 1988; 43:295–301.
14. Edwards OM, Clark JDA. Post-traulnatilc hypopituitarism. Medicine 1986; 65:281–290.
15. Asa SL, Bilbao JM, Kovacs K, Josser RG, Kreines K. Lymphocytic hypophysitis of pregnancy resulting in hypopituitarism: a distinct clinicopathologic entity. Ann Intern Med 1981; 95:166–171.
16. Miura M, Ushio Y, Kuratsu JI, Ikeda JI, Kai Y,. Yamashiro S. Lymphocytic adenohypophysitis: report of two cases. Surg Neurol 1989; 32:463–470.
17. Kelly TM, Edwards CQ, Meikle AW, Kushner JP. Hypogonadism in hemochromatosis: reversal with iron depletion. Ann Intern Med 1984; 101:629–632.
18. Ooi TC, Russell NA. Hypopituitarism resulting from an intrasellar carotid aneurysm. Canad J Neurol Sci 1986; 13:70–71.
19. Shone GR, Richards SH, Hourihan MD, Hall R. Thomazs JP, Scanlon MF. Non-secretory adenomas of the pituitary treated by trans-ethmoidal sellotomy. J R Soc Med 1991 ; 84: 140–143.
20. Constine LS, Woolf PD, Cann D, et al. Hypothalamic-pituitary dysfunction after radiation for brain tumors. N Engl J Med 1993; 328:87–94.
21. Snyder PJ, Fowble BF, Schatz NJ, Savino PJ, Gennarelli TA. Hypopituitarism following radiation therapy of pituitary adenomas. Am J Med 1986; 81:457–462.
22. Littley MD, Shalet SM, Beardwell CG, Ahmed SR, Applegate G, Sutton ML. Hypopituitarism following external radiotherapy for pituitary tumors in adults. Quart J Med 1989; 70:145–160.
23. Thapar K, Laws ER. Parasellar lesions other than pituitary adenomas. In: Management of Pituitary Tumours: A Handbook. M Powell, SL Lightman, eds. Churchill Livingston, London, 1996, pp. 175–222.
24. Rosén T. Bengtsson BA. Premature mortality due to cardiovascular disease in hypopituitarism. Lancet 1990; 336:285–288.
25. McGauley GA. Quality of life assessment before and after growth hormone treatment in adults with growth hormone deficiency. Acta Pediatr Scand [Suppl] 1989; 356:70–72.
26. Hall WA, Luciano MG, Doppman JL, Patronas NJ, Oldrileld EH. Pituitary magnetic resonance imaging in normal human volunteers: Occult adenomas in the general population. Ann Intern Med 1994; 120:817–820.
27. Elster AD. Modern imaging of the pituitary. Radiology 1993; 187:1–14.
28. Vance ML, Lipper M, Klibanski A, Biller BMK, Samaan NA, Molitch ME. Treatment of prolactin-secreting pituitary macroadenomas with the long-acting non-ergot dopamine agonist CV 205–502. Ann Intern Med 1990; 112:668–673.
29. Stevenaert A, Beckers A, Vandalem JL, Henen G. Early normalization of luteinizing hormone pulsatility after successful transsphenoidal surgery in women with microprolactinomas. J Clin Endocrinol Metab 1986; 62:1044–1047.
30. Sauder SE, Frager M, Case GD, Kelch RP, Marshall JC. Abnormal patterns of pulsatile luteinizing hormone secretion in women with hyperprolactinemia and amenorrhea: responses to bromocriptine. J Clin Endocrinol Metab 1984; 59:941–948.
31. Ebersold MJ, Quast LM, Laws ER Jr, et al. Long-term results in transsphenoidal removal of nonfunctioning pituitary adenomas. J Neurosurg 1986; 64:713–719.
32. Nelson PB, Goodman ML, Flickenger JC, Richardson DW, Robinson AG. Endocrine function in patients with large pituitary tumors treated with operative decompression and radiation therapy. Neurosurgery 1989; 24:398–400.
33. Arafah BM, Harrington JF, Madhoun ZT, Selman WR. Improvement of pituitary function after surgical decompression for pituitary tumor apoplexy. J Clin Endocrinol Metab 1990; 71 :323–328.

34. van Lindert EJ, Grotenhuis JA, Meijer E. Results of follow-up after removal of nonfunctioning pituitary adenomas by transcranial surgery. Br J Neurosurg 1991; 5:129–133.
35. Molitch ME, Elton RL, Blackwell RE, et al. Bromocriptine as primary therapy for prolactin-secreting macroadenomas: results of a prospective multicenter study. J Clin Endocrinol Metab 1985; 60:698–705.
36. Vance ML, Cragun JR, Reimnitz C, et al. CV 205502 treatment of hyperprolactinemia. J Clin Endocrinol Metab 1989; 68:336–339.
37. Kleinberg DL, Boyd AE, III, Wardlow S. et al. Pergolidle for the treatment of pituitary tumors secreting prolactin or growth hormone. N Engl J Med 1983; 309:704–709.
38. Arafah BM. Reversible hypopituitarism in patients with large nonfunctioning pituitary adenomas. J Clin Endocrinol Metab 1986; 62: 1173–1179.
39. Harris PE, Afshar F. Coates P. et al. The effects of transsphenoidal surgery on endocrine function and visual fields in patients with functionless pituitary tumours. Quart J Med 1989; 71:417–427.
40. Lukert BP, Raisz LG. Glucocorticoid-induced osteoporosis: pathogenesis and management. Ann Intern Med 1990; 112:352–364.
41. Greenspan SL, Oppenheim DS, Klibanski A. Importance of gonadal steroids to bone mass in men with hyperprolactinemic hypogonadism. Ann Intern Med 1989; 110:526–531.
42. Klibanski A, Neer RM, Beitins IZ, Ridgway EC, Zervas NT, McArthur JW. Decreased bone density in hyperprolactinemic women. N Engl J Med 1980; 303:1511–1514.
43. Matthews KA, Meilahn E, Kuller LH, Kelsey SF, Caggiula AW, Wing RR. Menopause and risk factors for coronary heart disease. N Engl J Med 1989; 321:641–646.
44. Findlay AC, Place VA, Snyder PJ. Transdermal delivery of testosterone. J Clin Endocrinol Metab 1987; 64:266–268.
45. Carey PO, Howards SS, Vance ML. Transdermal testosterone treatment of hypogonadal men. J Urology 1988; 140:76–79.
46. Mazer NA et al. Enhanced transdermal delivery of testosterone: a new physiologic approach for androgen replacement in hypogyonadal men. J Ctrl Rel 1992; 19:347–362.
47. Meikle AW et al. Enhanced transdermal delivery of testosterone across non-scrotal skin produces physiologic concentrations of testosterone and its metabolites in hypogonadal men. J Clin Endocrinol Metab 1992; 74:623–628.
48. Jorgensen JOL, Pedersen SA, Thuesen L, et al. Beneficial effects of growth hormone treatment in GH-deficient adults. Lancet 1989; II:1221–1225.
49. Salomon F, Cuneo RC, Hesp R, Sonksen PH. The effects of treatment with recombinant human growth hormone on body composition and metabolism in adults with growth hormone deficiency. N Engl J Med 1989; 321:797–803.
50. Cuneo RC, Salomon F, Wiles CM, Hesp R, Sonksen PH. Growth hormone treatment in growth hormone-deficient adults. I. Effects of muscle mass and strength. J Appl Physiol 1991; 70(2):688–694.
51. Cuneo RC, Salomon F, Wiles CM, Hesp R. Sonksen Pal. Growth hormone treatment in growth hormone-deficient adults. II. Effects on exercise performance. J Appl Physiol 1991; 70(2): 695–700.
52. Jorgensen JOL, Pedersen SA, Thuesen AL, et al. Long-term growth hormone treatment in growth hormone deficient adults. Acta Endocrinol (Copenh) 1991; 125:449–453.
53. Vance ML. Medical progress: hypopituitarism. New Engl J Med 1994; 330:1651–1662.

3 Prolactin

Normal Physiology

Virginia D. Sarapura, MD

Contents

INTRODUCTION

The lactogenic activity of anterior pituitary extracts was first discovered when their effect was observed in mammary glands of pseudopregnant rabbits *(1)*. A similar phenomenon was subsequently observed by several groups in guinea pig mammary glands and in pigeon crop sacs *(2,3)*, and in 1932, the hormone named prolactin was purified from sheep pituitaries *(4)*. However, human prolactin was not identified as distinct from human growth hormone until 1971 *(5,6)*. In 1980, the human prolactin gene was cloned, and later that decade Pit-1 was defined as a tissue-specific transcriptional activating factor for prolactin gene expression *(7)*. The regulation of prolactin synthesis and secretion has been extensively studied, particularly the inhibition by dopamine from the hypothalamus and the stimulation of release in response to suckling. Prolactin has multiple biological actions, including a recently recognized immunoregulatory role *(8)*. The identification of the prolactin receptor as a member of the family of structurally related hematopoietic cytokine receptors, as well as the cloning of receptor isoforms in rodents *(9)* and in humans *(10)*, may lead to a better understanding of the diversity of actions of prolactin at its target cells.

PROLACTIN GENE

Prolactin Gene Structure

The prolactin gene shares structural similarities with the growth hormone (GH) and chorionic somatomammotropin (CS) genes, and the concept of a common ancestor has

From: *Contemporary Endocrinology, Vol. 3: Diseases of the Pituitary: Diagnosis and Treatment*
Edited by M. E. Wierman Humana Press Inc., Totowa, NJ

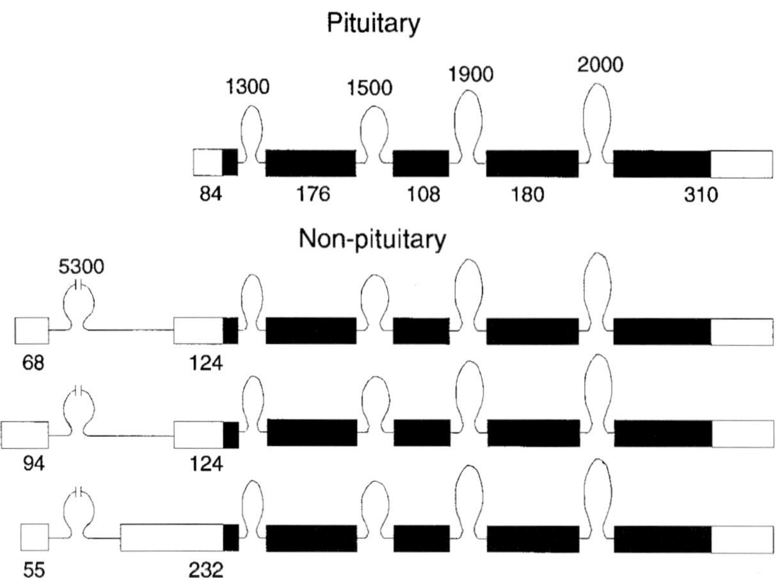

Fig. 1. Schematic representation of the human prolactin gene. The bars indicate exons and the lines, that are not drawn to scale, represent intronic DNA. The solid areas represent coding regions, the open areas represent untranslated regions. The intronic RNA is removed by splicing to form mature RNA. The numbers indicate the size in nucleotides of each exon or intron of the pituitary form, and differences in the nonpituitary variants are indicated. Note that the coding regions are identical in all forms.

been strengthened by the discovery of fish somatolactin that has a similar gene structure containing five exons and only a 24% amino acid homology with fish prolactin and growth hormone *(11)*. Whereas the human GH gene cluster contains five genes (pituitary GH-N and placental GH-V, CS-A, CS-B, and CS-L) located on chromosome 17, human prolactin shares 42% homology and is encoded by a single gene located on chromosome six. This contrasts with other species, such as rodents, that contain at least eight placental prolactin-related genes, including placental lactogens-I, -IV, and -II, prolactin-like proteins-A, -B, and -C, proliferin 1 and 2, and decidual prolactin-related protein *(12)*.

The human prolactin gene is approximately 7.5 kb in size and consists of five exons and four introns *(13)* (Fig. 1). The first exon contains the 5′ untranslated region (56 bp) and 28 bp of the coding region. The rest of the coding region is contained in the second (176 bp), third (108 bp), fourth (180 bp), and part of the fifth (189 bp) exons, and the 3′ untranslated region (121 bp) is contained in the fifth exon. The exons are separated by introns that are 1300, 1500, 1900, and 2000 bp in size. In nonpituitary tissues (decidualized endometrium and immune cells) an additional exon 1d of 55, 68, or 94 bp, depending on the transcription start site used, is located 5300 bp upstream and gives rise to alternatively spliced variants that also include an additional 40 or 148 bp upstream of the first exon (Fig. 1). These variant transcripts only differ in the length of the 5′ untranslated region so that the protein produced is identical to pituitary prolactin *(14–16)*.

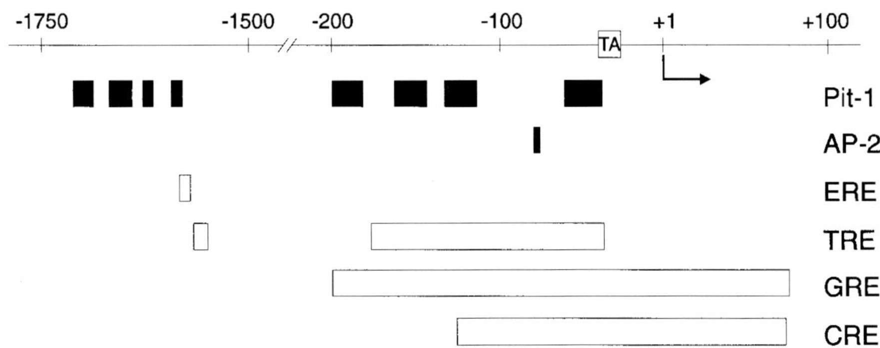

Fig. 2. Schematic representation of the rat pituitary prolactin promoter. The transcriptional start site (+1) is indicated by the arrow and the TATA box (TA) is shown. The numbers denote the position of the nucleotides relative to the transcriptional start site. The solid boxes indicate the binding sites for Pit-1 (−1718/−1694, −1670/−1645, −1636/−1619, −1586/−1578, −200/−180, −162/−142, −132/−115, and −62/−38) and AP-2 (−78/−71) and the open boxes indicate the regions important for the responses to estrogen (ERE: −1582/−1569), thyroid hormone (TRE: −1565/−1551 and −176/−38), glucocorticoids (GRE: −200/+75), and cAMP (CRE: −127/+73).

Prolactin Gene Promoter

As found in many other genes, sequences close to the transcriptional start site in the 5′ flanking sequence of the prolactin gene contain elements responsible for initiating transcription and regulating gene expression. The regulatory regions are therefore different for the two spliced variants described above, explaining the differences in the regulation of pituitary and nonpituitary prolactin gene expression. The pituitary promoter has been extensively studied in the rat *(12)* (Fig. 2). There is considerable species homology suggesting that important regulatory elements are likely to be conserved. The transcriptional initiation site (+1) defines the start of the first exon and a consensus TATA box is located at position −29. Four binding sites for Pit-1, a POU-homeodomain transcription factor that activates growth hormone and prolactin gene expression *(17)*, extend from −200 to −38 and constitute the proximal element, and another four Pit-1 binding sites extending from −1718 to −1578 constitute the distal element or enhancer. Both proximal and distal elements are necessary to confer pituitary-specific prolactin expression, as shown in transgenic mice *(18)*, but factors other than Pit-1 must be involved since the prolactin gene is not expressed in somatotropes. Other regulatory elements that have been localized on the prolactin promoter include a stimulatory estrogen response element (ERE) (−1582 to −1569) *(19)*, a stimulatory (−1565 to −1551) and an inhibitory (−176 to −38) thyroid hormone response element *(20)*, and an inhibitory glucocorticoid response element (−200 to +75) *(21)*. Dopamine is the major inhibitor of prolactin synthesis and its effect is mediated by a decrease in the levels of cyclic AMP. A cyclic AMP response element (CRE) located between −127 and +73 contains a binding site for activating protein 2 (AP2) *(22–24)*. However, the Pit-1 gene promoter also contains a CRE *(25)* and recent data suggests that the effect of cyclic AMP on the prolactin gene may be mediated primarily by modulating the transcriptional activity of Pit-1 *(26)*. Estrogen effects also appear to be mediated by Pit-1, but the Pit-1 promoter lacks an ERE, and other data suggest that estrogen may act by inhibiting dopaminergic input *(27)*. In addition, stimulatory thyrotropin releasing hormone and calcium responses may also be mediated by Pit-1, since those response regions have been mapped to the proximal Pit-1 element *(28)*.

The nonpituitary prolactin promoter has been studied more recently *(29)*. Progesterone response elements are present, although progesterone appears to regulate expression indirectly *(30)*. Pit-1 consensus sequences are also found, but there is no evidence for the action of Pit-1 in nonpituitary cells. Decidual prolactin releasing and prolactin-inhibitory factors have been purified *(31)*, but their mechanisms of action have yet to be elucidated.

BIOSYNTHESIS OF PROLACTIN

The major product of prolactin gene transcription in both pituitary and nonpituitary tissues has a molecular mass of 23 kDa *(32)*. Posttranscriptional and posttranslational modifications result in heterogeneous forms that may have important implications in the regulation of prolactin bioactivity in various physiological states.

Transcription

There are four transcriptional products of the prolactin gene, each resulting from specific activation of the pituitary and the non-pituitary promoters (Fig. 1). These transcripts differ at the 5′ untranslated region, but the aminoacid sequences are identical. In addition, a 21-kDa product has been described in rat and human pituitaries *(33)* that has been postulated to arise by alternative splicing, analogous to the 20-kDa form of GH *(34)*.

Regulation of Transcription

Pituitary prolactin transcription is influenced by various factors, including stimulation by estrogen, vasoactive intestinal peptide (VIP), and thyrotropin-releasing hormone (TRH), and inhibition by dopamine, glucocorticoids, and thyroid hormone. Whereas the effects of estrogen, glucocorticoids, and thyroid hormone appear to be directly mediated by binding of their receptors to the response elements on the promoter, VIP, TRH, and dopamine act on cell surface receptors that use signal transduction pathways and may exert their primary effect through their action on Pit-1, as described above. Dopamine mainly decreases intracellular cyclic AMP levels by inhibiting adenyl cyclase activity *(35)*. VIP increases intracellular cyclic AMP levels *(36)* and TRH activates the phosphoinositide-protein kinase C pathway that also increases intracellular calcium concentration *(37)*, although the physiological significance of these transcriptional effects is still unclear.

Translation and Posttranslational Modifications

The translation and processing of the prolactin protein is similar to other secreted proteins. The first product is preprolactin, containing a 28-amino acid signal peptide that is removed as the protein enters the rough endoplasmic reticulum, resulting in a 23-kDa product. The structure of the protein is similar to that of other helix bundle peptide hormones (growth hormone and hematopoietic cytokines) and consist of four α-helices connected by long nonhelical chains between the first and second and between the third and fourth helices, and a short nonhelical chain between the second and third helices *(38)*. In addition, disulfide bonds between cystein residues at positions 4 and 11, 58 and 174, and 191 and 199 result in the formation of a small amino-terminal loop, a large midmolecule loop, and a small carboxy-terminal loop *(38)*.

As it progresses into the Golgi apparatus, prolactin is partially (up to 25%) glycosylated at the asparagine residue at position 31, resulting in a 25-kDa product *(39)* that is less active in various assays *(40)* and is produced proportionally less in stimulated states, such as pregnancy *(41)*. Cleavage by an acid protease in the large midmolecule loop between the amino acid residues at position 145 and 146 results in the formation of 16-kDa and 8-kDa polypeptide chains linked by a disulfide bond *(42)*. This cleavage also occurs at the level of target tissues *(43)* and the identification of a unique receptor for the 16-kDa form in rat kidney, brain, liver, and endothelial cells *(44)* suggests an important physiological role for this cleavage product, that has been shown to inhibit angiogenesis *(45)*. In addition, the 16-kDa cleavage product may have a paracrine mitogenic effect on pituitary gonadotropes and thyrotropes *(42)*. Phosphorylation and deamidation also occur in the secretory granules and may modulate prolactin bioactivity *(46)*; however, a study of the differently charged isoforms that result from these modifications showed that, when prolactin secretion was stimulated, the relative abundance of these isoforms remained unchanged, suggesting that these two modifications may not be physiologically important *(47)*. Polymerization by disulfide bonding of up to 25% of prolactin stored in the secretory granules may result in the formation of dimers (45–50-kDa "big" prolactin) or multimers (150-kDa "big, big" prolactin) *(48)*, although the origin of"big, big" prolactin has been attributed to disulfide bonding to antiprolactin auto-antibodies *(49)*.

Biosynthesis of nonpituitary prolactin appears to differ from pituitary prolactin. Decidual prolactin is highly glycosylated, approximately 50% *(50)*, and is not stored in secretory granules *(51)*. These and other differences suggest distinct mechanisms for the regulation of nonpituitary prolactin secretion and bioactivity (*see* Secretion of Prolactin, below).

SECRETION OF PROLACTIN

The pituitary gland is the major source of circulating prolactin. Lactotropes comprise approximately 15–25% of the anterior pituitary cells in males and nonpregnant women *(52)*. Prolactin secretion occurs by exocytosis of secretory granules in which prolactin is stored along with chromogranin and secretogranin, which are storage proteins. Granules become electron dense and migrate to the cell surface. It was thought that only regulated secretion was carried out by secretory granules, but it has been shown that constitutive secretion is also carried out in this manner *(53)*. It appears that there are sparsely granulated lactotrope cells that rapidly turn over newly synthesized prolactin *(54)*. This heterogeneity in the lactotrope cell population may reflect different metabolic stages of the same cell or diverse secretory mechanisms may correspond to different lactotrope cell subpopulations.

The production rate of prolactin is 300–1200 μg/d with a plasma clearance rate of 60–100 mL/min and a half-life of 26–47 min *(55–57)*. The site of prolactin clearance in humans has not been determined, with the kidney aparently responsible for 33% of the clearance *(57)*, but prolactin uptake by the liver was not found *(58)*.

Measurement of Prolactin

Secretion of prolactin has been measured by reverse hemolytic plaque assay, a method that measures the secreted hormone from individual cells by the zone of hemolysis that results from the presence of an antibody to the hormone *(59)*. Sequentially using antiprolactin and anti-GH antibodies has allowed identification of individual cells that secrete prolactin alone (lactotropes) and others that cosecrete prolactin and GH (somatolactotropes) *(60)*.

Prolactin is commonly measured in serum and body fluids by a double antibody radioimmunoassay, using standardized prolactin preparations *(61)*. A method for directly measuring the nonglycosylated (more active) form of prolactin by an immunoradiometric assay has been developed *(41)*. A bioassay for prolactin based on the mitogenic effect on rat Nb2 node lymphoma cells after the addition of anti-GH antibody *(62)* has replaced the more cumbersome pigeon crop sac assay *(3)*, and a very sensitive mammary gland casein production assay has also been developed *(63)*. The normal serum prolactin level may vary from one laboratory to another but is usually less than 25 ng/mL.

Ontogeny of Prolactin Secretion

Immunoreactive prolactin cells have been observed in the human pituitary gland by 18 wk of gestation, comprising 8% of the anterior pituitary cells, with 70% of them cosecreting prolactin and growth hormone *(64)*. At birth, the prolactin levels are 10-fold increased, probably due to estrogen stimulation, and gradually decline to normal levels by 3 mo of age *(65)*.

Patterns of Prolactin Secretion

Pituitary prolactin is secreted in a pulsatile manner, similar to other pituitary hormones *(66)* (Fig. 3). Intrinsic pituitary prolactin pulses occur approximately every 8 min as shown by studies in rats in which the pituitary gland was transplanted under the kidney capsule *(67)* and in primate cultured pituitaries *(68)*. In humans with an intact pituitary under hypothalamic regulation, there are approximately 14 prolactin pulses occuring every 100 min, that appear to vary coordinately with gonadotropin pulses *(69)*, although the same pulsatile pattern was maintained in cases of hyperprolactinemia due to pituitary stalk interruption *(66)*.

Prolactin is secreted in a circadian pattern with lowest levels around noon and highest levels beginning 60–90 min after the onset of sleep *(70)*. The nocturnal rise results from increased pulse amplitude, but not pulse frequency *(71)*. Prolactin elevation has been found to coincide with rapid eye movement sleep in rats *(72)*. This circadian pattern of secretion was abolished in hyperprolactinemia due to pituitary stalk interruption *(66)*. Increases in prolactin levels also result from food intake, apparently caused by amino acids *(73)*, as well as stress *(74)*. The mechanism of stress-induced prolactin increase is still unclear *(75)* and has been attributed to β-endorphin *(76)* among other factors *(77)*.

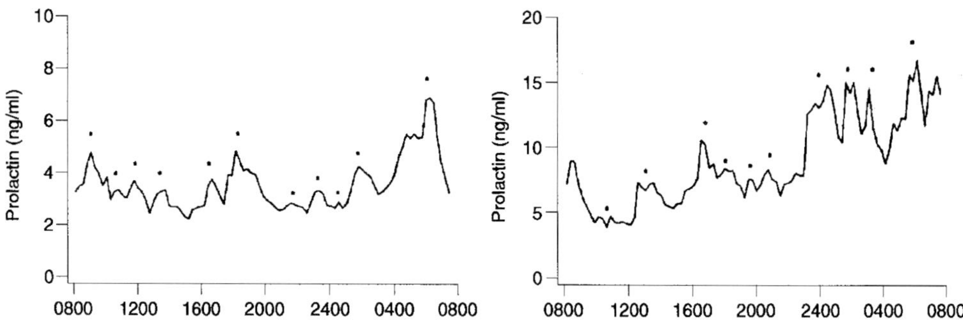

Fig. 3. Twenty-four hour prolactin levels in a representative healthy male (left panel) and healthy female (right panel). Note the difference in scale of the y-axes. *Significant prolactin pulses, located by cluster analysis. Reproduced with permission from Samuels et al. *(66)*.

Changes in Prolactin Secretion During the Menstrual Cycle, Pregnancy, and Lactation

Prolactin levels tend to be higher in women than in men *(66)* due to the stimulatory effect of estrogen (*see* Regulation of Prolactin Secretion, Peripheral Factors, below), and lower immunoreactive and bioactive levels have been observed after the menopause *(78)*. Daytime prolactin secretion is higher in the luteal than in the follicular phase of the menstrual cycle *(79)*. Serum prolactin levels gradually rise during pregnancy and reach levels over 200 ng/mL *(80)*. During labor, prolactin levels drop by 50% 2 h before delivery, then rise to a maximum 2 h after delivery, to decrease again 4 h later *(81)*. Subsequently, serum prolactin levels rise over the first 3–5 d postpartum to approximately 150 ng/mL and gradually fall to a mean of 24 ng/mL by 2 wk postpartum with continued lactation *(82)*. During lactation, prolactin is secreted following periods of suckling *(83)* and a mediating role for α-melanocyte stimulating hormone has been suggested *(84)*. Gradual decline in prolactin during lactation occurs in spite of continued suckling *(85)*, and has been attributed to refractoriness of the lactotropes to stimulatory factors *(86)*. However, the relationship between changes in prolactin levels and the recovery of gonadotropin pulses and ovulation is still controversial *(87)*. Similarities between the prolactin release in response to suckling and that due to vaginocervical stimulation in the rat *(88)* may lead to a better understanding of the neural pathways involved.

Regulation of Prolactin Secretion

Hypothalamic Factors

Prolactin Inhibitory Factors. The maintenance of prolactin secretion in the absence of any hypothalamic input to the pituitary gland, such as after transplantation under the kidney capsule *(89)*, indicates that the primary effect of the hypothalamus on prolactin secretion is inhibitory (Fig. 4). Dopamine is recognized as the physiologically important prolactin inhibitor *(90,91)*. Neurons of the tuberoinfundibular dopaminergic system arise in the arcuate nucleus of the medial basal hypothalamus and extend into the median eminence *(92)*. Dopamine is transported from the median eminence to the lactotropes in the anterior pituitary through the long pituitary portal vessels *(93)* and

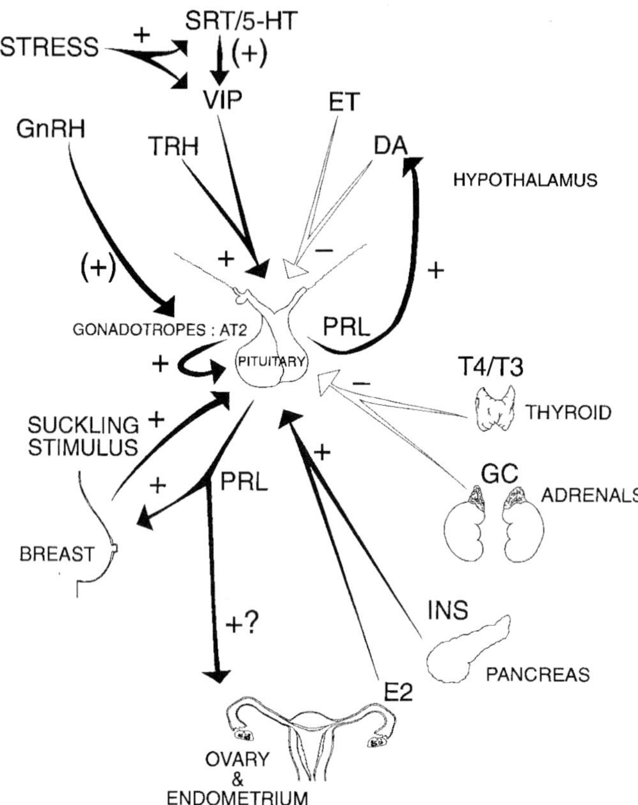

Fig. 4. Hypothalamic and peripheral control of pituitary prolactin secretion. Stimulatory effects are denoted with solid arrows and a plus sign, and inhibitory effects with open arrows and minus sign. (+) Denotes an indirect stimulatory effect; and +? denotes a possible stimulatory effect. PRL, prolactin; T4/T3, thyroid hormones; GC, glucocorticoids; INS, insulin; E2, estrogen; DA, dopamine; ET, endothelin; SRT, serotonin; 5-HT, 5-hydroxytryptamine; TRH, thyrotropin releasing hormone; VIP, vasoactive intestinal peptide; GnRH, gonadotropin releasing hormone; AT2, angiotensin II.

binds to the D2 receptor subtype *(94)* that is present in two isoforms generated by alternative splicing *(95)*. Interaction with each receptor isoform may differentially activate multiple signal transduction pathways, resulting in decreased intracellular cyclic AMP *(96)*, calcium *(97)*, and phosphoinositide *(98)* levels. Recent studies suggest that pulsatile stimulation of these pathways is necessary for prolactin activation *(99–101)*. As described above (*see* Prolactin Gene Promoter), although a direct effect on prolactin gene transcription at the AP2 binding site has been shown, an indirect effect mediated by Pit-1 may be primarily responsible for the inhibitory effect of dopamine on prolactin synthesis. Release of secretory granules is primarily affected by the reduction in intracellular calcium levels, since calcium is important in the process of exocytosis *(102)*. A recent study suggests that nitric oxide may mediate the inhibition of dopamine on prolactin release *(103)*.

γ-Aminobutyric acid (GABA) was found to inhibit rat prolactin in vivo and in vitro *(104)*, and a GABAergic system analogous to the tuberoinfundibular dopaminergic system has been described, as well as high affinity GABA receptors in the pituitary gland

(105–107). Gonadotropin releasing hormone-associated peptide (GAP) is a 56-amino acid polypeptide that has prolactin-inhibitory activity *(108)*. However, the potency of these two potential prolactin-inhibitory factors is 100-fold lower than that of dopamine, which raises questions about their physiological role. Recently, endothelin transcripts, protein, and receptors have been found in rat hypothalamus and pituitary gland *(109)*. Endothelin-1 and -2 have been found to be potent inhibitors of prolactin release in vitro, with effective doses in the range of 1 p*M*–1 n*M (110)*, but their physiologic role still needs to be defined.

Prolactin Releasing Factors. The acute prolactin release seen with suckling and stress cannot be fully explained by reversal of dopamine inhibition. Thyrotropin releasing hormone (TRH) was the first factor to be identified as a stimulator of prolactin release in rat pituitary cells *(111)* and humans *(112,113)*. TRH is produced by neurons of the parvocellular region of the paraventricular nucleus that extend to the median eminence. As described above (*see* Prolactin Gene Promoter), TRH exerts its effect via the phosphoinositide pathway, resulting in increased intracellular calcium concentrations and protein kinase C activation. Interestingly, the reverse hemolytic plaque assay described above has identified cells that respond to either dopamine or TRH, with a higher proportion of cells that only respond to TRH located near the periphery of the pituitary gland, where a higher proportion of somatolactotropes is also localized *(60)*. However, the physiologic role of TRH has been questioned by a number of studies, one of which showed that the immunoneutralization of TRH did not alter the prolactin response to suckling or to hypothalamic electrical stimulation *(114)*.

Vasoactive intestinal peptide (VIP) was found to stimulate prolactin release *(115)* and, subsequently, synthesis as well *(116)*. It is produced by neurons of the parvocellular region of the paraventricular nucleus *(117)*, as well as in the anterior pituitary *(118)*, and acts by increasing both intracellular cyclic AMP levels *(36)* and intracellular calcium concentrations *(119)*. Immunoneutralization of VIP altered the prolactin response to suckling and abolished the response to stress *(120)*. In addition, a peptide derived from the same precursor as VIP, peptide histidine-isoleucine, appears to have a similar activity to VIP *(121)* and its immunoneutralization results in an inhibitory effect on stress-induced prolactin release that is additive to the immunoneutralization of VIP *(122)*.

Serotonin and 5-hydroxytryptamine stimulate prolactin release through an indirect action on other hypothalamic factors, possibly VIP *(123)*. Gonadotropin releasing hormone (GnRH) was shown to stimulate lactotrope growth and prolactin release in culture only in the presence of gonadotropes *(124)*, and this effect is mediated by angiotensin II *(125)*. Studies of cultured human prolactinomas demonstrated GnRH binding and stimulation of prolactin secretion only if the tumors were also immunoreactive for gonadotropin α-subunit *(126)*. The physiological role of GnRH is supported by the finding of synchronous pulsatile secretion of prolactin and luteinizing hormone in ovariectomized primates that is suppressed by GnRH antagonists *(127)*. Other potential prolactin releasing factors include opioids, oxytocin, a vasopressin-cosynthesized 39 amino acid peptide, neurotensin, histamine, substance P, and others *(128)*. Recently, two prolactin releasing factors were isolated from intermediate lobe (melanotrope) tumors from transgenic mice *(129)*. The new factors were shown to differ from POMC-derivatives and other known prolactin releasing factors, and their physiological significance needs to be determined by further investigations.

Peripheral Factors

Estrogen. Estrogen is a potent stimulator of lactotrope differentiation and prolactin secretion. Rat somatotrope cells in culture have been induced to secrete prolactin with concomitant reduction in GH secretion by exposure to estradiol *(130)*. An increase in the proportion of somatotrope cells that produce prolactin has been found in pregnant women by both immunocytochemical and *in situ* hybridization studies *(131)*, explaining in part the marked lactotrope hyperplasia seen in pregnancy and lactation *(132)*.

The effect of estrogen occurs in part directly at the level of prolactin gene expression *(133)* resulting in a first phase independent of protein synthesis (0.5–2 h), followed by a second phase (6–48 h) that is blocked by the protein synthesis inhibitor cycloheximide. The latter is possibly mediated by modulation of other hypothalamic factors *(134)*, probably by inhibiting dopamine secretion and decreasing the number of dopamine receptors *(135,136)*. It has been proposed that the effects of estrogen on lactotrope proliferation and prolactin secretion may be mediated by galanin *(137)*, a peptide produced in the pituitary as well as other tissues. Thus, differential inhibition of estrogen-stimulated galanin but not prolactin gene transcription resulted in decreased plasma protein levels of both *(138)*.

Other Peripheral Factors. Glucocorticoids inhibit prolactin secretion probably by interfering with the binding of a transcriptional activator on the pituitary prolactin gene promoter *(139)*. Glucocorticoids also inhibit nonpituitary prolactin secretion, specifically from IM-9-P3 B-lymphocytes, by a decrease in mRNA stability (140).

As described above, the pituitary prolactin gene promoter contains both stimulatory and inhibitory thyroid hormone response elements, but the net effect is inhibitory on both prolactin transcription *(141)* and secretion *(142)*. Conversely, prolactin secretion is increased in hypothyroidism, with the concomitant effect of TRH contributing to this increase (*see* Hypothalamic Factors). However, total lack of thyroid hormone as seen after thyroidectomy in rats results in atrophy and hypofunction of lactotrope cells, as well as lack of response of prolactin to TRH, with thyroid hormone administration reversing these effects *(143)*.

Insulin stimulates pituitary prolactin secretion by a direct transcriptional effect *(144)*. Insulin stimulation is also observed in nonpituitary (decidual) prolactin expression *(145)*.

Feedback Control of Prolactin Secretion

Prolactin exerts an inhibitory effect on its own secretion by a short feedback loop, whereby prolactin acts on hypothalamic prolactin receptors *(146)* to stimulate dopamine synthesis *(147,148)*. A rat model for short feedback loop regulation is the intrahypothalamic anterior pituitary graft that has been shown to cause central but not peripheral elevation in prolactin levels and effectively inhibit prolactin secretion *(149)*. However, in late pregnancy this mechanism is nonfunctional *(150)*, and this loss of sensitivity to the prolactin feedback appears to be an adaptive mechanism to promote lactation. There is also evidence from studies of dwarf mice that prolactin acts as a neurotrophic factor for the development of the tuberoinfundibular dopaminergic neurons, and the deficit in this system may be reversed by prolactin replacement *(151)*.

ACTION OF PROLACTIN

Prolactin has a wide range of actions across different animal species *(152)*. These actions include effects on reproduction, immunomodulation, and osmoregulation. In humans, all these actions are secondary to the more important lactogenic effect *(153)*.

Prolactin Receptor

Prolactin acts by binding to a specific cell-surface receptor, although intracellular receptors have also been described *(154)*. Receptors have been detected in a wide variety of tissues *(155)*. The cDNA encoding the human prolactin receptor has recently been cloned *(156)*. The prolactin receptor consists of a single polypeptide chain of 622 amino acids that includes a 24-amino acid signal peptide, with a nonglycosylated molecular mass of 66.9 kDa. There are five cystein residues and three glycosylation sites in the extracellular domain (amino acid residues 1–210), a hydrophobic transmembrane domain (amino acid residues 211–234), and a long intracellular domain (amino acid residues 235–598). The gene is located on chromosome 5p 13–14, close to the localization of the growth hormone receptor gene *(157)*. Both of these receptors have a high sequence homology and belong to the hematopoietic cytokine receptor superfamily, which also includes the receptors for erythropoietin, interleukins, and granulocyte-macrophage colony stimulating factor *(158)*. In the rat, several isoforms have been described that vary in the length of the intracellular domain, as indicated: a long form with 357 amino acids *(159)*, an intermediate form with 159 amino acids produced in rat Nb2 lymphoma cells from a mutated prolactin receptor gene *(160)*, and a short form with 51 amino acids *(9)*. Yet another prolactin receptor isoform was identified in rat ovary, with only the 210 amino acid extracellular domain and a 20-amino acid unique carboxy terminus, that may be a soluble form of the receptor *(161)*. Only recently, an intermediate form of the prolactin receptor has been identified in human mammary gland tissue, consisting of a splice variant that removes 572 nucleotides that encode 191 amino acids close to the transmembrane domain, and also results in a frameshift that introduces a stop codon 13 amino acids after the splice site, resulting in an intracellular domain of 274 amino acids rather than the 364 amino acids of the long form *(10)*. A smaller protein, close in size to the rat short receptor isoform was also detected by immunoblotting, but its identity has not been established *(10)*. Specific physiologic roles for each isoform have yet to be defined.

High-affinity binding of prolactin to its receptor has been demonstrated, with a Kd of 10^{-10} *M* and a 50% saturation at a concentration of 7 ng/mL *(162)*. Receptor number in mammary glands and liver appears to increase in response to prolactin by both transcriptional and posttranscriptional effects *(163)*. Estrogens also produce the same effect indirectly, by increasing the release of prolactin from the pituitary gland, whereas progestins decrease prolactin receptor number *(164)*. Studies with antibodies to the prolactin receptor *(165,166)* and with growth hormone analogs *(167)* have indicated that dimerization of the prolactin receptor is required for receptor activation, resulting in a bell-shaped response curve in which high concentrations of receptor do not allow for dimerization to take place *(168)* (Fig. 5). Prolactin receptors, like the growth hormone and hematopoietic cytokine receptors, lack intrinsic tyrosine kinase activity and do not have the transmembrane domain structure of G protein-coupled receptors,

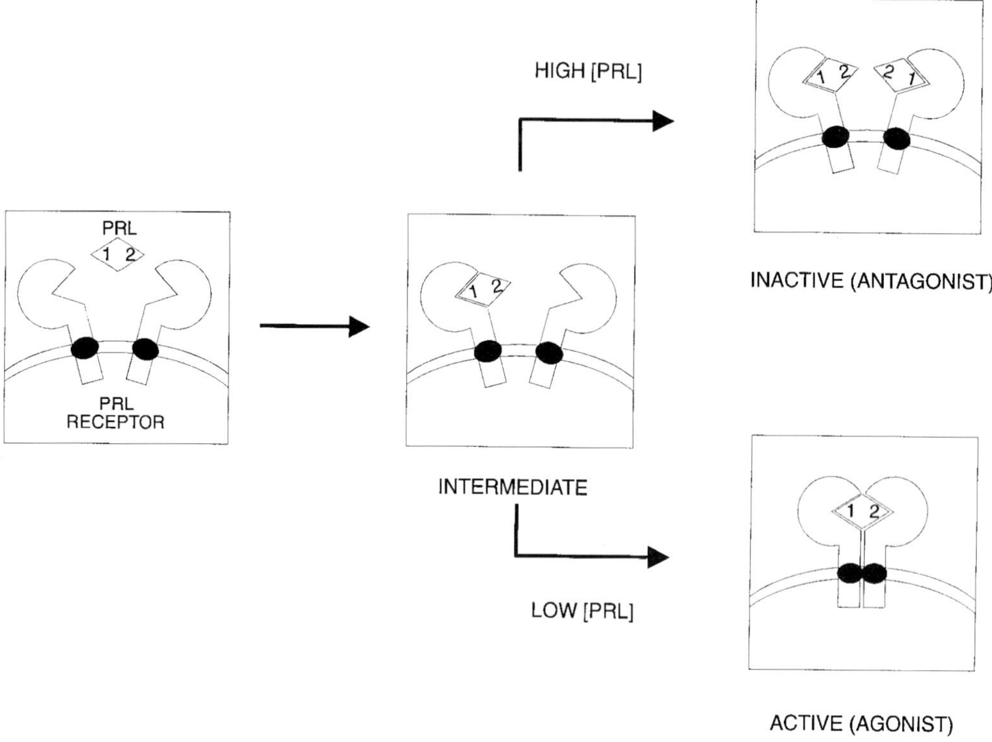

Fig. 5. Sequential dimerization model for activation of the prolactin receptor. At low concentrations, prolactin (PRL) binds first at site 1 and subsequently at site 2 (as indicated) to produce an active prolactin-(prolactin receptor)$_2$ complex. At high concentrations, prolactin saturates the receptor through site 1 interactions, therefore inhibiting dimerization and acting as an antagonist. Adapted with permission from Fuh et al. *(168)*.

so that the signal transduction pathways were not immediately evident when their structure was first determined. It appears that adenyl cyclase activation is not involved *(169)*. Rather, there is activation of protein kinases, such as the tyrosine kinase, Jak2, *(170)* and the serine/threonine kinase, Raf-1 *(171)*, any of which may activate MAP kinase and result in the nuclear translocation of transcription factors called STATs (signal transducers and activators of transcription) *(172)*. Subsequently, the prolactin-receptor complex is internalized *(173)*. Prolactin binding proteins that appear to be receptor cleavage products have been identified in rat serum *(174)* and rabbit milk *(175)*, and their significance is unknown.

It is interesting that human GH, but not that of other species, is able to interact with the human prolactin receptor. This interaction is dependent on the presence of Zn^{2+}, which does not appear to be necessary for the interaction between human GH or human prolactin with its own receptors *(12)*. Following that of the growth hormone receptor, crystallography of the prolactin receptor has recently been performed *(176)*, and further analysis of the structure of complexes formed between prolactin or growth hormone and their receptors will help elucidate the specificity of these interactions.

Effects of Prolactin

Effects on the Mammary Glands

The lactogenic effect, stimulation of milk production in the postpartum period, is the principal role of prolactin in humans. It has been well established that prolactin induces the transcription of casein and other milk proteins *(177)*, and recently it was shown that prolactin directly activates the mouse mammary gland factor, a nuclear transcription factor required for β-casein synthesis *(178)*. Prolactin also increases the activity of the glucose transporter GLUT1 *(179)*, whereas lipogenic enzymes and lipid uptake in mammary tissue are controlled by both prolactin and GH *(180)*, although other hormones such as insulin are also involved *(181)*. In bromocriptine-treated rats, thus prolactin-deficient, the fat content of milk remained unchanged, whereas protein and lactose content were reduced by 47 and 81%, respectively, whereas treatment with growth hormone antiserum caused only minor changes, suggesting a major role of prolactin in maintaining normal milk constitution *(182)*. Other effects of prolactin on the mammary gland include the synthesis of parathyroid hormone-related peptide *(183)*, which has been found in high concentrations in milk, possibly facilitating calcium transport *(184)*, and the induction of a secretory immune system for the production of IgA antibodies that are secreted in milk *(185)*.

The ability of normal and malignant human mammary epithelium to synthesize and secrete prolactin has been recently demonstrated *(10,186)*, suggesting an autocrine role of prolactin in the mammary gland. In addition, normal and malignant mouse mammary epithelium have been found to cleave prolactin and produce a 16-kDa product *(187)*, but the action of this product in the mammary gland has not been determined. In a recent study of prolactin secretion in human milk, multiple variants were detected ranging from 23 to >60 kDa and consisting of phosphorylated and glycosylated forms *(188)*. A high ratio of prolactin bioactivity to immunoreactivity in milk, 1.4 and 3.6 in mothers of term and preterm infants, respectively, contrasted with a ratio of 1 and 0.6 in the serum of the same mothers, suggesting that prolactin is activated in the mammary gland *(188)*. It is of note that the 16-kDa form of prolactin is only weakly immunoreactive, but it is bioactive on rat Nb2 node lymphoma cells *(189)*, so it is possible that secretion of this product into milk may explain that discrepancy.

It was thought that prolactin was also responsible for the mitogenic effect on mammary tissue, but this has now been found to be independent of the prolactin receptor and is possibly mediated by systemically or locally produced IGF-1 *(190)*. A 29-kDa IGF-binding protein that is induced by prolactin in mouse mammary epithelium has been described *(191)* that possibly plays a role in the growth of the mammary gland during gestation.

Effects on the Female Reproductive Organs

The role of prolactin in ovarian function differs among species. In rodents, prolactin is necessary to maintain the corpus luteum in early pregnancy *(192,193)* and a preovulatory prolactin surge is observed, apparently mediated by the posterior pituitary *(194)*. In humans, the disorder caused by elevated prolactin levels is well recognized clinically, resulting in inhibition of pulsatile gonadotropin secretion, at least in part by altering the function of the gonadotropin releasing hormone pulse generator *(195,196)*, as well as inhibition of estrogen and progesterone secretion directly from the ovary *(197–199)*. This results in a range of disorders from shortened luteal phases, to anovulation and amenorrhea. However, a physiologic role in human ovarian function is less well defined. Prolactin is present in ovarian follicular fluid, by both immunoreactive and bioactive assays, in levels higher than serum *(200)*, suggesting local synthesis or active transport. A case of isolated prolactin deficiency was reported to be associated with anovulation, but other cases of hypoprolactinemia with alactogenesis have not been associated with infertility *(201)*. Some investigators found that normally cycling women treated with bromocriptine, resulting in low normal prolactin levels, had low progesterone levels and shortened luteal phases *(202–204)*, correlating with a stimulatory effect of prolactin on progesterone production from human luteal cells observed in vitro *(205)*, but this was not observed by others *(206)*. A beneficial effect of prolactin on oocyte maturation was suggested by some studies of women undergoing in vitro fertilization. Follicular fluid prolactin levels were significantly higher in oocytes that were more mature (1.5- to 2-fold) and those that fertilized (fourfold) as well as in those associated with a successful pregnancy (twofold) *(207)*, agreeing with the finding in spontaneous cycles of a higher level of prolactin in follicular fluid associated with more mature oocytes *(208)*. In another study, women undergoing in vitro fertilization who received bromocriptine, resulting in a mean preovulatory prolactin level of 4 ng/mL, had a decreased rate of fertilization and cleavage, compared to untreated women whose preovulatory prolactin rose to a mean of 43 ng/mL *(209)*. On the other hand, some investigators have found no effect of transient hyperprolactinemia on the outcome of in vitro fertilization *(210–212)*, whereas others reported improvement in fertilization or cleavage rates by suppressing transient hyperprolactinemia with bromocriptine *(213,214)*.

The human endometrium contains high-affinity binding sites for prolactin, and in vitro studies have shown that the attachment and growth of isolated endometrial epithelial and stromal cells are stimulated by prolactin, with a bell-shaped dose–response suggestive of receptor dimerization *(215)* (*see* Prolactin Receptor and Fig. 5). This effect may be important in the process of implantation. In rodents and other species, a number placental prolactin-related genes have been described (*see* Prolactin Gene), and may have important effects in the uterus during pregnancy, possibly acting through prolactin receptors, whereas a specific placental lactogen receptor has recently been described in bovine endometrium *(216)*.

Effects on the Male Reproductive Organs

A direct physiologic role of prolactin in testicular function has also been postulated. In rodents, prolactin increased LH-stimulated spermatogenesis *(217)* and testosterone production *(218)*, apparently due to an increase in LH receptors *(219)*. Normal men treated with bromocriptine for 8 wk, with resulting reduced prolactin levels, exhibited lower basal and hCG-stimulated testosterone levels *(220)*. On the other hand, elevated prolactin levels resulted in decreased gonadotropin secretion and hypogonadism, with impotence and decreased libido as well as decreased sperm counts and motility. It has been noted that impotence and decreased libido are usually not reversible with testosterone treatment until prolactin levels are normalized *(221,222)*.

Studies in rodents have shown that prolactin enhances the effect of testosterone on the prostate gland, apparently by increasing the levels of nuclear androgen receptor, in addition to having testosterone-independent effects *(223)*. Citrate production, believed to be the primary function of the prostate, is directly increased by prolactin, through stimulation of synthesis and inhibition of degradation. Prolactin is required for prostate development *(224)* and also stimulates mature prostate growth *(225)*. A role in the development of benign prostate hyperplasia or prostate cancer has not been demonstrated.

Human semen contains high levels of prolactin, 1.6-fold higher than serum levels *(226)*, suggesting that it may be synthesized locally or actively transported from the serum. It appears to be secreted by both the testicular–epididimal unit and the prostate and seminal vesicles, since levels fall to approximately 50% after vasectomy *(227)*. Prolactin has been shown to stimulate metabolic functions of human spermatozoa, including fructose utilization and glycolysis *(228)*.

Effects on the Immune System

Information is accumulating to support an important role for prolactin as an immunomodulator *(229–231)*. In rodents, hypophysectomy was noted to result in the involution of the thymus, and this can be reversed by implantation of rat GH3 somatomammotropic tumor cells that secrete prolactin and growth hormone *(232)*. Hypophysectomy also resulted in decreased rejection of skin grafts and production of antibodies, as well as decreased DNA synthesis in lymphocytes, all of which were restored to normal by daily injections of growth hormone or prolactin *(233–235)*. Suppression of normal prolactin levels with bromocriptine resulted in similar effects that were also reversed by administration of prolactin *(236,237)*. In animal models of autoimmunity, bromocriptine was found to suppress disease activity *(238–240)*. Antagonism of prolactin action by cyclosporin was demonstrated in rodent *(241)* and human *(242)* T-lymphocytes, and may be the basis of its immunosuppressive effect. Activation of human B-lymphocytes by prolactin at physiologic concentrations was demonstrated in vitro *(243)*. In addition, increased serum prolactin levels have been found before rejection of transplanted human hearts *(244)* and in some human autoimmune diseases, for which treatment with bromocriptine has been proposed *(245–247)*. On the other hand, the markedly increased prolactin levels of pregnancy as well as other hyperprolactinemic states have been reported to suppress immunity *(248–250)*, suggesting a bell-shaped response of the immune function consistent with the concept of prolactin receptor dimerization (*see* Prolactin Receptors and Fig. 5).

The presence of prolactin receptors in human immune cells, including B- and T-lymphocytes, and monocytes *(251)* supports a direct effect of prolactin as an immunomodulator. In addition, prolactin receptor expression was found to be increased in rodent lymph nodes draining a site of immunization *(252)*. Moreover, it appears that T-lymphocytes are able to synthesize prolactin *(251,253)*, suggesting an autocrine/paracrine regulation. The mitogenic effect of prolactin on lymphoid cells was demonstrated by neutralization with antiprolactin antibodies, which inhibited the proliferative response to mitogens *(254)*. Studies have shown that the mitogen IL-2, a cytokine belonging to the family of helix bundle peptide hormones that includes prolactin, stimulates proliferation of rat Nb2 lymphoma cells by causing translocation of the prolactin receptor to the nuclear periphery and prolactin into the nucleus, and this effect was blocked with antiprolactin antibodies *(255)*. When Nb2 cells, which do not produce prolactin endogenously, were transfected with the prolactin gene, a similar effect was observed, but when transfected with a chimeric prolactin gene containing a signal peptide that directed nuclear localization, antiprolactin antibodies did not block IL-2-stimulated proliferation. This indicates that nuclear prolactin is important in mediating the proliferative effect of IL-2 and also that prolactin can function in the absence of its cell-surface receptor *(8)*. A short and long form of the prolactin receptor have recently been described in rodent lymphoid tissues, and the authors suggested that a possible function for the short form may be to translocate prolactin into the nucleus *(256)*. Tyrosine kinase phosphorylation was found to be necessary for prolactin internalization, but nuclear targetting appeared to require protein kinase C activation *(257)*, although others found that proliferation of Nb2 cells in response to prolactin, although still involving phosphorylation, was unaffected by TPA, an inhibitor of protein kinase C *(258)*.

Target genes for prolactin in lymphocytes include IRF-1, c-*fos*, c-*myc*, ODC, IFN-γ, Hsp70, gfi-1, and cyclins *(38)*. Expression of messenger RNA for GnRH, a truncated GnRH-associated peptide, and the GnRH receptor were detected by reverse transcriptase-polymerase chain reaction in rat Nb2 lymphoma cells, with a triphasic response to physiologic levels of prolactin *(259)*, but the significance of these findings is unclear.

In addition to its immunomodulatory effect, prolactin has been found to promote erythroid as well as myeloid differentiation *(260)*. Human hematopoietic progenitor cells were found to contain prolactin receptors, and prolactin was found to increase the number of erythropoietin receptors *(260)*. This effect may explain the increased erythropoiesis observed in pregnant women *(261)*.

Effects on Osmoregulation

The role of prolactin in osmoregulation is important in fish, amphibians, reptiles, birds, and rodents *(262)*. In these animals, prolactin causes increased absorption of water, sodium, and chloride from the intestinal tract and the kidney. In humans, a relationship between hyperprolactinemia and renal water metabolism was reported by some investigators *(263,264)* but not by others *(265,266)*, whereas evidence for the presence of prolactin receptors in the human kidney *(267)* suggests a physiologic role. Recently, a study of patients with cirrhosis showed a significant reduction in urinary sodium excretion in response to thyrotropin releasing hormone in a subset who had an exacerbated prolactin response *(268)*, but there was no proof that this indirect effect was due to prolactin. Modulation of chloride concentration in human sweat *(269)* and fetoplacental water diffusion *(270)* have also been attributed to prolactin.

A stimulatory effect of prolactin on intestinal calcium absorption and 1-α hydroxylation of 25-hydroxyvitamin D were described in rats *(271)*, but this was not demonstrated in human subjects with hyperprolactinemia *(272)*; however, the recent finding of prolactin receptors in human gastric and intestinal epithelia *(273)* suggests that prolactin may have a function in the human digestive system.

Effects on Behavior

Women with hyperprolactinemia have been noted to have higher indices of depression and hostility in psychometric testing, which improved when prolactin was normalized *(274)*. In men, decreased libido was not always corrected by treatment with testosterone until hyperprolactinemia was corrected as well *(221,222)*. However, whether prolactin exerts a physiologic effect on behavior is unclear. There is some indication that prolactin may play a role in the maternal behavior in rodents *(275,276)*, although the development of this behavior in hypophysectomized virgin rats exposed to pups was only delayed, not absent *(274)*. The relationship between stress and elevated prolactin levels has been documented in animals and humans, and interventions designed to increase active involvement in stressful situations, such as in the care of a sick relative, have been shown to decrease prolactin levels *(277)*. In human infants, a relationship was found between higher prolactin levels and abnormal affect, particularly unhappiness and withdrawal, suggesting that a characteristic neuroendocrine and behavioral response to stress involving changes in prolactin secretion may be observed early in life *(278)*.

REFERENCES

1. Stricker P, Grueter F. Action du lobe anterieure de l'hypophyse sur la montee laitesse. C R Soc Biol 1928; 99:1978–1980.
2. Corner GW. The hormonal control of lactation. I. Non-effect of the corpus luteum. II. Positive action of extracts of the hypophysis. Am J of Physiol 1980; 95:43–55.
3. Riddle O, Braucher FP. Studies on the physiology of reproduction in birds. Am J of Physiol 1931; 97:614–625.
4. Riddle O, Bates WR, Dykshorn WS. A new hormone of the anterior pituitary. Proc Soc Exp Biol Med 1983; 29:1211-1212.
5. Lewis UJ, Singh RNP, Seavey BK. Human prolactin: Isolation and some properties. Biochem Biophys Res Commun 1971; 44:1169-1176.
6. Hwang P, Guyda H, Friesen H. Purification of human prolactin. J Biol Chem 1972; 247:1955–1958.
7. Nelson C, Albert VR, Elsholtz HP, Lu LIW, Rosenfeld MG. Activation of cell-specific expression of rat growth hormone and prolactin genes by a common transcription factor. Science 1988; 239:1400–1405.
8. Clevenger CV, Altmann SW, Prystowsky MB. Requirement of nuclear prolactin for interleukin-2 stimulated proliferation of T lymphocytes. Science 1991; 253:77–79.
9. Kelly PA, Djiane J, Postel-Vinay M-C, Edery M. The prolactin/growth hormone receptor family. Endocrine Rev 1991; 12:235–251.
10. Clevenger CV, Chang W-P, Ngo W, Pasha TLM, Montone KT, Tomaszewski JE. Expression of prolactin and prolactin receptor in human breast carcinoma. Am J Pathol 1995; 146:695–705.
11. Takayama Y, Rand-Weaver M, Kawauchi H, Ono M. Gene structure of chum salmon somatolactin, a presumed pituitary hormone of the growth hormone/prolactin family. Mol Endocrinol 1991; 5:778–786.
12. Cooke NE, Liebhaber SA. Molecular biology of the growth hormone-prolactin gene system. Vitamins Hormones 1995; 50:385–459.
13. Truong AT, Duez C, Belayew A, Renard A. Isolation and characterization of the human prolactin gene. EMBO J 1984; 3:429–437.
14. Hiraoka Y, Tatsumi K, Shiozawa M, Aiso S, Fukasawa T, Yasuda K. A placenta-specific 5′ non-coding exon of human prolactin. Mol Cell Endocrinol 1991; 75:71–80.
15. Gellersen B, DiMattia GE, Friesen HG, Bohnet HG. Prolactin mRNA from human decidua differs from pituitary prolactin mRNA but resembles the IM-9-P3 lymphoblast prolactin transcript. Mol Cell Endocrinol 1989; 64:127–139.
16. DiMattia GE, Gellersen B, Duckworth ML, Friesen HG. Human prolactin gene expression. J Biol Chem 1990; 265:16412–16421.
17. Castrillo J-L, Theill LE, Karin M. Function of the homeodomain protein GHF-1 in pituitary cell proliferation. Science 1991; 253:197–199.
18. Crenshaw EB, Kalla D, Simmons DM, Swanson LW, Rosenfeld MG. Cell-specific expression of the prolactin gene in transgenic mice is controlled by synergistic interactions between promoter and enhancer elements. Genes & Dev 1989; 3:959–972.

19. Waterman ML, Adler S, Nelson C, Greene GL, Evans RM, Rosenfeld MG. A single domain of the estrogen receptor confers deoxyribonucleic acid binding and transcriptional activation of the rat prolactin gene. Mol Endocrinol 1988; 2:14–21.
20. Day RN, Maurer RA. Thyroid hormone-responsive elements of the prolactin gene: evidence for both positive and negative regulation. Mol Endocrinol 1989; 3:931–938.
21. Somasekhar MB, Gorski J. Two elements of the rat prolactin 5′ flanking region are required for its regulation by estrogen and glucocorticoids. Gene 1988; 69:13–21.
22. Keech CA, Gutierrez-Hartmann A. Analysis of rat prolactin promoter sequences that mediate pituitary-specific and 3′,5′-cyclic adenosine monophosphate-regulated gene expression in vivo. Mol Endocrinol 1989; 3:832–839.
23. Keech CA, Jackson SM, Siddiqui SK, Ocran KW, Gutierrez-Hartmann A. Cyclic adenosine 3′5′-monophosphate activation of the rat prolactin promoter is restricted to the pituitary-specific cell type. Mol Endocrinol 1992; 6:2059–2070.
24. Iverson RA, Day KH, d'Emden M, Day RN, Maurer RA. Clustered point mutation analysis of the rat prolactin promoter. Mol Endocrinol 1990; 4:1564–1571.
25. McCormick A, Brady H, Fukushima J, Karin M. The pituitary-specific regulatory gene GHF1 contains a minimal cell type-specific promoter centered around its TATA box. Genes & Dev 1991; 4:1490–1503.
26. Lew AM, Elsholtz HP. A dopamine-responsive domain in the N-terminal sequence of Pit-1. J Biol Chem 1995; 270:7156–7160.
27. Lee BJ, Kim JH, Lee CK, Kang HM, Kim HC, Kang SG. Changes in mRNA levels of a pituitary-specific trans-acting factor, Pit-1, and prolactin during the rat estrous cycle. Eur J Endocrinol 1995; 132:771–776.
28. Yan G-Z, Bancroft C. Mediation by calcium of thyrotropin-releasing hormone action on the prolactin promoter via transcription factor pit-1. Mol Endocrinol 1991; 5:1488–1497.
29. Gellersen B, Kempf R, Telgmann R, DiMattia GE. Nonpituitary human prolactin gene transcription is independent of pit-1 and differentially controlled in lymphocytes and in endometrial stroma. Mol Endocrinol 1994; 8:356–373.
30. Huang JR, Tseng L, Bischof P, Janne OA. Regulation of prolactin production by progestin, estrogen, and relaxin in human endometrial stromal cells. Endocrinology 1987; 121:2011–2017.
31. Handwerger S, Harman I, Golander A, Handwerger DA. Prolactin release from perifused human decidual explants; Effects of decidual prolactin-releasing factor (PRL-RF) and prolactin-release-inhibitory factor (PRL-IF). Placenta 1992; 13:55–62.
32. Cooke NE, Coit D, Shine J, Baxter JD, Martial JA. Human prolactin, cDNA structural analysis and evolutionary comparisons. J Biol Chem 1981; 256:4007–4016.
33. Sinha YN, Jacobsen BP. Structural and immunologic evidence for a small molecular weight ("21K") variant of prolactin. Endocrinology 1988; 123:1364–1370.
34. Estes PA, Cooke NE, Liebhaber SA. A native RNA secondary structure controls alternative splice-site selection and generates two growth hormone isoforms. J Biol Chem 1992; 267:14902–14908.
35. Maurer RA. Dopaminergic inhibition of prolactin synthesis and prolactin messenger RNA accumulation in cultured pituitary cells. J Biol Chem 1980; 255:8092–8097.
36. Onali P, Eva C, Olianas MC, Schwawrtz JP, Costa E. In GH3 pituitary cells, acetylcholine and vasoactive intestinal peptide antagonistically modulate adenylate cyclase, cyclic AMP content, and prolactin secretion. Mol Pharmacol 1983; 24:189–194.
37. Lamberts SWJ, MacLeod RM. Regulation of prolactin secretion at the level of the lactotroph. Physiol Rev 1990; 70:279–318.
38. Horseman ND, Yu-Lee L. Transcriptional regulation by the helix bundle peptide hormones: growth hormone, prolactin, and hematopoietic cytokines. Endocrine Rev 1994; 15:627–649.
39. Lewis UJ, Singh RNP, Sinha YN, Vanderlaan WP. Glycosylated human prolactin. Endocrinology 1985; 116:359–363.
40. Markoff E, Sigel MB, Lacour N, Seavey BK, Friesen HG, Lewis UJ. Glycosylation selectively alters the biological activity of prolactin. Endocrinology 1988; 123:1303–1306.
41. Brue T, Caruso E, Morange I, Hoffmann T, Evrin M, Gunz G, Benkirane M, Jaquet P. Immunoradiometric analysis of circulating human glycosylated and nonglycosylated prolactin forms: Spontaneous and stimulated secretions. J Clin Endocrinol Metab 1992; 75:1338–1344.
42. Andries M, Tilemans D, Denef C. Isolation of cleaved prolactin variants that stimulate DNA synthesis in specific cell types in rat pituitary cell aggregates in culture. Biochem J 1992; 281:393–400.

43. Clapp C. Analysis of the proteolytic cleavage of prolactin by the mammary gland and liver of the rat: characterization of the cleaved and 16K forms. Endocrinology 1987; 121:2055–2064.
44. Clapp C, Weiner RI. A specific high affinity saturable binding site for the 16-kilodalton fragment of prolactin on capillary endothelial cells. Endocrinology 1992; 130:1380–1386.
45. Clapp C, Martial JA, Guzman RC, Rentier-Delrue F, Weiner RI. The 16-kD N-terminal fragment of human prolactin is a potent inhibitor of angiogenesis. Endocrinology 1993; 133:1292–1299.
46. Oetting WS, Tuazon PT, Traugh JA, Walker AM. Phosphorylation of prolactin. J Biol Chem 1986; 261:1649–1652.
47. Mastro RM, Dannies PS. Lack of correlation of distribution of prolactin (PRL) charge isoforms with induction of PRL storage. Endocrinology 1995; 136:69–74.
48. Garnier PE, Aubert ML, Kaplan ASL, Grumbach MM. Heterogeneity of pituitary and plasma prolactin in man: Decreased affinity of "big" prolactin in a radioreceptor assay and evidence for its secretion. Endocrinology 41978; 7:1273–1279.
49. Hattori N, Ishihara T, Ikekubo K, Moridera K, Hino M, Kurahachi H. Autoantibody to human prolactin in patients with idiopathic hyperprolactinemia. J Clin Endocrinol Metab 1992; 75:1226–1229.
50. Lee DW, Markoff E. Synthesis and release of glycosylated prolactin by human decidua in vitro. J Clin Endocrinol Metab 1986; 62:990–993.
51. Handwerger S, Wilson S, Conn PM. Different subcellular storage sites for decidual- and pituitary-derived prolactin: Possible explanation for differences in regulation. Mol Cell Endocrinol 1984; 37:83–87.
52. Halmi S, Parson JA, Earlandsen SL, Duello T. Prolactin and growth hormone cells in the human hypophysis. A study with immunoenzyme histochemistry and differential staining. Cell Tissue Res 1975; 158:497–507.
53. Hinkel PM, Scammel JG, Shanshala ED II. Prolactin and secretogranin-II, a marker for the regulated pathway, are secreted in parallel by pituitary GH4C1 cells. Endocrinology 1992; 130:3503–3511.
54. Walker AM, Farquhar MG. Preferential release of newly synthesized prolactin granules is the result of functional heterogeneity among mammotrophs. Endocrinology 1980; 107:1095–1104.
55. Molitch ME, Raiti S, Baumann G, Belknap S, Reichlin S. Pharmacokinetic studies of highly purified human prolactin in normal human subjects. J Clin Endocrinol Metab 1987; 65:299–304.
56. Cooper BS, Ridgway EC, Kliman B. Metabolic clearance and production rates of prolactin in man. J Clin Invest 1979; 64:1669–1680.
57. Sievertsen GD, Lim VS, Nakawatase C, Frohman LA. Metabolic clearance and secretion rates of human prolactin in normal subjects and in patients with chronic renal failure. J Clin Endocrinol Metab 1980; 50:846–852.
58. Bratusch-Marrain P, Bjorkman O. Hepatic disposal of endogenous growth hormone and prolactin in man. Eur. J. Clin. Invest. 1979; 9:257–260.
59. Neill JD, Frawley LS. Detection of hormone release from individual cells in mixed populations using a reverse hemolytic plaque assay. Endocrinology 1983; 112:1135–1138.
60. Boockfor FR, Frawley SL. Functional variations among prolactin cells from different pituitary regions. Endocrinology 1987; 120:874–879.
61. Sinha YN, Selby FW, Lewis UJ, Vanderlaan WP. A homologous radioimmunoassay for human prolactin. J Clin Endocrinol Metab 1973; 36:509–516.
62. Tanaka T, Shiu RPC, Gout PW, Beer CT, Noble RL, Friesen HG. A new sensitive and specific bioassay for lactogenic hormones: Measurement of prolactin and growth hormone in human serum. J Clin Endocrinol Metab 1980; 51:1058–1063.
63. Frawley LS, Clark CL, Schoderbek WC. A novel bioassay for lactogenic activity. Demonstration that prolactin cells differ from one another in bio- and immuno-potencies of secreted hormone. Endocrinology 1986; 119:2867–2869.
64. Mulchahey JJ, Jaffe RB. Detection of a potential progenitor cell in the human fetal pituitary that secretes both growth hormone and prolactin. J Clin Endocrinol Metab 1988; 66:24-32.
65. Poindexter AN, Buttram VC, Besch P. Circulating prolactin levels, I. Normal females. Int J Fertil 1977; 22:1–5.
66. Samuels MH, Henry P, Kleinschmidt-DeMasters B, Lillehei K, Ridgway EC. Pulsatile prolactin secretion in hyperprolactinemia due to presumed pituitary stalk interruption. J Clin Endocrinol Metab 1991; 73:1289–1293.
67. Shin SH, Reifel CW. Adenohypophysis has an inherent property for pulsatile prolactin secretion. Neuroendocrinol 1981; 32:139–144.

68. Stewart JK, Clifton DK, Koerker DJ, Rogol AD. Pulsatile release of growth hormone and prolactin from the primate pituitary in vitro. Endocrinology 1985; 116:1–5.
69. Inaudi P, Genazzani AD, Reymond MJ, Lemarchand-Béraud T, Rey F. Pulsatile secretion of gonadotropins and prolactin during the follicular and luteal phases of the menstrual cycle: Analysis of instantaneous secretion rat and secretory concomitance. Fertil Steril 1992; 58:51–59.
70. Parker DC, Rossman LG, Vanderlaan EF. Relation of sleep-entrained human prolactin release to REM-nonREM cycles. J Clin Endocrinol Metab 1974; 38:646–651.
71. Veldhuis JD, Johnson ML. Operating characteristics of the hypothalamo-pituitary-gonadal axis in men: Circadian, ultradian, and pulsatile release of prolactin and its temporal coupling with luteinizing hormone. J Clin Endocrinol Metab 1988; 67:116–123.
72. Obal FJ, Payne L, Kacsoh B, Opp M, Kapas L, Grosvenor CE, Krueger JM. Involvement of prolactin in the REM sleep-promoting activity of systemic vasoactive intestinal peptide (VIP). Brain Res 1994; 645:143–149.
73. Carlson HE, Hyman DB, Blitzer MG. Evidence for an intracerebral action of phenylalanine in stimulation of prolactin secretion: Interaction of large neutral amino acids. J Clin Endocrinol Metab 1990; 70:814–816.
74. Noel GL, Suh HK, Stone SJG, Frantz AE. Human prolactin and growth hormone release during surgery and other conditions of stress. J Clin Endocrinol Metab 1973; 35:840–851.
75. Gala RR. The physiology and mechanisms of the stress induced changes in prolactin secretion in the rat. Life Sci 1990; 46:1407–1420.
76. Pontiroli AE, Baio G, Stella L, Crescenti A, Girardi AM. Effects of naloxone on prolactin luteinizing hormone, and cortisol responses to surgical stress in humans. J Clin Endocrinol Metab 1982; 55:378-380.
77. Kjaer A, Knigge U, Olsen L, Vilhardt H, Warberg J. Mediation of the stress-induced prolactin release by hypothalamic histaminergic neurons and the possible involvement of vasopressin in this response. Endocrinology 1991; 128:103-110.
78. Maddox PR, Jones DL, Mansel RE. Basal prolactin and total lactogenic hormone levels by microbioassay and immunoassay in normal human sera. Acta Endocrinol (Copenh) 1991; 125:621–627.
79. Tennekoon KH, Lenton EA. Early evening prolactin rise in women with regular cycles. J Reprod Fertil 1985; 73:523–527.
80. Rigg LA, Lein A, Yen SSC. Pattern of increase in circulating prolactin levels during human gestation. Am J Obstet Gynecol 1977; 129:454–456.
81. Rigg LA, Yen SSC. Multiphasic prolactin secretion during parturition in human subjects. Am J Obstet Gynecol 1977; 128:215–218.
82. Ostrom DM. A review of the hormone prolactin during lactation. Prog Food Nutr Sci 1990; 14:1–43.
83. Kremer JA, Borm G, Schellekens LA, Thomas CM, Rolland R. Pulsatile secretion of luteinizing hormone and prolactin in lactating and nonlactating women and the response to naltrexone. J Clin Endocrinol Metab 1991; 72:294–300.
84. Hill JB, Nagy GM, Frawley LS. Suckling unmasks the stimulatory effect of dopamine on prolactin release: possible role for alpha-melanocyte-stimulating hormone as a mammotrope responsiveness factor. Endocrinology 1989; 125:334–341.
85. Battin DA, Marrs RP, Fleiss PM, Mishell DR Effect of suckling on serum prolactin, luteinizing hormone, follicle-stimulating hormone and estradiol during prolonged lactation. Obstet Gynecol 1985; 65:785–788.
86. Shanti AS, Subramanian MG, Savoy-Moore RT, Kruger ML, Moghissi KS. Attenuation of the magnitude of suckling-induced prolactin release with advancing lactation: Mechanisms. Life Sci 1995; 56:259–266.
87. Tay CCK, Glasier AF, McNeilly AS. The 24 h pattern of pulsatile luteinizing hormone, follicle stimulating hormone and prolactin release during the first 8 weeks of lactational amenorrhoea in breastfeeding women. Hum Reprod 1992; 7:951–958.
88. Erskine MS. Prolactin release after mating and genitosensory stimulation in females. Endocrine Rev 1995; 16(4):508–528.
89. Everett J. Luteotrophic function of autografts of the rat hypophysis. Endocrinology 1954; 54:685–690.
90. Gibbs DM, Neill JD. Dopamine levels in hypophysial stalk blood in the rat are sufficient to inhibit prolactin secretion in vivo. Endocrinology 1978; 102:1895–1900.

91. Quigley ME, Judd SJ, Gilliland GB, Yen SC. Functional studies of dopamine control of prolactin secretion in normal women and women with hyperprolactinemic pituitary microadenoma. J Clin Endocrinol Metab 1980; 50:994–998.
92. Ben-Jonathan N. Dopamine: a prolactin-inhibiting hormone. Endocrine Rev 1985; 6:564–589.
93. Baertschi AJ. Portal vascular route from hypophysial stalk/neural lobe to adenohypophysis. Am Journal of Physiology 1980; 239:R463-R469.
94. Cronin MF, Roberts JM, Weiner RI. Dopamine and dihydroergocryptine binding to the anterior pituitary and other brain areas of the rat and sheep. Endocrinology 1978; 103:302–309.
95. Wood DF, Johnston JM, Johnston DG. Dopamine, the dopamine D2 receptor and pituitary tumours. Clin Endocrinol (Oxf) 1991; 35:455–466.
96. Swennen L, Denef C. Physiological concentrations of dopamine decrease adenosine 3′5′-monophosphate levels in cultured rat anterior pituitary cells and enriched populations of lactotrophs: Evidence for a causal relationship to inhibition of prolactin release. Endocrinology 1982; 111:398–405.
97. Drouva SV, Rerat E, Bihoreau C, Laplante A, Rasolonjanahary R, Clauser H, Kordon C. Dihydropyridine-sensitive calcium channel activity related to prolactin, growth hormone, and luteinizing hormone release from anterior pituitary cells in culture: interactions with somatostatin, dopamine, and estrogens. Endocrinology 1988; 123:2762–2773.
98. Jarvis WD, Judd AM, MacLeod RM. Attenuation of anterior pituitary phosphoinositide phosphorylase activity by the D2 dopamine receptor. Endocrinology 1988; 123:2793–2799.
99. Haisenleder DJ, Yasin M, Marshall JC. Regulation of gonadotropin, thyrotropin subunit, and prolactin messenger ribonucleic acid expression by pulsatile or continuous protein kinase-C stimulation. Endocrinology 1995; 136:13–19.
100. Haisenleder DJ, Yasin M, Marshall JC. Enhanced effectiveness of pulsatile cAMP in stimulating prolactin and alpha subunit gene expression. Endocrinology 1992; 131:3027–3033.
101. Haisenleder DJ, Yasin M, Marshall JC. The regulation of prolactin, thyrotropin and gonadotropin subunit gene expression by pulsatile or continuous calcium signals. Endocrinology 1993; 133:2055–2061.
102. Kidokoro Y. Spontaneous calcium action potentials in a clonal pituitary cell line and their relationship to prolactin secretion. Nature 1975; 258:741–742.
103. Duvilanski BH, Zambruno C, Seilicovich A, Pisera D, Lasaga M, Del C. Diaz M, Belova N, Rettori V, McCann SM. Role of nitric oxide in control of prolactin release by the adenohypophysis. Proc Natl Acad Sci USA 1995; 92:170–174.
104. Schally AV, Redding TW, Arimura A, DuPont A, Linthicum GL. Isolation of gamma-aminobutyric acid from pig hypothalami and demonstration of its prolactin release-inhibiting (PIF) activity in vivo and in vitro. Endocrinology 1977; 100:681–691.
105. Vincent SR, Hokfelt T, Wu JY. GABA neuron systems in the hypothalamus and the pituitary gland. Neuroendocrinol 1982; 34:117–125.
106. Mulchahey JJ, Neill JD. Gamma-aminobutyric acid (GABA) levels in hypophyseal stalk plasma of rats. Life Sci 1982; 32:453–456.
107. Grandison L, Guidotti A. Gamma-aminobutyric acid receptor function in rat anterior pituitary: Evidence for control of prolactin release. Endocrinology 1979; 105:754–759.
108. Nikolics K, Mason AJ, Szonyi E, Ramachandran J, Seeburg PH. A prolactin-inhibiting factor within the precursor for human gonadotropin-releasing hormone. Nature 1985; 316:511–517.
109. Takahashi K, Ghatei MA, Jones PM, Murphy JK, Lam H-C, O'Halloran AJ, Bloom SR. Endothelin in human brain and pituitary gland: presence on immunoreactive endothelin, endothelin messenger ribonucleic acid, and endothelin receptors. J Clin Endocrinol Metab 1991; 72:693–699.
110. Samson WK, Skala KD. Comparison of the pituitary effects of the mammalian endothelins: vasoactive intestinal contractor (endothelin–β, rat endothelin-2) is a potent inhibitor of prolactin secretion. Endocrinology 1992; 130:2964-2970.
111. Tashjian AHJ, Barowsky NJ, Jensen DK. Thyrotropin releasing hormone: direct evidence for stimulation of prolactin production by pituitary cells in culture. Biochem Biophys Res Commun 1971; 43:516–523.
112. Bowers CY, Friesen HG, Hwang P, Guyda HJ, Folkers K. Prolactin and thyrotropin release in man by synthetic pyroglutamyl-histidyl-prolinamide. Biochem Biophys Res Commun 1971; 45:1033–1041.
113. Jacobs LS, Snyder PJ, Utiger RD, Daughaday WH. Prolactin response to thyrotropin-releasing hormone in normal subjects. J Clin Endocrinol Metab 1973; 36:1069–1073.

114. Sheward WJ, Fraser HM, Fink G. Effect of immunoneutralization of thyrotrophin-releasing hormone on the release of thyrotrophin and prolactin during suckling or in response to electrical stimulation of the hypothalamus in the anaesthetized rat. J Endocrinol 1985; 106:113–119.
115. Kato Y, Iwasaki Y, Iwasaki J, Abe H, Yanaihara N, Imura H. Prolactin release by vasoactive intestinal polypeptide in rats. Endocrinology 1978; 103:554–558.
116. Carrillo AJ, Pool TB, Sharp ZD. Vasoactive intestinal peptide increases prolactin messenger ribonucleic acid content in GH3 cells. Endocrinology 1985; 116:202–206.
117. Mezey E, Kiss JZ. Vasoactive intestinal peptide-containing neurons in the paraventricular nucleus may participate in regulating prolactin secretion. Proc Natl Acad Sci USA 1985; 82:245–247.
118. Arnaout MA, Garthwaite TL, Martinson DR. Vasoactive intestinal polypeptide is synthesized in anterior pituitary tissue. Endocrinology 1986; 119:2052–2057.
119. Prysor-Jones RA, Silverlight JJ, Jenkins JS. Vasoactive intestinal peptide increases intracellular free calcium in rat and human pituitary tumour cells in vitro. J Endocrinol 1987; 114:119–123.
120. Abe H, Engler D, Molitch ME, Bollinger-Gruber J, Reichlin S. Vasoactive intestinal peptide is a physiological mediator of prolactin release in the rat. Endocrinology 1985; 116:1383–1390.
121. Werner S, Hulting AL, Hokfelt T. Effect of the peptide phi-27 on prolactin release in vitro. Neuroendocrinol 1983; 37:476–478.
122. Kaji H, Chihara K, Kita T, Kashio Y, Okimura Y, Fujita T. Administration of antisera to vasoactive intestinal polypeptide and peptide histidine isoleucine attenuates ether-induced prolactin secretion in rats. Neuroendocrinol 1985; 41:529–531.
123. Kaji H, Chihara C, Abe H, Kita T. Effect of passive immunization with antisera to vasoactive intestinal polypeptide and peptide histidine isoleucine amide on 5-hydroxy-1-tryptophan-induced prolactin release in rats. Endocrinology 1985; 117:1914–1919.
124. Denef C, Andries M. Evidence for paracrine interaction between gonadotrophs and lactotrophs in pituitary cell aggregates. Endocrinology 1983; 112:813–822.
125. Shinkai T, Ooka H. Effect of angiotensin II on the proliferation of mammotrophs from the adult rat anterior pituitary in culture. Peptides 1995; 16(1):25–29.
126. Brandi AM, Barrande G, Lahlou N, Crumeyrolle M, Berthet M, Leblanc P, Peillon F, Li JY. Stimulatory effect of gonadotropin-releasing hormone (GnRH) on in vitro prolactin secretion and presence of GnRH specific receptors in a subset of human prolactinomas. Eur J Endocrinol 1995; 132:163–170.
127. Gordon K, Williams RF, Danforth DR, Veldhuis JD, Hodgen GD. GnRH antagonists suppress prolactin release in non-human primates. Contraception 1992; 45:369–378.
128. Gunnett JW, Freeman ME. The mating-induced release of prolactin: A unique neuroendocrine response. Endocrine Rev 1983; 4:44–61.
129. Allen DL, Low MJ, Allen RG, Ben-Jonathan N. Identification of two classes of prolactin-releasing factors in intermediate lobe tumors from transgenic mice. Endocrinology 1995; 136:3093–3099.
130. Boockfor FR, Hoeffler JP, Frawley SL. Estradiol induces a shift in cultured cells that release prolactin or growth hormone. Am Journal of Physiology 1986; 250:103–106.
131. Stefaneanu L, Kovacs K, Lloyd RV, Scheithauer BW, Young WFJ, Sano T, Jin L. Pituitary lactotrophs and somatotrophs in pregnancy: a correlative in situ hybridization and immunocytochemical study. Virchows Archiv B Cell Pathol 1992; 62:291–296.
132. Scheithauer BW, Sano T, Kovacs KT, Young WJJ, Ryan N, Randall RV 1990 The pituitary gland in pregnancy. A clinicopathologic and immunohistochemical study of 69 cases. Mayo Clin Proc 1990; 65:461–474.
133. Maurer RA. Estradiol regulates the transcription of the prolactin gene. J Biol Chem 1982; 257:2133–2135.
134. Shull JD, Gorski J. The hormonal regulation of prolactin gene expression: An examination of mechanisms controlling prolactin synthesis and the possible relationship of estrogen to these mechanisms. Vitamins Hormones 1986; 43:197–249.
135. Raymond V, Beaulieu M, Labrie F, Biossier J. Potent antidopaminergic activity of estradiol at the pituitary level on prolactin release. Science 1978; 200:1173–1175.
136. Cramer OM, Parker CR, Porter JC. Estrogen inhibition of dopamine release into hypophysial portal blood. Endocrinology 1979; 104:419–422.
137. Nordstrom O, Melander T, Hokfelt T, Bartfai T, Goldstein M. Evidence for an inhibitory effect of the peptide galanin on dopamine release from the rat median eminence. Neurosci Lett 1987; 73:21–26.
138. Hyde JF, Howard G. Regulation of galanin gene expression in the rat anterior pituitary gland by the somatostatin analog SMS 201–995. Endocrinology 1992; 131:2097–2102.

139. Sakai DD, Helms S, Carlstedt-Duke J, Gustafsson J-A, Rottman FM, Yamamoto KR. Hormone-mediated repression: A negative glucocorticoid response element from the bovine prolactin gene. Genes & Dev 1988; 2:1144–1154.
140. Gellersen B, DiMattia GE, Friesen HG, Bohnet HG. Regulation of prolactin secretion in the human B-lymphoblastoid cell line IM-9-P3 by dexamethasone but not other regulators of pituitary prolactin secretion. Endocrinology 1989; 125:2853–2861.
141. Maurer RA. Thyroid hormone specifically inhibits prolactin synthesis and decreases prolactin messenger ribonucleic acid levels in cultured pituitary cells. Endocrinology 1982; 110:1507–1514.
142. Vale W, Blackwell R, Grant G, Guillemin R. Effects of TRF and thyroid hormones on prolactin secretion by rat anterior pituitary cells in vitro. Endocrinology 1973; 93:26–33.
143. Ozawa H, Kurosumi K. Morphofunctional study on prolactin-producing cells of the anterior pituitaries in adult male rats following thyroidectomy, thyroxine treatment and/or thyrotropin-releasing hormone treatment. Cell Tissue Res 1993; 272:41–47.
144. Stanley F. Stimulation of prolactin gene expression by insulin. J Biol Chem 1988; 263:13444–13448.
145. Thrailkill KM, Golander A, Underwood LE, Richards RG, Handwerger S. Insulin stimulates the synthesis and release of prolactin from human decidual cells. Endocrinology 1989; 124:3010–3014.
146. Chiu S, Koos RD, Wise PM. Detection of prolactin receptor (PRL-R) in the rat hypothalamus and pituitary gland. Endocrinology 1992; 130:1747–1749.
147. Perkins NA, Westfall TC, Paul CV, MacLeod R, Rogol AD. Effect of prolactin on dopamine synthesis in medial basal hypothalamus: Evidence for a short loop feedback. Brain Res 1979; 160:431–444.
148. Gudelsky GA, Porter JC. Release of dopamine from tuberoinfundibular neurons into pituitary stalk blood after prolactin or haloperidol administration. Endocrinology 1980; 106:526–529.
149. Grattan DR, Averill RLW. Intrahypothalamic pituitary grafts elevate prolactin in the cerebrospinal fluid and attenuate prolactin release following ether stress. Proc Soc Exp Biol Med 1991; 196:42–46.
150. Grattan DR, Averill RLW. Absence of short-loop autoregulation of prolactin during late pregnancy in the rat. Brain Res Bulletin 1995; 36(4):413–416.
151. Phelps CJ. Pituitary hormones as neurotrophic signals: anomalous hypophysiotrophic neuron differentiation in hypopituitary Dwarf mice. Proc Soc Exp Biol Med 1994; 206:6–23.
152. Nicoll CS. Ontogeny and evolution of prolactin's functions. Fed. Proc. 1980; 39:2563–2566.
153. Whitworth NS. Lactation in humans. Psychoneuroendocrinology 1988; 13:171–188.
154. Ymer SI, Stevenson JL, Herington AC. Differences in the developmental patterns of somatotrophic and lactogenic receptors in rabbit liver cytosol. Endocrinology 1989; 125:516–523.
155. Kelly PA, Djiane J, Katoh M, Ferland LH, Houdebine LM, Teyssot B, Dusanter-Fourt I. The interaction of prolactin with its receptors in target tissues and its mechanisms of action. Rec Prog Horm Res 1984; 40:379–439.
156. Boutin JM, Edery M, Shirota M, Jolicoeur C, Lesueur L, Ali S, Gould D, Djiane J, Kelly PA. Identification of a cDNA encoding a long form of prolactin receptor in human hepatoma and breast cancer cells. Mol Endocrinol 1989; 3:1455–1461.
157. Arden KC, Boutin J-M, Djiane J, Kelly PA, Cavenee WK. The receptors for prolactin and growth hormone are localized in the same region of human chromosome 5. Cytogenet Cell Genet 1990; 53:161–165.
158. Bazan JF. Structure, design and molecular evolution of a cytokine receptor superfamily. Proc Natl Acad Sci USA 1990; 87:6934–6938.
159. Shirota M, Banville D, Ali S, Jolicoeur C, Boutin JM, Edery M, Djiane J, Kelly PA. Expression of two forms of prolactin receptor in rat ovary and liver. Mol Endocrinol 1990; 4:1136–1143.
160. Ali S, Pellegrini I, Kelly PA. A prolactin-dependent immune cell line (Nb2) expresses a mutant form of prolactin receptor. J Biol Chem 1991; 266:20110–20117.
161. Zhang R, Buczko E, Tsai-Morris CH, Hu ZZ, Dufau ML. Isolation and characterization of two novel rat ovarian lactogen receptor cDNA species. Biochem Biophys Res Commun 1990; 168:415–422.
162. Kelly PA, Djiane J, Edery M. Different forms of the prolactin receptor. Insights into the mechanism of prolactin action. Trends Endocrinol Metab 1992; 3:54–59.
163. Jolicoeur C, Boutin JM, Okamura H. Multiple regulators of prolactin receptor gene expression in rat liver. Mol Endocrinol 1989; 3:895–900.
164. Jahn G, Edery M, Belair L, Kelly PA, Djiane J. Prolactin receptor gene expression in rat mammary gland and liver during pregnancy and lactation. Endocrinology 1991; 128:2976–2984.
165. Djiane J, Dusanter-Fourt I, Katoh M, Kelly PA. Biological activities of binding site monoclonal antibodies to prolactin receptors of rabbit mammary gland. J Biol Chem 1985; 21:11430–11435.

166. Rui H, Lebrun J-J, Kirken RA, Kelly PA, Farrar WL. JAK2 activation and cell proliferation induced by antibody-mediated prolactin receptor dimerization. Endocrinology 1994; 135:1299–1306.
167. Fuh G, Colosi P, Wood WI, Wells JA. Mechanism-based design of prolactin receptor antagonists. J Biol Chem 1993; 268:5376–5381.
168. Fuh G, Cunningham BC, Fukunaga R, Nagata S, Goeddel DV, Wells JA. Rational design of potent antagonists to the human growth hormone receptor. Science 1992; 256:1677–1680.
169. Kornberg LJ, Liberti JP. Nb2 cell mitogenesis: Effect of lactogens on cAMP and protein phosphorylation. Biochim Biophys Acta 1989; 1011:205–211.
170. David M, Petricoin EF 3rd, Igarashi K-I, Feldman GM. Prolactin activates the interferon-regulated p91 transcription factor and the Jak2 kinase by tyrosine phosphorylation. Biochemistry 1994; 91:7174–7178.
171. Clevenger CV, Torigoe T, Reed JC. Prolactin induces rapid phosphorylation and activation of prolactin receptor-associated RAF-1 kinase in a T-cell line. J Biol Chem 1994; 269:5559–5565.
172. Horseman ND. Editorial: famine to feast—growth hormone and prolactin signal transducers. Endocrinology 1994; 135:1289–1290.
173. Dunaif AE, Zimmerman EA, Friesen HG, Frantz AG. Intracellular localization of prolactin receptor and prolactin in the rat ovary by immunocytochemistry. Endocrinology 1982; 110:1465–1472.
174. Cohen H, Guillaumot P, Sabbagh I. Characterization of a prolactin binding protein in rat serum. Endocrinology 1993; 132:2601–2606.
175. Postel-Vinay M-C, Belair L, Kayser C, Kelly PA, Dijane J. Identification of prolactin and growth hormone binding proteins in rabbit milk. Proc Natl Acad Sci USA 1991; 88:6687–6690.
176. Ultsch M, de Vos AM. Crystals of human growth hormone-receptor complexes: Extracellular domains of the growth hormone and prolactin receptors and a hormone mutant designed to prevent receptor dimerization. J Mol Biol 1993; 231:1133–1136.
177. Rosen JM, Matusik RJ, Richards DA, Gupta P, Rodgers JR. Multihormonal regulation of casein gene expression at the transcriptional and posttranscriptional levels in the mammary gland. Rec Prog Horm Res 1980; 36:157–193.
178. Welte T, Garimorth K, Philipp S, Doppler W. Prolactin-dependent activation of a tyrosine phosphorylated DNA binding factor in mouse mammary epithelial cells. Mol Endocrinol 1994; 8:1091–1102.
179. Fawcett HAC, Baldwin SA, Flint DJ. Hormonal regulation of the glucose transporter GLUT1 in the lactating rat mammary gland. Biochem Soc Trans 1991; 20:17S.
180. Barber MC, Clegg RA, Finley E, Vernon RG, Flint DJ. The role of growth hormone,prolactin and insulin-like growth factors in the regulation of rat mammary gland and adipose tissue metabolism during lactation. J Endocrinol 1992; 135:195–202.
181. Da Costa THM, Williamson DH. Regulation of rat mammary-gland uptake of orally administered [1–14C]triolein by insulin and prolactin: evidence for bihormonal control of lipoprotein lipase activity. Biochem J 1994; 300:257–262.
182. Flint DJ, Gardner M. Evidence that growth hormone stimulates milk synthesis by direct action on the mammary gland and that prolactin exerts effects on milk secretion by maintenance of mammary deoxyribonucleic acid content and tight junction status. Endocrinology 1994; 135:1119–1124.
183. Thiede MA. The mRNA encoding a parathyroid hormone-like peptide is produced in mammary tissue in response to elevations in serum prolactin. Mol Endocrinol 1989; 3:1443–1447.
184. Khosla S, Johansen KL, Ory SJ, OBrien PC, Kao PC. Parathyroid hormone-related peptide in lactation and in umbilical cord blood. Mayo Clin Proc 1990; 65:1408–1414.
185. Weisz-Carrington P, Roux MF, McWilliams M, Phillips-Quagliata JM, Lamm ME. Hormonal induction of the secretory immune system in the mammary gland. Proc Natl Acad Sci USA 1978; 75:2928–2932.
186. Ginsburg E, Vonderhaar BK. Prolactin synthesis and secretion by human breast cancer cells. Cancer Res 1995; 55:2591–2595.
187. Baldocchi RA, Tan L, Hom YK, Nicoll CS. Comparison of the ability of normal mouse mammary tissues and mammary adencarcinoma to cleave rat prolactin. Proc Soc Exp Biol Med 1995; 208:283–287.
188. Ellis LA, Picciano MF. Bioactive and immunoreactive prolactin variants in human milk. Endocrinology 1995; 136:2711–2720.
189. Clapp C, Sears PS, Russell DH, Richards J, Levay-Young BK, Nicoll CS. Biological and immunological characterization of cleaved and 16 K forms of rat prolactin. Endocrinology 1988; 122:2892–2898.
190. Kleinberg DL, Ruan W, Catanese V, Newman CB, Feldman M 1990 Non-lactogenic effects of growth hormone on growth and insulin-like growth factor-I messenger ribonucleic acid of rat mammary gland. Endocrinology 1990; 126:3274–3276.

191. Fielder PJ, Thordarson G, English A, Rosenfeld RG, Talamantes F. Expression of a lactogen dependent insulin-like growth factor-binding protein in cultured mouse mammary epithelial cells. Endocrinology 1992; 131:261–267.
192. Richards JS, Williams JI. Luteal cell receptor content for prolactin (PRL) and luteinizing hormone (LH). Regulation by LH and PRL. Endocrinology 1976; 99:1571–1581.
193. Albarracin CT, Gibori G. Prolactin action on luteal protein expression in the corpus luteum. Endocrinology 1991; 129:1821–1830.
194. Murai I, Reichlin S, Ben-Jonathan N. The peak phase of the proestrus prolactin surge is blocked by either posterior pituitary lobectomy or antisera to vasoactive intestinal peptide. Endocrinology 1989; 124:1050–1055.
195. Klibanski A, Beitins IZ, Merriam GR, McArthur JW, Zervas NT, Ridgway EC. Gonadotropin and prolactin pulsations in hyperprolactinemic women before and during bromocriptine therapy. J Clin Endocrinol Metab 1984; 58:1141–1147.
196. Cohen-Becker IR, Selmanoff M, Wise PM. Hyperprolactinemia alters the frequency and amplitude of pulsatile luteinizing hormone secretion in the ovariectomized rat. Neuroendocrinol 1986; 42:328–333.
197. McNatty KP, Sawers RS, McNeilly AS. A possible role for prolactin in control of steroid secretion by the human Graafian follicle. Nature 1974; 250:653–655.
198. McNeilly AS, Glasier A, Jonassen J, Howie PW. Evidence for direct inhibition of ovarian function by prolactin. J Reprod Fertil 1982; 65:559–569.
199. Demura R, Ono M, Demura H, Shizume DK, Oouchi H. Prolactin directly inhibits basal as well as gonadotropin-stimulated secretion of progesterone and 17beta-estradiol in the human ovary. J Clin Endocrinol Metab 1982; 54:1246–1250.
200. Subramanian MC, Sacco AG, Moghissi KS. Prolactin size heterogeneity in human follicular fluid. Int J Fertil 1991; 36:367–371.
201. Falk RJ. Isolated prolactin deficiency: a case report. Fertil Steril 1992; 58:1060–1062.
202. Schulz KD, Geiger W, Del Pozo E, Kunzig HJ. Pattern of sexual steroids, prolactin, and gonadotropic hormones during prolactin inhibition in normally cycling women. Am J Obstet Gynecol 1978; 132:561–566.
203. Muhlenstedt D, Bohnet HG, Hanker JP, Schneider HPG. Short luteal phase and prolactin. Int J Fertil 1978; 23:214–218.
204. Kauppila A, Reinila M, Martikainen H, Roonberg L, Puistola U. Hypoprolactinemia and ovarian function. Fertil Steril 1988; 49:437–441.
205. Alila HW, Rogo KO, Gombe S. Effects of prolactin on steroidogenesis by human cells in culture. Fertil Steril 1987; 47:947–955.
206. Del Pozo E, Wyss H, Tolis G, Alcanız J, Campana A, Naftolin F. Prolactin and deficient luteal function. Obstet Gynecol 1979; 53:282–286.
207. Laufer N, Botero-Ruiz W, DeCherney AH, Haseltine F, Polan ML, Behrman HR. Gonadotropin and prolactin levels in follicular fluid of human ova successfully fertilized in vitro. J Clin Endocrinol Metab 1984; 58:430–434.
208. Seibel MM, Smith D, Dlugi AM, Levesque L. Periovulatory follicular fluid levels in spontaneous human cycles. J Clin Endocrinol Metab 1989; 68:1073–1077.
209. Oda T, Yoshimura Y, Takehara Y, Kohriyama S, Sano Y, Tanabe K, Kobayashi T, Nakamura Y, Ohno T, Nozawa S. Effects of prolactin on fertilization and cleavage of human oocytes. Horm Res 1991; 35:33–38.
210. Hofmann GE, Denis ALC, Scott RT, Muasher SJ. The incidence of transient hyperprolactinemia in gonadotropin-stimulated cycles for in vitro fertilization and its effect on pregnancy outcome. Fertil Steril 1989; 52:622–626.
211. Pattinson HA, Taylor PJ, Fleetham JA, Servis SA. Transient hyperprolactinemia has no effect on endocrine response and outcome in in vitro fertilization (IVF). J Vitro Fert Embryo Transfer 1990; 7:89–93.
212. Hummel WP, Clark MR, Talbert LM. Transient hyperprolactinemia during cycle stimulation and its inflence on oocyte retrieval and fertilization rates. Fertil Steril 1990; 53:677–681.
213. Reinthaller A, Bieglmayer C, Deutinger J, Csaicsich P. Transient hyperprolactinemia during cycle stimulation: influence on the endocrine repsonse and fertilization rate of human oocytes and effects of bromocriptine treatment. Fertil Steril 1988; 49:432–436.
214. Sopelak VM, Whitworth NS, Norman PF, Cowan BD. Bromocriptine inhibition of anesthesia-induced hyperprolactinemia: effect on serum and follicular fluid hormones, oocyte fertilization, and embryo cleavage rates during in vitro fertilization. Fertil Steril 1989; 52:627–632.

215. Negami AI, Tominaga T. Effects of prolactin on cultured human endometrial cells. Horm Res 1991; 35:50–57.
216. Galosy SS, Gertler A, Elberg G, Laird DM. Distinct placental lactogen and prolactin (lactogen) receptors in bovine endometrium. Mol Cell Endocrinol 1991; 78:229–236.
217. Bartke A. Effects of prolactin on spermatogenesis in hypophysectomized mice. Endocrinology 1971; 49:311–316.
218. Hafiez AA, Bartke A, Lloyd CW. The role of prolactin in the regulation of testis function: the synergistic effects of prolactin and luteinizing hormone on the incorporation of [1-14C] acetate into testosterone and cholesterol by testes from hypophysectomized rats in vitro. Endocrinology 1972; 53:223–230.
219. Aragona C, Bohnet HG, Friesen HG. Localization of prolactin binding in prostate and testis: the role of serum prolactin concentration on the testicular LH receptor. Acta Endocrinology 1977; 84:402–409.
220. Oseko F, Endo J, Nakano A, Taniguchi A, Morikawa K, Usui T. Effects of chronic bromocriptine-induced hyperprolactinemia on plasma testosterone responses to human chorionic gonadotropin stimulation in mormal men. Fertil Steril 1991; 55:355–357.
221. Carter JN, Tyson JE, Tolis G, Van Vliet S, Faiman C, Friesen HG. Prolactin-secreting tumors and hypogonadism in 22 men. N Engl J Med 1978; 299:847–852.
222. Drago F. Prolactin and sexual behavior. Neuroscience Biobehavioral Review 1984; 8:433–439.
223. Costello LC, Franklin RB. Effect of prolactin on the prostrate. Prostate 1994; 24:162–166.
224. Negro-Vilar A, Saad WA, McCann SM. Evidence for a role of prolactin in prostate and seminal vesicle growth in immature animals. Endocrinology 1977; 100:729–737.
225. Perez-Villamil B, Bordiu E, Puente-Cueva M. Involvement of physiological prolactin levels in growth and prolactin receptor content of prostate glands and testes in developing male rats. J Endocrinol 1992; 132:449–459.
226. Sheth AR, Mugatwala PP, Shah GV, Rao SS. Occurrence of prolactin in human semen. Fertil Steril 1975; 26:905–907.
227. Rui H, Torjesen PA, Jacobsen H, Purvis K. Testicular and glandular contributions to the prolactin pool in human semen. Arch Androl 1985; 15:129–136.
228. Shah GV, Desai RB, Sheth AR. Effect of prolactin on metabolism of human spermatozoa. Fertil Steril 1976; 27:1292–1294.
229. Gala RR. Prolactin and growth hormone in the regulation of the immune system. Proc Soc Exp Biol Med 1991; 198:513–527.
230. Hooghe R, Delhase M, Vergani P, Malur A, Hooghe-Peters EL. Growth hormone and prolactin are paracrine growth and differentiation factors in the haemopoietic system. Immunol Today 1993; 14:212–214.
231. Dardenne M, Savino W. Prolactin-mediated cellular interactions in the thymus. Ann NY Acad Sci 1994; 741:100–107.
232. Kelley KW, Brief S, Westly HJ, Novakofski J, Bechtel PJ, Simon J, Walker EB. GH3 pituitary adenoma cells can reverse thymic aging in mice. Proc Natl Acad Sci USA 1986; 83:5663–5667.
233. Nagy E, Berczi I. Immunodeficiency in hypophysectomized rats. Acta Endocrinol (Copenh) 1978; 89:530–537.
234. Nagy E, Berczi I, Friesen HG. Regulation of immunity in rats by lactogenic and growth hormones. Acta Endocrinol (Copenh) 1983; 102:351–357.
235. Berczi I, Nagy E, de Toledo AM, Matusik RJ, Friesen HG. Pituitary hormones regulate c-myc and DNA synthesis in lymphoid tissue. J Immunology 1991; 146:2201–2206.
236. Bernton EW, Meltzer MS, Holaday JW. Supression of macrophage activation and T-lymphocyte function in hypoprolactinemic mice. Science 1988; 239:401–404.
237. Compton CC, Rizk I, Regauer S, Burd E, Holaday J, Kenner J. The effect of bromocriptine-induced hypoprolactinemia on xenogenic and allogenic skin graft survival in a mouse model. J Burn Care Rehabil 1994; 15:393–400.
238. Whyte A, Williams RO. Bromocriptine suppresses postpartum exacerbation of collagen-induced arthritis. Arthritis Rheum 1988; 31:927–928.
239. Palestine AG, Muellenberg-Coulombre CG, Kim MK, Gelato MC, Nussenblatt RB. Bromocriptine and low dose cyclosporine in the treatment of experimental autoimmune uveitis in the rat. J Clin Invest 1987; 79:1078–1081.
240. McMurray R, Keisler D, Kanuckel K, Izui S, Walker SE. Prolactin influences autoimmune disease activity in the female B/W mouse. J Immunology 1991; 147:3780–3787.

241. Hiestand PC, Mekler P, Nordmann R, Grieder A, Permmongkol C. Prolactin as a modulator of lymphocyte responsiveness provides a possible menchanism of action for cyclosporine. Proc Natl Acad Sci USA 1985; 83:2599–2603.
242. Russell DH, Kibler R, Matrisian L, Larson DF, Poulos BM BE. Prolactin receptors on human T and B lymphocytes: antagonism of prolactin binding by cyclosporin. J Immunology 1985; 134:3027–3031.
243. Lahat N, Miller A, Shtiller R, Touby E. Differential effects of prolactin upon activation and differentiation of human B lymphocytes. J Neuro Immunol 1993; 47:35–40.
244. Carrier M, Russell DH, Wild JC, Emery RW, Copeland JG. Prolactin as a marker of rejection in human heart transplantation. J Heart Transplant 1987; 6:290–292.
245. Reber PM. Prolactin and Immunomodulation. Am J Med 1992; 95:637–644.
246. Buskila D, Sukenik S, Shoenfeld Y. The possible role of prolactin in autoimmunity. Am J Reprod Immunol 1991; 26:118–123.
247. Jara LJ, Lavalle C, Fraga A, Gomez-Sanchez C, Silveira LH, Martinez-Osuna P, Germain BF, Espinoza LR. Prolactin, immunoregulation, and autoimmune diseases. Semin Arthritis Rheumatism 1991; 20:273–284.
248. Harris RD, Kay NE, Seljeskog EL, Murray KJ, Douglas SD. Prolactin suppression of leukocyte chemotaxis in vitro. J Neurosurg 1979; 50:462–465.
249. Vidaller A, Llorente L, Larrea F, Mendez JP, Alcocer-Varela J, Alarcon-Segovia D. T cell dysregulation in patients with hyperprolactinemia: effect of bromocriptine treatment. Clin Immunol Immunopath 1986; 38:337–343.
250. Vidaller A, Guadarrama F, Llorente L, Mendez JP, Larrea F, Villa AR, Alarcon-Segovia D. Hyperprolactinemia inhibits natural killer (NK) cell function in vitro and its bromocriptine treatment not only corrects it but makes it more efficient. J Clin Immunol 1992; 12:210–215.
251. Pellegrini I, Lebrun J-J, Ali S, Kelly PA. Expression of prolactin and its receptor in human lymphoid cells. Mol Endocrinol 1992; 6:1023–1031.
252. Koh CY, Phillips JT. Prolactin receptor expression by lymphoid tissues in normal and immunized rats. Mol Cell Endocrinol 1993; 92:R21–R25.
253. Montgomery DW, LeFevre JA, Ulrich FD, Adamson CR, Zukoski CF. Identification of prolactin-like proteins synthesized by normal murine lymphocytes. Endocrinology 1990; 127:2601–2603.
254. Hartmann DP, Holaday JW, Bernton EW. Inhibition of lymphocyte proliferation by antibodies to prolactin. FASEB J 1989; 3:2194–2202.
255. Clevenger CV, Russell DH, Appasamv PM, Prystowsky MB. Regulation of interleukin 2-derived T-lymphocyte proliferation by prolactin. Proc Natl Acad Sci USA 1990; 87:6160–6464.
256. Touraine P, Kelly PA. Expression of the short and long forms of the prolactin receptor in murine lymphoid tissues. Rec Prog Horm Res 1995; 50:423–428.
257. Rao Y-P, Buckley DJ, Olson MD, Buckley AR. Nuclear translocation of prolactin: collaboration of tyrosine kinase and protein kinase C activation in rat Nb2 node lymphoma cells. J Cell Physiol 1995; 163:266–276.
258. Meyer N, Prentice DA, Fox MT, Hughes JP. Prolactin-induced proliferation of the Nb2 T-lymphoma is associated with protein kinase-C-independent phosphorylation of stathmin. Endocrinology 1992; 131:1977–1984.
259. Wilson TM, Yu-Lee L, Kelley MR. Coordinate gene expression of luteinizing hormone-releasing hormone (LHRH) and the LHRH-receptor after prolactin stimulation in the rat Nb2 T-cell line: implications for a role in immunomodulation and cell cycle gene expression. Mol Endocrinol 1995; 9:44–53.
260. Bellone G, Geuna M, Carbone A, Silvestri S, Foa R, Emanuelli G, Matera L. Regulatory action of prolactin in the in vitro growth of CD34+ve human hemopoietic progenitor cells. J Cell Physiol 1995; 163:221–231.
261. Widness JA, Clemons GK, Garcia JF, Schwartz R. Plasma immunoreactive erythropoietin in normal women studied sequentially during and after pregnancy. Am J Obstet Gynecol 1984; 149:646–650.
262. Loretz CA, Bern HA. Prolactin and osmoregulation in vertebrates. Neuroendocrinol 1982; 35:292–304.
263. Horrobin DF, Burstyn PG, Lloyd IJ, Durkin N, Lipton A, Muiruri KL. Actions of prolactin on human renal function. Lancet 1971; 2:352–354.
264. Buckman MT, Peake GT, Robertson G. Hyperprolactinemia influences renal function in man. Metabolism 1976; 25:509–516.
265. Berl T, Brautbar N, Ben-David M, Czaczkes W, Kleeman C. Osmotic control of prolactin release and its effect on renal water excretion in man. Kidney Int 1976; 10:158–163.

266. Baumann G, Marynick SP, Winters SJ, Loriaux L. The effect of osmotic stimuli on prolactin secretion and renal water excretion in normal man and in chronic hyperprolactinemia. J Clin Endocrinol Metab 1977; 44:199–202.
267. Mountjoy K, Cowden FA, Dobbie JW, Ratcliffe JG. Prolactin receptors in kidney. J Endocrinol 1980; 87:47–54.
268. Soupart A, Buisson L, Prospert F, Decaux G. Indirect evidence to suggest that prolactin induces salt retention in cirrhosis. J Hepatology 1994; 21:347–352.
269. Robertson MY, Bovajian MJ, Patterson K, Robertson WVB. Modualtion of the chloride concentration of human sweat by prolactin. Endocrinology 1986; 119:2439–2444.
270. Tyson JE. The evolutionary role of prolactin in mammalian osmoregulation: Effects on fetoplacental hydromineral transport. Semin Perinatol 1982; 6:216–228.
271. Pahuja DN, DeLuca HF. Stimulation of intestinal calcium transport and bone calcium mobilization by prolactin in vitamin D-deficient rats. Science 1981; 214:1038–1039.
272. Kumar R, Abboud CF, Riggs BL. The effect of elevated prolactin levels on plasma 1,25-dihydroxivitamin D and intestinal absorption of calcium. Mayo Clin Proc 1980; 55:51–53.
273. Nagano M, Chaster E, Choquet A, Bara J, Gespach C, Kelly PA. Expression of prolactin and growth hormone receptor genes and their isoforms in the gastrointestinal tract. Am Journal of Physiology 1995; 268:431–432.
274. Sobrinho LG. The psychogenic effects of prolactin. Acta Endocrinol (Copenh) 1993; 129 (suppl) 1:38–40.
275. Bridges RS, Mann PE. Prolactin-brain interactions in the induction of maternal behavior in rats. Psychoneuroendocrinology 1994; 19:611–622.
276. McCarthy MM, Curran GH, Siegel HI. Evidence for the involvement of prolactin in the maternal behavior of the hamster. Physiol Behav 1994; 55:181–184.
277. Theorell T. Prolactin—a hormone that mirrors passiveness in crisis situations. Integr Physiol Behav Sci 1992; 27:32–38.
278. Lozoff B, Felt BT, Nelson EC, Wolf AW, Meltzer HW, Jimenez E. Serum prolactic levels and behavior in infants. Biol Psychiatry 1995; 37:4–12.

4 Differential Diagnosis and Management of Hyperprolactinemia

Janet A. Schlechte, MD

CONTENTS

INTRODUCTION

Hyperprolactinemia is a common pituitary disorder and a leading cause of reproductive dysfunction in females. Unlike other hormones from the anterior pituitary, which are stimulated by hypothalamic releasing factors, prolactin (PRL) secretion is under inhibitory control. Dopamine produced by tuberoinfundibular neurons is the major factor controlling PRL synthesis and release *(1)*. Prolactin is secreted episodically with a marked increase after the onset of sleep and a peak around 5:00–7:00 AM *(2)*. Serum levels are usually <20 ng/mL in females and <10 ng/mL in males and higher levels in females are due to the effects of estrogen on PRL gene expression *(3)*. In animals, PRL plays a role in the regulation of salt and water balance, has prominent behavioral effects, and is involved in regulation of the immune response.

In humans, the primary action of PRL is to stimulate development of mammary tissue and synthesis of lactalbumin, but it is the effect of PRL on the reproductive system, which is responsible for the clinical syndromes that accompany PRL hypersecretion. This chapter will highlight the differential diagnosis of hyperprolactinemia and the management of hyperprolactinemia associated with PRL secreting pituitary tumors.

DIFFERENTIAL DIAGNOSIS

The causes of hyperprolactinemia are diverse (Table 1). Prolactin-secreting pituitary adenomas are the most common cause of hyperprolactinemia, but elevated PRL can also be seen with growth hormone and ACTH secreting tumors and with large "non-

From: *Contemporary Endocrinology, Vol. 3: Diseases of the Pituitary: Diagnosis and Treatment*
Edited by M. E. Wierman Humana Press Inc., Totowa, NJ

Table 1
Causes of Hyperprolactinemia

Causes
Central nervous system
Pituitary tumors (PRL, GH, ACTH, nonsecreting)
Hypothalamic tumors (craniopharyngioma)
Granulomatous disease
Pinealoma
Aneurysm
Meningioma
Medications
Histamine blockers
Metoclopromide
Neuroleptic agents
Estrogen
Amitriptyline
Primary hypothyroidism
Chronic Renal Failure
Chest Trauma
Stress
Idiopathic

functioning" pituitary tumors. Any process that disrupts the hypothalamus or pituitary stalk or alters dopamine synthesis or action will lead to hyperprolactinemia. Extrapituitary central nervous system lesions associated with hyperprolactinemia include: craniopharyngioma, meningioma, ectopic pinealoma, third ventricle tumor, and aneurysm *(4)*. Hypothalamic tumors and granulomatous disease will also lead to hyperprolactinemia.

Drugs

A variety of medications cause hyperprolactinemia by altering the dopaminergic inhibition of PRL secretion. Neuroleptic agents act as dopamine receptor antagonists to cause rapid elevation of serum PRL with levels that may reach 200 ng/mL. After drug withdrawal, serum PRL returns to normal within 48–96 h *(5)*. Other dopamine antagonists that cause PRL elevation include derivatives of procainamide, such as metaclopromide, which may be associated with a 15-fold increase in PRL concentrations *(6)*. Peripheral decarboxylase inhibitors such as carbidopa and benserazide interfere with dopamine biosynthesis, and reserpine and alpha methyl dopa stimulate PRL secretion by depleting central catecholamine levels *(7,8)*. Histamine type 2 receptor blockers like cimetidine and ranitidine also produce hyperprolactinemia via a central mechanism *(9)*.

There are substantial data supporting the role of estrogen in inducing hyperprolactinemia. Administration of estrogen to normal women stimulates PRL secretion and is associated with lactotroph hyperplasia *(10)*. Prolactin levels may increase during the midphase of the menstrual cycle, and PRL levels increase 10-fold during pregnancy *(11,12)*. Approximately one-third of women taking oral contraceptive agents have mild hyperprolactinemia *(13)*. Estrogen appears to act by decreasing the inhibitory potential of dopamine or may alter the release of PRL via increased hypothalamic TRH secretion *(14,15)*.

Hypothyroidism

Patients with longstanding primary hypothyroidism may develop hyperprolactinemia because of hypothalamic TRH secretion, which stimulates PRL release. Restoration of normal thyroid function will normalize serum PRL *(16)*.

Chronic Renal Failure

Mild elevation of PRL is also seen in patients with chronic renal insufficiency. Inhibition of PRL release in these patients is abnormal, but the precise mechanism by which hyperprolactinemia occurs has not been elucidated. Prolactin levels are not affected by peritoneal or hemodialysis *(17)*.

Stress

Prolactin has been shown to increase after surgery, anesthesia, exercise, burns, and herpes zoster infections, and chest trauma and chronic nipple stimulation may elevate PRL by stimulation of afferent nerves *(18–20)*. Psychic stress has a variable effect on PRL secretion and higher indices of depression and hostility have been reported in hyperprolactinemic women *(21)*.

PROLACTINOMAS

Prolactin secreting tumors comprise nearly 80% of functioning pituitary tumors (40–50% of all tumors) and are the most common cause of hyperprolactinemia due to a tumor *(22)*. In women, most prolactinomas are smaller than 1 cm, and visual loss and hypopituitarism rarely occur. Tumors larger than 1 cm occur in only 30% of hyperprolactinemic women. In men, prolactinomas are usually large tumors that are associated with neurological defects and visual loss *(23)*.

The diagnosis of a prolactinoma is confirmed by sustained hyperprolactinemia and radiographic evidence of a pituitary tumor. There is no PRL level that is absolutely diagnostic of a pituitary tumor and there is, in general, poor correlation between serum PRL and tumor size *(24)*. Magnetic resonance imaging and high resolution computed tomography scans are equally effective in demonstrating PRL tumors, but the magnetic resonance imaging technique is superior in visualizing large tumors that may have lateral or suprasellar extension. A variety of stimulation tests have been proposed to differentiate between tumoral and nontumoral causes of hyperprolactinemia. Provocative tests using thyrotrophin releasing hormone, chlorpromazine, and insulin-induced hypoglycemia are insensitive and are of little practical use in the evaluation of the patients with hyperprolactinemia *(25)*.

Clinical Presentation

Women with PRL secreting pituitary tumors usually present with amenorrhea, galactorrhea, and infertility. Amenorrhea may occur without galactorrhea, galactorrhea may occur alone, and some hyperprolactinemic women have no menstrual dysfunction *(26)*. Hyperprolactinemic women who have regular menses may have a large molecular weight PRL molecule with decreased biologic activity *(27)*. In males, hyperprolactinemia is associated with impotence and decreased libido but more common presenting symptoms are headaches, visual loss, and neurological deficits. Up to one-third of men with hyperprolactinemia may have galactorrhea and nearly half will have visual impairment *(28)*.

Hyperprolactinemia exerts effects on the reproductive system by interfering with pulsatile gonadotrophin release and altering gonadotrophin action in the ovary *(29,30)*. In males, hyperprolactinemia also alters testosterone metabolism and affects sperm synthesis, morphology, and metabolism. Prolactin may also alter the rate of fructose utilization and glucose oxidation in human spermatozoa *(31)*.

Therapy

The two established indications for treatment of hyperprolactinemia are restoration of fertility and the presence of a macroadenoma. The high rate of recurrence of hyperprolactinemia after surgery and the delayed effects of radiation therapy make them unacceptable options for primary therapy *(32)*. The treatment of choice for prolactinomas, irrespective of size, is a dopamine agonist.

By direct stimulation of neuronal and pituitary dopamine receptors, dopamine agonists cause a rapid decline in PRL levels and decrease in tumor size *(33)*. After treatment with a dopamine agonist, 80–90% of women with PRL secreting microadenomas will have normal serum PRL, regular menstrual periods, and restoration of fertility *(33)*. Suppression of serum PRL occurs rapidly and gonadal function may normalize as early as 3 mo after treatment. Normalization of PRL occurs in only 60% of patients with macroadenomas, and tumor size will be reduced by one-half in approximately 46% of female patients with large tumors *(34)*. Reduction in tumor size may occur as early as 6 wk after treatment and results from a reduction in individual tumor cells and cell necrosis *(35)*.

Bromocriptine, 2-br-alpha-ergocryptine mesylate, is the prototype for all dopamine agonists. Others include pergolide, lergotrile, emsulergine, cabergoline, and terguride. Cabergoline can be given once per week and pergolide and quinagolide (cv 205–502) have a longer duration of action than bromocriptine *(36)*. Therapy is begun with a dose of 1.25 mg of bromocriptine at bedtime. At weekly intervals, the drug can be slowly increased until the PRL normalizes. Normalization of PRL and restoration of menses rarely require more than 5–7.5 mg of bromocriptine in women with microadenomas. Higher doses are required to lower serum PRL and decrease tumor size in males. Normalization of serum PRL does not always accompany normalization of serum testosterone or restoration of potency. After pregnancy is achieved, bromocriptine should be discontinued. Whereas bromocriptine is not associated with an increased risk of congenital defects, it does cross the placenta *(37)*.

All of the dopamine agonists may cause nausea, vomiting, nasal stuffiness, and orthostatic hypotension, but the side-effects are lessened if the drug is started at a very low dosage at bedtime. Monthly injections of a long acting dopamine agonist (Parlodel-lar, Sandoz, Basel, Switzerland) have been associated with transient side-effects and transvaginal administration of bromocriptine has been reported to be associated with fewer gastrointestinal side-effects *(38,39)*.

Dopamine agonist therapy is not associated with permanent lowering of PRL, and withdrawal of the drug is associated with tumor regrowth and return to pretreatment PRL levels *(40)*. There appear to be no long-term adverse effects of therapy with bromocriptine; however, eight patients taking bromocriptine in doses of 20–50 mg/d for Parkinson's disease developed pulmonary fibrosis *(41)*.

The effects of estrogen on PRL secretion and the increase in pituitary size that occurs during pregnancy raised early concerns about tumor expansion during pregnancy in women with prolactinomas. However, <5% of women with PRL microadenomas showed radiographic evidence of tumor expansion during pregnancy and <2% had clinical symptoms suggestive of tumor growth *(42)*. Women with PRL macroadenomas, however, may develop significant visual field defects during pregnancy, and 13 in one study required surgery during pregnancy *(42)*. In women with large prolactinomas the tumor should be debulked before pregnancy is attempted.

Most prolactinomas in women have a benign clinical course. In a prospective analysis of 30 women with untreated hyperprolactinemia followed for 5 yr, Schlechte et al. showed that none developed a macroadenoma or pituitary hypofunction. Fifteen percent of women who had a normal pituitary X-ray on presentation had no radiographic abnormalities at the end of the study. In this study, serum PRL did not correlate with changes in tumor size and was not a reliable indicator of tumor progression *(43)*.

PRL and the Skeleton

The hypogonadism that accompanies hyperprolactinemia also has effects on the skeleton. Hyperprolactinemic women have 25% lower spinal bone mineral than that seen in healthy control women *(44)*. Normalization of PRL and restoration of menses is associated with an increase in spinal bone density, but bone mass does not return to normal *(45)*. Klibanski et al. have shown that estrogen deficiency is the major factor leading to osteopenia as hyperprolactinemic patients with regular menses do not demonstrate low bone mass *(46)*.

There is conflicting information as to the *rate* of bone loss in amenorrheic women with increased PRL. In women followed prospectively, Schlechte et al. demonstrated no significant decline in spinal or forearm bone mineral and no fractures over 5 yr *(47)*. In a shorter study of similar design, Biller et al. reported that hyperprolactinemic women lost spinal bone at a rate of 3.8% per yr *(48)*. These data suggest that there may be a subset of patients with hyperprolactinemia who are at risk for accelerated bone loss.

Unresolved Issues

When fertility is not an issue, estrogen therapy would appear to be an attractive option for treatment of women with hyperprolactinemic amenorrhea. However, the standard of practice is to avoid estrogen in hyperprolactinemic women because estrogen increases PRL, has been associated with tumor formation in animals, and may lead to tumor growth in humans *(10,49,50)*. Estrogen and a dopamine agonist could be administered simultaneously, but this combination is expensive and the dopamine agonist has significant side-effects.

To assess the safety of administration of estrogen to women with increased PRL, Schlechte et al. performed serial magnetic resonance imaging scans in 20 amenorrheic women with hyperprolactinemic amenorrhea. After 1 yr of therapy, none of the tumors had changed in size by more than 1 mm, and no tumors developed in women who had normal MRI scans at entry into the study *(51)*. These preliminary data suggest that estrogen administration may not be associated with rapid tumor induction or expansion, but only long-term studies will confirm its safety. For now, estrogen should only be used in hyperprolactinemic women in conjunction with frequent radiographic monitoring or with a dopamine agonist.

REFERENCES

1. Yeo T, Thorner MO, Jones A, et al. The effects of dopamine, bromocriptine, lergotrile and metoclopramide on prolactin release from continuously perfused columns of isolated rat pituitary cells. Clin Endocrinol 1979; 10:123–130.
2. Sassin JF, Frantz AG, Weitzman ED, Kapen S. Human prolactin: 24-hour pattern with increased release during sleep. Science 1972; 177:1205–1207.
3. Shupnik MA, Baxter LA, French LR, et al. In vivo effects of estrogen on ovine pituitaries: prolactin and growth hormone biosynthesis and messenger ribonucleic acid translation. Endocrinology 1979; 104:729–735.
4. Balagura S, Frantz AG, Housepain EM, Carmel PW. The specificity of serum prolactin as a diagnostic indicator of pituitary adenoma. J Neurosurg 1979; 51:42–46.
5. Rubin RT, Hays SE. The prolactin secretory response to neuroleptic drugs: mechanisms, applications and limitations. Psychoneuroendocrinology 1980; 5:121.
6. Perez-Lopez FR, Abos MD: Pituitary hormonal response to the orthopramides clebopride, bromopride, metoclopramide and sulpiride. Fertil Steril 1982; 37:445.
7. Polleri A, Masturzo P, Murialdo G, et al. Dose and sex related effects of aromatic amino acids decarboxylase inhibitors on serum prolactin in humans. Acta Endocrinol 1980; 93:7.
8. Camanni E, Strumia E, Portaleone P, et al. Prolactin secretion during reserpine and syrosingopine treatment. Eur J Clin Pharmacol 1981; 20:347.
9. Pasquali R, Corinaldesi R, Miglioli M, et al. Effect of prolonged administration of ranitidine on pituitary and thyroid hormones, and their response to specific hypothalamic-releasing factors. Clin Endocrinol 1981; 15:457.
10. Yen SSC, Ehara Y, Siler TM. Augmentation of prolactin secretion by estrogen in hypogonadal women. J Clin Invest 1974; 53:652–655.
11. Tyson JE, Hwang P, Guyda H, Friesen HG. Studies of prolactin secretion in human pregnancy. Am J Obstet Gynecol 1972; 113:14–20.
12. Backstrom CT, McNeilly AS, Leask RM, Baird DT. Pulsatile secretion of LH, FSH, prolactin, oestradiol and progesterone during the human menstrual cycle. Clin Endocrinol 1982; 17:29–42.
13. Reyniak JV, Wenof M, Aubert JM, et al. Incidence of hyperprolactinemia during oral contraceptive therapy. Obstet Gynecol 1980; 55:8.
14. Raymond V, Beaulieu M, Labrie F, Boissier J. Potent antidopaminergic activity of estradiol at the pituitary level on prolactin release. Science 1978; 200:1173.
15. Veldhuis JD, Evans WS, Stumpf PG. Mechanisms that subserve estradiol's induction of increased prolactin concentrations: Evidence of amplitude modulation of spontaneous prolactin secretory busts. Am J Obstet Gynecol 1989; 161:1149–1158.
16. Edwards CRW, Forsyth IA, Besser GM. Amenorrhea, galactorrhoea and primary hypothyroidism with high circulating levels of prolactin. Br Med J 1971; 111:462–464.
17. Nagel TC, Freinkel N, Bell RH, et al. Gynecomastia, prolactin and other peptide hormones in patients undergoing chronic hemodialysis. J Clin Endocrinol Metab 1973; 36:428–432.
18. Noel GL, Suh HK, Stone JG, et al. Human prolactin and growth hormone release during surgery and other conditions of stress. J Clin Endocrinol Metab 1972; 35:840.
19. Brisson GR, Ledoux M, Peronnet F, et al. Prolactinemia in exercising male athletes. Horm Res 1981; 15:218.
20. Morley JE, Dawson M, Hodgkinson H, et al. Galactorrhea and hyperprolactinemia associated with chest wall injury. J Clin Endocrinol Metab 1977; 45:931.
21. Miyabo S, Asato T, Mizushima N. Prolactin and growth hormone responses to psychological stress in normal and neurotic subjects. J Clin Endocrinol Metab 1977; 44:947.
22. Randall RV, Laws Jr ER, Trautmann JC. Results of transsphenoidal microsurgery for pituitary adenoma in 892 patients. In: *Pituitary Hyperfunction: Pathophysiology and Clinical Aspects* (Camanni F, Muller EE, eds). New York, Raven Press, 1984; pp. 417–419.

23. Wilson C, Dempsey L: Transsphenoidal microsurgical removal of 250 pituitary adenomas. J Neurosurg 58:13, 1978.
24. Randall RV, Laws Jr ER, Abboud CF, et al. Transsphenoidal microsurgical treatment of prolactin-producing pituitary adenomas. Results in 100 patients. Mayo Clin Proc 1983; 58:108–121.
25. Ferrari C, Rampini P, Benco R, et al. Functional characterization of hypothalamic hyperprolactinemia. J Clin Endocrinol Metab 1982; 55:897–901.
26. Schlechte JA, Sherman BM, Halmi N, VanGilder J, Chapler FK, Dolan K, Granner DK, Duello T, Harris C: Prolactin-secreting pituitary tumors in amenorrheic women: A comprehensive study. Endocrine Rev 1980; 1:295–308.
27. Jackson RD, Wortsman J, Malarkey WB. Characterization of a large molecular weight prolactin in women with idiopathic hyperprolactinemia and normal menses. J Clin Endocrinol Metab 1985; 61:258–264.
28. Carter JN, Tyson JE, Tolis G, et al. Prolactin-secreting tumors and hypogonadism in 22 men. N Engl J Med 1978; 299:847–852.
29. Dorrington J, Gore-Langton RE. Prolactin inhibits oestrogen synthesis in the ovary. Nature 1981; 290:600–602.
30. Moult PJA, Rees LH, Besser GM. Pulsatile gonadotropin secretion in hyperprolactinemic amenorrhea and the response to bromocriptine therapy. Clin Endocrinol (Oxf) 1982; 16:153–162.
31. Wong TW, Jones TM. Hyperprolactinemia and male infertility. Arch Pathol Lab Med 1984; 108:35.
32. Schlechte JA, Sherman BM, Chapler FK, et al. Long-term follow-up of women with surgically treated prolactin-secreting pituitary tumors. J Clin Endocrinol Metab 1986; 62:1296–1301.
33. Thorner MO, Schran HF, Evans WS, et al. A broad spectrum of prolactin suppression by bromocriptine in hyperprolactinemic women: A study of serum prolactin and bromocriptine levels after a cure and chronic administration of bromocriptine. J Clin Endocrinol Metab 1980; 50:1026–1033.
34. Molitch ME, Elton RL, Blackwell RE, et al. Bromocriptine as primary therapy for prolactin-secreting macroadenomas: Results of a prospective multicenter study. J Clin Endocrinol Metab 1985; 60:698–705.
35. Mori H, Shintaro M, Saitoh Y, et al. Effects of bromocriptine on prolactin-secreting pituitary adenomas. Mechanism of reduction in tumor size evaluated by light and electron microscopic, immunohistochemical, and morphometric analysis. Cancer 1985; 56:230–238.
36. Melis GB, Mais V, Gambacciani M, Sghedoni D, Paoletti AM, Floretti P. Reduction in the size of prolactin-producing tumor after cabergoline administration. Fertil Steril 1989; 52:412.
37. Tarkalj I, Braun P, Krupp P. Surveillance of bromocriptine in pregnancy. JAMA 1982; 247:1589–1591.
38. Van't Verlaat JW, Lancranjan I, Hendriks MJ, Croughs RJM. Primary treatment of macroprolactinomas with Parlodel LAR. Acta Endocrinol (Copenh) 1988; 119:51.
39. Kletzky OA, Vermesh M. Effectiveness of vaginal bromocriptine in treating women with hyperprolactinemia. Fertil Steril 1989; 51:269.
40. Vance ML, Evans WS, Thorner MO, et al. Bromocriptine. Ann Intern Med 1984; 100:78–91.
41. McElvaney NG, Wilcox PG, Churg AM, et al. Pleuropulmonary disease during promocriptine treatment of Parkinson's disease. Arch Intern Med 1988; 148:2231–2236.
42. Molitch ME. Pregnancy and the hyperprolactinemic woman. N Engl J Med 1985; 312:1364–1370.
43. Schlechte J, Dolan K, Sherman B, et al. The natural history of untreated hyperprolactinemia: A prospective analysis. J Clin Endocrinol Metab 1989; 68:412–418.
44. Schlechte J, El-Khoury G, Kathol M, Walkner L. Forearm and vertebral bone mineral in treated and untreated hyperprolactinemic amenorrhea. J Clin Endocrinol Metab 1987; 64:1021–1026.
45. Klibanski A, Greenspan SL. Increase in bone mass after treatment of hyperprolactinemic amenorrhea. N Engl J Med 1986; 315:542–546.
46. Klibanski A, Biller BMK, Rosenthal DI, et al. Effects of prolactin and estrogen deficiency in amenorrheic bone loss. J Clin Endocrinol Metab 1988; 67:124–130.
47. Schlechte J, Walkner L, Kathol M. A longitudinal analysis of premenopausal bone loss in healthy women and women with hyperprolactinemia. J Clin Endocrinol Metab 1992; 75:698–703.
48. Biller BMK, Baum HBA, Rosenthal DI, et al. Progressive trabecular osteopenia in women with hyperprolactinemic amenorrhoea. J Clin Endocrinol Metab 1992; 75:692–697.
49. Lloyd RV. Estrogen-induced hyperplasia and neoplasia in the rat anterior pituitary gland: An immunohistochemical study. Am J Pathol 1983; 113:198–206.
50. Bevan JS, Sussman J, Roberts A, et al. Development of an invasive macroprolactinoma: A possible consequence of prolonged oestrogen replacement. Case report. Br J Obstet Gynaecol 1989; 96:1440–1444.
51. Schlechte J, Tullis M. The effect of estrogen therapy on pituitary tumor growth and bone density in amenorrheic women with hyperprolactinemia. (Abstract) Endocrinology 1995; 131:51.

5 Growth Hormone
Normal Physiology

Ian M. Chapman, MBBS, PhD, *and*
Michael O. Thorner, MB, DSc

Contents

SOMATOTROPHS AND THE ANTERIOR PITUITARY GLAND

Growth hormone (GH) is an anabolic growth promoting hormone that is synthesized, stored, and secreted by somatotroph cells of the anterior pituitary gland. In addition to GH, some somatotrophs also produce prolactin and the glycoprotein alpha-subunit. Somatotrophs comprise approximately 35–50% of human anterior pituitary cells and are distributed throughout the gland, with a possible preponderance in the lateral portions. The human anterior pituitary contains 5–15 mg of GH *(1)*. Both

From: *Contemporary Endocrinology, Vol. 3: Diseases of the Pituitary: Diagnosis and Treatment*
Edited by M. E. Wierman Humana Press Inc., Totowa, NJ

somatotrophs and prolactin producing lactotrophs are acidophilic on standard H&E staining. Somatotrophs can be specifically identified by a number of techniques, including immunohistochemical staining for GH, *in situ* hybridization, and by characteristic features on electron microscopy examination. Electron microscopy reveals several subsets of somatotrophs. Cells of the predominant subset contain abundant, large (500 nm or greater) secretory granules and a lesser number of small granules (200 nm or less), whereas cells of the minority subset are sparsely granulated *(2)*.

GH STRUCTURE

Growth hormone belongs to a family of single-chain polypeptide hormones that also includes prolactin and human chorionic somatomammotropin (hCS, also known as human placental lactogen). These hormones are thought to have evolved from a common ancestral protein by gene duplication at least 500 million years ago, at or before the earliest vertebrate stage *(3)*. The gene for human pituitary GH, hGH-N, is located on the long arm of chromosome 17, as part of a five-gene complex *(4)* that also includes two genes for chorionic somatomammotropin (hCS-A and -B), hCS-L, which is probably not expressed, and hGH-V, which codes for placental GHs *(5,6)*. Each of these genes has four introns separating five exons *(4)*. The hGH-N gene is expressed only in the somatotrophs of the anterior pituitary. This specificity results, at least in part, from the interaction of the GH gene with Pit-1, a protein transcription factor that is unique to pituitary cells, and acts as a promoter of GH gene expression *(7–9)*.

Human GH has considerable structural heterogeneity, as a result of pretranslational, posttranslational and postsecretory modifications to the hGH-N gene product. Approximately 75% of pituitary GH is a nonglycosylated, single chain, 191-amino acid, 22-kDa protein with two intrachain disulfide bonds *(10)*. Five to ten percent of pituitary GH is in the form of a 20-kDa protein, produced by an alternate splicing of the second exon of the gene that results in a 15 amino acid deletion between amino acids 32 and 46 in the GH molecule *(6,11)*. Smaller amounts of other GH variants, including dimers and oligomers of the 22- and 20-kDa forms, are also found in the pituitary *(12)*. The relative proportions of circulating GH variants are similar to those in the pituitary, except for an approximate twofold increase in the abundance of the 20-kDa form. This increase results from slower clearance of the 20-kDa than the 22-kDa form from the circulation *(12)*. Both 22- and 20-kDa forms circulate as dimers and as oligomers of up to five molecules *(13,14)*. Low molecular weight forms are also present in the circulation, and may represent secreted or degradation products *(15,16)*. The relative proportions of the different circulating GHs do not seem to be affected by the nature of the secretory stimulus, age, gender, or a variety of pathological conditions *(17–19)*.

GH RECEPTOR AND GH BINDING PROTEIN

Growth hormone exerts its actions by binding to transmembrane GH receptors on the plasma membranes of hepatocytes, adipocytes, fibroblasts, lymphocytes, heart, kidney, muscle, and other cell types, and also to cytosolic receptors that may represent internalized or newly formed receptors *(20)*. The GHR is a member of a family of single transmembrane cytokine receptors that includes receptors for prolactin, interleukin-2 to -7, granulocyte macrophage-colony stimulating factor (GM-CSF), granulocyte colony stimulating factor (G-CSF), and erythropoietin *(21,22)*. In adipose tissue, GHR mRNA levels are modulated by circulating GH levels; they fall with hypophysectomy and rise again with GH replacement *(23)*. It has not been established if receptor levels are regulated by GH in other tissues.

The extracellular amino terminal amino acid sequence of the GHR is identical to the amino acid sequence of a circulating 60-kDa high affinity, low capacity, GH binding protein (GHBP), which has been identified in a number of species, including humans *(11,24–29)*. In humans and rabbits, the high affinity 60-kDa GHBP arises by proteolysis of the GHR, whereas in rodents it is produced by alternative RNA splicing and contains a unique carboxyterminal end *(30)*. In humans the relationship between the GHR and this GHBP is further supported by the finding that both are absent in individuals with Laron-type dwarfism *(31,32)*.

A second, 100-kDa, low affinity GHBP has also been identified in the circulation *(33)*. It does not appear to be related to the GHR. The affinity of the major 60-kDa GHBP is greater for 22-kDa than for 20-kDa GH, whereas 20-kDa GH preferentially binds to the low affinity GHBP *(34)*. Under basal conditions, when circulating GH concentrations are less than about 15 μg/L, approximately 50% of 22-kDa GH and 25% of 20-kDa GH are bound to these binding proteins, with over 80% of this binding being to the high affinity GHBP *(35)*. As GH concentrations increase further, the proportion of GH that is bound decreases.

The exact function and significance of these GHBPs is unclear. Circulating concentrations of the high affinity form increase during childhood *(36)*, but then remain fairly constant throughout adulthood, with little diurnal variation. There is wide variation between individuals, but little within individuals. GH itself does not regulate concentrations of either type of GHBP *(26,37)*; normal levels are found in both hypopituitarism and acromegaly *(26,37)*. The overall effect of these binding proteins may be to dampen the effects of pulsatile GH and flatten the hormone profiles at the target tissue level. GH binding protein complexes are too big to be filtered by the kidney, and in rat experiments, protein bound GH is cleared 10 times more slowly than free GH *(38)*. The binding protein also acts to reduce circulating unbound GH concentrations during GH secretory bursts *(39)* and inhibits GH binding to GHR by competing for this binding *(38)*.

INTRACELLULAR MECHANISMS OF GH ACTION

The binding of GH to its receptor leads to receptor dimerization, followed by hormone-receptor internalization and degradation *(24)*. The subsequent intracellular signal transduction mechanisms have not been fully defined. Whereas the GHR and the other members of its cytokine receptor family share homology in their extracellular domains, their intracellular domains share no homology with each other or with other receptors with already defined signaling mechanisms *(22)*. Growth hormone stimulates tyrosine phosphorylation of multiple intracellular proteins *(40,41)*, including a GHR-associated kinase Jak 2 *(42,43)*. Phosphorylation of Jak 2 in turn results in the phosphorylation of STAT proteins (signal transducers and activators of transcription) including STATS 1, 3, and 5 *(44)*. The STAT proteins are then translocated to the nucleus where they bind to DNA and activate transcription of target genes (Fig. 1).

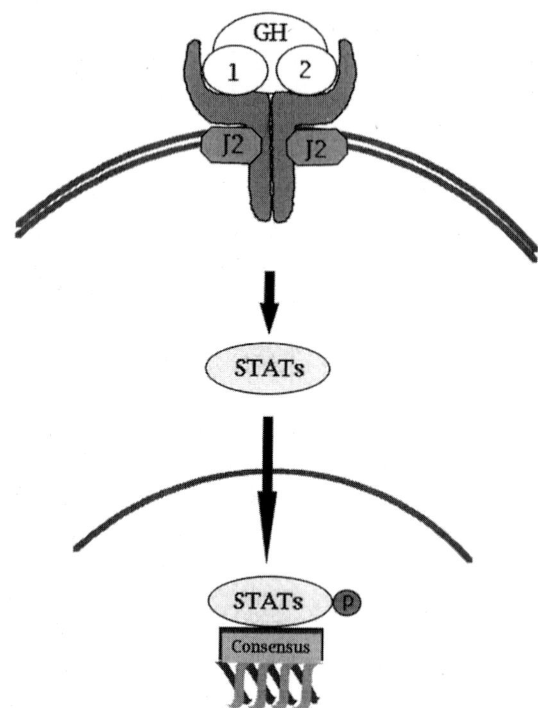

Fig. 1. Schematic overview of the intracellular mechanisms of growth hormone action. Growth hormone binding to its transmembrane receptor results in dimerization of the receptor (1 and 2), which in turn stimulates tyrosine phosphorylation of the kinase Jak 2 (J2). This phosphorylation stimulates phosphorylation of the STAT proteins (signal transducers and activators of transcription), which are then transported to the nucleus and bind to consensus DNA sequences to activate gene transcription. (Courtesy of C. M. Silva.)

INTERACTION OF GH AND INSULIN-LIKE GROWTH FACTOR-I

Currently available evidence indicates that GH induces local as well as hepatic insulin-like growth factor (IGF)-I production, that GH has direct actions independent of IGF-I, and that GH and IGF-I act synergistically to stimulate growth. This synergism between GH and IGF-I has been termed the "dual effector theory" of GH action *(45)*; *see* Fig. 2). In 1957, Salmon and Daughaday proposed the "somatomedin hypothesis" of GH action, according to which GH exerts its effects indirectly, by stimulating hepatic production of IGF-I (previously called somatomedin-C) *(46)*. This hypothesis arose from a study in which these investigators demonstrated that cartilage proliferation in hypophysectomized rats was stimulated in vitro by serum from normal rats, but not by either GH or serum from other hypophysectomized rats. Within 24–72 h of hypophysectomized rats being started on GH treatment, their serum had acquired the ability to stimulate cartilage proliferation. The GH-dependent growth factor in the serum responsible for cartilage proliferation was later identified as IGF-I.

Subsequent studies have confirmed the importance of circulating IGF-I in mediating the actions of GH, and circulating IGF-I and GH concentrations across the range from GH deficiency to acromegaly are significantly correlated. However, evidence has also

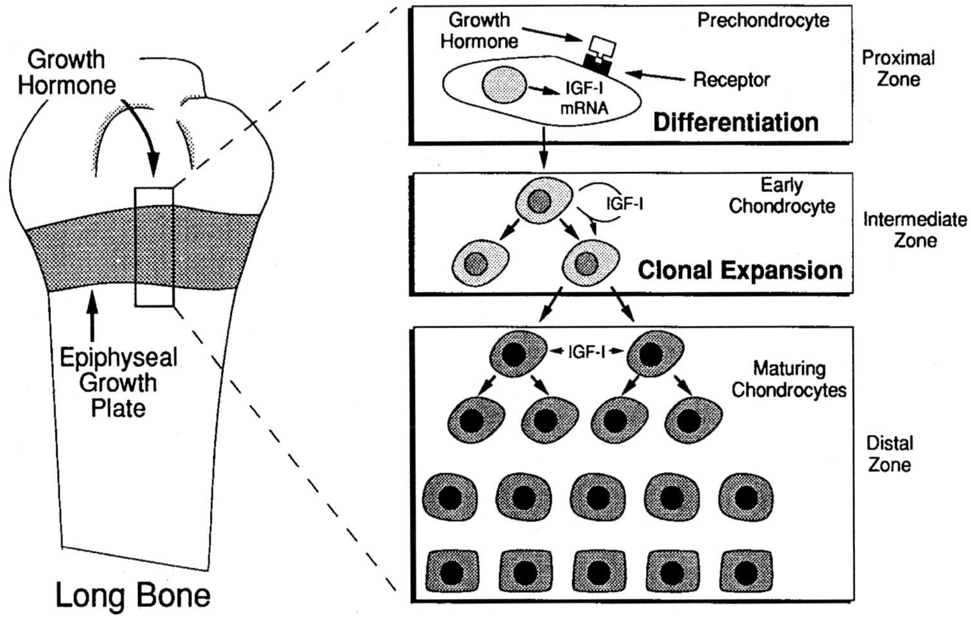

Fig. 2. Schematic representation of the dual-effector hypothesis proposed by Green *(45)*. Growth hormone acts directly at the epiphyseal plate to stimulate linear growth. The GH stimulates differentiation of prechondrocytes into early chondrocytes, which then secrete IGF-I. In turn, IGF-I stimulates clonal expansion and maturation of chondrocytes. (Modified from ref. *45a*.)

accumulated that circulating IGF-I of hepatic origin is not the only mediator of GH action. Unilateral injections of GH into the tibial growth plate of hypophysectomized rats have been shown to produce bone growth on the ipsilateral side *(47)*, an effect that is blocked by passive immunization with IGF-I antibodies *(48)*. The administration of GH to hypophysectomized rats results in increased IGF-I levels in nonhepatic tissues some hours before the increase in circulating levels *(49)*. When IGF-I and GH are separately administered to hypophysectomized rats, in doses that produce comparable circulating IGF-I concentrations, the rats given IGF-I grow less than those given GH, suggesting a GH action independent of IGF-I *(50,51)*. There is evidence that GH directly stimulates the early differentiation of prechodrocyte stem cells in the epiphyseal growth plate, and these cells then undergo clonal expansion. The IGF-I (either hepatic or local in origin) then induces clonal expansion of the committed, more highly differentiated chondrocytes *(52)*.

INSULIN-LIKE GROWTH FACTORS (IGFS)

The major forms of insulin-like growth factors (IGFs) are IGF-I and IGF-II. They are closely related single-chain polypeptide molecules with three intrachain sulfide bridges *(53)*. IGF-I, most important in mediating the actions of GH, comprises 70 amino acids and has a molecular weight of 7.64 kDa. IGF-II is composed of 67 amino acids and has a molecular weight of 7.47 kDa. The sequence homology between IGF-I and IGF-II is 62%, and both share approximately 40% homology with proinsulin

(54,55). The liver is the major source of circulating IGFs, but the IGF genes are located in most tissues *(56)*, and the autocrine and paracrine actions of locally produced IGFs are thought to be important in the regulation of growth and differentiation *(57)*. Because of this, and the complex effects of the IGF binding proteins (*see below*), considerable caution must be exercised when inferring IGF actions at the tissue level from circulating IGF concentrations.

The IGFs bind to two known receptors. The IGF-I receptor (type I IGF receptor) mediates most of the biological actions of IGF-I and IGF-II and has a high degree of homology with the insulin receptor. It is found in a wide variety of tissues including the pituitary and hypothalamus and has an affinity for IGF-I of approximately 1 n*M* *(57)*. Its affinity is two- to 10-fold lower for IGF-II, and 100- to 500-fold lower for insulin *(58–61)*. The insulin receptor has a 100-fold higher affinity for insulin than IGF-I. The IGF-II receptor (type 2 IGF receptor) is identical to the mannose 6-phosphate receptor, and has no known IGF signaling function.

IGF BINDING PROTEINS (IGFBPs)

In both the circulation and the tissues, IGF-I and IGF-II are associated with specific binding proteins, 200–300 amino acids in length. Six IGFBPs have been described, and IGFBPs 3–6 are glycoslyated, which may aid their adherence to cell surfaces. The IGFBPs bind most of the circulating IGFs; in the basal state only approximately 1% of IGF-I is free. The IGFBP-3, -2, and -1 are responsible for most of this binding. Their serum concentrations are approximately 5 mg/L, 250 ug/L, and 50 ug/L, respectively *(57)*. Approximately 75% of IGF-I and IGF-II circulates as part of a 150-kDa ternary complex that consists of IGF-I or IGF-II, plus IGFBP-3 and an 85-kDa acid-labile subunit. This ternary complex is unable to leave the vascular compartment, and binding of the IGFs in this complex leads to a dramatic prolongation of circulating IGF half-life; from about 10 min to 12–15 h for IGF-I *(62)*. A 40-kDa complex containing IGFBPs-1, -2, -4, and -6 is also present in the circulation. It carries much smaller amounts of IGF than the 150-kDa complex, but contains most of the unsaturated binding sites in serum *(63,64)*.

Circulating concentrations of the IGFBPs are regulated by hormonal and nutritional factors (*see* ref. *57* for review, and Table 1). Serum IGFBP-3 concentrations correlate with GH levels and are increased by GH administration. Growth hormone is essential for the maintenence of normal acid-labile subunit levels and the development of the 150-kDa ternary complex *(65)*. IGF-I may mediate some of the stimulatory effects of GH on IGFBP-3 levels, at least in the rat, as IGF-I treatment of GH-deficient rats increases levels of IGBP-3 but not the acid-labile subunit or ternary complex *(65)*. The IGF-I treatment of GHR-deficient humans (Laron type dwarfs) has been reported to have no effect on IGFBP-3 levels *(66)*. Serum IGFBP-3 levels are increased in acromegaly and decreased in hypopituitarism *(67)* and measurement of IGFBP-3 has been recommended as a diagnostic test for GH-deficiency in both children *(68)* and adults *(69)*. In contrast, GH and IGF-I appear to exert opposite effects on IGFBP-2. Blood concentrations of IGFBP-2 are inversely related to GH status and decrease with GH administration *(59,70)*, whereas IGFBP-2 concentrations are increased by IGF-I administration and in conditions of IGF-II excess *(64)*. Serum concentrations of IGFBP-2 and -3 are relatively constant over the day.

Table 1
Modulation of Circulating IGF Binding Protein Concentrations by GH, IGF-I, and Fasting

	Percentage of IGF-I bound[a]	*Effect of GH*	*Effect of IGF-I*	*Effect of fasting*
IGFBP-1	?	Decreased	Increased	Increased
IGFBP-2	?	Decreased	Increased	Increased
IGFBP-3	75%	Increased	Increased	Decreased
IGFBP-4	?	?	Decreased	?
IGFBP-5	?	Increased	Increased	?
IGFBP-6	?	?	?	?

?, unknown or uncertain.
[a]It can be predicted from the abundance and affinity constants of the different IGFBPs that the hierarchy for binding in serum would be: IGFBP-3, -2, -1, -4, -6, -5.

Circulating IGFBP-1 concentrations show marked variations during the day, because they are tightly linked to blood glucose and insulin concentrations. IGFBP-1 is inversely regulated by both insulin and GH, with insulin having the predominant effect *(71)*. Insulin appears to inhibit IGFBP-1 synthesis by directly decreasing gene transcription *(72)*. Concentration of IGFBP-1 is increased in insulin-dependent diabetes and normalized by insulin treatment *(73)*. After glucose ingestion, normal subjects have a decrease in IGFBP-1 concentration that correlates inversely with the rise in insulin concentration *(74)*. The fall in circulating insulin concentration with fasting is associated with increased circulating IGFBP-1 concentration *(75–77)*, and energy restriction has the same effect *(78)*. Fasting and protein restriction also increase IGFBP-2 concentration *(78,79)*, but lower the concentration of IGFBP-3.

The physiological role of the IGF binding proteins is unclear. The concept of unbound or "free" hormone as active hormone, useful in considering the actions of other protein-bound hormones such as the thyroid hormones, appears inadequate to describe the actions of the IGFs. Binding of IGF in the 150-kDa complex may act to dampen the metabolic actions of the IGFs, by trapping them in the circulation, and by preventing binding to receptors. IGF-I has a hypoglycemic potency approximately 7% that of insulin *(80)*, and plasma concentrations of total IGF-I are approximately 1000 times greater than those of insulin. The binding of IGF-I to IGFBPs prevents it from exerting this full hypoglycemic effect *(71,81,82)*. There is also evidence that binding to IGFBPs can *enhance* the biological action of IGF-I in cells such as fibroblasts, by binding to the target cell surface and potentiating the binding of IGF-I to adjacent receptors, and by aiding the transport of IGFs out of the circulation to target tissues *(83,84)*. The situation is further complicated by the existence of specific IGFBP proteases, which act to produce IGFBP fragments with reduced affinity for IGFs *(61,85)*, and by the current absence of a convenient and accurate assay for unbound IGF-I.

GH ACTIONS

GH is not essential for normal intrauterine development and growth, as indicated by the normal size of infants born with congenital absence of the pituitary. As childhood progresses, GH becomes an increasingly important stimulant of longitudinal growth. The interaction of GH with circulating and locally produced IGF-I produces linear growth by a process of chondrocyte proliferation and differentiation in the epiphyseal growth plate of long bones followed by calcification and incorporation into metaphyseal bone *(86–88)*.

Growth hormone also exerts a number of metabolic effects. Unlike the stimulation of linear growth, these persist throughout life. Continuous or intermittent high dose GH administration results in hyperinsulinemia accompanied by varying degrees of glucose intolerance, the major cause of which is hepatic postreceptor insulin resistance *(89–93)*. The insulin-antagonistic effects of increased nocturnal GH secretion (*see* Sleep section) have been implicated as a cause of the morning hyperglycemia often present in people with type I diabetes mellitus (dawn phenomenon). By contrast, GH-deficient children have decreased insulin levels and increased insulin sensitivity, accompanied by decreased fasting glucose levels and occasionally symptomatic hypoglycemia *(94)*.

Growth hormone is anabolic. Administration of GH to GH-deficient children *(95)*, normal and obese adults *(96)*, and adults with a variety of catabolic states including burns *(97,98)*, high dose glucocorticoid treatment *(99)*, and chronic obstructive lung disease *(100)*, results in positive nitrogen balance. Muscle mass is increased in GH-deficient children given GH *(101,102)*, and GH treatment produces significant increases in lean body mass in GH-deficient adults *(103)*, and healthy elderly subjects chosen on the basis of low circulating IGF-I concentrations *(104)*. Growth hormone administration has been found to increase muscle size in highly trained non-GH-deficient adult athletes *(105)*, but the effects on muscle strength in such GH-sufficient subjects have not been reported. Indeed, such treatment might even reduce muscle strength in some individuals, as myopathy and muscle weakness are features of acromegaly.

Growth hormone deficiency is associated with an increase in percentage of body fat, and redistribution of that fat to central sites. The net effect of GH on fat metabolism is lipolytic, with a decrease in fat deposition and an increase in fat mobilization. GH replacement therapy reduces body fat in GH-deficient subjects. In addition, GH deficiency is associated with abnormalities in circulating lipid profiles, including decreases in high density lipoprotein (HDL) and increases in low density lipoprotein (LDL) and total cholesterol levels, that favor the development of atherosclerosis *(103,106,107)*. These effects are reversible with GH therapy *(103,108,109)*.

A number of studies have shown that bone mineral density is increased by GH treatment in GH-deficient subjects, although these effects are rather small *(104,110)*, and most GH-deficient subjects are not osteoporotic. The effects of GH on bone are most likely mediated via increases in gastrointestinal calcium absorption and stimulatory effects of systemic and locally produced IGFs *(111)*.

Growth hormone exerts a number of effects on the immune system, apparently via production of IGFs. These include stimulatory effects on thymic development and natural killer cell activity. However, no clinical symptoms or syndromes associated with immune dysfunction have been described in GH-deficient humans *(112,113)*.

GH SECRETION

Mammalian GH secretion is pulsatile. The significance of this pulsatility has not been established, but there is evidence that it maximizes the growth promoting ef-

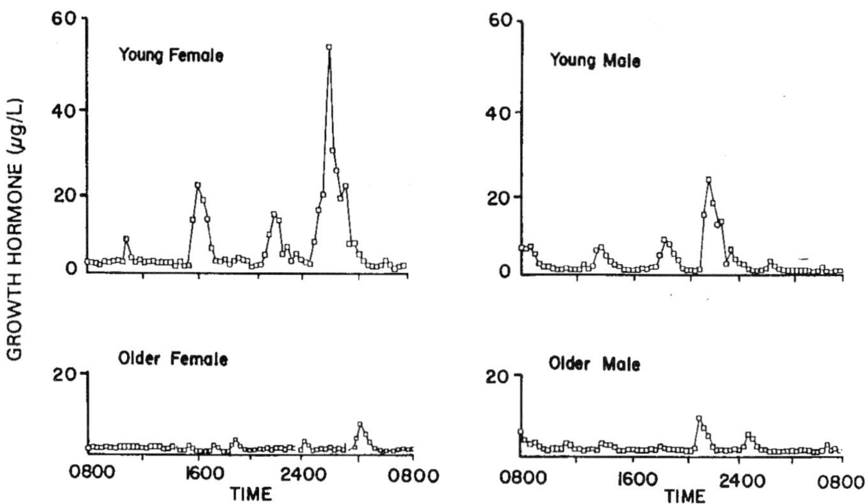

Fig. 3. Serum GH concentration profiles from a young woman, young man, older woman, and older man sampled every 20 min for 24 h. (Reprinted with permission from ref *237*.)

fects of GH and enhances its metabolic actions *(114–116)*. As a result of this pulsatility, and the relatively short half-life of GH, in the range 10–20 min *(14,117–120)*, GH concentrations can vary by as much as three orders of magnitude (e.g., 0.04–40 ug/L) over a 24-h period in normal young adults. Typical profiles of GH concentrations in normal men and women are shown in Fig. 3, and characteristics of GH secretion and pulsatility as estimated by deconvolution analysis in Table 2. It must be emphasized that mean GH concentrations are dependent on the assay used, particularly on its sensitivity, as many GH values between peaks fall below the limit of detection of current standard GH assays (0.1–0.5 ug/L). Estimates of characteristics of pulsatile GH release, such as the number and size of pulses and secretion rate, are affected not only by the assay used, but also by the blood sample collection frequency and by the pulse detection method used *(121)*. Normal ranges need to be established for each assay and subject population. Accurate comparisons between results obtained from different GH assays, or by using different GH pulse detection methods, are not usually possible. Recently a variety of ultrasensitive assays have been developed that can detect GH concentrations as low as 1 pg/mL *(21,22,122,123)*. These assays reveal that basal GH concentrations fall to approximately 15–25 pg/mL in fed, healthy adults *(122)*. We have recently used a modified ultra-sensitive chemiluminescence assay to measure GH in blood collected from a variety of subjects, including the elderly and GH-deficient young adults, under basal conditions and following an oral glucose load to suppress GH secretion, and GH was detectable in all samples assayed *(123,124)*. The ability to detect GH in all samples is essential for the study of low-level secretion and promises to provide new insights into the mechanisms underlying GH release.

Sleep, gender, age, body composition, nutrition, and exercise are all physiological variables that modulate GH secretion. These variables most likely exert their effects by altering the activity and interactions of the stimulatory and inhibitory hypothalamic hor-

Table 2
Deconvolution Analysis-Derived Attributes of GH Secretion in Man

	GH secreted, μg/24 h[a]	*No. secretory burst/24 h*	*Mass of GH secreted per burst, μg*[a]	*Half-life, min*
Normal young men *(121)*[b]	540 ± 44	12 ± 1.2	45 ± 3.7	17 ± 1.7
Fasted men *(303)*[b]	2171 ± 333	32 ± 2.4	64 ± 9.4	18 ± 2.2
Obese men *(300)*[c]	77 ± 20	3.2 ± 0.5	24 ± 4.6	12 ± 1.6
Normal middle-aged men *(300)*[c]	196 ± 65	9.7 ± 0.7	20 ± 6.3	16 ± 0.8

Data are given as mean ± SE.
[a]Assuming mean GH volume of distribution of 7.9% body weight.
[b]Samples obtained at 5-min intervals; age of subjects = 22–28; BMI = 21–29 kg/m^2.
[c]Samples obtained at 10-min intervals; mean age of obese subjects = 40 ± 3.1 yr; normal subjects = 48 ± 4.7 yr; mean BMI obese = 46 ± 1.6 kg/m^2; mean BMI normals = 28 + 1.3 kg/m^2.
(Reprinted with permission from ref *35*.)

mones, growth hormone releasing hormone (GHRH), and somatostatin (SRIH), respectively, and the feedback effects of IGF-I and GH.

Although there is evidence that some constitutive *(125)* and possibly episodic *(126)* pituitary GH release occurs in the absence of hypothalamic inputs, pulsatile GH release is largely produced and modulated by interacting stimulatory and inhibitory inputs from the hypothalamus. Growth hormone releasing hormone is the most important stimulator of GH secretion. Other GH stimulating factors identified in the hypothalamus include galanin *(127–130)*, motilin *(131,132)*, substance P *(133,134)*, neurotensin *(133)*, vasoactive intestinal peptide (VIP) *(135,136)*, and pituitary adenylate cyclase activating polypeptide (PACAP) *(137,138)*. The physiological significance of these non-GHRH factors is not yet known, and may be minor. In addition, thyrotropin releasing hormone (TRH) induces GH secretion in a majority *(139)*, and gonadotropin releasing hormone (GnRH or LHRH) in a minority of subjects with acromegaly *(140)*. Pharmacological doses of the pancreatic hormone glucagon stimulate GH release in most normal subjects *(141,142)*. A potent hexapeptide that stimulates GH secretion, growth hormone releasing peptide (GHRP), has been developed from the enkephalins *(143,144)*. It acts through a unique receptor that has recently been characterized *(143,145)*. An endogenous ligand for this substance may exist, but has not been identified.

Somatostatin (SRIH) is the principal hypothalamic inhibitor of GH release, although other peptides including corticotrophin releasing hormone (CRF) have some GH inhibiting effects *(146)*.

GROWTH HORMONE RELEASING HORMONE

Human GHRH exists in two forms, one with 40 and the other with 44 amino acids *(147,148)*. Both forms are found in the hypothalamus, and the full biological activity resides in the first 29 amino acids at the amino-terminal end. The gene for human GHRH spans 10 kb, consists of five exons, and is located on chromosome 20 *(149)*. It codes for a 108-amino acid preprohormone for GHRH *(150,151)*. In humans and other primates, GHRH cell bodies are located in the infundibular and ventromedial (arcuate) hypothalamic nuclei *(152–154)* and project to the external layer of the median eminence. The GHRH is also synthesized in a wide variety of tissues outside the hypothalamus; it was first isolated from pancreatic neuroendocrine tumors that had caused acromegaly by inducing somatotroph hyperplasia *(155,156)*.

GHRH binds to receptors on the somatotroph membrane. The receptor for GHRH has recently been cloned, and belongs to the family of seven transmembrane receptors that includes receptors for secretin, vasoactive intestinal peptide, parathyroid hormone, and calcitonin *(157,158)*. The GHRH-receptor binding stimulates adenylate cyclase, thus increasing intracellular cAMP levels *(159,160)*, and also increases intracellular calcium concentrations *(161)*. These intracellular events stimulate transcription of GH mRNA *(162)* and increased GH synthesis and secretion. GHRH is specific in its actions on GH release. Apart from a small increase in blood prolactin concentrations *(163)*, it does not affect other pituitary hormones.

SOMATOSTATIN

Somatostatin (SRIH) exists in two biologically active forms, SRIH-14 and SRIH-28 *(164)*, which are derived from a 116-amino acid prohormone precursor *(165)*. The predominant form released by the hypothalamus in response to normal stimuli is probably SRIH-14 *(166)*, although both SRIH-14 and SRIH-28 inhibit GH release, and the 28-amino acid form has a longer lasting inhibitory effect on GH secretion *(167)*. In the hypothalamus, cell bodies of SRIH neurons that project to the median eminence are mainly located in the anterior periventricular region *(168)*. Somatostatin is widely distributed and is found outside the hypothalamus in the pancreas, gut, and elsewhere in the brain *(169)*. Somatostatin has a short half-life of about 2–3 min in the peripheral blood *(164)*.

Somatostatin binds to specific receptors on the somatotrophs, and several receptor subtypes have been described *(170)*. This binding results in inhibition of adenylate cyclase and reduction of intracellular calcium concentrations *(171)* (i.e., effects opposite to GHRH), actions that are mediated via Gi, which is coupled to the somatostatin receptors. Somatostatin does not inhibit GH gene transcription *(172)* and reduces GH release without blocking ongoing synthesis. Administration of SRIH to humans blocks both basal GH release and the GH release induced by a variety of stimuli, including GHRH, sleep, exercise, arginine, and insulin-induced hypoglcycemia. Somatostatin is less specific in its actions than GHRH, and also inhibits release of TRH, prolactin, insulin, and a number of other extrapituitary hormones *(168)*.

Growth hormone releasing hormone and SRIH are secreted at the median eminence into the hypothalamic-pituitary portal circulation for transport to the anterior pituitary. Under physiological conditions, most of the GHRH and SRIH acting on the pituitary is of hypothalamic origin. However, it is not possible to deduce hypothalamic GHRH or SRIH release from concentrations of these hormones in the peripheral circulation, because of their extensive extrahypothalamic production.

SOMATOSTATIN AND GHRH INTERACTIONS TO PRODUCE THE GH PULSE

Simultaneous measurements of serum GH concentrations and hypothalamic-pituitary portal SRIH and GHRH concentrations have not been performed in humans. Knowledge of the way in which GHRH and SRIH interact to produce pulsatile GH release is therefore based on portal sampling studies performed in other species, and on studies using less direct techniques. Somatostatin-GHRH interactions are complex and occur in both the pituitary and hypothalamus.

Secretion of GHRH is clearly necessary for GH release. In rats, systemic and intracerebroventricular administration of GHRH antiserum abolishes GH pulsatility and, in humans, GHRH antagonist administration inhibits both spontaneous and GHRH-stimulated GH release *(173)*. In anesthetized male rats, the episodic GH concentration peaks that occur every 3–3.5 h are associated with increases in GHRH secretion, coincident with a fall in SRIH secretion *(174)*. Studies in conscious sheep have not yielded such clear-cut results. In one study, a highly significant relationship was demonstrated between portal GHRH peaks and peripheral plasma GH peaks, but no association between GH pulses and either SRIH peaks or troughs *(175)*. In another study, 48% of GH concentration peaks were associated with concurrent increases in portal GHRH and decreases in SRIH, 18.5% with increases in *both* GHRH and SRIH, and 12.9% with decreases in SRIH without accompanying changes in GHRH *(176)*. It is not clear whether pulsatile (rather than continuous) GHRH secretion is necessary to generate pulsatile GH release in humans. Persistent pulsatile GH release has been demonstrated in a man with acromegaly caused by an ectopic GHRH secreting tumor *(177)* and in healthy adults and short children given continuous GHRH infusions for at least a week *(177–179)*.

Continuous infusions of SRIH abolish GH pulsatility, and there is a rebound secretion of GH when SRIH is discontinued *(180)*, as GHRH stimulated GH synthesis is not inhibited by SRIH (*see above*). When SRIH antiserum was administered as a single injection, GH release persisted *(174,181)*, perhaps owing to delivery of insufficient doses. Total or near total depletion of SRIH by antisera infusion elevates basal GH levels and inhibits GH pulsatility *(182)*, and some *(183)* but not all *(184)* in vitro studies have shown that SRIH withdrawal is needed for GHRH-induced GH release. Pulsatile SRIH release also protects the pituitary from desensitization and exhaustion under the stimulatory effects of GHRH *(185,186)*. The most likely interpretation of these results may be that periodic reductions in SRIH secretion determine the timing of major GH pulses and prime the somatotroph to subsequently respond to GHRH.

In addition to interactions at the pituitary level, there is evidence that SRIH and GHRH also each influence the release of the other via ultrashort feedback effects in the hypothalamus, where there are anatomical connections between SRIH and GHRH neurons *(187,188)*. Although the significance of intracerebral injection study results are not always clear, they support the existence of stimulatory effects of GHRH on SRIH release *(189)*, inhibitory effects of SRIH on its own release *(190)*, and, perhaps surprisingly, stimulatory effects of SRIH on GHRH release *(191)*. An overview of the regulation of GH secretion is shown in schematic form in Fig. 4.

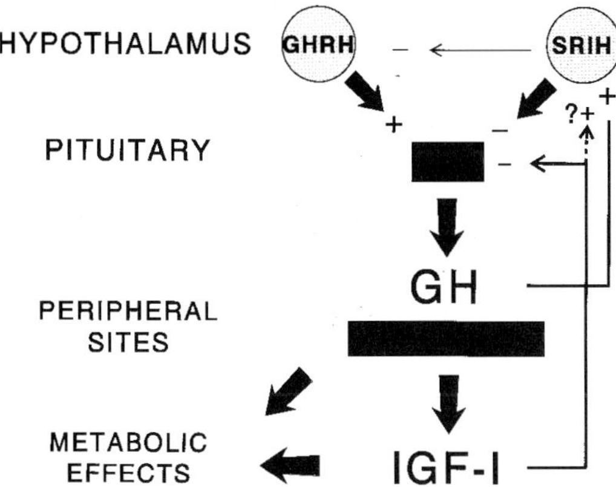

Fig. 4. Schematic illustration of Growth hormone secretion. GH is secreted in a pulsatile fashion under coordinate regulation by hypothalamic somatostatin (SRIH) and GHRH. GH acts on multiple tissues to regulate metabolic functions and growth. Peripheral tissues produce IGF-I, which is secreted into the circulation and acts as a paracrine factor. Circulating and hypothalamic- or pituitary-derived IGF-I may also inhibit GH at the pituitary and/or hypothalamic levels. GH also regulates its own secretion by short-loop feedback.

GROWTH HORMONE AND IGF-I NEGATIVE FEEDBACK EFFECTS ON GH SECRETION

In humans and other species, the administration of GH by various routes reduces endogenous GH secretion *(192–194)*. Available evidence indicates that this short-loop feedback effect is exerted predominantly, if not entirely, at the level of the hypothalamus, most likely by stimulation of SRIH release *(195–198)*.

Insulin-like growth factor I appears to exert long-loop negative feedback effects on GH secretion. In humans, exogenous IGF-I suppresses GH secretion when hypoglycemia (which stimulates GH secretion) is prevented *(80,199–201)*. There are a number of conditions, including starvation/malnutrition, type 1 diabetes mellitus, and Laron type dwarfism, in which circulating IGF-I levels are decreased as a result of GH resistance at the receptor or postreceptor level *(202–207)*. In these conditions, GH concentrations are elevated, consistent with a reduction of IGF-I negative feedback, and decrease following IGF-I administration *(200,208,209)*. The suppressive effects of IGF-I are exerted at the level of the pituitary *(210,211)*, and possibly also the hypothalamus, where IGF-I has been reported to increase the production and secretion of SRIH, to decrease production and secretion of GHRH, or both *(201,210,212–214)*.

NEUROTRANSMITTER CONTROL OF GH RELEASE

Virtually every neurotransmitter system has been implicated in the neural control of GH release, and a thorough review is beyond the scope of this chapter (*see* ref. *215* for review). In general, opioidergic *(216–218)*, cholinergic *(215)*, serotoninergic *(219,220)*, and dopaminergic *(221,222)* inputs are stimulatory, whereas the effects of catecholamines are complex and determined by the balance of the receptor subtypes to which they bind. Alpha-2 receptor agonists are stimulatory, alpha-1 agonists inhibitory, beta-2 agonists inhibitory, and beta-blockers probably stimulatory *(223–225)*.

PHYSIOLOGICAL FACTORS CONTROLLING GH SECRETION

Sleep

Unstimulated GH release in humans is greatest at night *(226,227)*. This nocturnal increase, characterized by increased pulse amplitudes, is partly a result of the loss of inhibition by nutrients (*see* Nutrition section), but is more strongly related to sleep. Delay in the onset of sleep usually delays the onset of the major GH peak. Release of GH is most strongly linked to slow wave sleep (stages III and IV), particularly the onset of the first episode in the night, which usually occurs within an hour of sleep onset *(228,229)*. Thirty second blood sampling for GH during simultaneous electroencephalographic monitoring of young men has indicated that GH secretion rates maximally correlate with slow wave sleep with a lag of 4.5 min *(229)*. Rapid eye movement (REM) sleep is negatively correlated with, and may terminate, GH secretion *(230)*. Growth hormone responses to GHRH are augmented during slow wave sleep, compared to those during REM sleep or in the waking state *(231)*. This suggests that the increased GH associated with slow wave sleep may result from reduced hypothalamic SRIH secretion, and the reduced GH secretion during REM sleep from increased SRIH secretion.

It is not known whether slow wave sleep directly stimulates GH secretion, or whether a common underlying factor stimulates both. Such a factor may be GHRH, as acute administration of GHRH to young men at times of reduced sleep propensity significantly increases slow wave sleep as well as GH release *(232,233)*. Somatostatin administration has little if any effect on sleep *(233,234)*, though a trend to increased REM sleep has been reported *(233)*.

Gender

Sex hormones modulate the release of GH in humans and other species. The rat, the most popular subject of animal GH studies, displays dramatic gender differences. In the conscious, unstressed, adult male rat, distinct GH peaks, in which concentrations of several hundred nanograms per mL are often achieved, occur at intervals of 3–3.5 h, irrespective of the light-dark cycle and whether or not the animal is asleep or awake. Between peaks, GH levels are low or undetectable *(235)*. Plasma GH concentration profiles are not as regular in female rats, which have smaller peaks at more frequent intervals, and higher basal interpulse concentrations *(236)*.

The gender differences in humans are less dramatic, and are largely quantitative rather than qualitative (Fig. 3). A person's gender cannot be confidently predicted from an inspection of their GH concentration profile, as is possible in the rat. Premenopausal women have mean GH concentrations and GH secretion rates approximately 20–50% higher than those of age-matched men *(237–240)*. Differences in the characteristics of pulsatile GH release between men and women have not been clearly defined; women have variously been reported to have larger, but not more frequent, pulses than men *(241)*, and more frequent pulses of the same size *(242)*.

Studies of the variation of GH concentrations across the menstrual cycle have produced conflicting results, most likely due to varying study designs and assay sensitivities. Whereas a number of studies have found no differences between follicular, midcycle, and luteal phases *(243,244)*, others have detected significant variations *(245–247)*. Growth hormone concentrations have been reported to increase significantly around the time of the midcycle LH surge *(246)*, and change across the cycle in parallel with endogenous estrogen levels, with an approximately twofold increase in serum GH concentrations in the late follicular phase *(247)*. In view of the known stimulatory actions of estrogen on GH secretion, it seems likely that GH concentrations do vary across the menstrual cycle, though the extent and significance of these changes is unclear. These variations should be considered when studying GH secretion in premenopausal women.

Numerous studies have examined gender differences in the GH response to secretagogues. Some stimuli, such as exercise *(248)*, glucagon *(249)*, and GHRP *(250)*, exert equal effects in men and women. Others, such as arginine *(251)*, and possibly pyridostigmine *(252)* and insulin *(251)*, produce greater GH release in women. Clonidine *(253)* and baclofen *(254)* produce greater GH release in men. The response to GHRH is not clear. Different studies report a greater *(255,256)* or lesser *(257)* response in women, or no difference between men and women *(258,259)*. Using an ultrasensitive GH assay, oral glucose suppresses GH to a significantly lower nadir in young adult men than women of similar age *(123)*. Such findings highlight the importance of considering gender differences when administering suppressive and stimulatory agents, particularly as part of a diagnostic test.

Stimulatory effects of endogenous estrogen appear to be the major cause of gender differences in GH secretion. Testosterone also stimulates GH release and serum testosterone levels correlate with measures of GH secretion in adult men *(260)*. However, it appears that testosterone stimulates GH release only after aromatization to estrogens *(261,262)*. Serum levels of endogenous estradiol correlate with the increased GH secretion in girls during puberty *(263)*, and serum-free and total estradiol (but not testosterone) concentrations largely account for the higher 24-h integrated GH concentrations in adult women than men *(237)*. Anovulatory women have reduced GH responses to various stimuli *(264)*, and therapeutic reduction of endogenous estrogen levels is associated with reduced basal and stimulated GH secretion *(265,266)* and IGF-I concentrations *(267)*. Moreover, oral estrogen treatment produces a sustained two- to threefold increase in basal GH secretion in girls with Turner's syndrome *(268)*, and oral estrogen treatment also increases basal and stimulated GH serum concentrations in postmenopausal women *(269,270)*. It is of interest that integrated 24-h GH concentrations were recently reported to be approximately 50% higher in black men than in white men matched for age and body weight, a difference that was attributed to the higher circulating 17 beta-estradiol levels in the black men *(271)*.

The mechanisms underlying the gender-related differences in GH secretion apparently act at several levels. Higher circulating estrogen concentrations in women most likely act to reduce the negative feedback effects of IGF-I on GH secretion. In standard replacement doses, oral estrogen decreases circulating IGF-I concentrations *(269,270)*, probably due to a direct suppressive effect of estrogen in the portal circulation on hepatic IGF-I synthesis. Several gender-related differences at the hypothalamic-pituitary level have been identified in rats, and similar differences may exist in humans. Somatotrophs of male rats release more GH in response to GHRH than those of female rats *(272)*, and somatotrophs of female rats are more sensitive to the inhibitory effects of SRIH *(273)*. There is evidence that higher peak GH levels in male rats are caused by increased hypothalamic GHRH release at the onset of peaks, combined with a greater somatotroph sensitivity to GHRH, and lower interpeak GH levels in male rats to greater interpeak hypothalamic SRIH release and lower basal GHRH release *(151,186,274,275)*. In female rats there is more continuous release of both GHRH and SRIH than in male rats, although superimposed GHRH bursts probably also occur *(276,277)*.

Another cause of the higher circulating GH concentrations in premenopausal women than age-matched men may be a lower rate of GH clearance, with a consequent increase in half-life. Reduced GH clearance has been reported in women *(277,278)*, though differences in half-life have not. The reduced clearance in women may result from increased binding of GH to GH-binding proteins; although gender differences in GHBP concentrations have not been reported in adults under 40 yr *(279,280)*, GH has been reported to have a greater binding affinity for these binding proteins in female than male rats *(281)*.

Age

Growth hormone is detectable in fetal serum at the end of the first trimester, and it peaks at 100–150 µg/L at about 20 wk of gestation, before falling to about 30 µg/L at birth, and falling further in the early postnatal months *(282)*. During childhood, circulating GH concentrations are similar to those in adulthood, then increase during the pubertal growth spurt, before returning to previous levels. Increasing age is associated with declining GH secretion, and parallel reductions in circulating GH and IGF-I concentrations *(104,237,283,284)*. A substantial number of elderly people are GH-deficient by young adult standards. Much of this decrease occurs between the ages of 20 and 40 yr (Fig. 5), and mean GH concentrations of adults 60–80 yr of age are reported to be, on average, one-fourth to two-thirds those of adults in their twenties *(237,244,283,284)*. It has been estimated, using deconvolution analysis, that the GH production rate decreases by 14% with each advancing decade during adulthood *(283)*. In the same study, GH half-life was calculated to decline by 6% per decade, suggesting that increased GH clearance may be another cause of reduced circulating GH concentrations in the elderly. Growth hormone secretion is reduced proportionally across the day in the elderly; nocturnal release, although lower than in young subjects, is still more than twice the daytime GH release *(284,285)*.

Responses to stimuli of GH release are variably affected by aging. The acute GH response to exercise is reduced *(286,287)*. Most, but not all, studies report a reduced GH response to GHRH *(288)*, and the response to insulin-induced hypoglycemia is either reduced or unchanged *(289,290)*. The acute GH response to arginine, an amino acid postulated to stimulate GH secretion by inhibiting SRIH action *(291)*, is unaltered *(292,293)*.

The mechanisms responsible for the decline in GH secretion of aging have not been determined, and may be multiple. Reduced pituitary function is probably a cause, though not likely to be a major one. Although people 40–55 yr of age were found to have significantly fewer and smaller somatotrophs than people 16–37 yr of age in one autopsy study *(294)*, somatotroph function appears to be relatively intact in the elderly. This is indicated by the ability of arginine, which is thought to act at the hypothalamic

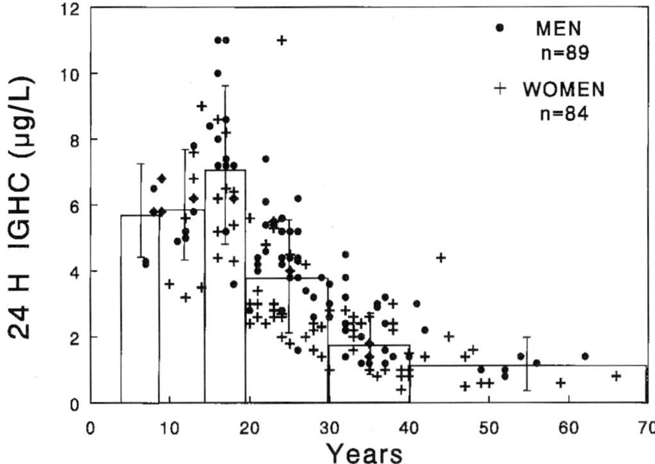

Fig. 5. The relationship between 24-h integrated growth hormone concentration (IGHC) and age in 89 normal men (solid circle) and 84 normal women (+). (Reprinted with permission from ref. *244*.)

and not the pituitary level, to restore the GH response to GHRH in elderly adults to that of young adults *(293)*. The effects of aging are probably exerted mainly at the hypothalamic level. There is evidence from both animal and human studies (including the above-mentioned arginine study), to suggest that SRIH tone increases with age. Growth hormone releasing hormone input to the pituitary may also be reduced, as indicated by the partial reversal of the reduced GH response to GHRH in elderly subjects by repetitive administration of GHRH *(295,296)*, and the increased serum GH and IGF-I concentrations observed in older men after 14 d of sc GHRH treatment *(284)*. In view of the evidence that GHRH can induce slow wave sleep, the phase most strongly associated with GH release, it is possible that the decreased GH secretion and sleep fragmentation that accompany aging are both related to decreased GHRH activity. Little is known about the effect of age on the sensitivity to negative feedback effects of inhibitory factors such as circulating free fatty acids, insulin, and GH itself, but there is evidence that the sensitivity to the negative feedback effects of endogenous IGF-I does not increase with age *(124)*.

Aging is associated with significant changes in body composition; between the ages 30–75 yr the mean percentage body fat increases up to 100%, muscle mass decreases 20–50%, and bone mass decreases by 20% *(297)*. In addition, fat is redistributed from peripheral to central sites and total body water decreases. The same qualitative body composition changes are present in younger adults who are GH-deficient as a result of pituitary or hypothalamic disease, and these changes can be at least partially reversed by GH treatment *(103,298)*. It has been proposed that GH-deficient adults have a greater overall mortality rate than non-GH-deficient adults, owing to death from cardiovascular disease *(299)*. By analogy from these younger adults with "true" GH-deficiency, it has been suggested that functional GH-deficiency may be a cause of the changes in body composition and increased risk of cardiovascular disease that accompany normal aging *(297)*. These body composition changes have been partially reversed by GH administration in selected elderly men *(104)*. Both increased adiposity

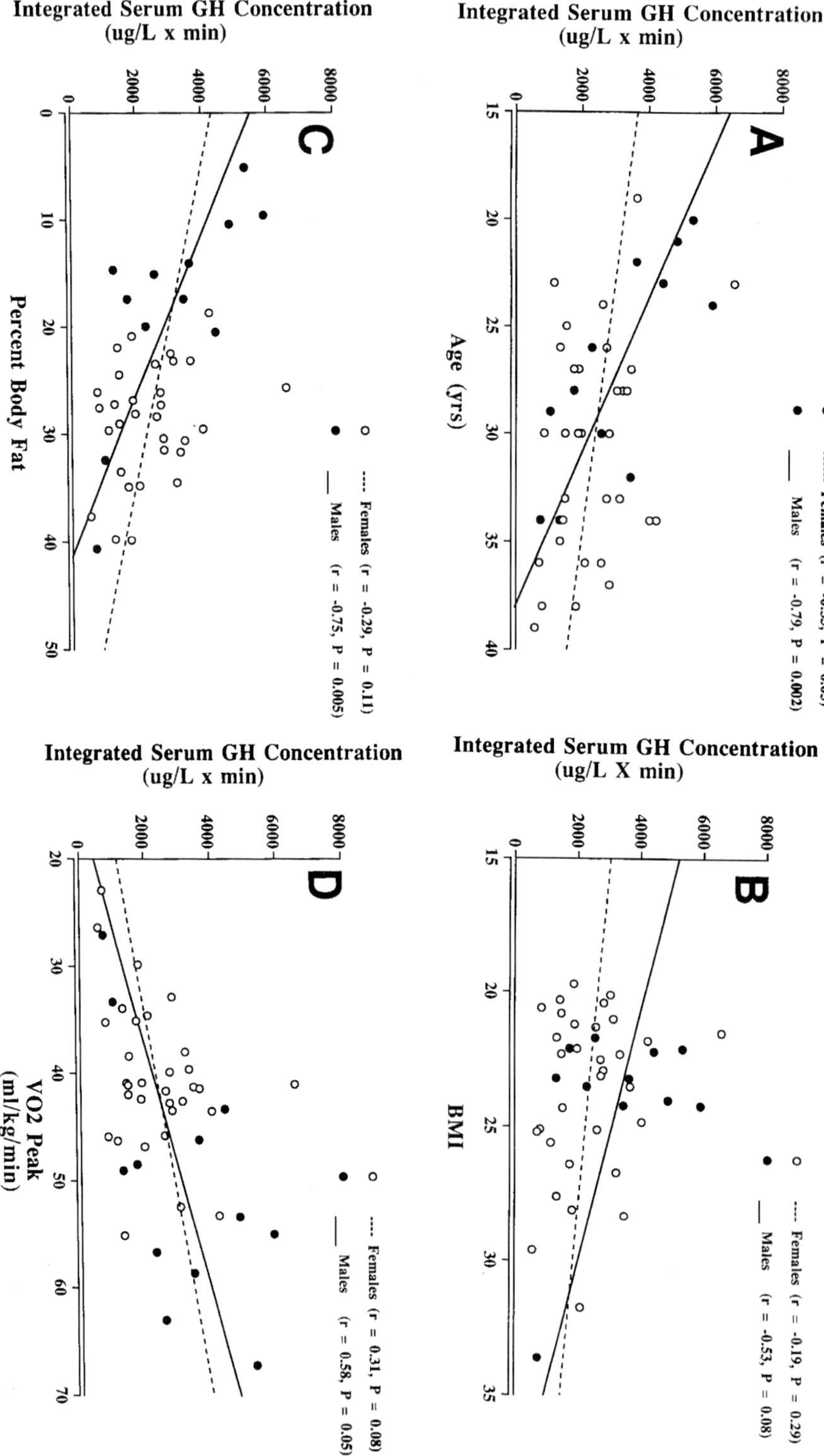

Fig. 6. The relationship between 24-h integrated serum GH concentration and age **(A)**, BMI **(B)**, percentage body fat **(C)**, and peak oxygen consumption (VO2 peak), a measure of physical fitness **(D)** in men ($n = 12$) and women ($n = 32$). (Reprinted with permission from ref. *238*.)

and decreased activity levels are independently associated with decreased GH secretion (*see below*), and both changes tend to accompany aging in western societies. It is not known whether obesity and reduced activity levels precede and cause the decline in GH secretion that accompanies aging, or whether the decline in GH secretion itself is a major cause of the body composition changes and possibly also the reduced activity levels (by reducing energy levels for example). A number of centers are actively investigating this question and are exploring means of preventing or reversing the declining GH secretion that accompanies aging.

BODY COMPOSITION

Increased adiposity is associated with decreased circulating GH concentrations. Percentage body fat, as measured by a variety of methods, has been consistently found to independently and negatively correlate with GH levels in men and women across the age range from young adulthood to old age *(238,283,300,301)*. This relationship has been reported to be stronger for young men than young women (Fig. 6), with a one standard deviation increase in percentage body fat, as measured by hydrostatic weighing, associated with 42 and 16% reductions in 24-h integrated GH concentrations in young men and women, respectively *(238)*.

The reduced circulating GH concentrations in obesity have been reported to result from a combination of decreased GH secretion, owing to decreased pulse amplitude without significant effects on pulse frequency *(283)*, and increased metabolic clearance of GH *(300)*. The mechanisms that underlie these effects are unknown, but may include inhibition by the increased levels of circulating insulin and free fatty acids *(302)* that accompany obesity.

NUTRITION

Growth hormone secretion is profoundly affected by nutrient intake in humans. Fasting from food for 2 5 d increases mean 24-h mean GH concentrations three- to fivefold in normal weight and obese individuals *(203,303,304)*, owing to increased size and frequency of GH secretory episodes, without changes in clearance *(303)*. Fasting-enhanced GH secretion is suppressed within 60 min of refeeding with a mixed meal *(305)*. Several mechanisms probably underlie this fast-induced increase. Circulating IGF-I concentrations fall during fasting *(202)*, and negative feedback inhibition by IGF-I is therefore reduced. Fasting also suppresses circulating insulin concentrations, and there is evidence that insulin inhibits GH secretion. Under most conditions, insulin concentrations are inversely associated with GH concentrations. Insulin directly inhibits GH secretion in vitro *(306)*, and reduces IGFBP-1 concentrations, thus possibly increasing free IGF-I concentrations and enhancing IGF-I negative feedback effects *(200)*. In sheep, the fast-induced increase in GH secretion is associated with reduced SRIH levels in the hypothalamic-portal circulation, without changes in GHRH levels *(307)*. It has been hypothesized that fast-induced increases in human GH secretion result from a combination of reduced SRIH and increased GHRH secretion *(308)*.

Acute administration of carbohydrates suppresses both GH secretion *(123)* and the GH response to GHRH *(309)*, whereas administration of amino acids such as arginine and lysine stimulates GH release *(310)*. These responses are reliable and reproducible and form the basis of the standard arginine and oral glucose tolerance tests used in the diagnosis of GH deficiency and acromegaly, respectively. Free fatty acids acutely suppress the GH secretory response to GHRH *(310)*, and prior ingestion of meals high in fat (but not glucose) reduces the acute GH response to exercise, in association with increased circulating SRIH levels *(311)*. The overall effect of a mixed meal is most likely to inhibit acute GH release. In contrast to these data on the acute effects of diet and various nutrients on GH release, the effects of long-term variations in diet on stimulated and unstimulated GH secretion are not known.

EXERCISE AND PHYSICAL FITNESS

Acute exercise stimulates GH release, probably via cholinergic mechanisms *(312)*, and this secretion is probably dependent on the increases in core body temperature that accompany exercise *(313)*. Blood GH concentrations usually peak 10–20 min after the onset of aerobic exercise. There is wide variation between subjects in the GH secretory response to a given exercise stimulus *(314)*, and factors such as the intensity *(315,316)*, and duration *(317)* of the exercise, mode of exercise *(318,319)*, aerobic vs anaerobic exercise *(320)*, the fitness level *(321)* and gender *(322)* of the individual, and food intake prior to exercise *(311)*, all influence the GH response. Acute GH responses to aerobic and resistance exercise correlate positively with the physical fitness level, both in young and older adults *(286)*. Older adults have a lower GH response to exercise than young adults *(286,323)*, possibly due to the reduced fitness levels that accompany normal aging. There is also evidence that physical fitness influences the GH secretion at times not associated with exercise. After controlling for the effects of age and body fat, physical fitness, as measured by peak oxygen consumption (VO_2 peak), significantly correlates with basal GH secretion in young men, and the correlation in young women approaches significance *(306)* (Fig. 6). One year of exercise training at an intensity above the lactate threshold doubled 24-h mean GH concentrations on nonexercise days in young women despite little change in body composition *(316)*. In view of the blunted GH response to exercise in the elderly, it might be expected that spontaneous GH secretion would not be increased as much by increases in physical fitness in elderly as in young adults. Indeed, one group of elderly men and women who completed a resistance exercise training program, in which they performed weightlifting exercises three times per week for 1 yr, showed no increase in basal or stimulated GH release during this time *(324)*. Further studies in this area are needed.

ACKNOWLEDGMENTS

Thanks to D.R. Clemmons for information regarding IGF binding proteins, and to S.S. Pezzoli for proofreading and assistance with the figures; thanks also to D.R. Clemmons for help in compiling Table 1.

REFERENCES

1. Cryer PE, Daughaday WH. Growth hormone. In: Martini L, Besser GM, ed. Clinical Neuroendocrinology. Academic, New York, 1977; pp. 243–247
2. Pelletier G, Robert F, Hardy J. Identification of human anterior pituitary cells by immunoelectron microscopy. J Clin Endocrinol Metab 1978; 46:534–542.
3. Moore DD, Walker MD, Diamond DJ, Conkling MA, Goodman HM. Structure, expression and evolution of growth hormone genes. Recent Prog Horm Res 1982; 38:197–225.

4. Miller WL, Eberhardt NL. Structure and evalutation of growth hormone gene family. Endocr Rev 1983; 4:97–130.
5. Frankenne F, Closset J, Gomez F, Scippo ML, Smal J, Hennen G. The physiology of growth hormones (GHs) in pregnant women and partial characterization of the placental GH variant. J Clin Endocrinol Metab 1988; 66:1171–1180.
6. Cooke NE, Ray J, Watson MA, Estes PA, Kuo BA, Liebhaber SA. Human growth hormone gene and the highly homologous growth hormone variant gene display different splicing patterns. J Clin Invest 1988; 82:270–275.
7. Lefevre C, Imagawa M, Dana S, Grindlay J, Bodner M, Karin M. Tissue-specific expression of the human growth hormone gene is conferred in part by the binding of a specific trans-acting factor. Embo J 1987; 6:971–981.
8. Simmons DM, Voss JW, Ingraham HA, et al. Pituitary cell type phenotypes involve cell-specific Pit-1 mRNA translation and synergistic interactions with other classes of transcription factors. Genes Dev 1990; 4:696–711.
9. Voss JW, Yao FP, Rosenfeld MG. Alternative translation initiation site usage results in two structurally distinct forms of Pit-I. J Biol Chem 1991; 266:12832–12835.
10. Li CH, Dixon JS, Liu WK. Human pituitary growth hormone. Arch Biochem Biophys. 133:70–91.
11. DeNoto FM, Moore DD, Goodman HM. Human growth hormone DNA sequence and mRNA structure: possible alternative splicing. Nucleic Acids Res 1981; 9:3719–3730.
12. Baumann G Molecular variants of human growth hormone in serum and circulating growth hormone binding proteins. In: Hormonal regulation of growth. Frish, Thorner Mo, ed. Serono Symp Public/Raven, New York, pp. 175–184
13. Baumann G, Stolar MW, Buchanan TA. The metabolic clearance, distribution and degradation of dimeric and monomeric growth hormone (GH): implications for the pattern of circulating GH forms. Endocrinology 1986; 119:1497–1501.
14. Hendricks CM, Eastman RC, Takeda S, Asakawa K, Gorden P. Plasma clearance of intravenously administered pituitary human growth hormone: gel filtration studies of heterogeneous components. J Clin Endocrinol Metab 1985; 60:864–867.
15. Stolar MW, Baumann G. Big growth hormone forms in human plasma: immunochemical evidence for their pituitary origin. Metabolism 1986; 35:75–77.
16. Baumann G, Vance ML, Shaw MA. Plasma transport of human growth hormone in vivo. J Clin Endocrinol Metab 1990; 71:470–473.
17. Stolar MW, Baumann G, Vance ML, Thorner MO. 1984 Circulating growth hormone forms after stimulation of pituitary secretion with growth hormone-releasing factor in man. J Clin Endocrinol Metab 1984; 59:235–239.
18. Baumann G, Stolar MW. Molecular forms of human growth hormone secreted in vivo: nonspecificity of secretory stimuli. J Clin Endocrinol Metab 1986; 62:789–790.
19. Baumann G, Winter RJ, Shaw M. Circulating molecular variants of growth hormone in childhood. Pediatr Res 1987; 22:21–22.
20. Roupas P, Herington AC. Cellular mechanisms in the processing of growth hormone and its receptor. Mol Cell Endocrinol 1989; 61:1–12.
21. Kelly PA, Djiane J, Postel-Vinay M-C, Edery M. The prolactin/growth hormone receptor family. Endocr Rev 1991; 12:235–251.
22. Bazan JF. A novel family of growth factor receptors: a common binding domain in the growth hormone, prolactin, erythropoietin and IL-6 receptors, and the p75 IL-2 receptor beta-chain. Biochem Biophys Res Commun 1989; 164:788–795.
23. Vikman K, Carlsson B, Billig H, Eden S. Expression and regulation of growth hormone (GH) receptor messenger ribonucleic acid (mRNA) in rat adipose tissue, adipocytes, and adipocyte precurser cells: GH regulation of GHR mRNA. Endocrinology 1991; 129:1155–1161.
24. Leung DW, Spencer SA, Cachianes G, et al. Growth hormone receptor and serum binding protein: purification, cloning and expression. Nature 1987; 330:537–543.
25. Spencer SA, Hammonds RG, Henzel WJ, Rodriguez H, Waters MJ, Wood WI. Rabbit liver growth hormone receptor and serum binding protein. Purification, characterization, and sequence. J Biol Chem 1988; 263:7862–7867.
26. Baumann G, Stolar MW, Amburn K, Barsano DP, DeVries BC. A specific growth hormone-binding protein in human plasma: initial characterization. J Clin Endocrinol Metab 1986; 62:134–141.

27. Massa G, Mulumba N, Ketelslegers J-M, Maes M. Initial characterization and sexual dimorphism of serum growth hormone-binding protein in adult rats. Endocrinology 1990; 126:1976–1980.
28. Peeters S, Friesen HG. A growth hormone binding factor in the serum of pregnant mice. Endocrinology 1977; 101:1164–1183.
29. Ymer SI, Herington AC. Evidence for specific binding of growth hormone to a receptor-like protein in rabbit serum. Mol Cell Endocrinol 1985; 41:153–161.
30. Baumbach WR, Horner DL, Logan JS. The growth hormone-binding protein in rat serum is an alternatively spliced form of the rat growth hormone receptor. Genes Dev 1989; 3:1199–1205.
31. Baumann G, Shaw MA, Winter RJ. Absence of the plasma growth hormone-binding protein in Laron-type dwarfism. J Clin Endocrinol Metab 1987; 65:814–816.
32. Daughaday WH, Trivedi B. Absence of serum growth hormone binding protein in patients with growth hormone receptor deficiency (Laron dwarfism). Proc Natl Acad Sci U S A 1987; 84:4636–4640.
33. Baumann G, Shaw MA. A second, lower affinity growth hormone-binding protein in human plasma. J Clin Endocrinol Metab 1990; 70:680–686.
34. Baumann G, Shaw MA. Plasma transport of 20,000-Dalton variant of hGH. Evidence for a 20K-specific binding site. J Clin Endocrinol Metab 1990; 71:1335–1343.
35. Thorner MO, Vance ML, Horvath E, Kovacs K The anterior pituitary. In: Williams Textbook of Endocrinology 1992; Wilson JD, Foster DW, ed. W.B.Saunders & Co., Philadelphia, pp. 221–310
36. Daughaday WH, Trivedi B, Andrews BA. The ontogeny of serum GH binding protein in man: a possible indicator of hepatic GHR development. J Clin Endocrinol Metab 1987; 65:1072–1074.
37. Baumann G, Shaw MA, Amburn K. 95 Regulation of plasma growth hormone-binding proteins in health and disease. Metabolism 1995; 38:683–689.
38. Baumann G, Amburn KD, Buchanan TA. The effect of circulating growth hormone-binding protein on metabolic clearance, distribution, and degradation of human growth hormone. J Clin Endocrinol Metab 1987; 64:657–660.
39. Lim L, Spencer SA, McKay P, Waters MJ. Regulation of growth hormone (GH) bioactivity by a recombinant human GH-binding protein. Endocrinology 1990; 127:1287–1291.
40. Campbell GS, Christian LJ, Carter-Su C. 1993 Evidence for involvement of the growth hormone receptor-associated tyrosine kinase in actions of growth hormone. J Biol Chem 1993; 268:7427–7434.
41. Moller C, Hansson A, Enberg B, Lobie PE, Norstedt G. Growth hormone (GH) induction of tyrosine phosphorylation and activation of mitogen-activated protein kinases in cells transfected with rat GHR cDNA. J Biol Chem 1992; 267:23403–23408.
42. Argetsinger LS, Campbell GS, Yang X. et al. 1993 Identification of JAK2 as a growth hormone receptor-associated kinase. Cell 1993; 74:237–244.
43. Silva CM, Lu H, Weber MJ, Thorner MO. Differential tyrosine phosphorylation of JAK1, JAK2, and STAT1 by growth hormone and interferon-gamma in IM-9 cells. J Biol Chem 1994; 269:27532–27539.
44. Waxman DJ, Ram PA, Park S-H, Choi HK. Intermittent plasma growth hormone triggers tyrosine phosphorylation and nuclear transcription of a liver-expressed, stat 5-related DNA binding protein. J Biol Chem 1995; 22:13262–13270.
45. Green H, Morikawa M, Nixon T. A dual effector theory of growth-hormone action. [Review]. Differentiation 1985; 29:195–198.
45a. Isaksson OGP, Isgaard J, Nilsson A, et al, Direct actin of growth hormone. In: Bercu BB, ed, Basic and Clinical Aspects of Growth Hormone. Plenum, New York, 1988; pp. 1992–211.
46. Salmon WD,Jr., Daughaday WH. 1957 A hormonally controlled serum factor which stimulates sulfate incorporation by cartilage in vitro. J Lab Clin Med 1957; 49:825.
47. Isaksson OGP, Jansson JO, Clark RG, Gause IAM. Growth hormone stimulates longitudinal bone growth directly. Science 1982; 216:1237–1239.
48. Schlechter NL, Russell SM, Spencer EM, Nicoll CS. Evidence suggesting that the direct growth-promoting effect of growth hormone on cartilage in vivo is mediated by local production of somatomedin. Proc Natl Acad Sci U S A 1986; 83:7932–7934.
49. D'Ercole AJ, Stiles AD, Underwood LE. 1984 Tissue concentrations of somatomedin C: further evidence for multiple sites of synthesis and paracrine or autocrine mechanisms of action. Proc Natl Acad Sci U S A 1984; 81:935–939.
50. Skottner A, Clark RG, Robinson IC, Fryklund L. Recombinant human insulin-like growth factor: testing the somatomedin hypothesis in hypophysectomized rats. J Endocrinol 1987; 112:123–132.

51. Guler HP, Zapf J, Scheiwiller E, Froesch ER. Recombinant human insulin-like growth factor I stimulates growth and has distinct effects on organ size in hypophysectomized rats. Proc Natl Acad Sci U S A 1988; 85:4889–4893.
52. Lindahl A, Isgaard J, Carlsson L, Isaksson OGP. Differential effects of growth hormone and insulin-like growth factor-I on colony formation of epiphyseal chondrocytes in suspension culture in rats of different ages. Endocrinology 1987; 121:1061–1069.
53. Humbel RE Insulin-like growth factors, somatomedins and multiplication stimulating activity: chemistry. In: Hormonal Proteins and Peptides 1986; LiCH, ed. Academic Press, Orlando, pp. 57–79.
54. Rinderknecht E, Humbel RE. The amino acid sequence of human insulin-like growth factor I and its structural homology with proinsulin. J Biol Chem 1978; 253:2769–2776.
55. Rinderknecht E, Humbel RE. Primary structure of human insulin like growth factor II. Febs Lett 1987; 89:283–286.
56. Han VKM, D'Ercole AJ, Lund PK. Cellular localization of somatomedin (insulin-like growth factor) messenger RNA in the human fetus. Science 1987; 236:193–197.
57. Cohick WS, Clemmons DR. 1993 The insulin-like growth factors. Annu Rev Physiol 1993; 55:131–153.
58. Camacho-Hubner C, McCusker R, Clemmons DR. Secretion and biological actions of insulin-like growth factor binding proteins in two human tumor-derived cell lines in vitro. J Cell Physiol 1991; 148:281–289.
59. Clemmons DR, Snyder DK, Busby WHJr. Variables controlling the secretion of insulin-like growth factor binding protein-2 in normal human subjects. J Clin Endocrinol Metab 1991; 73:727–733.
60. Clemmons DR, Thissen JP, Maes M, Ketelslegers JM, Underwood LE. Insulin-like growth factor-I (IGF-I) infusion into hypophysectomized or protein-deprived rats induces specific IGF-binding proteins in serum. Endocrinology 1989; 125:2967–2972.
61. Jones JI, Clemmons DR. Insulin-like growth factors and their binding proteins: biological actions. Endocr Rev 1985; 16:3–34.
62. Guler HP, Zapf J, Schmid C, Froesch ER. Insulin-like growth factors I and II in healthy man. Estimations of half-lives and production rates. Acta Endocrinol 1989; 121:753–758.
63. Keifer MC, Masiarz FR, Bauer DM, Zapf J. Identification and molecular cloning of two new 30-kDa insulin-like growth factor binding proteins isolated from adult human serum. J Biol Chem 1991; 266:9043–9049.
64. Zapf J, Kiefer M, Merriweather J, Musiarz F, Bauer D. Isolation from adult human serum of four insulin-like growth factor (IGF) binding proteins and molecular cloning of one of them that is increased by IGF I administration and in extrapancreatic tumor hypoglycemia. J Biol Chem 1990; 265:14892–14898.
65. Gargosky SE, Tapaniainen P, Rosenfeld RC. Administration of growth hormone (GH), but not insulin-like growth factor-I (IGF-I), by continous infusion can induce the formation of the 150-kilodalton IGF-binding protein-3 complex in GH-deficient rats. Endocrinology 1994; 134:2267–2276.
66. Wilson KF, Fielder PJ, Guevara-Aguirre J, et al. Long-term effects of insulin-like growth factor (IGF)-I treatment on serum IGFs and IGF binding proteins in adolescent patients with growth hormone receptor deficiency. Clin Endocrinol (Oxf) 1995; 42:399–407.
67. Baxter RC, Martin JL. Radioimmunoassay of growth hormone-dependent insulin-like growth factor binding protein in human plasma. J Clin Invest 1986; 78:1504–1512.
68. Blum WF, Ranke MB. Use of insulin-like growth factor-binding protein 3 for evaluation of growth disorders. Horm Res. 1990; 33(Suppl):31–37.
69. de Boer H, Blok G-J, Van Der Veen EA. Clinical aspects of growth hormone deficiency in adults. Endocr Rev 1995; 16:63–86.
70. Cohick WS, McGuire MA, Clemmons DR, Baumann DE. Regulation of insulin-like growth factor-binding proteins in serum and lymph of lactating cows by somatotropin. Endocrinology 1992; 130:1508–1514.
71. Busby WH, Snyder DK, Clemmons DR. Radioimmunoassay of a 26000 dalton plasma insulin like growth factor binding protein: control by nutritional variables. J Clin Endocrinol Metab 1988; 67:1225–1230.
72. Unterman TG, Oehler DT, Murphy LJ, Lacson RG. Multihormonal regulation of insulin-like growth factor-binding protein-I in rat H4IIE hepatoma cells: the dominant role of insulin. Endocrinology 1991; 128:2693–2701.
73. Suikkari AM, Koivistinen VA, Rutanen EM, Yki-Jarvinen J, Karonen SL, Seppala M. Insulin regulates serum levels of low molecular weight insulin-like growth factor binding protein. J Clin Endocrinol Metab 1988; 66:266–272.

74. Suikkari AM, Koivisto VA, Koistinen R, Seppala M, Yki-Jarvinen H. Dose-response characteristics for suppression of low molecular weight plasma insulin-like growth factor-binding protein by insulin. J Clin Endocrinol Metab 1989; 68:135–140.
75. Ooi GT, Orlowski CC, Brown AL, Becker RE, Unterman TG. Different tissue distribution and hormonal regulation of messenger RNAs encoding rat insulin-like growth factor binding proteins-1 and -2. Mol Endocrinol 1992; 4:321–328.
76. Orlowski CC, Brown AL, Ooi GT, Yang YW, Tseng LY. Tissue, developmental, and metabolic regulation of messenger ribonucleic acid encoding a rat insulin-like growth factor binding protein. Endocrinology 1990; 126:644–652.
77. Straus DS, Ooi GT, Orlowski CC, Rechler MM. Expression of the genes for insulin-like growth factor-I (IGF-I), IGF-II, and IGF-binding proteins-1 and -2 in fetal rat under conditions of intrauterine growth retardation caused by maternal fasting. Endocrinology 1991; 128:518–525.
78. Straus DS, Takemoto CD. Effect of dietary protein deprivation on insulin-like growth factor (IGF)-I and -II, IGF binding protein-2, and serum albumin gene expression in rat. Endocrinology 1990; 127:1849–1860.
79. McCusker RH, Cohick WS, Busby WH, Clemmons DR. Evaluation of the developmental and nutritional changes in porcine insulin-like growth factor-binding protein-1 and -2 serum levels by immunoassay. Endocrinology 1991; 129:2631–2638.
80. Guler HP, Zapf J, Froesch ER. Short-term metabolic effects of recombinant human insulin-like growth factor in healthy adults. N Engl J Med 1987; 317:137–140.
81. Lewitt M, Denyer GS, Cooney GJ, Baxter RC. Insulin-like growth factor-binding protein-1 modulates glucose effects. Endocrinology 1991; 129:2254–2256.
82. Zapf J, Hauri C, Waldvogel M. Recombinant human insulin-like growth factor I induces its own specific carrier protein in hypophysectomized and diabetic rats. Proc Natl Acad Sci U S A 1989; 86:3813–3817.
83. Elgin RG, Busby WH, Clemmons DR. An insulin-like growth factor binding protein enhances the biologic response to IGF-I. Proc Natl Acac Sci U S A 1987; 84:3254–3258.
84. Blum WF, Jenne EW, Reppin F, Kietzmann K, Ranke MB, Bierich JR. Insulin-like growth factor I (IGF-I) binding protein complex is a better mitogen than free IGF-I. Endocrinology 1989; 125:766–772.
85. Binoux M, Roghani M, Hossenlopp. P, Hardouin S, Gourmelen M. Molecular forms of human IGF binding proteins: physiological implications. Acta Endocrinol 1991; 124(Suppl 2):41–47.
86. Kember NF, Walker DVR. 1971 Control of bone growth in rats. Nature 1971; 229:428–429.
87. Kember NF, Sissons HA. 1976 A quantitative histology of the human growth plate. J Bone Joint Surg 1976; 58B:426–435.
88. Kember NF. Cell kinetics and the control of growth in long bones. Cell Tissue Kinet 1978; 11:477–485.
89. Sherwin RS, Schulman GA, Hendler R, Walesky M, Belous A, Tamborlane W. Effect of growth hormone on oral glucose tolerance and circulating metabolic fuels in man. Diabetologia 1983; 24:155–161.
90. Rosenfeld RG, Wilson DM, Dollar LA, Bennett A, Hintz RL. Both human pituitary growth hormone and recombinant DNA- derived human growth hormone cause insulin resistance at a postreceptor site. J Clin Endocrinol Metab 1982; 54:1033–1038.
91. Bratusch-Marrain PR, Smith D, DeFronzo RA. The effect of growth hormone on glucose metabolism and insulin secretion in man. J Clin Endocrinol Metab 1982; 55:973–982.
92. Metcalfe P, Johnston DG, Nosadini R, Orksov H, Alberti KG. Metabolic effects of acute and prolonged growth hormone excess in normal and insulin-deficient man. Diabetologia 1981; 20:123–128.
93. Orskov L, Schmitz O, Jorgensen JO, et al. Influence of growth hormone on glucose-induced glucose uptake in normal men as assessed by the hyperglycemic clamp technique. J Clin Endocrinol Metab 1989; 68:276–282.
94. Lippe BM, Kaplan SA, Golden MP, Hendricks SA, Scott ML. Carbohydrate tolerance and insulin receptor binding in children with hypopituitarism: responses after acute and chronic growth hormone administration. J Clin Endocrinol Metab 1981; 53:507–513.
95. Dahms WT, Owens RP, Kalhan SC, Kerr DS, Danish RK. Urea synthesis, nitrogen balance and glucose turnover in growth deficient children before and after GH administration. Metabolism 1989; 38:197–203.
96. Manson JM, Wilmore DW. Positive nitrogen balance with human growth hormone and hypocaloric intravenous feeding. Surgery 1986; 100:188–197.
97. Soroff HS, Pearson E, Green NL, Artz CP. 1960 The effect of growth hormone on nitrogen balance at various levels of intake in burned patients. Surg Gynecol Obstet 1960; 111:259–273.

98. Wilmore DW, Moylan JA,Jr., Bristow BF, Mason AD,Jr., Pruitt BA,Jr.. 1974 Anabolic effects of human growth hormone and high caloric feedings following thermal injury. Surg Gynecol Obstet 1974; 138:875–884.
99. Horber FF, Haymond MV. Human growth hormone prevents the protein catabolic side effects of prednisone in humans. J Clin Invest 1990; 86:265–272.
100. Pape GS, Friedman M, Underwood LE, Clemmons DR. The effect of growth hormone on weight gain and pulmonary function in patients with chronic obstructive lung disease. Chest 1991; 99:1495–1500.
101. Cheek DB, Hill DE. 1970 Muscle and liver cell growth: role of hormone and nutritional factors. Fed Proc 1970; 29:1503–1509.
102. Tanner JM, Hughes PCR, Whitehouse RN. Comparitive rapidity of response of height, limb muscle and limb fat to treatment with human growth hormone in patients with and without growth hormone deficiency. Acta Endocrinol 1977; 84:681–696.
103. Salomon F, Cuneo RC, Hesp R, Sonksen PH. The effects of treatment with recombinant human growth hormone on body composition and metabolism in adults with growth hormone deficiency. N Engl J Med 1989; 321:1797–1803.
104. Rudman D, Feller AG, Nagraj HS, et al. Effects of human growth hormone in men over 60 years old. N Engl J Med 1990; 323:1–6.
105. Crist DM, Peake GT, Egan PA, Waters DL. Body composition response to exogenous GH during training in highly conditioned adults. J Appl Physiol 1988; 65:579–584.
106. Rosen T, Eden S, Larson G, Wilhelmsen L, Bengtsson BA. Cardiovascular risk factors in adult patients with growth hormone deficiency. Acta Endocrinol 1993; 129:195–200.
107. de Boer H, Blok GJ, Voerman HJ, Phillips M, Schouten JA. Serum lipid levels in growth hormone-deficient men. Metabolism 1994; 43:199–203.
108. Blackett PR, Weech PK, McConathy WJ, Fesmire JD. Growth hormone in the regulation of hyperlipidemia. Metabolism 1982; 31:117–120.
109. Asayama K, Amemiya S, Kusano S, Kato K. Growth hormone-induced changes in postheparin plasma lipoprotein lipase and hepatic triglyceride lipase activties. Metabolism 1984; 33:129–131.
110. Baum HBA, Biller BMK, Oppenheim DS, Baker KE, Lord J, Klibanski A. Long-term physiologic growth hormone (GH) replacement improves bone density and body composition in men with adult-onset GH deficiency. Prog 77th Meeting of the Endocrine Society 1995; P2–261:356. (Abstract)
111. Bouillon R. Growth hormone and bone [Review]. Horm Res 1991; 36(Suppl.):49–55.
112. Gala RR. Prolactin and growth hormone in the regulation of the immune system [Review]. Proc Soc Exp Biol Med 1991; 198:513–527.
113. Wit JM, Kooiijman R, Riskers GT, Zegers BJ. 1993 Immunological findings in growth hormone-treated patients [Review]. Horm Res 1993; 39:107–110.
114. Jansson JO, Isaksson OG, Eden S, Isgaard J, Carlsson L, Ekberg S. Effects of plasma GH pattern on growth factors and body growth. In: Hormonal regulation of growth. Serono Symp 1989; Vol 58. Frisch H, Thorner MO, ed. Raven Press, New York, pp. 185–199
115. Isgaard J, Carlsson L, Isaksson OGP, Jansson JO. Pulsatile intravenous growth hormone (GH) infusion to hypophysectomized rats increases insulin-like growth factor I messenger ribonucleic acid in skeletal tissues more effectively than continuous GH infusion. Endocrinology 1988; 123:2605–2610.
116. Jansson JO, Albertsson-Wikland K, Eden S, Thorngren K-G, Isaksson O. Circumstantial evidence for a role of the secretory pattern of growth hormone in the control of body growth. Acta Endocrinol 1982; 99:24–30.
117. Faria AC, Veldhuis JD, Thorner MO, Vance ML. Half-time of endogenous growth hormone (GH) disappearance in normal man after stimulation of GH secretion by GH-releasing hormone and suppression with somatostatin. J Clin Endocrinol Metab 1989; 68:535–541.
118. Hindmarsh PC, Matthews DR, Brain CE, et al. The half-life of exogenous growth hormone after suppression of endogenous growth hormone secretion with somatostatin. Clin Endocrinol (Oxf) 1989; 30:443–450.
119. Veldhuis JD, Iranmanesh A, Ho KK, Waters MJ, Johnson ML, Lizarralde G. Dual defects in pulsatile growth hormone secretion and clearance subserve the hyposomatotropism of obesity in man. J Clin Endocrinol Metab 1991; 72:51–59.
120. Hindmarsh PC, Matthews DR, Brain C, Pringle PJ, Brook CG. The application of deconvolution analysis to elucidate the pulsatile nature of growth hormone secretion using a variable half-life of growth hormone. Clin Endocrinol (Oxf) 1990; 32:739–747.

121. Hartman ML, Faria ACS, Vance ML, Johnson ML, Thorner MO, Veldhuis JD. Temporal structure of in vivo growth hormone secretory events in man. Am J Physiol 1991; 260:E101–E110.
122. Iranmanesh A, Grisso B, Veldhuis JD. Low basal and persistent pulsatile growth hormone secretion are revealed in normal and hyposomatotropic men studied with a new ultrasensitive chemiluminescence assay. J Clin Endocrinol Metab 1994; 78:526–535.
123. Chapman IM, Hartman ML, Straume M, Johnson ML, Veldhuis JD, Thorner MO. Enhanced sensitivity growth hormone (GH) chemiluminescence assay reveals lower postglucose nadir GH concentrations in men than women. J Clin Endocrinol Metab 1994; 78:1312–1319.
124. Chapman IM, Hartman ML, Pezzoli SS, Thorner MO. Evidence against increased sensitivity to IGF-I negative feedback as a cause of the aging-associated decline in GH secretion. Prog 77th Meeting Endocrine Society 1995; OR20–5:73. (Abstract)
125. Fletcher TP, Thomas GB, Willoughby J0, Clarke IJ. Constitutive growth hormone secretion in sheep after hypothalamopituitary disconnection and the direct in vivo pituitary effect of growth hormone releasing peptide 6. Neuroendocrinology 1994; 60:76–86.
126. Stewart JK, Clifton DK, Koerker DJ, Rogol AD, Jaffe T, Goodner CJ. Pulsatile release of growth hormone and prolactin from the primate pituitary in vitro. Endocrinology 1985; 116:1–5.
127. Niimi M, Takahara J, Sato M, Kawanishi K. Immunohistochemical identification of galanin and growth hormone-releasing factor-containing neurons projecting to the median eminence of the rat. Neuroendocrinology 1990; 51:572–575.
128. Ottlecz A, Samson WK, McCann SM. Galanin: Evidence for a hypothalamic site of action to release growth hormone. Peptides 1986; 7:51–53.
129. Bauer FE, Ginsberg L, Venetikou M, MacKay DJ, Burrin JM, Bloom SR. Growth hormone release in man induced by galanin, a new hypothalamic peptide. Lancet 1986; 2:192–195.
130. Maiter DM, Hooi SC, Koenig JI, Martin JB. Galanin is a physiological regulator of spontaneous pulsatile secretion of growth hormone in the male rat. Endocrinology 1990; 126:1216–1222.
131. O'Donohue TL, Beinfield MC, Chey WY, et al. Identification, characterization and distribution of motilin immunoreactivity in the rat central nervous system. Peptides 1981; 2:467–477.
132. Samson WK, Lumpkin MD, Nilaver G, McCann SM. 1984 Motilin: A novel growth hormone releasing agent. Brain Research Bulletin 1984; 12:57–62.
133. Rivier C, Brown M, Vale W. Effect of neurotensin, substance P and morphine sulphate on secretion of prolactin and growth hormone in the rat. Endocrinology 1977; 100:751–754.
134. Vijayan E, McCann SM. Effects of substance P and neurotensin on growth hormone and TSH release in vivo and in vitro. Life Sci 1980; 26:321–327.
135. Vijayan E, Samson WK, Said SI, McCann SM. VIP: evidence for a hypothalamic site of action to release growth hormone, luteinizing hormone and prolactin in conscious ovariectomized rats. Endocrinology 1979; 104:53–57.
136. Chihara K, Iwasaki J, Minamitani H, et al. Effect of vasoactive intestinal polypeptide on growth hormone secretion in perifused acromegalic pituitary adenoma tissue. J Clin Endocrinol Metab 1982; 54:773–779.
137. Miyata A, Arimura A, Dahl RR, et al. Isolation of a novel 38 residue-hypothalamic polypeptide which stimulates adenylate cyclase in pituitary cells. Biochem Biophys Res Commun 1989; 164(1):567–574.
138. Goth MI, Lyons CE, Canny BJ, Thorner MO. Pituitary adenylate cyclase activating polypeptide, GH-releasing peptide and GH-releasing hormone stimulate GH release through distinct pituitary receptors. Endocrinology 1992; 130:939–944.
139. Irie M, Tsushima T. 1972 Increase of serum growth hormone concentration following thyrotropin-releasing hormone injection in patients with acromegaly or gigantism. J Clin Endocrinol Metab 1972; 35:97–100.
140. Merola B, Colao A, Cataloi M, et al. Evaluation of GH paradoxical responses to TRH and LHRH in acromegalic patinets during long-term treatment with octreotide. Horm Res 1992; 37:18–22.
141. Martin JB. 1973 Neural regulation of growth hormone secretion. Medical progress report. N Engl J Med 1973; 228:1384–1393.
142. Kanaley JA, Hartman ML. A continuous glucagon infusion enhances 24-hour pulsatile growth hormone (GH) release in young men. Prog 77th Meeting of the Endocrine Society 1995; P1–181:158. (Abstract)
143. Bowers CY, Momany FA, Reynolds GA, Hong A. 1984 On the in vitro and in vivo activity of a new synthetic hexapeptide that acts on the pituitary to specifically release growth hormone. Endocrinology 1984; 114:1537–1545.

144. Bowers CY, Reynolds GA, Durham D, Barrera CM, Pezzoli SS, Thorner MO. Growth Hormone (GH)-releasing peptide stimulates GH release in normal men and acts synergistically with GH-releasing hormone. J Clin Endocrinol Metab 1990; 70:975–982.
145. Pong SS, Chaung LYP, Dean DC, Nargund RP, Patchett AA, Smith RG. Identification of a new G-protein-linked receptor for growth hormone secretagogues. Mol Endocrinol 1996; 10:57–61.
146. Rivier C, Vale W. Corticotropin-releasing factor (CRF) acts centrally to inhibit growth hormone secretion in the rat. Endocrinology 1984; 114:2409–2411.
147. Ling N, Esch F, Bohlen P, Brazeau P, Wehrenberg WB, Guillemin R. Isolation, primary structure, and synthesis of human hypothalamic somatocrinin: growth hormone-releasing factor. Proc Natl Acac Sci U S A 1984; 81:4302–.
148. Thorner MO. On the discovery of growth hormone-releasing hormone. Acta Pediatr Suppl 1993; 388:2–7.
149. Mayo KE, Vale W, Rivier J, Rosenfeld MG, Evans RM. Expression-cloning and sequence of a cDNA encoding human growth hormone-releasing factor. Nature 1983; 306:86–88.
150. Gubler U, Monahan JJ, Lomedico PT, et al. Cloning and sequence analysis of cDNA for the precursor of human growth hormone-releasing factor, somatocrinin. Proc Natl Acac Sci U S A 1983; 80:4311–4314.
151. Wehrenberg WB, Ling N, Bohlen P, Esch F, Brazeau P, Guillemin R. Physiological roles of somatocrinin and somatostatin in the regulation of growth hormone secretion. Biochem Biophys Res Commun 1982; 109:562–567.
152. Bloch B, Brazeau P, Bloom F, Ling N. Topographical study of the neurons containing hpGRF immunoreactivity in monkey hypothalamus. Neurosci Lett 1983; 37:23–28.
153. Bloch B, Brazeau P, Ling N, et al. Immunohistochemical detection of growth hormone-releasing factor in brain. Nature 1983; 301:607–608.
154. Bloch B, Gaillard RC, Brazeau P. Topographical and ontogenetic study of the neurons producing growth hormone releasing factor in human hypothalamus. Regul Pept 1984; 8:21–31.
155. Guillemin R, Brazeau P, Bohlen P, Esch F, Ling N, Wehrenberg WB. Growth hormone-releasing factor from a human pancreatic tumor that caused acromegaly. Science 1982; 218:585–587.
156. Rivier J, Spiess J, Thorner M, Vale W. Characterization of a growth hormone-releasing factor from a human pancreatic islet tumour. Nature 1982; 300:276–278.
157. Mayo KE. Molecular cloning and expression of a pituitary-specific receptor for growth hormone-releasing hormone. Mol Endocrinol 1992; 6:1734–1744.
158. Gaylinn BD, Harrison JK, Zysk JR, Lyons CE, Lynch KR, Thorner MO. Molecular cloning and expression of a human anterior pituitary receptor for growth hormone-releasing hormone. Mol Endocrinol 1993; 7:77–84.
159. Cronin MJ, Rogol AD, Dabney LG, Thorner MO. Selective growth hormone and cyclic AMP stimulating activity is present in human pancreatic islet cell tumor. J Clin Endocrinol Metab 1982; 55:381–383.
160. Cronin MJ, Hewlett EL, Evans WS, Thorner MO, Rogol AD. Human pancreatic tumor growth hormone (GH) - releasing factor and cyclic adenosine 3′,5′- monophosphate evoke GH release from anterior pituitary cells: the effects of pertussis toxin, cholera toxin, forskolin, and cycloheximide. Endocrinology 1984; 114:904–913.
161. Holl RW, Thorner MO, Leong DA. Intracellular calcium concentration and growth hormone secretion in individual somatotropes: effects of growth hormone-releasing factor and somatostatin. Endocrinology 1988; 122:2927–2932.
162. Barinaga M, Yamonoto G, Rivier C, Vale W, Evans R, Rosenfeld MG. Transcriptional regulation of growth hormone gene expression by growth hormone-releasing factor. Nature 1983; 306:84–86.
163. Goldman JA, Molitch ME, Thorner MO, Vale W, Rivier J, Reichlin S. Growth hormone and prolactin responses to bolus and sustained infusions of GRH-1-40-OH in man. J Endocrinol Invest 1987; 10:397–406.
164. Reichlin S. Somatostatin. [Review]. N Engl J Med 1983; 309:1495–1501.
165. Shen LP, Picket RL, Rutter WJ. Human somatostatin I: Sequence of the cDNA. Proc Natl Acad Sci U S A 1982; 79:4575–4579.
166. Harmar AJ, Pierotti AR. The patterns of molecular forms of somatostatin released by the rat median eminence differs from that released by the hypothalamus as a whole. J Physiol (London) 1984; 357:95.
167. Tannenbaum GS, Ling N, Brazeau P. Somatostatin 28 is longer acting and more selective than somatostatin 14 on pituitary and pancreatic hormone release. Endocrinology 1982; 111:101–107.
168. Patel YC, Srikant CB. Somatostatin mediation of adenohypophyseal secretion. Annu Rev Physiol 1986; 48:551–567.

169. Finley JWC, Maderchut JL, Roger LJ, Petrusz P. The immunocytochemical localization of somatostatin-containing neurons in the rat central nervous system. Neuroscience 1981; 6:2173–2192.
170. Yamada Y, Post SR, Wang K, Tager H, Bell GI, Seino S. Cloning and functional characterization of a family of human and mouse somatostatin receptors expressed in brain, gastrointestinal tract and kidney. Proc Natl Acad Sci U S A 1992; 89:251–255.
171. Holl RW, Thorner MO, Mandell GL, Sullivan JA, Sinha YN, Leong DA. Spontaneous oscillations of intracellular calcium and growth hormone secretion. J Biol Chem 1988; 263:9682–9685.
172. Herman V, Weiss M, Becker D, Melmed S. Hypothalamic hormonal regulation of human growth hormone gene expression in somatotroph adenoma cell cultures. Endocr Pathol 1990; 1:236–244.
173. Jaffe CA, Friberg RD, Barkan AL. Suppression of growth hormone (GH) secretion by a selective GH-releasing hormone (GHRH) antagonist. Direct evidence for involvement of endogenous GHRH in the generation of GH pulses. J Clin Invest 1993; 92:695–701.
174. Plotsky PM, Vale W. Patterns of growth hormone-releasing factor and somatostatin secretion into the hypophysial-portal circulation in the rat. Science 1985; 230:461–463.
175. Frohman LA, Downs TR, Clarke IJ, Thomas GB. Measurement of growth hormone-releasing hormone and somatostatin in hypothalamic-portal plasma of unanesthetized sheep. Spontaneous secretion and response to insulin-induced hypoglycemia. J Clin Invest 1990; 86(1):17–24.
176. Cataldi M, Magnan E, Guillaume V, et al. Relationship between hypophyseal portal GHRH and somatostatin and peripheral GH levels in the conscious sheep. J Clin Invest 1994; 17:717–722.
177. Vance ML, Kaiser DL, Evans WS, et al. Pulsatile growth hormone secretion in normal man during a continuous 24-hour infusion of human growth hormone releasing factor (1-40). Evidence for intermittent somatostatin secretion. J Clin Invest 1985; 75:1584–1590.
178. Brain C, Hindmarsh PC, Brook CG, Matthews DR. Continuous subcutaneous growth hormone releasing factor analogue. Clin Endocrinol (Oxf) 1988; 28:543–549.
179. Ross RJ, Kirk JM, Tsagarakis S, et al. Subcutaneous growth hormone-releasing hormone augments pulsatile nocturnal GH release in GH-insufficient children, but may also raise basal GH secretion. Clin Endocrinol (Oxf) 1990; 33:239–248.
180. Clark RG, Carlsson LMS, Robinson ICAF. The rebound release of growth hormone (GH) following somatostatin in rats involves hypothalamic GH-releasing factor release. J Endocrinol 1988; 119:397–404.
181. Ferland L, Labrie F, Jobin M. 1976 Physiological role of somatostatin in the control of growth hormone and thyrotrin secretion. Biochem Biophys Res Commun 1976; 68:149–156.
182. Frohman LA, Downs RT, Katakami H. The interaction of growth hormone-releasing hormone and somatostatin in the regulation of growth hormone secretion. In: Growth hormone—Basic and Clinical Aspects 1987; Isaksson O, Binder A, Hall R, Hokfelt T. ed. Excerpts Medica, Amsterdam, pp. 63–77
183. Kracier J, Lussier B, Moor B, Cowan JS. Failure of growth hormone (GH) to feedback at the level of the pituitary to alter the response of the somatotrophs to GH-releasing factor. Endocrinology 1988; 122:1511–1514.
184. Weiss J, Cronin MJ, Thorner MO. Periodic interactions of GH-releasing factor and somatostatin can augment GH release in vitro. Am J Physiol 1987; 253:E508–E514.
185. Wehrenberg WB, Brazeau P, Ling N, Textor G, Guillemin R. Pituitary growth hormone response in rats during a 24 hour infusion of growth hormone releasing factor. Endocrinology 1984; 114:1613–1616.
186. Wehrenberg WB. Continuous infusion of growth hormone-releasing factor: effects on pulsatile growth hormone secretion in normal rats. Neuroendocrinology 1986; 43:391–396.
187. Horvath S, Palkovits M, Gorcs T, Arimura A. Electron microscopic immunoctochemical evidence for the existence of bidirectional synaptic connections between growth hormone releasing hormone and somatostatin neurons in the hypothalamus of the rat. Brain Res 1989; 481:8–15.
188. McCarthy GF, Beaudet A, Tannenbaum GS. Colocalization of somatostatin receptors and growth hormone-releasing factor immunoreactivity in neurons of the rat arcuate nucleus. Neuroendocrinology 1992; 56:18–24.
189. Katakami H, Arimura A, Frohman LA. Growth hormone (GH)-releasing factor stimulates hypothalamic somatostatin release: an inhibitory feedback effect on GH secretion. Endocrinology 1986; 118:1872–1877.
190. Willoughby JO, Brogan M, Kapoor R. Intrahypothalamic actions of somatostatin and growth hormone releasing factor neurons. Neuroendocrinology 1989; 50:592–596.

191. Murakami Y, Kato Y, Kabayama Y, Inoue T, Koshiyama H, Imura H. Involvement of hypothalamic growth hormone (GH)-releasing factor in GH secretion induced by intracerebroventricular injection of somatostatin in rats. Endocrinology 1987; 120:311–316.
192. Abe H, Molitch ME, Van W, Underwood LE. Human growth hormone and somatomedin C suppress the spontaneous release of growth hormone in unanesthetized rats. Endocrinology 1983; 113:1319–1324.
193. Abrams RL, Grumbach MM, Kaplan SL. The effect of administration of human growth hormone on the plasma growth hormone, cortisol, glucose and free fatty acid response to insulin: evidence for growth hormone autoregulation in man. J Clin Invest 1971; 50:940–950.
194. Rosenthal J, Hulse JA, Kaplan SL. Exogenous growth hormone inhibits growth hormone releasing factor-induced growth hormone secretion in normal men. J Clin Invest 1986; 77:176–180.
195. Berelowitz M, Firestone SL, Frohman LA. Effects of growth hormone excess and deficiency on hypothalamic somatostatin content and release and on tissue somatostatin distribution. Endocrinology 1981; 109:714–719.
196. Chihara K, Minamitani N, Kaji H, Arimura A, Fujita T. Intraventricularly injected growth hormone stimulates somatostatin release into rat hypophyseal portal blood. Endocrinology 1981; 109:2279–2281.
197. Richman RA, Weiss JP, Hochberg Z, Florini JR. Regulation of growth hormone release: evidence against negative feedback in rat pituitary cells. Endocrinology 1981; 108:2287-2297.
198. Voogt JL, Clemens JA, Negro-Vilar A, Welsch C, Meites J. 1971 Pituitary GH and hypothalamic GHRF after median eminence implantation of ovine or human GH. Endocrinology 1971; 88:1155–1161.
199. Zenobi PD, Graf S, Ursprung H, Froesch ER. Effects of insulin-like growth factor I on insulin secretion and renal function in normal human subjects. Proc Natl Acad Sci U S A 1992; 86:2868–2872.
200. Hartman ML, Clayton PE, Johnson ML, et al. A low dose euglycemic infusion of recombinant human insulin-like growth factor I rapidly suppresses fasting-enhanced pulsatile growth hormone secretion in humans. J Clin Invest 1993; 91:2453–2462.
201. Bermann M, Jaffe CA, Tsai W, DeMott-Friburg R, Barkan AL. Negative feedback regulation of pulsatile growth hormone secretion by insulin-like growth factor I. Involvement of hypothalamic somatostatin. J Clin Invest 1994; 94:138–145.
202. Clemmons DR, Klibanski A, Underwood LE, et al. Reduction of plasma immunoreactive somatomedin-C during fasting in humans. J Clin Endocrinol Metab 1981; 53:1247–1250.
203. Ho KY, Veldhuis JD, Johnson ML, et al. Fasting enhances growth hormone secretion and amplifies the complex rhythms of growth hormone secretion in man. J Clin Invest 1988; 81:968–975.
204. Straus DS, Takemoto CD. Effect of fasting on insulin-like growth factor-I (IGF-I) and growth hormone receptor mRNA levels and IGF-I gene transcription in rat liver. Mol Endocrinol 1990; 4:91–100.
205. Guevara-Aguirre J, Rosenbloom AL, Vaccarello MA, et al. Growth hormone receptor deficiency (Laron Syndrome): Clinical and genetic characteristics. Acta Paediatr Scand [Suppl] 1991; 377:96–103.
206. Dunger DB, Edge JA, Pal R, Taylor AM, Holly JMP, Matthews DR. Impact of increased growth hormone secretion on carbohydrate metabolism in adolescents with diabetes. Acta Paediatr Scand [Suppl] 1995; 377:69–77.
207. Lanes R, Recker B, Fort P, Lifschitz F. Impaired somatomedin generation test in children with insulin-dependent diabetes mellitus. Diabetes 1985; 34:156–160.
208. Vaccarello MA, Diamond FB,Jr., Guevara-Aguirre J, et al. Hormonal and metabolic effects and pharmacokinetics of recombinant insulin-like growth factor-I in growth hormone receptor deficiency syndrome/Laron syndrome. J Clin Endocrinol Metab 1993; 77:273–280.
209. Cheetham TD, Jones J, Taylor AM, Holly J, Matthews DR, Dunger DB. The effects of recombinant insulin-like growth factor I administration on growth hormone levels and insulin requirements in adolescents with Type I (insulin-dependent) diabetes mellitus. Diabetologia 1993; 36:678–681.
210. Berelowitz M, Szabo M, Frohman LA, Firestone S, Chu L, Hintz RL. Somatomedin-C mediates growth hormone negative feedback by effects on both the hypothalamus and the pituitary. Science 1981; 212:1279–1281.
211. Yamashita S, Melmed S. Insulin-like growth factor 1 action on rat anterior pituitary cells: suppression of growth hormone secretion and messenger ribonucleic acid levels. Endocrinology 1986; 118:176–182.
212. Aquila MC. Insulin-like growth factor I (IGF-I) regulates somatostatin (SRIF) release, messenger ribonucleic acid levels in the rat hypothalamus. Prog 73rd Meeting of The Endocrine Society 1991; A1580:(Abstract)

213. Karbonits M, Little JA, Besser GM, Grossman AB, Trainer PJ. IGF-I and IGF-II act synergistically to inhibit GHRH secretion from rat hypothalamic explants. Prog 76th Meeting of The Endocrine Society 1994; A1122:(Abstract)
214. Sato M, Frohman LA. Differential effects of central and peripheral administration of growth hormone (GH) and insulin-like growth factor on hypothalamic GH-releasing hormone and somatostatin gene expression in GH-deficient dwarf rats. Endocrinology 1993; 133:793–799.
215. Muller EE. Neural control of somatotropic function. Physiol Rev 1987; 67:962–1053.
216. Chihara K, Arimura A, Coy DH, Schally AV. Studies on the interaction of endorphins, substance P and endogenous somatostatin in growth hormone and prolactin release in rats. Endocrinology 1978; 102:281–289.
217. Katakami H, Kato Y, Matsushita N, Hiroto S, Shimatsu A, Imura H. Involvement of alpha-adrenergic mechanisms in growth hormone release induced by opioid peptides in conscious rats. Neuroendocrinology 1981; 33:129–135.
218. Morley JE, Baranesky NG, Wingert TD, et al. Endocrine effects of naloxone-induced opiate receptor blockade. J Clin Endocrinol Metab 1980; 50:251–257.
219. Arnold MA, Fernstrom JD. L-tryptophan injection enhances pulsatile growth hormone secretion in the rat. Endocrinology 1983; 108:331–335.
220. Smythe GA, Lazarus L. Growth hormone regulation by melatonin and serotonin. Nature 1973; 244:230, 231.
221. Boyd AE, Lebovitz HE, Pfeiffer JB. 1Stimulation of growth hormone secretion by L-dopa. N Engl J Med 1970; 283:1425–1429.
222. Huseman CA, Hassing JM. Evidence for dopaminergic stimulation of growth velocity in some hypopituitary children. J Clin Endocrinol Metab 1984; 58:419–425.
223. Kreig RJ, Perkins SN, Johnson JH, Rogers JP, Arimura A, Cronin MJ. Beta-adrenergic stimulation of growth hormone (GH) release in vivo, and subsequent inhibition of GH-releasing factor-induced GH secretion. Endocrinology 1988; 122:531–537.
224. Mazza E, Ghigo E, Bellone J, et al. Effects of alpha- and beta-adrenergic agonists and antagonists on growth hormone secretion in man. Endocrinol Exp 1990; 24:211–219.
225. Krulich L, Mayfield MA, Steele MK, McMillen BA, McCann SM, Koenig JI. Differential effects of pharmacological manipulations of central alpha-1 and alpha-2 adrenergic receptors on the secretion of thyrotropin and growth hormone in male rats. Endocrinology 1982; 110:796–804.
226. Hunter WM, Friend JAR, Strong JA. The diurnal pattern of plasma growth hormone concentration in adults. J Endocrinol 1966; 34:139–146.
227. Takahashi Y, Kipnis DM, Daughaday WH. Growth hormone secretion during sleep. J Clin Invest 1968; 47:2079–2090.
228. Illig R, Stahl M, Henrichs I, Hecker A. Growth hormone release during slow-wave sleep: comparison with insulin and arginine provocation in children with small stature. Helv Paediatr Acta 1971; 26:665–672.
229. Holl RW, Hartman ML, Veldhuis JD, Taylor WM, Thorner MO. 30-second-sampling of plasma growth hormone (GH) in man: correlation with sleep stages. J Clin Endocrinol Metab 1991; 72:854–861.
230. Golstein J, Van Cauter E, Desir D, et al. Effects of "jet lag" on hormonal patterns. IV. Time shifts increase growth hormone release. J Clin Endocrinol Metab 1983; 56:433–440.
231. Van Cauter E, Kerkhofs M, Van Onderbergen A, Caufriez A, Copinschi G. Modulation of spontaneous and GHRH-stimulated GH secretion by sleep. Prog 71st Meeting of the Endocrine Soc 1989; p 220. (Abstract)
232. Kerkhofs M, Van Cauter E, Van Onderbergen E, Caufriez A, Thorner MO, Copinschi G. Sleep promoting effects of growth hormone-releasing hormone in normal men. Am J Physiol 1993; 264:E594–E598.
233. Steiger A, Guldner J, Hemmeter U, Rothe B, Wiedemann K, Holsboer F. Effects of growth hormone-releasing hormone and somatostatin on sleep EEG and nocturnal hormone secretion in male controls. Neuroendocrinology 1992; 56:566–573.
234. Kupfer DJ, Jarrett DB, Ehlers CL. The effect of SRIF on the EEG sleep of normal men. Psychoneuroendocrinology 1992; 17:37–43.
235. Tannenbaum GS, Martin JB. Evidence for an endogenous ultradian rhythm governing growth hormone secretion in the rat. Endocrinology 1976; 98:562–570.
236. Clark RG, Carlsson LMS, Robinson ICAF. Growth hormone secretory profiles in conscious female rats. J Endocrinol 1976; 114:399–407.

237. Ho KY, Evans WS, Blizzard RM, et al. Effects of sex and age on the 24-hour profile of growth hormone secretion in man: importance of endogenous estradiol concentrations. J Clin Endocrinol Metab 1987; 64:51–58.
238. Weltman A, Weltman JY, Hartman ML, et al. Relationship between age, percentage body fat, fitness, and 24-hour growth hormone release in healthy young adults: effects of gender. J Clin Endocrinol Metab 1994; 78:543–548.
239. Asplin CM, Faria AC, Carlsen EC, et al. Alterations in the pulsatile mode of growth hormone release in men and women with insulin-dependent diabetes mellitus. J Clin Endocrinol Metab 1989; 69:239–245.
240. Thompson RG, Rodriguez A, Kowarski A, Blizzard RM. Growth hormone: metabolic clearance rates, integrated concentrations, and production rates in normal adults and the effect of prednisone. J Clin Invest 1972; 51:3193–3199.
241. Veldhuis JD, Pincus S, Van Den Berg G, Roelfsema F. An amplitude-specific divergence in the pulsatile mode of GH secretion underlies the gender difference in mean GH concentrations in men and women. Prog 76th Meeting End Soc. Abst 1994;564:341. (Abstract)
242. Jaffe CA, Ocampo-Lim I, Sugahara DT, Mauger R, DeMott Friberg R, Barkan AL. Sexual dimorphism of growth hormone (GH) secretion in humans. Prog 77th Meeting Endocrine Soc 1995; P1–170:155. (Abstract)
243. Holst N, Jenssen TG, Burhol PG, Haug E, Forsdahl F. Plasma gastrointestinal hormones during spontaneous and induced menstrual cycles. J Clin Endocrinol Metab 1989; 68:1160–1166.
244. Zadik Z, Chalew SA, McCarter RJ,Jr., Meistas M, Kowarski AA. The influence of age on the 24-hour integrated concentration of growth hormone in normal individuals. J Clin Endocrinol Metab 1985; 60:513–516.
245. Frantz AG, Rabkin MT. Effects of estrogen and sex difference on secretion of human growth hormone. J Clin Endocrinol Metab 1965; 25:1470–1480.
246. Genazzini AR, Lemarchand-Beraud Th, Aubert ML, Felberg JP. Pattern of plasma ACTH, hGH, and cortisol during menstrual cycle. J Clin Endocrinol Metab 1975; 41:431–437.
247. Faria ACS, Bekenstein LW, Booth RA,Jr., et al. Pulsatile growth hormone release in normal women. Clin Endocrinol (Oxf) 1992; 36:591–596.
248. Kanaley JA, Boileau RA, Bahr JA, Misner JE, Nelson RA. Substrate oxidation and GH response to exercise are independent of menstrual phase and status. Med Sci Sports Exerc 1992; 24:873–880.
249. Rao RH, Spathis GS. Intramuscular glucagon as a provocative stimulus for the assessment of pituitary function: growth hormone and cortisol responses. Metab Clin Exp 1987; 36:658–663.
250. Penalva A, Pombo M, Carballo A, Barriero J, Casanueva FF, Dieguez C. Influence of sex, age, and adrenergic pathways on the growth hormone response to GHRP-6. Clin Endocrinol (Oxf) 1993; 38:87–91.
251. Merimee TJ, Rabinowtitz D, Fineberg SE. Arginine-initiated release of human growth hormone. Factors modifying the response in normal man. N Engl J Med 1969; 280:1434–1438.
252. Corsello SM, Tofani A, Della Casa S, et al. Effects of sex and age on pyridostigmine potentiation of growth hormone-releasing hormone-induced growth hormone release. Neuroendocrinology 1992; 56:208–213.
253. Tulandi T, Lal S, Guyda H. Effect of estrogen on the growth hormone response to the alpha adrenergic ag onist clonidine in women with menopausal flushing. J Clin Endocrinol Metab 1987; 65:6–10.
254. Monteleone P, Maj M, Iovino M, Steardo L. Evidence for a sex difference in the basal growth hormone response to GAGAergic stimulation in humans. Acta Endocrinol 1988; 119:353–357.
255. Benito P, Avila L, Corpas MS, Jimenez JA, Cacicedo L, Franco FS. Sex differences in growth hormone response to growth hormone-releasing hormone. J Endocrinol Invest 1991; 14:265–268.
256. Lang I, Schernthaner G, Pietschmann P, Kurz R, Stephenson JM, Templ H. Effects of sex and age on growth hormone response to growth hormone-releasing hormone in healthy individuals. J Clin Endocrinol Metab 1987; 65:535–540.
257. Smals AEM, Pieters GFFM, Smals AGH, Benraad TJ, van Laarhoven J, Kloppenborg PWC. Sex difference in human growth hormone (GH) response to intravenous human pancreatic GH-releasing hormone administration in young adults. J Clin Endocrinol Metab 1986; 62:336–341.
258. Lima L, Arce V, Lois N, et al. Growth hormone (GH) responsiveness to GHRH in normal adults is not affected by short-term gonadal blockade. Acta Endocrinol 1989; 120:31–36.
259. Arat E, Cappa M, Casanueva FF, et al. Pyridostigmine potentiates growth hormone (GH)-releasing hormone-induced GH release in both men and women. J Clin Endocrinol Metab 1993; 76:374–377.

260. Iranmanesh A, Lizarralde G, Veldhuis JD. Age and relative adiposity are specific negative determinants of the freqency and amplitude of growth hormone (GH) secretory bursts and the half-life of endogenous GH in healthy men. J Clin Endocrinol Metab 1991; 73:1081–1088. (Abstract)
261. Weissbeger AJ, Ho KK. Activation of the somatotropic axis by testosterone in adult males: evidence for the role of aromatization. J Clin Endocrinol Metab 1993; 76:1407–1412.
262. Metzger DL, Kerrigan JR. Estrogen receptor blockade with tamoxifen diminishes growth hormone secretion in boys: evidence for a stimulatory role of endogenous estrogens during male adolescence. J Clin Endocrinol Metab 1994; 79:513–518.
263. Plotnick LP, Thompson RG, Beitins I, Blizzard RM. Integrated concentrations of growth hormone correlated with stage of puberty and estrogen levels in girls. J Clin Endocrinol Metab 1974; 38:436–439.
264. Ovesen P, Christiansen JS, Moller J, Orskov H, Moller N, Jorgensen JOL. Growth hormone secretory capacity and serum insulin-like growth factor I levels in primary infertile, anovulatory women with regular menses. Fertil Steril 1992; 57:97–101.
265. Word RA, Odom MJ, Byrd W, Carr BR. The effect of gonadotropin-releasing hormone agonists on growth hormone secretion in adult premenopausal women. Fertil Steril 1990; 54:73–78.
266. De Leo V, Lanzetta D, D'Antona D, Danero S. Growth hormone secretion in premenopausal women before and after ovariectomy: effect of hormone replacement therapy. Fertil Steril 1993; 60:268–271.
267. Harris DA, van Vliet G, Egli CA, et al. Somatomedin-C in normal puberty and in true precocious puberty before and after treatment with potent lutenizing hormone-releasing hormone agonist. J Clin Endocrinol Metab 1985; 61:152–159.
268. Mauras N, Rogol AD, Veldhuis JD. Increased hGH production rate after low-dose estrogen therapy in prepubertal girls with Turner's syndrome. J Clin Endocrinol Metab 1990; 28:626–630.
269. Dawson Hughes B, Stern D, Goldman J, Reichlin S. Regulation of growth hormone and somatomedin-C secretion in postmenopausal women: effect of physiological estrogen replacement. J Clin Endocrinol Metab 1986; 63:424–432.
270. Weissberger AJ, Ho KKY, Lazarus L. Contrasting effects of oral and transdermal routes of estrogen replacement therapy on 24-hour growth hormone (GH) secretion, insulin-like growth factor I, and GH-binding protein in postmenopausal women. J Clin Endocrinol Metab 1991; 72:374–381.
271. Wright NM, Reanault J, Willi S, et al. Greater secretion of growth hormone in black than in white men: possible factor in greater bone mineral density—a clinical research center study. J Clin Endocrinol Metab 1995; 80:2291–2297.
272. Cronin MJ, Rogol AD. Sex differences in the cyclic adenosine 3′:5′-monophosphate and growth hormone response to growth hormone-releasing factor in vitro. Biol Reprod 1984; 31:984–988.
273. Kerrigan JR, Martha PM,Jr., Krieg RJ,Jr., Rogol AD, Evans WS. Somatostatin inhibition of growth hormone secretion by somatotropes from male, female, and androgen receptor-deficient rats: evidence for differing sensitivities. Endocrinology 1989; 125:3078–3083.
274. Painson JC, Tannenbaum GS. Sexual dimorphism of somatostatin and growth hormone-releasing factor secretion in the rat. Endocrinology 1991; 128:2858–2866.
275. Ge F, Tsagarakis S, Rees LH, Besser GM, Grossman A. Relationship between growth hormone-releasing hormone and somatostatin in the rat: effects of age and sex on content and in-vitro release from hypothalamic explants. J Endocrinol 1989; 123:53–58.
276. Maiter D, Underwood LE, Martin JB, Koenig JI. Neonatal treatment with monosodium glutamate: Effects of prolonged growth hormone (GH)-releasing hormone deficiency on pulsatile GH secretion and growth in female rats. Endocrinology 1991; 128:1100–1106.
277. Rosenbaum M, Gertner JM. Metabolic clearance rates of synthetic human growth hormone in children, adult women, and adult men. J Clin Endocrinol Metab 1989; 69:821–824.
278. Gupta SK, Krishnan RR, Ellinwood EH, Ritchie JC, Nemeroff CB. Pharmacokinetics of growth hormone secretion in humans induced by growth hormone releasing hormone. Life Sci 1990; 47:1887–1893.
279. Hattori N, Kurahachi H, Ikekubo K, et al. Effects of sex and age on serum GH binding protein levels in normal adults. Clinical Endocrinology 1991; 35:295–297.
280. Snow KJ, Shaw MA, Winer LM, Baumann G. Diurnal pattern of plasma growth hormone-binding protein in man. J Clin Endocrinol Metab 1990; 70:417–420.
281. Kwekkeboom DJ, de Jong FH, Lamberts SWJ. Gonadotropin release by clinically nonfunctioning and gonadotroph pituitary adenomas in vivo and in vitro: relation to sex and effects of thyrotropin-releasing hormone, gonadotropin- releasing hormone, and bromocriptine. J Clin Endocrinol Metab 1989; 68:1128–1135.

282. Gluckman PD, Grumbach MM, Kaplan SL. The neuroendocrine regulation and function of growth hormone and prolactin in the mammalian fetus. Endocr Rev 1981; 2:363–395.
283. Iranmanesh A, Lizzarralde G, Veldhuis JD. Age and relative adiposity are specific determinants of the frequency and amplitude of GH secretory bursts and the half-life of endogenous GH in healthy men. J Clin Endocrinol Metab 1991; 73:1081–1088.
284. Corpas E, Harman SM, Pineyro MA, Roberson R, Blackman MR. GHRH 1-29 twice daily reverses the decreased GH and IGF-I levels in old men. J Clin Endocrinol Metab 1992; 75:530–535.
285. Vermeulen A. Nyctohemeral growth hormone profiles in young and aged men: correlation with somatomedin-C levels. J Clin Endocrinol Metab 1987; 64:884–888.
286. Hagberg JM, Seals DR, Yerg JE, et al. Metabolic responses to exercise in young and old athletes and sedentary men. J Appl Physiol 1988; 65:900–908.
287. Craig BW, Brown R, Everhart J. Effects of progressive resistance training on growth hormome and testosterone levels in young and elderly subjects. Mech Ageing Dev 1989; 49:159–169.
288. Corpas E, Harman SM, Blackman MR. Human growth hormone and human aging. Endocr Rev 1993; 14:20–39.
289. Kalk WJ, Vinik AI, Pimstone BL, Jackson PU. Growth hormone response to insulin hypoglycemia in the elderly. J Gerontol 1973; 28:431–433.
290. Muggeo M, Fedele D, Tiengo A, Molinari M, Crepaldi G. Human growth hormone and cortisol response to insulin stimulation in aging. J Gerontol 1975; 30:546–551.
291. Ghigo E, Bellone J, Mazza E, et al. Arginine potentiates the GHRH- but not the pyridostigmine-induced GH secretion in normal short children. Further evidence for a somatostatin suppressing effect of arginine. Clin Endocrinol (Oxf) 1990; 32:763–767.
292. Blichert-Toft M. Stimulation of the release of corticotrophin and somatotrophin by metyrapone and arginine. Acta Endocrinol 1975; 195(Suppl.):65–85.
293. Ghigo E, Goffi E, Nicolosi M, et al. Growth hormone (GH) responsiveness to combined administration of arginine and GH-releasing hormone does not vary with age in man. J Clin Endocrinol Metab 1990; 71:1481–1485.
294. Sun YK, Xi YP, Fenoglio CM, et al. The effect of age on the number of pituitary cells immunoreactive to growth hormone and prolactin. Hum Pathol 1984; 15:169–180.
295. Iovino M, Monteleone P, Steardo L. Repetitive growth hormone-releasing hormone administration restores the attenuated growth hormone (GH) response to GH-releasing hormone testing in normal aging. J Clin Endocrinol Metab 1989; 69:910–913.
296. Franchimont P, Urbain-Choffray D, Lambelin P, Fontaine MA, Frangin G, Reginster JY. Effects of repetitive administration of growth hormone-releasing. Acta Endocrinol 1989; 120:121–128.
297. Rudman D. Growth hormone, body composition, and aging. [Review]. J Am Geriatr Soc 1985; 33:800–807
298. Johannsson G, Rosen T, Bosaeus L, Bengtsson BA. The effects of 2 years treatment with recombinant human growth hormone on body composition and metabolism in adults with growth hormone deficiency. Prog 76th Meeting of The Endocrine Society 1994; A18:(Abstract)
299. Rosen T, Bengtsson BA. Premature mortality due to cardiovascular disease in hypopituitarism. Lancet 1990; 336:285–288.
300. Veldhuis JD, Iranmanesh A, Ho KK, Waters MJ, Johnson ML, Lizarralde G. Dual defects in pulsatile growth hormone secretion and clearance subserve the hyposomatotropism of obesity in man. J Clin Endocrinol Metab 1991; 72:51–59.
301. Williams T, Berelowitz M, Joffe SN, et al. Impaired growth hormone responses to growth hormone-releasing factor in obesity. A pituitary defect reversed with weight reduction. N Engl J Med 1984; 311:1403–1407.
302. Pontiroli AE, Malighetti ME, Manzoni MF, Lanzi R. Acute reduction of plasma free fatty acid levels restores growth hormone responsiveness to GH-releasing hormone in elderly and obese subjects. Prog 77th Meeting Endocrine Soc 1995; OR20–4:72. (Abstract)
303. Hartman ML, Veldhuis JD, Johnson ML, et al. Augmented growth hormone (GH) secretory burst frequency and amplitude mediate enhanced GH secretion during a two day fast in normal men. J Clin Endocrinol Metab 1992; 74:757–765.
304. Clasey JL, Hartman ML, Pezzoli SS, Weltman A, Veldhuis JD, Thorner MO. The hyposomatotropism associated with obesity is reversed by five days of fasting. Prog 77th Meeting Endocrine Soc 1995; P1–172:155. (Abstract)

305. Hartman ML, Thorner MO. Fasting-induced enhancement of pulsatile growth hormone (GH) secretion is rapidly abolished by refeeding. Prog 72nd Meeting of the Endocrine Soc 1990; A123. (Abstract)
306. Yamashita S, Melmed S. Effects of insulin on rat anterior pituitary cells: inhibition of growth hormone secretion and mRNA levels. Diabetes 1986; 35:440–447.
307. Thomas GB, Cummins JT, Francis H, Sudbury AW, McCloud PI, Clarke IJ. Effect of restricted feeding on the relationship between hypophysial portal concentrations of growth hormone (GH)-releasing factor and somatostatin, and jugular concentrations of GH in ovariectomized ewes. Endocrinology 1991; 128:1151–1158.
308. Hartman ML, Kanaley JA, Weltman A Growth hormone economy in menopausal women: effects of age. In: The somatotrophic axis and the reproductive process in health and disease. Adashi EY, Thorner MO, ed. 1995; Springer-Verlag, New York, pp. 142–159
309. Masuda A, Shibasaki T, Nakahara M, et al. The effect of glucose on growth hormone (GH)-releasing hormone- mediated GH secretion in man. J Clin Endocrinol Metab 1985; 60:523–526.
310. Reichlin S. Regulation of somatotropic hormone secretion. In: Handbook of Physiology 1974; Am Physiol Society, Washington, pp. 405–407
311. Cappon JP, Ipp. E, Brasel JA, Cooper DM. Acute effects of high fat and high glucose meals on the growth hormone response to exercise. J Clin Endocrinol Metab 1993; 76:1418–1422.
312. Casanueva FF, Villanueva L, Cabranes JA, Cabezas-Cerrato, Fernandez-Cruz A. Cholinergic mediation of growth hormone secretion elicited by arginine, clonidine and physical exercise in man. J Clin Endocrinol Metab 1984; 59:526–530.
313. Christensen SE, Jorgensen OL, Moller N, Orskov H. Characterization of growth hormone release in response to external heating: comparison to exercise induced release. Acta Endocrinol 1984; 107:295–301.
314. Raynaud J, Capderou A, Martineaud JP, Bordachar J, Durand J. Intersubject viability in growth hormone time course during different types of work. J Appl Physiol 1983; 55:1682–1687.
315. Felsing NE, Brasel JA, Cooper DM. Effect of low and high intensity exercise on circulating growth hormone in men. J Clin Endocrinol Metab 1992; 75:157–162.
316. Weltman A, Weltman JY, Schurrer R, Evans WS, Veldhuis JD, Rogol AR. Endurance training amplifies the pulsatile release of growth hormone: effects of training intensity. J Appl Physiol 1992; 72:2188–2196.
317. Karagiorgos A, Garcia JF, Brooks GA. Growth hormone response to continuous and intermittent exercise. Med Sci Sports 1979; 11:302–307.
318. Kozowski S, Chwalbinska-Moneta J, Vigas M, Kaciuba-Usciko H, Nazar K. Greater serum GH response to arm than to leg exercise performed at equivalent oxygen uptake. Eur J Appl Physiol 1983; 52:131–135.
319. VanHelder WP, Casey K, Goode RC, Radomski WM. Growth hormone regulation in two types of aerobic exercise of equal oxygen uptake. Eur J Appl Physiol 1986; 55:236–239.
320. VanHelder WP, Goode RC, Radomski MW. Effect of anaerobic and aerobic exercise of equal duration and work expenditure on plasma growth hormone levels. Eur J Appl Physiol 1984; 52:255–257.
321. Chang FE, Dodds WG, Sullivan M, Kim MH, Malarkey WB. The acute effects of exercise on prolactin and growth hormone secretion: comparison between sedentary women and women runners with normal and abnormal menstrual cycles. J Clin Endocrinol Metab 1986; 62:551–556.
322. Bunt JC, Boileau RA, Bahr JM, Nelson RA. Sex and training differences in human growth hormone during prolonged exercise. J Appl Physiol 1986; 61:1796–1801.
323. Pyka G, Wiswell RA, Marcus R. Age-dependent effect of resistance exercise on growth hormone secretion in people. J Clin Endocrinol Metab 1992; 75:404–407.
324. Pyka G, Taaffe DR, Marcus R. Effect of a sustained program of resistance training on the acute growth hormone response to resistance exercise in older adults. Horm Metab Res 1994; 26:330–333.

6 Growth Hormone Deficiency

Differential Diagnosis and Treatment

Maya K. Hunter, MD, *and Ron G. Rosenfeld,* MD

CONTENTS

NORMAL GROWTH

Growth is a fundamental part of childhood and reflects the complex interactions of environmental, hormonal, and genetic factors. Assessment of growth is an essential component in monitoring childhood health and development. During the first few years of life, a child's height can cross percentile lines on a growth chart, reflecting, at least in part, his or her genetic makeup. After this time, children grow in a relatively predictable manner and deviation from a normal growth pattern may reflect an underlying chronic disorder. Accurate growth measurements should therefore be a part of the routine pediatric examination.

MEASUREMENTS OF GROWTH

Height

Accurate serial measurements of height are vital to the evaluation of a child or adolescent with a question of abnormal growth. It is best to measure supine length of children 2 yr of age or younger, using a firm horizontal surface with a permanently attached rule. Older children can be measured by means of a wall-mounted stadiometer with a

From: *Contemporary Endocrinology, Vol. 3: Diseases of the Pituitary: Diagnosis and Treatment*
Edited by M. E. Wierman Humana Press Inc., Totowa, NJ

perpendicular sliding plate ("Harpenden" stadiometer). It is important to record the position the child was measured in, since standing height is approximately 1.25 cm less than supine height. Transitioning from supine to standing height measurements may falsely suggest a decreased growth velocity when the position of measurement is not recorded. Positioning of the child is critical for accurate measurement and height determination should be performed by an experienced member of the staff.

Diurnal variation in height has been observed with small decreases (2 mm) in height noted between morning and early afternoon *(1)*. Serial measurements of height should, therefore, be obtained at the same time of day. Seasonal variation in growth has also been documented, with greater growth rates occurring in the spring and summer. It is not uncommon for a child to demonstrate a slow-down in growth over a 3-mo interval during the fall or winter.

Evaluation of height for any individual is based upon the comparison to normal standards. Most American pediatricians use the National Center for Health Statistics (NCHS) standards for cross-sectional growth data (Figs. 1 and 2). This database was developed after surveying a large group of children in the United States and is invaluable for assessing children between the 5th and 95th percentile. Standard deviation (SD) charts are also available and are based on the distribution of the NCHS data above and below a mean value. The SD scores are helpful in identifying an individual with abnormalities of growth. Tanner and colleagues have developed longitudinal charts for both British and North American children, which depict curves 2.5 SD on either side of the mean and illustrate the pubertal growth spurt more accurately than do cross-sectional charts.

Height velocity (growth per year), which is based on serial measurements, is a more sensitive reflection of growth than is height determination at a single time-point. Growth velocity standards have been derived from both cross-sectional and longitudinal growth data (Figs. 3 and 4). Children tend to grow rapidly in the first year of life and then slow to a more constant growth rate between 2 yr and the onset of puberty. Abnormal height velocity within this interval warrants further investigation.

Body Proportions

Variability in body proportions occurs from fetal to adult life. Abnormal growth disturbances may be characterized by disproportionate or proportionate growth. Certain growth states have characteristic changes in proportional size of the head, trunk, and extremities. The following measurements should be included in the evaluation of abnormal growth: upper body segment (sitting height), lower body segment (distance from the top of the symphysis pubis to the floor), arm span, and occipitofrontal head circumference. Standard charts are available for measurements of body proportion. These values vary relative to the child's age. For example, upper segment:lower segment ratios range from 1.7 in the newborn to just below 1.0 in the adult.

Skeletal Age

Skeletal maturation is a reflection of physiologic development and is distinct from chronologic age. In normal children, the ossification centers of the skeleton appear and progress in a predictable manner, allowing the degree of skeletal maturation to be used as an indicator of remaining growth available. One method to determine skeletal age is

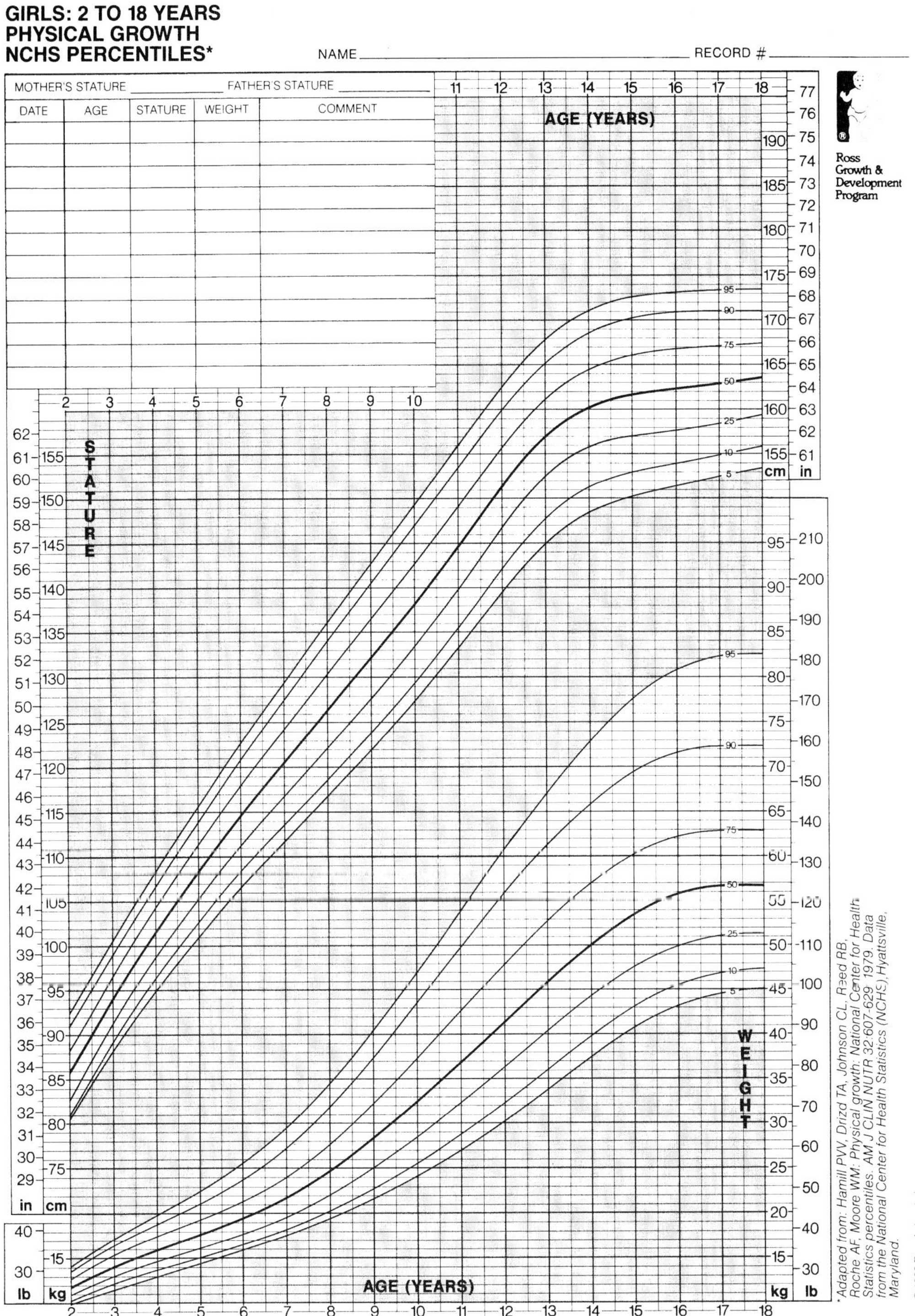

Fig. 1. NCHS centiles for stature and weight for age: females, 2–18 yr (From Ross Laboratories, Columbus, OH).

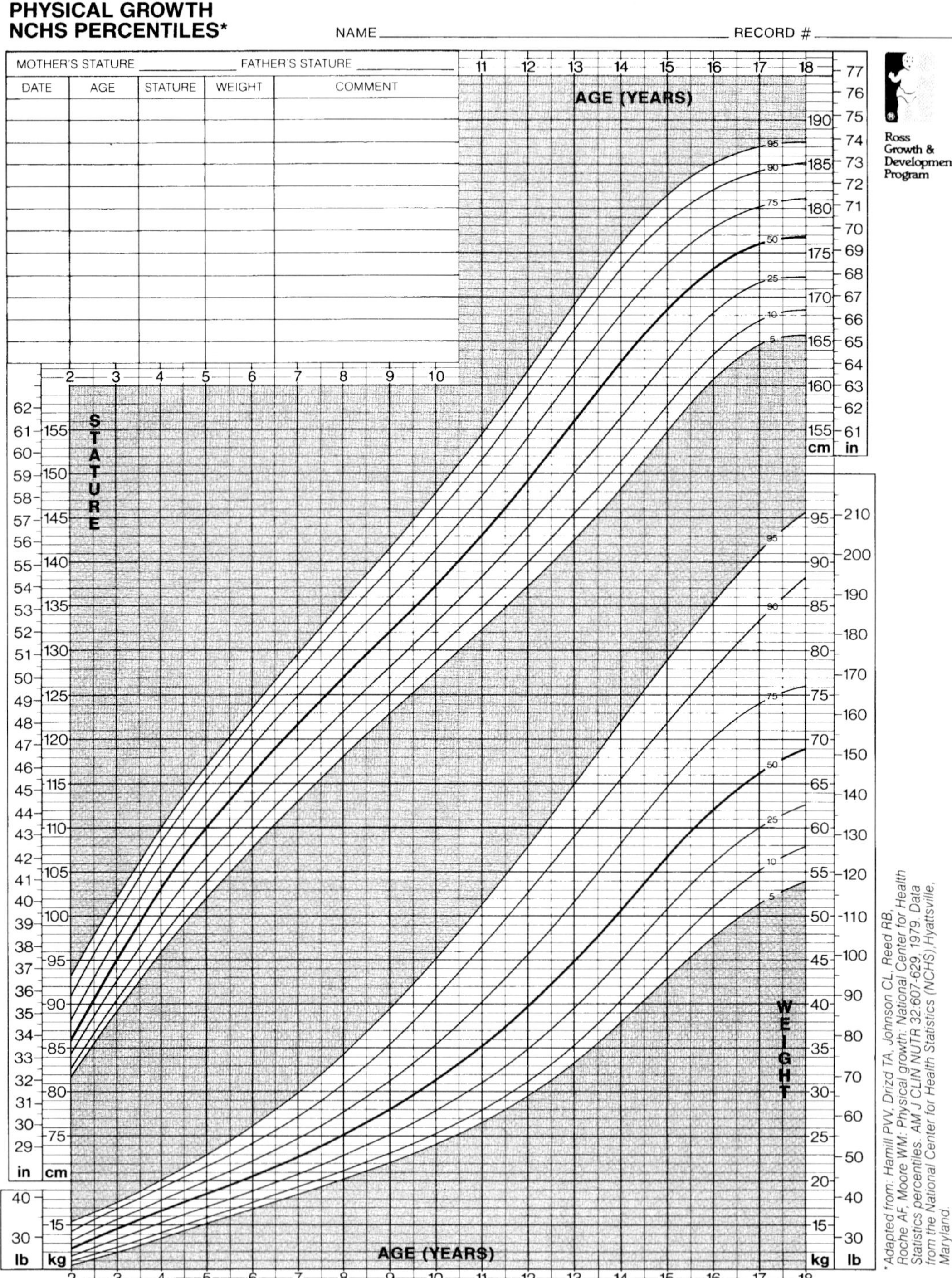

Fig. 2. NCHS centiles for stature and weight for age: males, 2–18 yr (From Ross Laboratories, Columbus, OH).

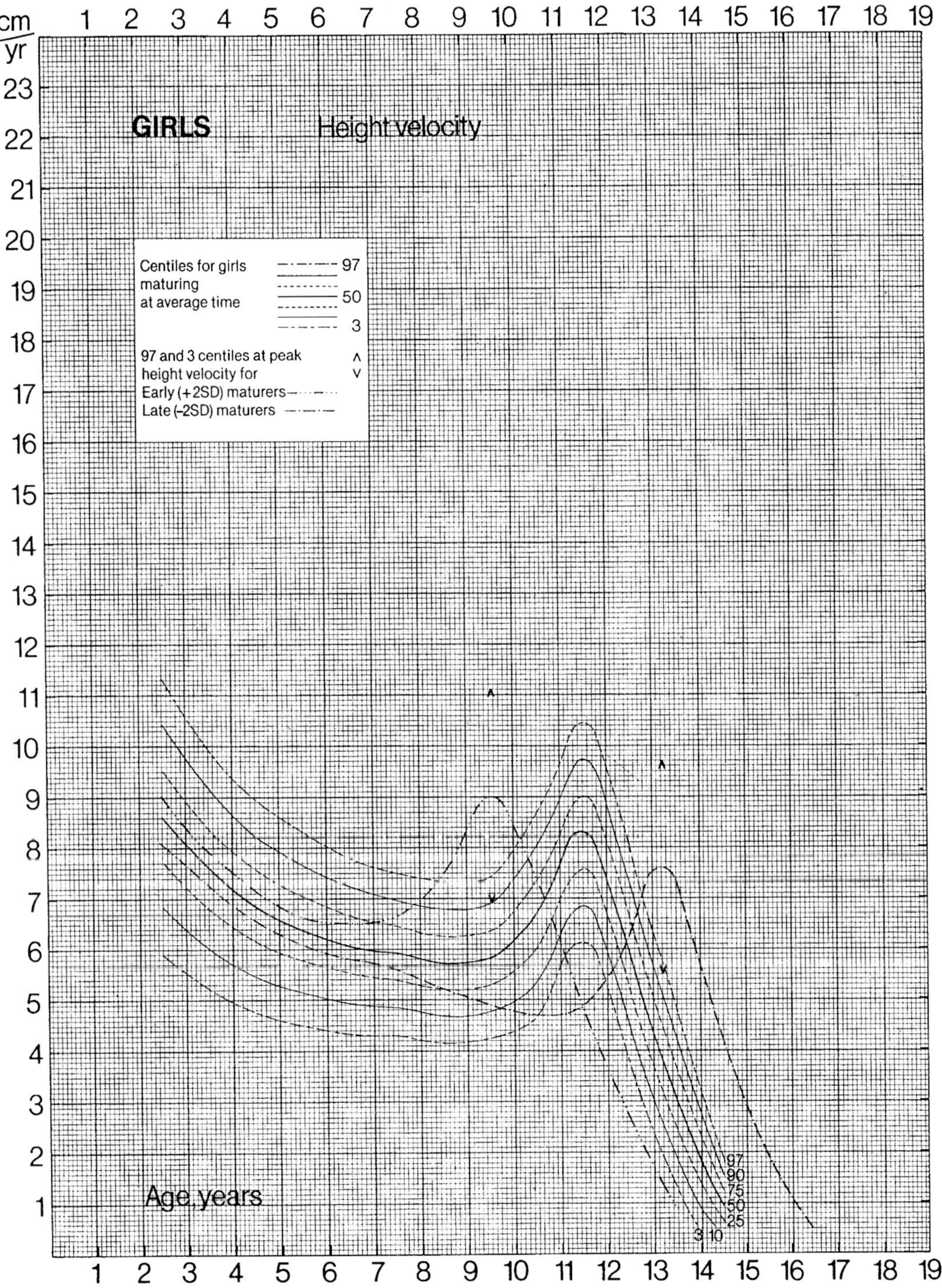

Fig. 3. Height velocity chart for females 0–19 yr of age (Tanner, Davies, J Pediatr 1985; 107:312–319).

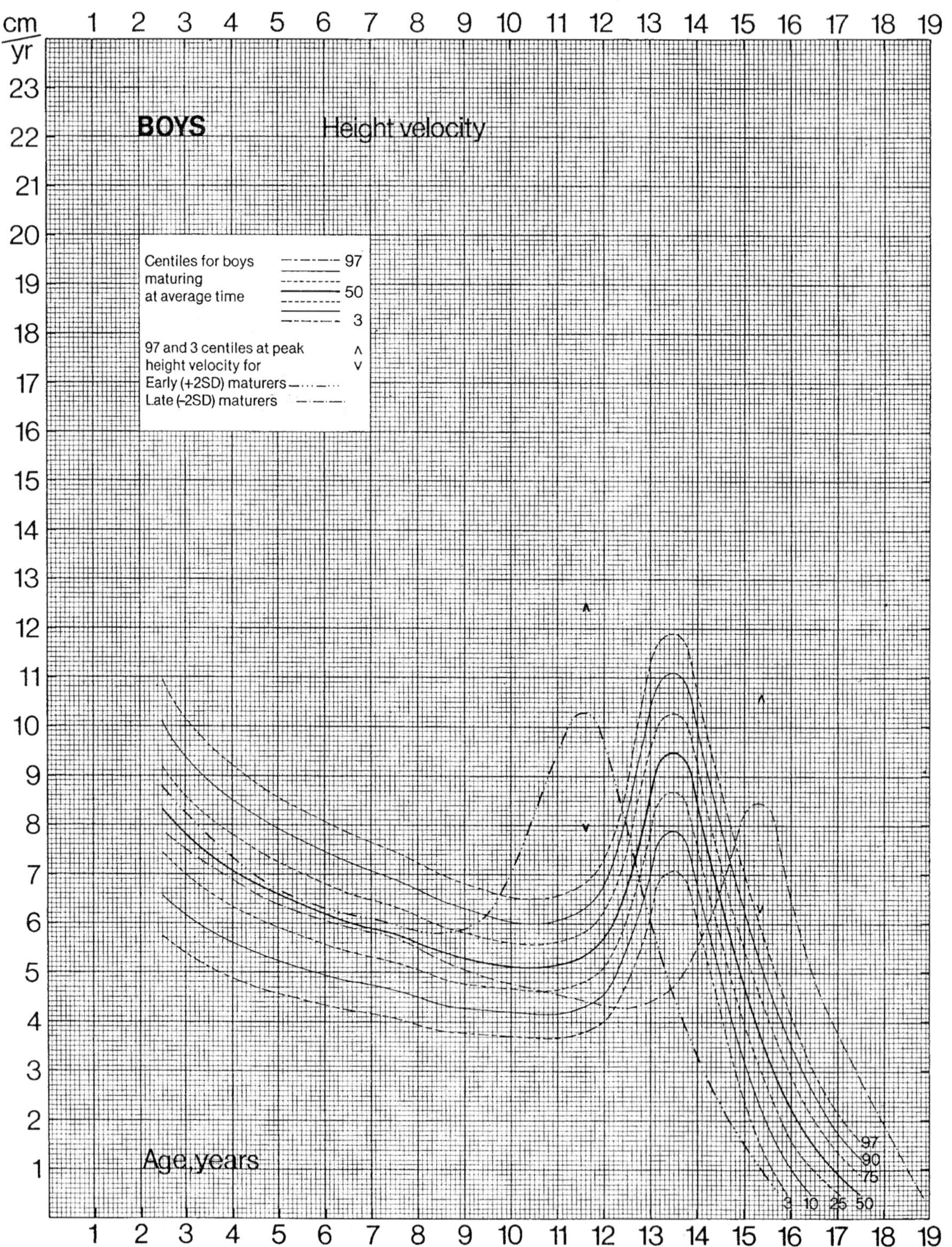

Fig. 4. Height velocity chart for males 0–19 yr of age (Tanner, Davies, J Pediatr 1985; 107:312–319).

by comparison of the left hand and wrist radiograph to the published standards of Greulich and Pyle *(2)*. Hemiskeleton radiographs to include the foot and knee are used for children younger than 2 yr. Skeletal maturation is reached when epiphyseal fusion and calcification is complete. Height prediction tables developed by Bayley and Pinneau *(3)* rely on a child's current bone age and height, and can be used to estimate final adult height. Height prediction is more accurate with a more advanced bone age.

Target Height

The parental target height is easily obtained by calculation of the mid parental height and adding or subtracting 6.5 cm for male and female children, respectively. A child's target height (mid parental height ± 2 SD) will estimate the child's final height within a wide range (± 10 cm).

REGULATION OF GROWTH

The regulation of growth is a complex process involving many hormonal and nonhormonal factors. The hormonal factors are primarily under the control of the hypothalamic-pituitary axis (HPA). This chapter will concentrate on the growth hormone-insulin-like growth factor(GH-IGF) axis (Fig. 5), which includes the hypothalamic neuropeptide hormones: growth hormone releasing hormone (GHRH) and somatostatin, growth hormone (GH), the insulin-like growth factors (IGFs), the insulin-like growth factor binding proteins (IGFBPs), which regulate IGF availability to the receptors, and two different insulin-like growth factor receptors.

Growth hormone is produced by the pituitary and is a single-chain peptide composed of 191 amino acids and two intramolecular disulfide bonds. Its pulsatile secretion is under the dual control of two hypothalamic regulatory neuropeptides, GHRH and somatostatin (somatotropin release inhibiting factor, SRIF). In addition to these neuropeptides, GH secretion is also controlled and influenced by a variety of other factors including, but not limited to, IGF I, GH itself, glucocorticoids, androgens, estrogens, thyroxine, and metabolic substances such as glucose or fatty acids.

The secretion of GH begins late in the first trimester and by 3 mo of age, maximal daily production is associated with sleep. In prepubertal children, GH secretion is episodic, with approximately 6–8 secretory pulses occurring in a 24-h period. Maximal GH secretion occurs during adolescence, in response to rising sex hormone levels. Estradiol has been reported to be the dominant sex steroid affecting GH secretion *(4)*. Growth hormone levels decline throughout late adolescence and adult life. Growth hormone circulates in serum primarily bound to a highly specific binding protein (GHBP), which is the cleaved extracellular portion of the growth hormone receptor. Fewer than 5% of patients with GH deficiency will have GHBP levels below –2 SD; this marker is, thus, of little utility in the diagnosis of GHD *(5)*.

The direct effects of GH are on carbohydrate and lipid metabolism. It is antagonistic to insulin action and stimulatory towards lipolysis of adipose tissue, where it increases the free fatty acid concentration. The majority of the stimulatory effects of GH on growth and anabolism are mediated through peptides called somatomedins or insulin-like growth factors. The synthesis of these proteins is initiated by the binding of GH to its receptor.

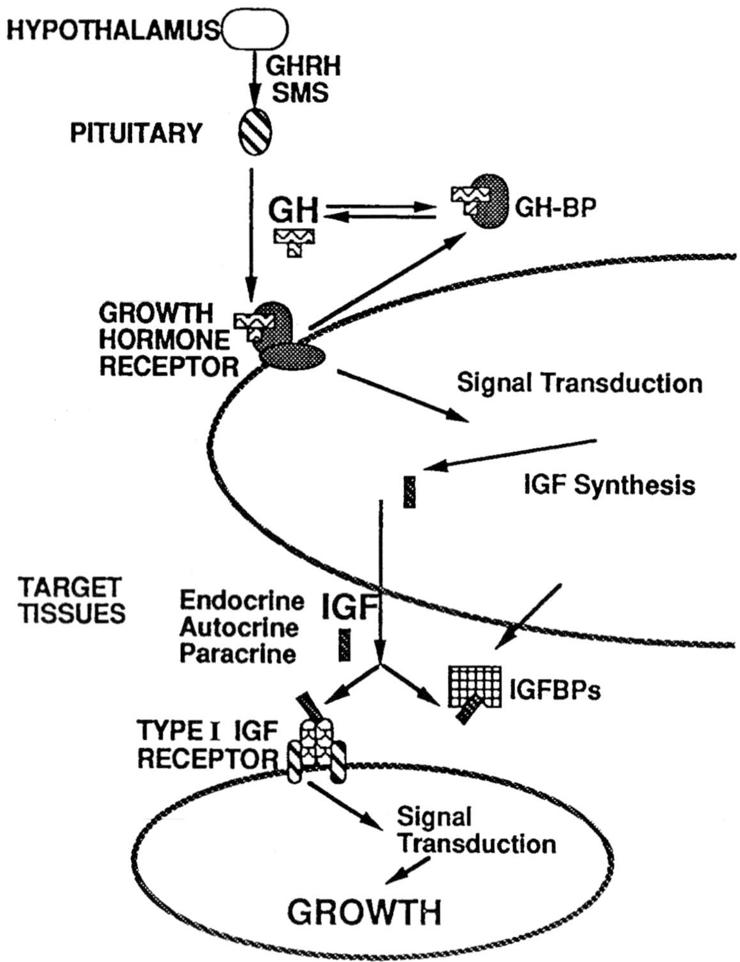

Fig. 5. The IGF axis.

Insulin-Like Growth Factors

IGF-I, previously known as somatomedin-C, and IGF-II peptides are believed to mediate many of the actions of GH. Initially identified in 1957 by Salmon and Daughaday *(6)*, the IGFs have been heavily investigated over the last 35 yr. Both of the IGF peptides are able to bind to the insulin receptor, an observation consistent with their strong structural homology to insulin. They have approximately 50% of their amino acids in common with insulin *(7,8)*. The gene for IGF-I has been located on the long arm of chromosome 12 and the gene for IGF-II has been localized to the short arm of chromosome 11, contiguous with the insulin gene *(9,10)*. The structures for these genes are complex, containing several exons, introns, and multiple potential initiation sites. Different mRNA species exist for both IGF-I and IGF-II, giving rise to complex regulation of gene expression.

IGF-I levels in serum are positively correlated with the rate of GH secretion. In the newborn, IGF-I levels are approximately 30–50% of adult levels. Similar to GH

Table 1
Plasma IGF-I and IGF-II Levels by Age and Sex

	Normal			Normal short stature			GH deficiency		
Age, yr	*n*	*IGF-I*	*IGF-II*	*n*	*IGF-I*	*IGF-II*	*n*	*IGF-I*	*IGF-II*
Boys									
<3	10	77 ± 33	480 ± 85	3	38 ± 39	477 ± 640	0		
3–5	9	157 ± 103	573 ± 259	5	80 ± 75	244 ± 100[a]	9	28 ± 17[a]	288 ± 277[a]
6–8	15	211 ± 112	607 ± 135	9	99 ± 41[a]	339 ± 139[a]	9	38 ± 20[a]	271 ± 137[a]
9–11	10	301 ± 173	505 ± 139	8	148 ± 109	580 ± 380	11	101 ± 94[a]	409 ± 380
12–14	38	466 ± 188	500 ± 114	5	207 ± 94	490 ± 171	5	92 ± 76[a]	352 ± 164
>15	14	516 ± 139	531 ± 107	1	252	384	4	73 ± 75[a]	603 ± 201
Girls									
<3	10	134 ± 53	419 ± 145	0			0		
3–5	15	247 ± 175	526 ± 201	3	103 ± 52	300 ± 129	7	31 ± 35[a]	273 ± 145[a]
6–8	20	298 ± 151	601 ± 228	4	198 ± 42[a]	704 ± 119	8	47 ± 67[a]	452 ± 144
9–11	16	366 ± 109	522 ± 135	4	196 ± 126[a]	412 ± 220	7	60 ± 59[a]	286 ± 138[a]
12–14	26	521 ± 164	498 ± 116	1	90	231	7	54 ± 23[a]	509 ± 361
>15	14	464 ± 141	466 ± 145	1	122	824	1	25[a]	669

Values expressed as mean ± SD nanograms per milliliter. Means were compared by repeated analysis of variance for each age group.

[a]Significantly different from normal patients ($p < 0.05$). IGF-I and IGF-II levels in normal short and GH-deficient children were not significantly different from each other in any age group. Table reproduced with permission from ref. *32*.

secretion, IGF-I levels are age-related, being relatively low in infancy and childhood, peaking in adolescence and then declining with age, after the late adolescent period *(11)*.

In the human newborn, levels of IGF-II are generally 50% of adult levels. The levels of IGF-II are less age-dependent and a relatively constant adult level is reached after one year of age *(12)*. Measurement of these peptides, especially IGF-I, can aid in the evaluation of growth hormone status. The IGF-I levels more closely reflect GH secretory patterns, but are also affected by age, degree of sexual maturation, and nutritional status (Table 1).

Two receptor types have been described for the IGFs. The type I IGF receptor is closely related to the insulin receptor; both are heterotetramers with two extracellular α-subunits containing the binding regions and two β-subunits containing a tyrosine phosphokinase domain. The type I receptor is capable of binding IGF-I, IGF-II, and insulin with decreasing affinity, respectively *(13,14)*. The type II IGF receptor has been shown to be identical to the cation-independent mannose-6-phosphate receptor *(15)*. The receptor binds IGF-II with high affinity and has poor affinity for IGF-I and no affinity for insulin *(16)*. Currently, the biological role of IGF-II binding to its type II mannose-6-phosphate receptor in the control of growth remains unresolved.

In the last few years, six IGF binding proteins (BP) have been identified and characterized. These proteins are structurally similar to each other and act as carrier proteins that extend the half-life of the IGF peptides and modulate the interaction of the IGFs with their receptors *(17)*. The most abundant form of IGF binding protein in human serum is IGF BP-3. This BP is GH-dependent and its serum concentration is correlated with total IGF-I and II levels *(18)*. It is the only BP that circulates as part of a ternary complex, consisting of IGFBP-3, an IGF peptide, and an acid-labile subunit *(19)*. In many conditions, the IGFBPs appear to inhibit the biological actions of IGF peptides, suggesting that the active IGF is the free protein. It is clear that the regulation of somatic growth during infancy through adolescence is highly complex and is under the integrated control of the GH-IGF axis. Thus the evaluation of a child with a growth disorder would be incomplete without the measurement of the various components of the GH-IGF axis. This would include investigation of GH secretion and an evaluation of the IGF peptides and the IGFBPs, especially IGFBP3.

GROWTH FAILURE

Deviation from a normal pattern of growth may be the first clue to a wide variety of underlying chronic disease processes. A child is considered to have growth failure if any of the following four criteria are met:

1. Short stature (severe) in the absence of an alternative explanation (Turner syndrome, intrauterine growth retardation, and so on); height >3 SD below mean.
2. Short stature (moderate: height -2 to -3 SD) and growth deceleration (height velocity < 25%).
3. Severe growth deceleration.
4. Predisposing condition (tumor, radiation, and so on) and growth deceleration (height velocity < 25%).

A child with growth failure warrants further evaluation.

SHORT STATURE

The differential diagnosis for a child with short stature is extensive and there are numerous different systems for classifications of growth disorders. Table 2 classifies growth retardation into three broad categories:

1. Primary growth abnormalities, in which the defect(s) appears to be intrinsic to the growth plate.
2. Genetic short stature.
3. Secondary growth disorders, where growth failure is owing to an underlying chronic disease or an endocrine disorder.

The skeletal dysplasias and chondrodystrophies represent a heterogeneous group of disorders associated with growth retardation. These disorders are owing to intrinsic abnormalities of cartilage and/or bone *(20)* and are characterized by genetic transmission, skeletal abnormalities that are usually evident on physical and/or radiologic exam, and disproportionate body segments. Family history is usually helpful, although many cases represent new mutations.

There are a variety of chromosomal abnormalities, which may involve both autosomes and sex chromosomes, that are associated with poor linear growth. Many of these disorders are evident from characteristic dysmorphic features and mental retardation, such as trisomy 13, 18, or 21. Girls with Turner syndrome (45X or variants) may present with classic phenotypic findings, which include delayed puberty, webbing of the neck, and cubitus valgus. Many patients, however, may present with growth failure as their only feature. Consequently, all girls with unexplained poor linear growth should have a karyotype included in their evaluation.

Intrauterine growth retardation (IUGR) is another large category included in the primary growth disorders. The category IUGR can be further divided into intrinsic fetal abnormalities, placental abnormalities, and maternal disorders (*see* Table 1). Children who are small for gestational age at birth frequently have poor postnatal growth, particularly when their growth retardation is associated with a specific syndrome.

Genetic or familial short stature is a common cause of short stature in children. Typically, the parents' heights are in the lower normal percentiles as adults. These children have normal growth velocities, a bone age representative of their calculated age, and a normal pubertal growth spurt. They generally fall into their projected target height based on genetic potential. It is important to remember, however, that short parents may have a pathologic explanation for their short stature (especially if their heights fall greater than 2 SD below the mean targeted height), and the child could have inherited the same disorder.

Secondary growth abnormalities, on a worldwide basis, account for the majority of children, with malnutrition and major organ system disease being the largest categories. Many of these patients will be identified by history and physical exam, although subtle underlying abnormalities, such as renal or gastrointestinal disorders, often require further laboratory evaluation. Endocrine disorders are another broad diagnostic category under secondary growth abnormalities. The most consistent feature of hypothyroidism is growth failure associated with delayed bone age. When the diagnosis is made and appropriate replacement therapy is given, children often have a period of rapid catch-up

Table 2
Differential Diagnosis of Short Stature

- **Primary growth abnormality**
  - Skeletal dysplasia
    - Osteochondrodysplasia
      - Achondroplasia (autosomal dominant)
      - Achondrogenesis
      - Hypochondroplasia (autosomal dominant)
      - Camptomelic dysplasia (autosomal recessive)
      - Metaphyseal chondroplasia
      - Multiple epiphyseal dysplasia (autosomal dominant)
      - Osteogenesis imperfecta
      - Osteopetrosis (autosomal recessive/autosomal dominant)
    - Dysostoses affecting face, cranium, axial skeleton, and/or extremities
  - Chromosomal abnormalities
    - Trisomies 13, 18, 21
    - Gonadal dysgenesis (45X and variants)
  - Intrauterine growth retardation
    - Syndromes associated with primary growth failure
      - Russell-Silver syndrome
      - Seckel syndrome
      - Noonan syndrome
      - Progeria
      - Cockayne syndrome
      - Bloom syndrome
      - Prader-Willi syndrome
      - Rubenstein-Taybi syndrome
    - Congenital infections
    - Congenital anomalies
    - Placental abnormalities
    - Maternal disorders
      - Malnutrition
      - Constraints on uterine growth
      - Vascular disorders
      - Uterine malformations
      - Drug ingestion: tobacco, alcohol, and/or narcotics
- **Genetic short stature**
- Secondary growth disorders
  - Psychosocial
  - Nutritional
  - Gastrointestinal
  - Cardiac
  - Pulmonary
  - Renal
  - Endocrine
    - Hypothyroidism
    - Pseudohypoparathyroidism
    - Hyposphatemic, vitamin D-resistant rickets

Table 2 (*Continued*)

- Insulin-dependent diabetes mellitus
- Cushing's syndrome
- Precocious puberty
- Constitutional growth delay
- IGF deficiency
  - Hypothalamic dysfunction
    - Genetic abnormality of hypothalamic factors
    - Congenital malformation involving the hypothalamus
    - Trauma to brain or hypothalamus (birth injury, child abuse)
    - Inflammation of brain or hypothalamus (autoimmune, infection)
    - Irradiation of the brain or hypothalamus
  - Pituitary GH deficiency
    - Genetic abnormality of GH production and/or secretion
    - Congenital absence or hypoplasia of pituitary
    - Trauma
    - Inflammation
    - Tumors
      - Craniopharyngioma
      - Histiocytosis
    - Psychosocial dwarfism
    - GH neurosecretory dysfunction
  - GH insensitivity
    - Primary GH insensitivity syndrome (Laron syndrome)
      - GH receptor deficiency
      - Abnormalities of GH signal transduction (postreceptor defects)
      - Primary defects of synthesis of IGF-I
    - Secondary GH insensitivity syndromes
      - Circulating antibodies to GH that inhibit GH action
      - Antibodies to the GH receptor
      - GH insensitivity caused by malnutrition
      - GH insensitivity caused by liver disease
      - Other conditions that cause GH insensitivity

growth. If there is a long duration of hypothyroidism prior to treatment, a deficit in final height relative to predicted adult height is often seen *(21)*. Patients with pseudohypoparathyroidism have hypocalcemia associated with a characteristic phenotype, which includes short stature. Hypophosphatemic, vitamin D-resistant rickets is an X-linked condition with decreased renal tubular reabsorption of phosphate. Clinical features include short stature and prominent bowing of the legs.

Poorly controlled insulin-dependent diabetes mellitus may be associated with poor linear growth, although, the correlation between glycemic control and skeletal maturation is unreliable. Cortisol excess, regardless of its etiology, has a profound effect on skeletal growth *(22)* and will result in short stature. Children with cortisol excess, or Cushing's syndrome, have poor linear growth velocity, delayed bone age, and typical cushingoid features, which include truncal obesity, purple striae, thin skin, proximal muscle weakness, increased dorsal fat pad, and moon facies. Ultimate height can be compromised, even after the source of excess cortisol is removed. Children with untreated precocious puberty may be short as adults, compared to their target height, secondary to advancement of skeletal maturation. The rapid growth of these children during childhood is thus counterbalanced by premature epiphyseal fusion and compromised adult heights.

Constitutional growth delay (CGD) is another common cause of short stature. It is considered a variant of normal growth, and is characterized by constitutional slow growth with delayed puberty and adolescence. It is seen more often in boys than girls and there is often a positive family history. These children have a delayed onset of puberty and, therefore, a late adolescent growth spurt, but eventually achieve normal adult heights.

GH deficiency is a category that has undergone considerable changes in recent years due to advances in IGF research. An alternative method for approaching the diagnostic category of growth hormone deficiency is through re-evaluation under the new category of "IGF deficiency." This category can be further subdivided into IGF deficiency resulting from hypothalamic dysfunction, pituitary growth hormone deficiency, or growth hormone insensitivity. The clinical diagnosis of IGF-I deficiency will be discussed later in this chapter.

DIAGNOSIS OF GROWTH HORMONE DEFICIENCY

The diagnosis of growth hormone deficiency (GHD) continues to be a controversial area. Nevertheless, it is clear that the foundation for diagnosis must be subnormal growth velocity for age. Testing of growth hormone (GH) secretion is not necessary in a child who displays a normal growth pattern in the absence of associated pituitary dysfunction or underlying chronic disorder. A child who undergoes growth deceleration, even if remaining within the normal growth curve, warrants further evaluation, however.

Random serum growth hormone levels are unreliable in the diagnosis of GHD owing to the episodic nature of GH secretion. Between pulses, GH levels are typically below the sensitivity of most conventional assays. Provocative (stimulated) GH tests have been the hallmark of diagnostic procedures for assessing GHD for the past 30 yr. Both physiological stimuli (including sleep, fasting, and exercise) and pharmacological stimuli (including clonidine, L-dopa, propranolol, insulin, arginine, and glucagon) have been used. No single provocative test has been able to unfailingly identify children with GHD. Variables that are known to falsely lower GH levels include hypothyroidism, obesity, cortisol excess, oral carbohydrate load, and emotional disorders. Approximately 10% of normal short children have subnormal GH levels in response to a single stimulus. Thus, to improve specificity, two provocative tests *(23–25)* are often administered in combination. Although the stimulation tests remain the backbone to the diagnosis of GHD, several limitations exist, prompting further searches for improved screening methods *(26)*. First, the cutoff point for distinguishing GH-deficient states is largely arbitrary and has gradually climbed to 10 ng/mL. Values of 7–10 ng/mL are often referred to as partial GHD, if observed in combination with growth failure. No definitive data exist to support these cutoff levels. Second, wide variability exists in the assays used for the measurement of GH levels *(27)*. Heterogeneity of circulating GH, differences in GH standards, and use of monoclonal vs polyclonal antibodies all play a part in the discrepancies seen. Third, the provocative tests do not satisfactorily mimic the normal GH secretory pattern and a child who responds normally to pharmacological stimuli may still not secrete GH normally on a daily basis *(28)*. Fourth, GH responsiveness to provocative stimuli is age dependent and is increased after administration of estrogens or androgens *(29)*. Priming with sex steroids prior to a GH stimulation test is not universally done and it has been shown that without sex steroid pretreatment, 61% of normal prepubertal children will fail to raise their GH level above 7 ng/mL *(30)*. Fifth, provocative GH tests are poorly reproduced and have limited ability to diagnose children with partial GHD. Finally, many of the GH tests require multiple sequential blood draws and are uncomfortable and not totally risk free. The procedures are expensive and virtually all of the pharmacological agents used have adverse effects, including nausea, hypotension, and insulin-induced hypoglycemia.

Despite these limitations, no universally accepted "gold standard" has been identified to replace provocative tests. An alternative approach would be to include an evaluation of key components of the GH-IGF axis in conjunction with accurate documentation of growth velocity to identify children with GH or IGF-I deficiency.

Serum levels of the GH-dependent peptide, IGF-I, appear to accurately reflect the GH status of the patient *(29)*. IGF-I levels are influenced by the pubertal and nutritional status of the patient, as well as the age. Other chronic disorders, such as hypothyroidism, diabetes, and renal failure may be associated with a reduction in IGF-I levels. When IGF-II levels were measured in addition to IGF-I concentrations, there was improved correlation with GH-status *(32)*. The measurement of IGFBP-3, the major serum carrier protein for IGF-I and II peptides, reflects the circulating serum levels of both of these peptides, and is of great promise in identifying children with GHD and IGF deficiency. It is less nutritionally dependent and varies only modestly with age. Although recent research of the various components of the GH-IGF axis is promising, the measurements of these elements do not correlate perfectly with established provocative GH testing. This may more reflect the discrepancies in direct GH secretion testing, than limitations of the IGF/IGFBP assays. The role of direct GH measurements remains important for the identification of impaired hypothalamic-pituitary function. This information would eliminate GH insensitivity as the etiology of poor growth and be helpful in interpreting the overall clinical picture of the patient. Clinical evaluation remains the most important and useful parameter in assessing the child with growth failure. When coupled with appropriate measures of the IGF axis, this provides an effective way to evaluate the GH status of a patient with short stature. An algorithm incorporating both provocative GH testing and evaluation of GH-IGF axis is illustrated in Fig. 6.

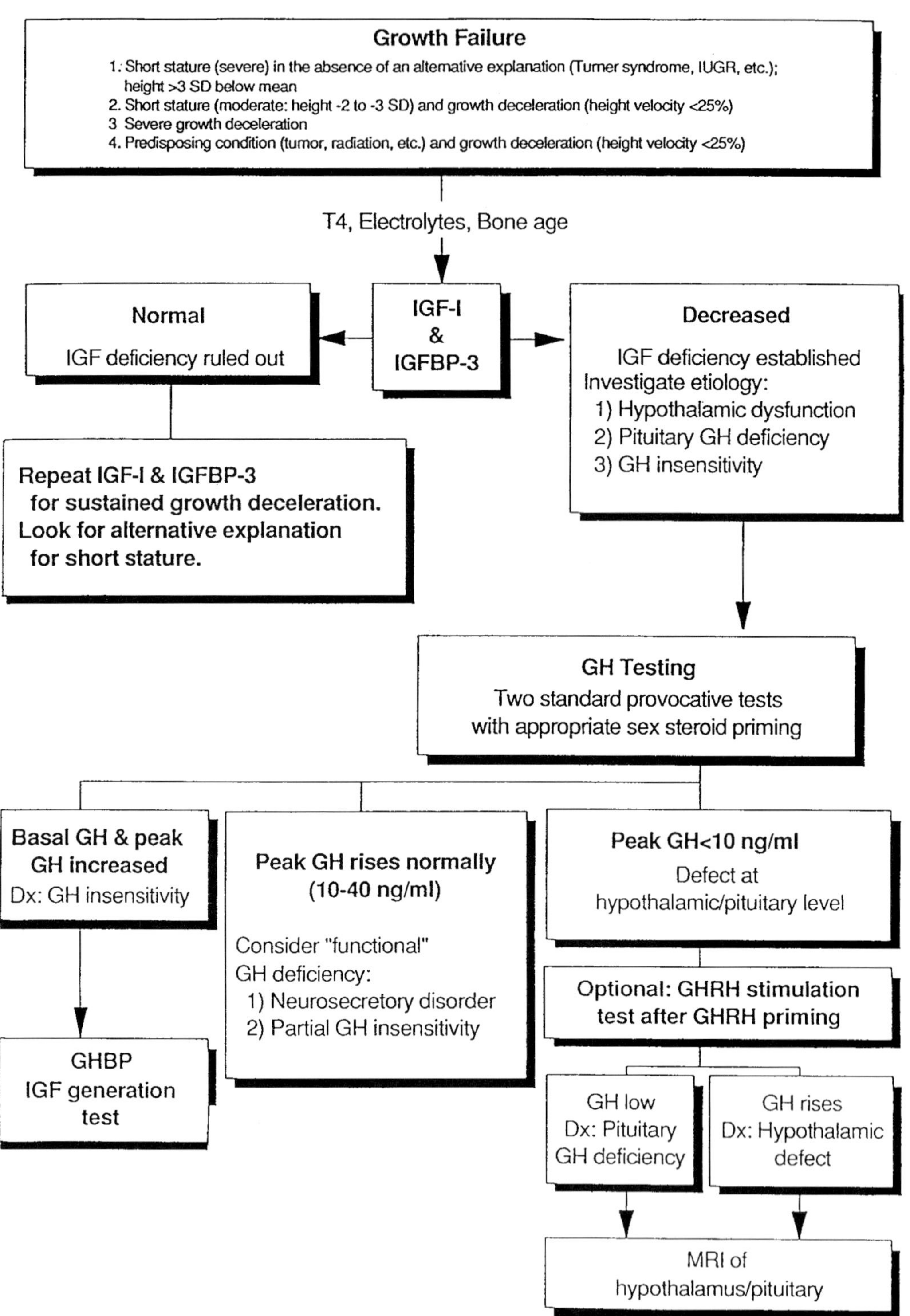

Fig. 6. Biochemical evaluation of growth failure: algorithm.

IGF DEFICIENCY

Given the difficulties inherent to establishing a diagnosis of GHD, it may be preferable to consider the diagnostic category of IGF defiency. The clinical presentation and etiology of IGF-I deficiency is varied, although growth failure remains the consistent finding. Deficiency of IGF-I may result from hypothalamic dysfunction, pituitary GH deficiency, or GH insensitivity (Table 1). It is not always possible, however, to easily differentiate between hypothalamic and pituitary dysfunction. IGF-I deficiency can also be divided into a congenital or acquired deficit (primary or secondary defects).

Hypothalamic dysfunction may be due to a decreased or abnormal production of several hypothalamic factors that normally act to stimulate GH secretion from the anterior pituitary. These include GHRH, pituitary adenyl cyclase activating peptide (PACAP), galanin, and Pit-1 (GHF-I). Pit-1 is a member of a large group of transcription factors termed POU-domain proteins, that regulate the expression of GH, prolactin, and TSH genes *(33)*. Mutations in the Pit-1 gene have been identified in patients with hypopituitarism *(34)*.

Congenital malformations associated with hypothalamic dysfunction include anencephaly, holoprosencephaly, and schizencephaly. De Morsier's syndrome, or septo-optic dysplasia, is associated with abnormalities of the septum pellucidum and/or corpus callosum, optic nerve hypoplasia, and frequently, hypothalamic insufficiency. Many pathological processes may involve both the hypothalamus and pituitary. Trauma to the brain due to child abuse or birth injury; inflammation resulting from bacterial, viral or fungal infections; and tumors of the central nervous system can result in hypothalamic deficiency. The risk of deficiency is especially high in midline defects, such as meningiomas, germinomas, and optic nerve gliomas. Cranial irradiation may directly impair function of the hypothalamus and/or pituitary, resulting in subnormal GH secretion. Younger children are at greater risk for radiation-induced GH deficiency.

IGF-I deficiency can also occur owing to defects in pituitary function. These include "idiopathic" GH deficiency, pituitary dysplasia, and certain forms of familial GH deficiency. Up to 30% of children with pituitary GH deficiency have been reported to have an affected family member. Four familial forms of isolated GHD have been reported, with varying degrees of severity and modes of transmission (autosomal recessive, autosomal dominant, and X-linked). Familial hypopituitarism owing to defects in the Pit-1 gene have also been identified. Congenital absence or hypoplasia of the pituitary, trauma, inflammation, irradiation, and surgery can also result in pituitary dysfunction. Tumors that affect hypothalamic function may also affect the pituitary. Craniopharyngiomas arise from remnants of Rathke's pouch, which gives rise to cells located at the junction of the adeno- and neurohypophysis. Most children present with symptoms of increased intracranial pressure, such as headache and visual disturbances. Infiltrating disorders such as histiocytosis X, psychosocial dwarfism, and GH neurosecretory dysfunction may all lead to IGF-I deficiency.

Primary GH insensitivity, classically known as Laron syndrome, describes patients who appear to have GH deficiency, with decreased levels of IGF-I, IGF-II, and IGFBP-3, but display normal or elevated serum GH levels. Abnormalities of the GH receptor, postreceptor signaling defects, and defects in IGF-I biosynthesis all result in primary GH insensitivity. Secondary causes of GH insensitivity include acquired conditions, such as antibodies to circulating GH or to its receptor, malnutrition, and liver disease.

The clinical features of IGF-I deficiency are similar regardless of where the defect occurs. Mild variation in presentation occurs based on whether the defect is congenital or acquired or if it is isolated or associated with other abnormalities. Children with deficiency of IGF-I production are near-normal size at birth. Children with congenital deficiency may present in the neonatal period with hypoglycemia, microphallus, cryptorchidism, and prolonged jaundice. Postnatal growth deviates from normal during infancy and childhood. Body proportions are typically in line with skeletal age, which is delayed. Classically, GH deficient children have an increased weight/height ratio, "cherubic" or "doll-like" appearance, high pitched voices resulting from hypoplasia of the larynx, and immature facial appearance. The skull tends to grow at a normal rate compared to the facial bones, leading to the appearance of hydrocephalus. Children with acquired IGF-I deficiency tend to exhibit features of the primary underlying defect combined with growth failure.

Therapy

Treatment of growth disorders is dependent on the cause. Growth failure owing to a chronic disease, such as malabsorption, poorly controlled insulin-dependent diabetes mellitus, or cystic fibrosis, requires treatment directed at improving the underlying condition. Hypothyroidism, Cushing's syndrome, rickets, and pseudohypoparathyroidism should all be treated based on the specific hormonal defect. Constitutional growth delay is a normal variant of growth that requires only reassurance and yearly follow-up. However, there are cases of constitutional delay where short stature and delayed pubertal maturation may be psychologically disabling *(35)*. In males with poor self-image owing to the stigmata of growth delay, a short course of depot testosterone enanthate, 100–200 mg im every 3–4 wk for a total of four injections, will usually "jump-start" patients into puberty. Secondary sex characteristics together with accelerated growth are typically seen by the fourth injection. In girls with constitutional growth delay who desire treatment, a short-term course of estrogen therapy can be employed. Chronic use of either androgens or estrogens is to be avoided, however, since it will promote epiphyseal fusion.

Recombinant human GH (hGH) is the treatment of choice in children with GH deficiency. Current recommended doses range from 0.025–0.05 mg/kg/d sc. Alternatively, the same total weekly dose may be given as a 3 or 6 d/wk schedule. The greatest effect of GH therapy is generally seen in the first year of treatment. A child, on average, accelerates from a pretreatment growth rate of 3–4 cm/yr to 10–12 cm/yr on therapy. In years 2 and 3 of treatment, growth remains at approximately 7–9 cm/yr *(36)*. The GH therapy in GH deficient patients increases muscle mass and reduces adipose tissue, in addition to promoting growth. Treatment of any other associated pituitary deficiency should also be addressed.

The following possibilities must be considered in situations of poor clinical response to hGH therapy: poor compliance, improper measurement of dosage, incorrect injection technique, subclinical hypothyroidism, underlying chronic disease, spinal irradiation, epiphyseal fusion, incorrect diagnosis of GH deficiency, and, rarely, the development of anti-GH antibodies. Obtaining optimal final adult height is dependent on early diagnosis and treatment, combined with careful follow-up. In the past, children received GH treatment until epiphyseal fusion and/or the beneficial growth promoting effects were no longer seen. Recently, studies of adults with GH deficiency have found that these individuals have increased cardiovascular risk *(37)*, increased body fat, increased cholesterol, decreased lean body mass, and reduced bone mineral density. Adult GH-deficient patients also had impaired quality of life and reduced energy and vitality. Several current hGH trials in adults have noted improved emotional well-being, enhanced exercise tolerance and muscle mass, and reduction in fat distribution and serum lipids. Whether it will be optimal to continue hGH therapy after the cessation of growth remains under investigation.

Recombinant hGH therapy has been accepted for growth disorders other than IGF-I or GH deficiency. Children with chronic renal failure and girls with Turner syndrome benefit from receiving GH therapy. In Turner syndrome, treatment with hGH accelerates growth, although not to the degree observed in GHD, and results in an 8–10 cm improvement in mean final height. Multiple studies are currently looking at the growth promoting effects of GH therapy in other disorders, such as Down syndrome, IUGR, the osteochondrodysplasias, and normal short children. The anabolic effects of GH are being investigated in several catabolic states, such as burns, AIDS, and tumor cachexia. Approval and wide acceptance of GH therapy in the above disease states remains to be determined.

Recombinant hGH has eliminated the risk of Creutzfeldt-Jacob disease *(38)*, which was associated with cadaveric pituitary GH use. Currently, serious side-effects appear relatively uncommon and extensive research with recombinant GH is encouraging. Adverse effects include glucose intolerance, diabetes, pancreatitis, pseudotumor cerebri, gynecomastia, slipped capital femoral epiphysis, allergic reactions, lipoatrophy at injection sites, and formation of antibodies to GH *(39)*. The increased risk of leukemia has been a concern after cases of leukemia associated with GH therapy were reported in Japan *(40)*. Extensive research in the United States has suggested a possible small increase, at most, in leukemia among GH recipients who have received chemotherapy or irradiation. Several cases of leukemia have occurred in untreated GH-deficient patients, however, suggesting that GH deficiency, by itself, may be a risk factor in the development of leukemia. This issue should be discussed with all patients prior to receiving GH therapy. All patients receiving GH should be carefully monitored for side-effects throughout the time of therapy.

Recombinant IGF peptides have now been available for clinical trials. Initial studies noted hypoglycemia to occur after an iv injection of IGF-I to healthy male subjects *(41)*. Subsequent studies using sc IGF-I in GH receptor-deficient (GHRD) patients at a dose of 150 mcg/kg/d resulted in no symptomatic hypoglycemia *(42)*. Laron et al. *(43)* reported acceleration of growth in response to IGF-I therapy. Several recent studies *(44–46)* have continued to note a good growth promoting response to IGF-I therapy despite the lack of elevation in IGFBP-3 levels after IGF-I administration. Adverse effects with this treatment include hypoglycemia, seizures, headache, and papilledema, and possible pseudotumor cerebri. The long-term anabolic effects, optimal dosing, and frequency of injection are still being investigated. These recent studies have established the groundwork for possible therapeutic uses of IGF peptides in multiple conditions of growth failure, catabolic states, aging, and diabetes mellitus.

FUTURE DIRECTIONS

With the recent advancements in the field of insulin-like growth factors, alternative methods for both diagnosing and categorizing children with GH deficiency (or IGF deficiency) are becoming available. Appropriate measures of the IGF axis, combined with auxological criteria for growth failure, may become more important in the diagnosis of IGF-deficient patients, as the limitations of provocative GH testing become more apparent. Clinical evaluation and careful auxological measurements remain the foundation for the diagnosis of growth disorders, such as IGF deficiency.

REFERENCES

1. Whitehouse RH, Tanner JM, Healy MJR. Diurnal variation in stature and sitting height in 12–14 year old boys. Ann Hum Biol 1974; 1:103–106.
2. Greulich WW, Pyle SI. Radiographic Atlas of Skeletal Development of the Hand and Wrist. 2nd ed. Stanford University Press, Stanford, CA, 1959.
3. Bayley N, Pinneau SR. Tables for predicting adult height from skeletal age: revised for use with the Greulich-Pyle hand standards. J Pediatr 1952; 40:423–441.
4. Ho KY, Evans WS, Blizzard RM, et al. Effects of sex and age on the 24-hour profile of growth hormone secretion in man: importance of endogenous estradiol concentrations. J Clin Endocrinol Metab 1987; 64:51–58.
5. Carlsson LMS, Attie KM, Compton PG, et al. Reduced concentrations of serum GHBP in children with idiopathic short stature. J Clin Endocrinol Metab 1994; 78:1325–1330.
6. Salmon WD Jr, Daughaday WH. A hormonally controlled serum factor which stimulates sulfate incorporation by cartilage in vitro. J Lab Clin Med 1957; 49:825–836.
7. Rinderknecht E, Humbel RE. The amino sequence of human insulin-like growth factor I and its structural homology with proinsulin. J Biol Chem 1978; 253:2769–2776.
8. Rinderknecht E, Humbel RE. Primary structure of human insulin-like growth factor II. FEBS Lett 1978; 89:283–286.
9. Brissenden JE, Ullrich A, Francke U. Human chromosomal mapping of genes for insulin-like growth factors I and II and epidermal growth factor. Nature 1984; 310:781–784.
10. Tricoli JV, Rall LB, Scott J, et al. Localization of human insulin-like growth factor genes to human chromosomes 11 and 12. Nature 1984; 310:784–785.
11. Luna AM, Wilson DM, Wibbelsman CJ, et al. Somatomedins in adolescence: a cross-sectional study of the effect of puberty on plasma insulin-like growth factor I and II Levels. J Clin Endocrinol Metab 1983; 57:258–271.
12. Hintz RL, Liu F. A radioimmunoassay for insulin-like growth factor-II specific for the C-peptide region. J Clin Endocrinol Metab 1982; 54:442–446.
13. Massague J, Czech MP. The subunit structures of two distinct receptors for insulin-like growth factors I and II and their relationship to the insulin receptor. J Biol Chem 1982; 257:5038–5045.
14. Rosenfeld RG, Hintz RL. Somatomedin receptors: structure, function and regulation. In: Conn M, ed. The Receptors. Academic, New York, 1986; pp. 281–329.
15. MacDonald R, Pfeffer SR, Coussens L, et al. A single receptor binds both insulin-like growth factor II and mannose-6-phosphate. Science 1988; 239:1134–1137.
16. Rosenfeld RG, Conover CA, Hodges D, et al. Heterogeneity of insulin-like growth factor-I affinity for the insulin-like growth factor-II receptor: comparisonm of natural, synthetic and recombinant DNA derived insulin-like growth factor I. Biochem Biophys Res Commum 1987; 143:195–205.
17. Cohen P, Rosenfeld RG. Physiologic and clinical relevance of the insulin-like growth factor binding proteins (review). Cur Opinion Peds 1994; 6:462–467.
18. Martin GL, Baxter RC. Insulin-like growth factor binding protein from human plasma. Purification and characterization. J Biol Chem 1986; 261:8754–8760.
19. Baxter RC. Characterization of the acid-labile subunit of the growth hormone-dependent insulin-like growth factor binding howmone complex. J Clin Endocrinol Metab 1988; 67:265–272.
20. Spranger J. International classification of osteochondrodysplasias. Eur J Pediatr 1992; 151:407–415.

21. Rivkees SA, Bode HH, Crawford JD. Long-term growth in juvenile acquired hypothyroidism. N Engl J Med 1988; 318:599–602.
22. Magiakou MA, Mastorakos G, Oldfield EH, et al. Cushing's syndrome in children and adolescents. Presentation, diagnosis and therapy. N Engl J Med 1994; 331:629–636.
23. Katz HP, Youlton R, Kaplan SL, et al. Growth and growth hormone. III. Growth hormone release in children with primary hypothyroidism and thyrotoxicosis. J Clin Endocrinol Metab 1969; 29:346.
24. Fratz AG, Rabkin MT. Human growth hormone. Clinical measurement, response to hypoglycemia and suppression by corticosteroids. N Engl J Med 1964; 271:1375.
25. Thompson RG, Rodriguez A, Kowarski A, et al. Growth hormone: metabolic clearance rates in normal adults and effect of prednisone. J Clin Invest 1972; 51:3193–3199.
26. Rosenfeld RG, Albertsson-Wikland K, Cassorla F, et al. Diagnostic Controversy: The diagnosis of childhood growth hormone deficiency revisited. J Clin Endocrinol Metab 1995; 80:1532–1540.
27. Reiter EO, Morris AH, MacGillivray MH, et al. Variable estimates of serum growth hormone concentrations by different radioassay systems. J Clin Endocrinol Metab 1988; 66:68–71.
28. Spiliotis BE, August GP, Hung W, et al. Growth neurosecretory dysfunction : a treatable cause of short stature. JAMA 1984; 252:2223–2230.
29. Deller, Jr JJ, Boulis MW, Hariss WE, et al. Growth hormone response patterns to sex hormone administration in growth retardation. Am J Med Sci. 1970; 259:292–296.
30. Marin G, Domene HM, Barnes KM, et al. The effects of estrogen priming and puberty on the growth hormone response to standardized treadmill exercise and arginine-insulin in normal girls and boys. J Clin Endocrinol Metab 1994; 79:537–541.
31. Underwood LE, D'Ercole AJ, Van Wyk JJ. Somatomedin-C and the assessment of growth. Pediatric Clin North Am. 1980; 27:771–782.
32. Rosenfeld RG, Wilson DM, Lee PDK, et al. Insulin-like growth factors I and II in evaluation of growth retardation. J Pediatr. 1986; 109:428–433.
33. Magalam HJ, Albert VR, Ingraham HA, et al. A pituitary POU domain protein, pit-1, activates both growth hormone and prolactin promoters transcriptionally. Genes Dev 1989; 3:946–958.
34. Pfaffle RW, DiMattia E, Parks JS, et al. Mutations of the POU-specific domain of Pit-1 and hypopituitarism without pituitary hypoplasia. Science 1992; 257:1118–1121.
35. Rosenfeld RG, Northcraft GB, Hintz RL. A prospective, randomized trial of testosterone treatment of constitutional short stature in adolescent males. Pediatrics 1982; 69:681–687.
36. Frasier SD. Human pituitary growth hormone (hGH) therapy in growth hormone deficiency. Endocr Rev 1983; 4:155–170.
37. Rosen T, Bengtsson BA. Premature mortality due to cardiovascular disease in hypopituitarism. Lancet 1990; 336:285–288.
38. Fradkin JE. Creutzfeldt-Jacob disease in pituitary growth hormone recipients. Endocrinologist 1993; 3:108–114.
39. Hintz RL. Untoward events in patients treated with growth hormone in the USA. Horm Res 1992; 38(suppl 1):44–49.
40. Fisher DA, Job JC, Preece M, et al. Leukemia in patients treated with growth hormone. Lancet 1988; 1:1159–1160.
41. Guler HP, Schmid C, Zapf J, et al. Effects of recombinant insulin-like growth factor-I on insulin secretion and renal function in normal human subjects. Proc Natl Acad Sci USA 1989; 86:2868–2872.
42. Laron Z, Klinger B, Jensen JT, et al. Biochemical and hormonal changes induced by one week of administration of rIGF-I to patients with Laron type dwarfism. Clin Endocrinol (Oxf) 1991; 35:145–150.
43. Laron Z, Anin S, Klipper-Auerbach Y, et al. Effects of insulin-like growth factor-I on linear growth, head circumference, and body fat in patients with Laron-type dwarfism. Lancet 1992; 339:1258–1261.
44. Walker J, Van Wyk JJ, Underwood LE. Stimulation of statural growth by recombinant insulin-like growth factor-I in a child with growth hormone insensitivity syndrome (Laron type). J Pediatr 1992; 121:641–646.
45. Savage MO, Wilton P, Ranke MB, et al. Therapeutic response to recombinant IGF-I in thirty-two patients with growth hormone insensitivity. Pediatr Res 1993; 33:S5 (abstract).
46. Guevara-Aguirre J, Vasconez O, Martinez V, et al. A randomized, doulbe-blind, placebo controlled trial on safety and efficacy of recombinant human insulin-like growth factor-I in children with growth hormone receptor deficiency. J ClinEndocrinol Metab 1995; 80(4):1393–1398.

7 Acromegaly

Differential Diagnosis and Treatment

Ilan Shimon, MD
and Shlomo Melmed, MD

Contents

INTRODUCTION

Acromegaly, a clinical syndrome of acral enlargement and metabolic disturbances, is usually caused by the autonomous secretion of growth hormone (GH) by a monoclonal pituitary adenoma. Elevated GH and insulin-like growth factor-I (IGF-I) levels, if left untreated, lead to disfigurement, severe morbidity, and increased mortality. Early diagnosis and aggressive treatment will ameliorate or reverse symptoms and improve patient outcome.

ETIOLOGY

Most patients with acromegaly have a GH secreting pituitary adenoma (Table 1). Pure somatotrope tumors exclusively producing GH account for 60% of these cases. These tumors contain either dense or sparse cytoplasmic GH granules. The former tumors grow slowly with insidious clinical progression, whereas sparsely granulated adenomas are rapidly growing and often locally invasive. Mixed GH-cell and prolactin (PRL)-cell adenomas (25%) consist of two different cell populations *(1)*, leading to acromegaly with moderately elevated serum PRL levels. In contrast, monomorphous mammosomatotrope cell adenomas are composed of a single mature cell expressing both GH and PRL. Acidophil stem cell adenomas consist of one cell type derived from the common immature precursor of GH and PRL cells, are often rapidly growing and

From: *Contemporary Endocrinology, Vol. 3: Diseases of the Pituitary: Diagnosis and Treatment*
Edited by M. E. Wierman Humana Press Inc., Totowa, NJ

Table 1
Etiology of Acromegaly

Excess GH secretion
Pituitary (98%)
Densely or sparsely granulated GH-cell adenoma (60%)
Mixed GH-cell and PRL-cell adenoma (25%)
Mammosomatotrope cell adenoma (10%)
Plurihormonal adenoma
GH-cell carcinoma
Multiple endocrine neoplasia-I (GH-cell adenoma)
McCune-Albright syndrome (rarely, adenoma)
Ectopic sphenoid or parapharyngeal sinus pituitary adenoma
Extrapituitary tumor
Pancreatic islet-cell tumor (one case)
Excess GHRH Secretion (Somatotrope Hyperplasia)
Central-eutopic (<1%)
Hypothalamic hamartoma, choristoma, glioma, ganglioneuroma
Peripheral-ectopic (1%)
Bronchial carcinoid, pancreatic islet-cell tumor, small-cell lung cancer, adrenal adenoma, medullary thyroid carcinoma, pheochromocytoma
Excess growth factor activity
Acromegaloidism (very rare)

Adapted with permission from ref. *27*.

invasive tumors. However, hyperprolactinemia rather than acromegaly is the predominant feature in patients with this primitive tumor. Clinical features of acromegaly are common in patients with plurihormonal tumors, which express GH with any combination of PRL, thyroid-stimulating hormone (TSH), adrenocorticotrophic hormone (ACTH), or α-subunit *(2)*. In addition to GH oversecretion, other pituitary hormones may be elevated in these patients. The GH-cell pituitary adenoma causing acromegaly is a component of the autosomal dominant multiple endocrine neoplasia I (MEN-I) syndrome, and acromegaly occurring in association with the sporadic McCune-Albright syndrome is usually the result of somatotrope hyperplasia, but somatotrope adenomas have been reported in some patients *(3)*. Rare cases of acromegaly are caused by ectopic GH-cell adenoma arising in the sphenoid or parapharyngeal sinuses *(4)*. GH-cell pituitary carcinomas are exceedingly rare, aggressive, and rapidly growing tumors *(5–7)*. Malignancy is only diagnosed with well-documented extracranial metastasis, and rarely acromegaly is caused by functional metastatic tumor tissue *(7)*.

A GH secreting pancreatic islet-cell tumor with clinical evidence of acromegaly, GH gene expression by the tumor tissue, marked arteriovenous gradient in GH levels across the tumor, and a rapid fall of GH and IGF-I after tumor resection has been documented in a single patient *(8)*. In contrast to this ectopic GH secreting tumor, in other tumors, including bronchial carcinoids, and lung, breast, and gastric carcinomas, GH immunoreactivity is expressed without evidence of acromegaly or clinically excessive GH secretion.

Somatotrope hyperplasia is usually associated with acromegaly resulting from pituitary stimulation by ectopic growth hormone releasing hormone (GHRH) secreting tumors. This rare cause of acromegaly, indistinguishable clinically, and difficult to differentiate histologically from a GH-cell pituitary adenoma, has been reported in patients with carcinoid tumors *(9)*, pancreatic islet-cell tumors *(10)*, small-cell lung cancers, adrenal adenomas, and pheocromocytomas. Growth hormone releasing hormone with reduced biologic activity may also be secreted by these ectopic tumors. Eutopic hypothalamic GHRH secreting tumors, including hamartomas, choristomas, gliomas, and ganglioneuromas are also rarely associated with pituitary somatotrope hyperplasia or adenoma and GH hypersecretion *(11,12)*.

Acromegaloidism is a condition characterized by clearly acromegalic features without demonstrable pituitary or extrapituitary tumor or elevated GH and IGF-I levels. Some of these patients produce a circulating erythroprogenitor growth factor, distinct from other growth factors *(13)*, which may be demonstrated by bioassay.

CLINICAL MANIFESTATIONS (TABLE 2)

Acromegaly frequency is similar in both sexes, and the mean age at diagnosis is 40–45 yr. Symptoms usually progress slowly, and the delay until diagnosis is approximately 7–10 yr *(14)*. About 25% of acromegalic patients harbor microadenomas (<10 mm), whereas most patients have macroadenomas when first diagnosed, many with parasellar or suprasellar invasion *(15)*. Headaches, reported in more than half of patients, hypopituitarism, and visual field defects occurring secondary to the expanding tumor mass correlate well with tumor size. Cosecretion of PRL with GH by the tumor cells results in hyperprolactinemia in 30% of patients. Amenorrhea or impotence are common, and galactorrhea may be diagnosed even in patients with normal PRL levels, as elevated GH may act as an agonist for breast PRL receptors. Moreover, hyperprolactinemia may result from pituitary stalk compression by large somatotrope adenomas.

The most common sign, acral and soft tissue overgrowth, occurs in virtually all acromegalic patients. Increased hand, feet, and heel pad thickness results in increased shoe and glove size, and ring tightening. Characteristic coarse facial features include mandibular enlargement with prognathism, frontal bossing, large fleshy nose, and wide spacing of the lower teeth. Degenerative arthropathy, involving the knee and other peripheral joints, back pain, and kyphosis occur in half of patients. Voice deepening, carpal tunnel syndrome, proximal muscle weakness and fatigue, oily skin, hyperhidrosis, acanthosis nigricans, skin tags, and affective disorders are also components of the clinical syndrome. Generalized visceromegaly with enlargement of soft organs, including the tongue, thyroid, and salivary glands occur commonly.

Rarely, GH hypersecretion is associated with pituitary gigantism, when the disease preceeds epiphyseal closure of the long bones in children. Upper airway obstruction and sleep apnea may be diagnosed in half of patients, but these patients do not have higher GH and IGF-I levels. Central sleep apnea is encountered in 20% of patients who have significantly increased hormone levels compared to those with obstructive sleep apnea *(16)*.

Cardiovascular disease, a major determinant of mortality and morbidity, includes left ventricular hypertrophy, diastolic dysfunction, arrhythmias, and ischemic heart disease. Hypertension, commonly diagnosed, also contributes to cardiomyopathic changes.

Table 2
Risks of Long-Term Exposure to Elevated GH

1. Musculoskeletal involvement
   - Unrelated to age of onset or to GH levels
   - Usually occurs with long duration
   - Reversibility
     - Rapid symptomatic improvement of acral enlargement and arthralgia
     - Irreversibility of bone and cartilage lesions
2. Neuropathy
   - Peripheral nerves: intermittent anesthesia, paresthesias, sensorimotor polyneuropathy
   - Reversibility
     - Onion bulbs (whorls) do not regress
3. Cardiovascular disease
   - Cardiomyopathy: Increased LV mass, LV diastolic dysfunction, arrhythmias
   - Hypertension: exacerbates cardiomyopathy
   - Reversibility
     - Rapid decrease of LV mass, hypertension usually does not regress
4. Respiratory disease
   - Upper airway obstruction: soft tissue overgrowth
   - Central sleep apnea
   - Reversibility
     - Responds to treatment, even when biochemical cure is not achieved
5. Malignancy
   - Increased risk of gastrointestinal cancer
   - Increased risk of soft tissue polyps (colon, skin tags)
   - Reversibility
     - Effect of therapy on risk unknown
6. Carbohydrate intolerance
   - 50%: glucose intolerance, 25%: diabetes, family history
   - Reversibility
     - Rapid improvement with reduced GH

Adapted with permission from ref. *31*.

Metabolic disturbances including glucose intolerance, hypertriglyceridemia or hypercalciuria are also found frequently. One-fourth of acromegalic patients have frank diabetes, often associated with a family history of glucose intolerance.

Acromegaly is associated with increased risk of gastrointestinal polyps and cancer (Table 3). The GH-IGF-I axis involvement in normal and disordered regulation of cellular proliferation contributes to this phenomenon. Premalignant adenomatous colonic polyps are identified by colonoscopy in 30% of patients *(17,18)*, and approximately 10% develop malignant tumors, including adenocarcinomas of the colon, stomach, esophagus, and melanoma *(19,20)*.

Increased overall mortality in acromegaly, about two to three times higher than normal *(14,21)*, is primarily associated with cardiovascular and cerebrovascular disorders, malignancy, and respiratory disease (Table 4). Reduced survival (by 10 yr on average) is significantly correlated with higher GH levels, and the presence at diagnosis of cardiovascular disease, hypertension, or diabetes mellitus *(22*; Table 4).

Table 3
Common Cancers Occurring in 1041 Acromegalic Male Patients with no Evidence for Cancer at Diagnosis

Cancer	*Observed (n)*	*Expected (n)*	*O/E*	*95% CI*
All	116	72	1.6	1.3–1.9
Colon	13	4.2	3.1	1.7–5.1
Esophagus	7	2.3	3.1	1.3–6.0
Stomach	4	1.6	2.5	0.8–6.0
Melanoma	3	0.9	3.3	0.7–9.7

Adapted with permission from ref. *20*.

Table 4
Acromegaly: Survival Determinants

Survival determinants[a]	
Last known GH	$p < 0.0001$
Hypertension	$p < 0.02$
Cardiac disease	$p < 0.03$
Diabetes mellitus	$p < 0.03$
Symptom duration	$p < 0.04$
Causes of death[b]	
Cardiovascular	38–62%
Respiratory	0–25%
Malignancy	9–25%

[a]Adapted with permission from ref. *22*.
[b]Based on refs. *15,21,22*, and *34*.

DIAGNOSIS

The biochemical diagnosis of acromegaly is established by demonstrating excessive GH and IGF-I secretion with failure to suppress circulating GH levels by glucose loading.

Random GH Levels

Random GH measurement is not recommended as a criterion for the diagnosis or exclusion of acromegaly, and correlates poorly with disease activity. The pulsatile nature of pituitary GH secretion, and its relatively short serum half-life (approximately 20 min) decrease its cost effectiveness for screening, and integrated measurements over time (at least every 20 min) are more accurate, but expensive. In addition, uncontrolled diabetes, malnutrition, renal failure, and states of physical and emotional stress may enhance random GH levels. When GH is sampled every 5 min in healthy subjects, levels are undetectable in about half of samples, whereas in acromegaly, all samples collected over 24 h contain detectable GH levels (> 2 μg/L) *(23)*. Although most laboratories consider 5 μg/L (by RIA) the upper limit of random GH levels in the normal population, this criterion is not acceptable today. Normal subjects have basal GH values of <1 μg/L, below the sensitivity of most RIAs, and only the new sensitive GH immunoradiometric assays (IRMA), employing two MAbs, detect these levels, and indicate normal integrated GH levels to be < 0.5 μg/L.

IGF-I Levels

In contrast to GH, IGF-I clearance from the circulation takes hours (half-life of 12 h in association with insulin-like growth factor binding protein 3 [IGFBP-3]), and its levels do not fluctuate significantly during the course of the day and are not affected by physical exercise or stress. Serum IGF-I levels are invariably high in acromegaly *(24)*, correlate well with 24-h GH secretion, and correlate better with the clinical manifestations of hypersomatotropism than single random GH measurements *(25,26)*. Therefore, single elevated IGF-I levels, measured by a commercial RIA, are highly specific for diagnosing acromegaly, and may help in monitoring the progress of therapy. IGF-I levels are affected by nutritional status, age (values are normally low in infants and elderly subjects, and elevated in late puberty), and estrogens (pregnancy is often associated with high levels).

Oral Glucose Tolerance Test (OGTT)

This dynamic test establishes the diagnosis of active acromegaly when morning oral glucose load (50–100 g; after overnight fasting) fails to suppress GH levels to <1 μg/L during 1–2 h. Some acromegalic patients may even have a paradoxic GH rise after 30–60 min *(27)*. This classic suppression test is also useful in monitoring long-term response to therapy.

Thyrotropin Releasing Hormone (TRH) Test

In 50% of patients iv TRH (200–500 μg) increases GH levels, unlike normal subjects who have no GH response *(28)*. GH response to TRH may also indicate the continued presence of adenomatous tissue after unsuccessful transsphenoidal surgery. However, this test is not specific, as TRH may also stimulate GH release in renal failure, liver disease, and depression, and is therefore rarely used to establish the diagnosis of acromegaly.

IGFBPs

IGFBP-3 levels are significantly elevated in acromegaly, even in patients with normal GH suppression to glucose *(29)*, and correlate well with IGF-I levels. IGFBP-I levels are low in acromegaly, are inversely correlated with GH levels, and may in the future become useful in determining responses to therapy *(30)*. However, using these binding proteins as accurate clinical tests in acromegaly still requires further confirmation.

Thus, determining plasma IGF-I level and the GH response to glucose load are the preferred and most cost effective strategy for biochemical diagnosis of acromegaly, and subsequent monitoring of therapeutic interventions *(31)*.

DIFFERENTIAL DIAGNOSIS—TUMOR LOCALIZATION

The approach to diagnosis of the different possible forms of acromegaly is depicted in Fig. 1. Magnetic resonance imaging (MRI) (with the paramagnetic contrast agent gadolinium) should identify the GH-secreting adenoma in almost all patients with pitu-

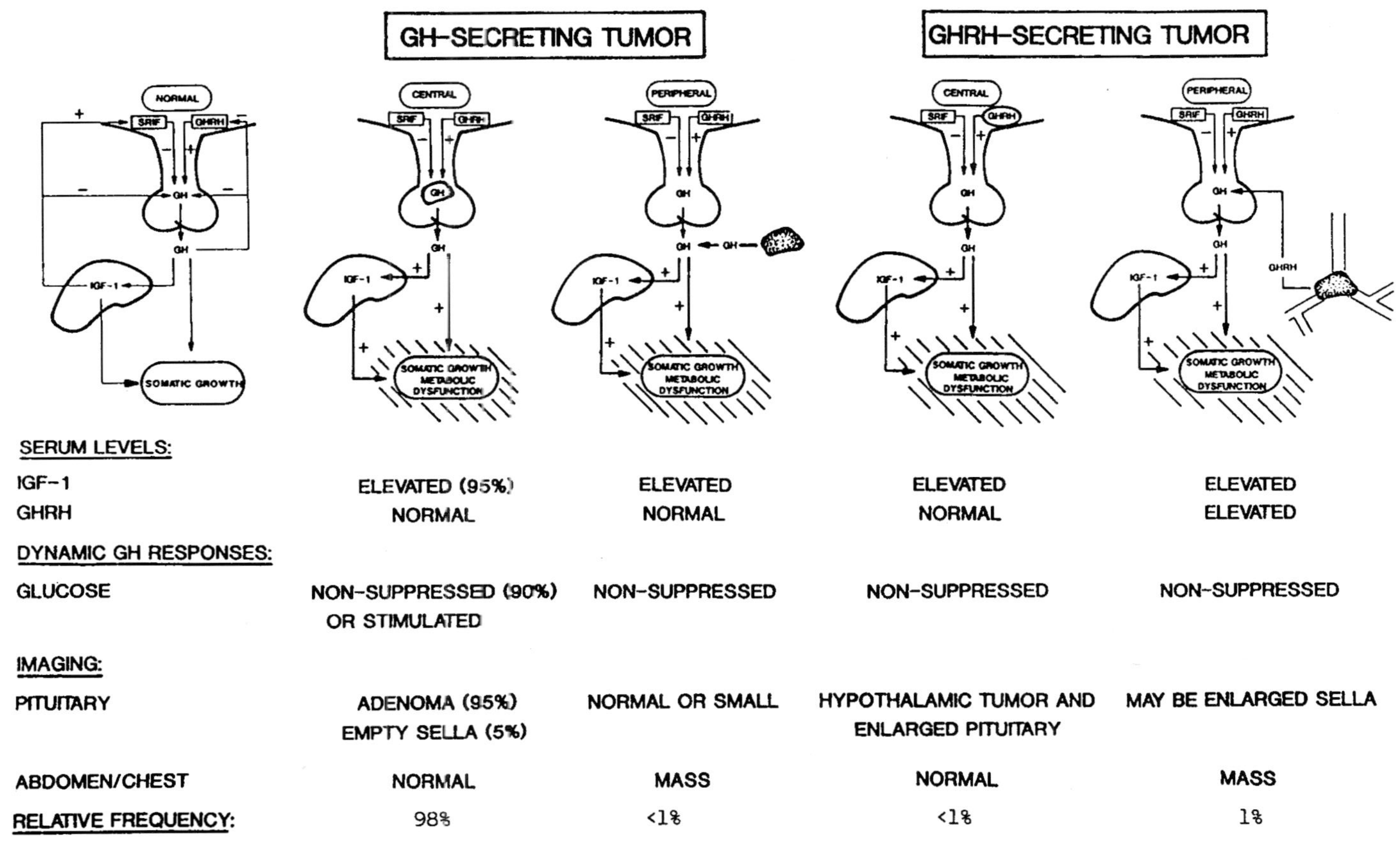

Fig. 1. Differential diagnosis of acromegaly. Adapted with permission from ref. *27*.

itary acromegaly. True acromegaly with normal GH and IGF-I levels and no evidence for extrapituitary tumor may represent a "burned out" adenoma, i.e., an infarcted, previously active pituitary tumor.

If sellar tumor is not evident, the rare possibility of GHRH secretion by an ectopic tumor with somatotrope hyperplasia and hypersomatotropism should be considered. An enlarged pituitary is, however, often found on MRI of patients with ectopic GHRH secreting tumors, and somatotrope adenoma formation has also been reported in some patients with ectopic GHRH secretion *(32)*. The presence of a hypothalamic GHRH secreting tumor may be excluded by MRI of the suprasellar region.

GH secretion in ectopic acromegaly is similar to that seen in pituitary acromegaly, and dynamic pituitary tests (GH response to GHRH or TRH) cannot distinguish pituitary tumors from extrapituitary tumors. Plasma GHRH levels are usually elevated in patients with peripheral GHRH secreting tumors *(33)*, compared with barely measurable concentrations in patients with pituitary acromegaly. However, hypothalamic GHRH secreting tumors do not raise circulating GHRH levels, as the excess eutopic hypothalamic GHRH is secreted directly into the hopophyseal portal system without entering the systemic circulation.

Unique and unexpected clinical features and biochemical markers in acromegaly, related to carcinoid syndrome (respiratory wheezing, flushing), islet-cell tumors (peptic ulcers and hypergastrinemia, hypoglycemia, with hyperinsulinemia) or small-cell lung cancer (hypercortisolism) may be associated with the ectopic GHRH secreting tumor. The presence of these specific clinical signs should be an indication for abdominal and chest imaging, including X-ray, computerized tomography, MRI, arteriography, endoscopic ultrasound, bronchoscopy, and radiolabeled octreotide scan (*see* Octreotide section), to localize the ectopic tumor.

TREATMENT

Reduced quality of life, shorter life expectancy, and increased risk of malignancy are associated with acromegaly. In addition, large and invasive somatotrope adenomas may compress and destroy adjacent sellar structures, and result in visual decompensation and hypopituitarism. Thus, early diagnosis and aggressive medical intervention may improve patient outcome *(34)*, even when the symptoms are mild and GH excess is minimal. The tumor secreting excess GH (or GHRH) should be identified, and the goal of management is either to remove it or suppress its hypersecretion. Surgery, irradiation, and medical treatment are the three therapeutic options currently available. Effective treatment should restore soft tissue overgrowth, and ameliorate other signs of hypersomatotropism. Suppressed postglucose GH (to < 1 µg/L) and normal IGF-I levels *(31)*, restored circadian rhythm, and appropriate responses of GH to provocative stimuli, should ideally be achieved to ensure that acromegaly is cured. In addition, residual anterior pituitary function should not be compromised after tumor resection or shrinkage. Unfortunately, using these maximal biochemical and clinical criteria, cure of acromegaly is not attained in many treated patients, even after combination therapy.

Transsphenoidal Surgery

Selective transsphenoidal surgical resection for well localized GH secreting pituitary adenoma should be the first treatment modality considered *(35–38)*. Harvey Cushing already used this surgical approach in 1909 when operating on an acromegalic patient. This procedure has yielded vastly improved results in the last decade when performed by experienced neurosurgeons using accurate MRI localization, microinstrumentation, and sophisticated head immobilization techniques. Sellar structure compression, compromised pituitary trophic hormone secretion, soft tissue swelling, and metabolic derangements are often immediately restored after successful tumor resection. The GH levels return to normal within 1 h, and IGF-I levels are usually normalized after 1 wk, but may remain elevated for several months despite GH remitting to cured values. A transcranial surgical approach is rarely indicated, and reserved only for large invasive tumors, with optic tract compression, or contiguity with major blood vessels.

Precise interpretation and comparison of surgical results in acromegaly is difficult, as most series do not provide the results of postglucose levels or IGF-I measurements but only random GH levels or mean percentage reductions, and long-term data are often not reported. In his series, Fahlbusch reports that 72% of patients with intrasellar microadenomas had postglucose GH levels of < 2 µg/L (81% had random levels of < 5 µg/L) in the early postoperative period *(36)*, whereas only 50% of all-sized macroadenomas had GH levels < 2 µg/L after glucose load *(36)*. Most large surgical series report that 60% of operated patients had random GH levels < 5 µg/L after surgery *(35–39*; Fig. 2A), and success rates were even lower with macroadenomas. The IGF-I levels usually fall to within the normal range in half of operated acromegalics. However, despite reduction of GH levels to < 5 µg/L, patients may have increased IGF-I levels, or have increased GH secretion when retested several years after surgery. Thus, recurrences occurring in up to 10% of operated patients despite normal dynamic GH response shortly after surgery, are reported in different series with long-term follow-up data. This probably also reflects incomplete tumor resection, and if residual tumor is documented by MRI, reoperation may be indicated.

Surgical removal of ectopic GHRH or GH producing tumors will cure patients with benign ectopic acromegaly if GHRH, GH, and IGF-I are normalized together with GH suppressibility to glucose *(40)*. Alternative therapeutic strategies are used in patients with inoperable metastatic disease (i.e., malignant carcinoid or lung cancer), including pituitary surgery (ineffective in most GHRH producing tumors) and octreotide administration.

Side-Effects

Postoperative new onset hypopituitarism with the need for permanent hormonal replacement therapy occurs in about 15% of patients *(36)*, and this risk correlates with size and invasiveness of the operated tumors. Permanent diabetes insipidus, cerebrospinal fluid rhinorrhea, hemorrhage, meningitis, and central nervous system damage are rarely seen. A mortality rate of <1% is associated with resection of large invasive tumors.

Radiotherapy

The anterior pituitary should be considered as the target for external beam irradiation therapy in acromegalic patients uncontrolled by surgery or medical treatment. Before the introduction of octreotide as effective treatment, sellar irradiation was commonly used. Tumor localization by MRI, beam direction and field size simulation, head immobilization, and isocentral rotational techniques result in maximal tumor irradiation

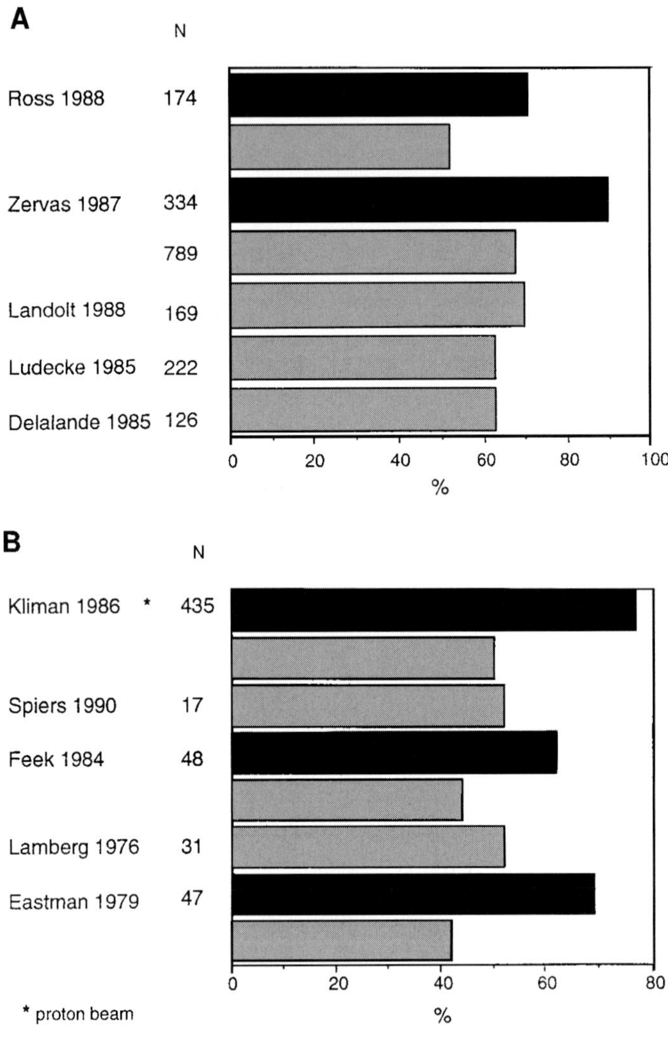

Fig. 2. Percentage of acromegalic patients with GH levels below 5 (gray bars) or 10 μg/L (black bars) in different series **(A)** after transsphenoidal surgery; **(B)** 10 yr after radiotherapy. Adapted with permission from ref. *39*.

and minimal damage to normal surrounding tissue. The conventional megavoltage X-irradiation generated by cobalt-60 or linear accelerators is a common method of treatment. The recommended total dose is 4500–5000 rad given during 5–6 wk in treatment fractions not exceeding 180 rad/d *(41)*. Proton beam (heavy particle, the recommended dose is 15,000 rad) therapy decreases GH levels to normal faster compared to conventional radiotherapy, but is contraindicated in patients with suprasellar tumor extension as the optic tract can be exposed to the radiation field. Stereotactic ablation of GH secreting adenomas by the gamma knife radiosurgery is highly promising, but is performed only in specialized centers, and long-term results are not yet available.

Table 5
Comparison of Treatment Modalities for Acromegaly: Success Rates and Complications

	Transsphenoidal surgery				
	Microadenoma	*Macroadenoma*	*Radiotherapy*	*Bromocriptine*	*Octreotide,%*
GH < 5 μg/L	80%	50–60%	77% (15 yr)	20%	65
GH < 2 μg/L	70%	40%	nd	nd	40
Normal IGF-I	~50%[a]		nd	10%	50
Tumor shrinkage	>95%	70%	95%	10%	50
Disadvantages	Recurrence 5–10%		Late response	Low efficacy	3 sc injections/d
	Persistent GH↑ 40%				
Complications:					
New hypopituitarism	15%		>50%	No	No
Others	Diabetes insipidus 2.6%		Neurological deficits	Nausea, dizziness	Asymptomatic gallstones

nd, no data.
[a]Data derived from our experience.
Adapted with permission from ref. *61*.

The slow rate of response is the main disadvantage of radiotherapy, and high levels of circulating GH and IGF-I continue to expose many acromegalic patients to enhanced morbidity and mortality for several years after irradiation. The GH levels begin falling gradually during the first year, drop to < 10 μg/L after 5–10 yr, and values < 5 μg/L are encountered between 10–15 yr after treatment (Fig. 2B), with up to 77 and 90% of patients falling below 5 μg/L after 15 and 20 yr, respectively *(41–43)* (Table 5). Tumor growth is arrested, over 95% of GH-cell adenomas shrink, and headaches improve *(41,44)*.

Side-Effects

Hypopituitarism develops in about half of acromegalic patients receiving radiotherapy within 10 yr after treatment *(41)*, and the incidence increases thereafter. Prior surgery also increases the risk of postirradiation damage to the anterior pituitary. Hypogonadism and hypocortisolism are the common trophic hormone deficits encountered, and pituitary hypothyroidism occurs in 10% of patients after irradiation. Other postirradiation complications including cranial-nerve palsies, vision loss, memory deficits, and brain necrosis are very rare and are usually associated with larger doses than currently recommended.

Secondary intracranial tumors occurring following sellar radiation have been reported in 1.3–1.7% of patients within the first 10 yr after radiotherapy, with a relative risk of up to 16 times greater as compared to a control population *(45,46)*. These brain tumors include astrocytoma, glioblastoma, meningioma, and, rarely, sarcoma.

Octreotide

The introduction of the somatostatin analog, octreotide, as an efficient therapy for acromegaly 10 yr ago has resulted in important therapeutic progress, and the first time acromegaly could be controlled by a drug. Octreotide treatment is indicated in acromegalic patients who have inadequate response to surgery or irradiation, or cannot be treated by these modalities; to improve severe symptoms, including headaches and sleep apnea, while awaiting for transsphenoidal adenomectomy; and to control acromegaly after radiotherapy as clinical remission is delayed.

This 8-amino acid analog inhibits GH secretion with at least 40-fold greater potency than the naturally occurring hypothalamic somatostatin, and has a serum half-life of approximately 2 h after sc injection, compared with the short duration of action of human somatostatin (serum half-life of about 2 min). Furthermore, rebound GH hypersecretion seen following somatostatin infusion is not encountered after octreotide, and prolonged use of the analog is not associated with desensitization. The inhibitory therapeutic response to octreotide is mediated via specific membrane receptors on the tumor cells *(47)*, and correlates directly with the density of pituitary tumor-ssomatostatin receptors *(48)*, and with the presence of receptors demonstrated clinically by radiolabeled octreotide scan *(49)*. Acute decrease of GH secretion in response to a test dose of octreotide is demonstrated only in those acromegalics who have visible in vivo receptors shown by the scan, and also predicts long-term response to octreotide. Octreotide exerts its GH-suppression effect through receptor subtypes 2 and 5, both of which are expressed by GH secreting tumors *(50,51)*.

A single sc injection of 50–100 μg octreotide suppresses GH secretion in over 90% of acromegalic patients whithin 1 h, usually lasting for 4–6 h *(52)*. The drug is administered in three daily injections (100–200 μg each), and the daily dose can be increased up to 1500 μg. A long-acting injectable formulation of somatostatin analog (Sandostatin LAR) that produces slow release of octreotide from microspheres is currently under clinical investigation. Comparable GH suppression occurs in acromegalic patients for as long as 6 wk after a single 30-mg im injection of this compound *(53)*. Octreotide administered sc every 8 h significantly suppresses integrated GH levels over 5 h after injection to < 5 μg/L in 50% of patients, to < 2 μg/L in 25% *(52)*, and normalizes IGF-I levels in 47% of treated patients *(39)* (Table 5, Fig. 3). The drug is less effective in larger adenomas, whereas in patients treated for microadenomas, integrated GH and IGF-I levels are almost invariably normalized *(52)*. Long-term octreotide treatment in 103 patients was recently reported to suppress GH levels 2 h after injection to < 5 μg/L in 65% of the patients and to 2 μg/L or less in 40% *(54)* (Table 5). Significant tumor shrinkage, assessed by MRI or CT scan, occurs in up to 50% of patients *(52)*, but this effect is reversible if treatment is stopped. Over two-thirds of patients experience rapid relief of soft tissue swelling, hyperhidrosis, headache, arthralgia, and paresthesias within several days of treatment initiation *(52)*.

The rapid reduction in GH levels associated with octreotide administration results in marked enhancement of insulin sensitivity and a dramatic decrease of insulin requirement in diabetic patients.

Sleep apnea improves frequently in acromegalics treated with octreotide *(55)*, even if biochemical remission is not achieved. Somatostatin analog usually does not cure

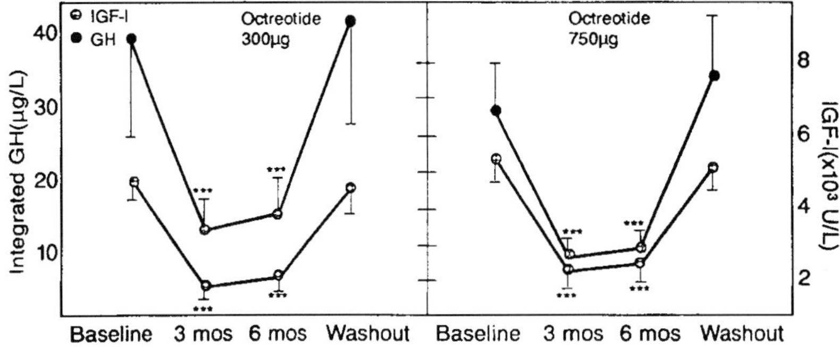

Fig. 3. Effect of low (100 μg every 8 h, $n = 50$, left panel) and high-dose octreotide (250 μg every 8 h, $n = 54$, right panel) on integrated GH and IGF-I levels in acromegalic patients treated with subcutaneous octreotide for 6 months. *** $p < 0.001$ vs baseline. Adapted with permission from ref. *52*.

Table 6
Octreotide Side-Effects

Gallbladder	Asymptomatic gallstones or sludge
Gastrointestinal	Nausea, abdominal discomfort, flatulence, diarrhea (transient)
Glucose	Hypoglycemia, hyperglycemia
Thyroid	Hypothyroxinemia
Other	Headache, local pain on injection, depression, asymptomatic sinus bradycardia

Adapted with permission from ref. *61*.

hypertension, but biochemiacal remission is associated with significantly decreased left ventricular mass *(56)* and improved left ventricular function.

Octreotide also suppresses GHRH secretion by ectopic GHRH-producing tumors, while decreasing pituitary GH hypersecretion and, thus, can be used to ameliorate clinical and biochemical manifestations of acromegaly in patients harboring these rare tumors *(57)*.

Side-Effects (Table 6)

Octreotide treatment is well tolerated in most patients. Most side-effects are short-lived and related to drug-induced suppression of gastrointestinal motility and secretion *(31)*. These include nausea, abdominal discomfort, fat malabsorption, diarrhea, and flatulence occurring in one-third of the patients; side-effects usually remit within 2 wk, even if treatment continues. Mild glucose intolerance may rarely occur due to transient suppression of insulin secretion. The most significant side-effect, both in acromegalic and nonacromegalic patients, involves the gallbladder. Octreotide attenuates postprandial gallbladder contractility and delays gallbladder emptying, and up to 35% of long-term treated patients in the United States develop asymptomatic cholesterol gallstones or sludge, as assessed by ultrasound. The incidence of gallstones is geographically variable, with the highest rates observed in China. Other side-effects include mild asymptomatic bradycardia, depression, hypothyroxinemia, local pain at the injection site, and rarely, drug dependence triggered by striking headache relief.

Bromocriptine

Administration of bromocriptine, an ergot derivative dopamine agonist, to healthy subjects results in acute GH release, but usually suppresses GH secretion by neoplastic somatotropes. Thus, bromocriptine was commonly used to treat patients before octreotide approval for acromegaly, and it still serves as primary or adjuvant therapy, in combination with octreotide or irradiation, or before surgery. Usually patients require > 20 mg/d, far higher than the dose needed to normalize PRL in patients with prolactinoma. In addition, the duration of GH suppression is shorter in acromegaly, compared with the effect on PRL in hyperprolactinemia, and instead of two daily doses, three to four daily doses are required to suppress GH levels. Among 549 acromegalic patients reported in 31 different studies treated with bromocriptine, random GH levels decreased below 10 μg/L and 5 μg/L in 53 and 20%, respectively *(58)* (Table 5). However, IGF-I levels were normalized in only 10% of patients, and < 20% of tumors shrank during therapy. Most patients experience subjective clinical improvement while taking the drug, including improved fatigue, arthralgias, perspiration, and headache, usually with no correlation with objective clinical changes, and commonly without GH or IGF-I normalization. Thus, it has been proposed that bromocriptine may have a beneficial clinical effect by impairing GH bioactivity unrelated to the direct effect on hormone secretion. In contrast to the morphologic changes found in prolactinomas after long-term bromocriptine treatment, where decrease in tumor size is frequently associated with fibrosis, fibrotic changes are rarely demonstrated in pure GH secreting tumors that decrease in size during bromocriptine therapy *(58)*.

Combined therapy with bromocriptine and octreotide induces a significantly additive suppression of GH and IGF-I compared with separate administration of similar doses of either drug *(59)*. Other dopamine agonists including pergolide, lisuride, and the long-acting preparation, cabergoline, also suppress GH and IGF-I secretion in acromegaly.

Side-Effects

Bromocriptine may cause gastointestinal upset, nausea, orthostatic hypotension, lightheadedness, and dizziness at the beginning of therapy, but most of these side-effects resolve with continued drug use. Other side-effects including nasal stuffiness, psychosis, nightmares, hallucinations, insomnia, and vertigo are reversible after decreasing the drug dose.

Novel drugs

Growth hormone analogs behaving as antagonists to the action of endogenous GH at the receptor level *(60)* are currently being developed, and, hopefully, will block the peripheral effects of GH hypersecretion in acromegalic patients. GHRH antagonists block GHRH effects in the hypothalamus and pituitary, and thus will prevent GH secretion and hypersomatotropism in acromegaly.

MANAGEMENT STRATEGY (FIG. 4)

1. Transsphenoidal surgery should be the primary treatment for acromegaly, both for microadenomas and macroadenomas. If biochemical remission is achieved after surgery, no additional treatment is indicated.

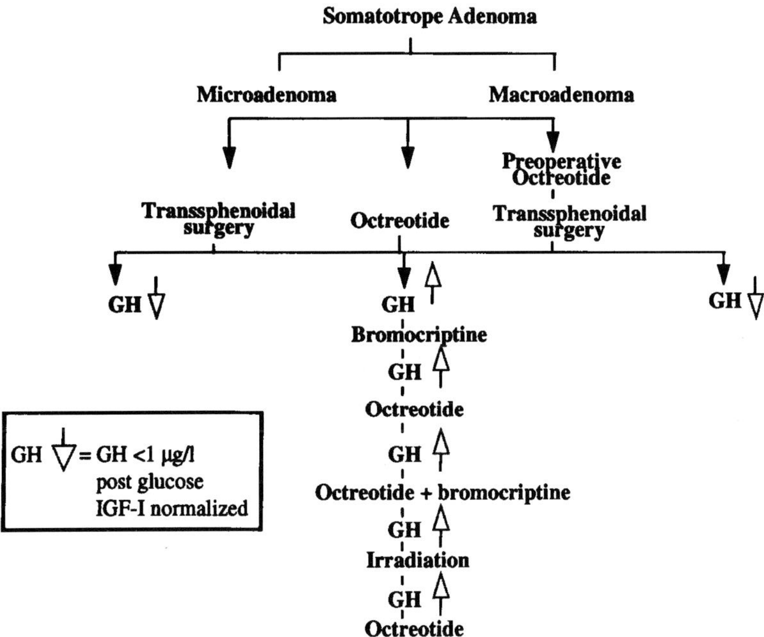

Fig. 4. Management strategy of acromegaly caused by a pituitary adenoma. Adapted with permission from ref. *61*.

2. Octreotide treatment may be tried before surgery in patients harboring invasive macroadenomas to shrink the tumor and improve postsurgical results. If surgery fails to control the disease, medical management with octreotide and/or bromocriptine should be initiated. For elderly asymptomatic patients, therapy may be withheld, but for symptomatic elderly patients, octreotide is the preferred primary treatment *(31)*. Octreotide is also used for immediate control of symptoms in the case of recurrent disease or until surgery is performed.
3. Radiotherapy of the pituitary is selected when surgery and/or medical treatment fail to normalize GH hypersecretion.

FOLLOW-UP

1. *Biochemical remission.* After treatment, patients should be followed quarterly to achieve postglucose GH of <1 μg/L and normal IGF-I levels, the criteria for biochemical cure. However, even cured acromegalic patients usually have abnormal patterns of GH secretion, and experience most of their secretion basally and not during pulses, as normal subjects do.
2. *Anterior pituitary function.* To monitor residual anterior pituitary function, hormone evaluation should be performed semiannually, and if a hormone deficit is identified, replacement therapy should be instituted.
3. *Tumor mass.* MRI should be repeated every year in the first years following successful therapy. Semiannual visual field assessment by perimetry is mandatory in patients with residual extrasellar tumor, in those treated by octreotide or bromocriptine, and in patients requiring hormone replacement.

4. *Gastrointestinal malignancy*. Frequent colonoscopic evaluation is recommended in patients over 50 yr old, for early detection and treatment of premalignant colonic polyps.

REFERENCES

1. Lloyd RV, Cano M, Chandler WF, Barkan AL, Horvath E, Kovacs K. Human growth hormone and prolactin secreting pituitary adenomas analyzed by in situ hybridization. Am J Pathol 1989;134:605–613.
2. Kovacs K, Horvath E, Asa SL, Stefaneanu L, Sano T. Pituitary cells producing more than one hormone. Trends Endocrinol Metab 1989;1:104–107.
3. Weinstein LS, Shenker A, Gejman PV, Merino MJ, Friedman E, Spiegel AM, Activating mutations of the stimulatory G protein in the McCune-Albright syndrome. N Engl J Med 1991;325:1688–1695.
4. Rasmussen P, Lindholm J. Ectopic pituitary adenomas. Clin Endocrinol 1979;11:69–74.
5. Mountcastle RB, Roof BS, Mayfield RK, Mordes DB, Sagel J, Biggs PJ, Rawe SE. Case report: pituitary adenocarcinoma in an acromegalic patient: response to bromocriptine and pituitary testing: a review of the literature on 36 cases of pituitary carcinoma. Am J Med Sci 1989;298:109–118.
6. Stewart PM, Carey MP, Graham CT, Wright AD, London DR. Growth hormone secreting pituitary carcinoma: a case report and literature review. Clin Endocrinol 1992;37:189–195.
7. Greenman Y, Woolf P, Congilio J, O'Mara R, Pei L, Said JW, Melmed S. Remission of acromegaly caused by pituitary carcinoma after surgical excision of growth hormone secreting metastasis detected by 111-indium pentetreotide scan. J Clin Endocrinol Metab 1996;81:1628–1633.
8. Melmed S, Ezrin C, Kovacs K, Goodman RS, Frohman LA. Acromegaly due to secretion of growth hormone by an ectopic pancreatic islet-cell tumor. N Engl J Med 1985;312:9–17.
9. Scheithauer BW, Carpenter PC, Bloch B, Brazeau P. Ectopic secretion of a growth hormone-releasing factor. Report of a case of acromegaly with bronchial carcinoid tumor. Am J Med 1984;76:605–615.
10. Schulte HM, Benker G, Windeck R, Olbricht T, Reinwein D. Failure to respond to growth hormone releasing hormone (GHRH) in acromegaly due to a GHRH secreting pancreatic tumor: dynamics of multiple endocrine testing. J Clin Endocrinol Metab 1985;61:585–587.
11. Asa SL, Scheithauer BW, Bilbao JM, Horvath E, Ryan N, Kovacs K, Randall RV, Laws ER Jr., Singer W, Linfoot JA, Thorner MO, Vale W. A case for hypothalamic acromegaly: a clinicopathological study of six patients with hypothalamic gangliocytomas producing growth hormone-releasing factor. J Clin Endocrinol Metab 1984;58:796–803.
12. Asa SL, Bilbao JM, Kovacs K, Linfoot JA. Hypothalamic neuronal hamartoma associated with pituitary growth hormone cell adenoma and acromegaly. Acta Neuropathol 1980;53:231–234.
13. Ashcraft MW, Hartzband PI, Van Herle AJ, Bersch N, Golde DW. A unique growth factor in patients with acromegaloidism. J Clin Endocrinol Metab 1983;57:272–276.
14. Molitch ME. Clinical manifestations of acromegaly. Endocrinol Metab Clin North Am 1992;21:597–614.
15. Nabarro JDN. Acromegaly. Clin Endocrinol 1987;26:481–512.
16. Grunstein RR, Ho KY, Sullivan CE. Sleep apnea in acromegaly. Ann Intern Med 1991;115:527–532.
17. Klein I, Parveen G, Gavaler JS, Vanthiel DH. Colonic polyps in patients with acromegaly. Ann Intern Med 1982;97:27–30.
18. Ezzat S, Storm C, Melmed S. Colon polyps in acromegaly. Ann Intern Med 1991;114:754–758.
19. Ituarte EA, Petrini J, Hershman JM. Acromegaly and colon cancer. Ann Intern Med 1984;101:627–628.
20. Ron E, Gridley G, Hrubec Z, Page W, Arora S, Fraumeni JJ. Acromegaly and colon cancer. Cancer 1991;68:1673–1677.
21. Bengtsson B-A, Eden S, Ernest I, Oden A, Sjogren B. Epidemiology and long-term survival in acromegaly. Acta Med Scand 1988;223:327–335.
22. Rajasoorya C, Holdaway MI, Wrightson P, Scott DJ, Ibbertson HK. Determinants of clinical outcome and survival in acromegaly. Clin Endocrinol 1994;41:95–102.
23. Hartman ML, Veldhuis JD, Vance ML, Faria AC, Furlanetto RW, Thorner MO. Somatotropin pulse frequency and basal concentrations are increased in acromegaly and are reduced by successful therapy. J Clin Endocrinol Metab 1990;70:1375–1384.
24. Clemmons DR, Van Wyk JJ, Ridgway EC, Kliman B, Kjellberg RN, Underwood KE. Evaluation of acromegaly by radioimmunoassay of somatomedin-C. N Engl J Med 1979;301:1138–1142.
25. Rieu M, Girard F, Bricaire H, Binoux M. The importance of insulin-like growth factor (somatomedin) measurements in the diagnosis and surveillance of acromegaly. J Clin Endocrinol Metab 1982;55:147–153.

26. Chang-DeMoranville BM, Jackson IM. Diagnosis and endocrine testing in acromegaly. Endocrinol Metab Clin North Am 1992;21:649–668.
27. Melmed S. Acromegaly. N Engl J Med 1990;322:966–977.
28. Irie M, Tsushima T. Increase of serum growth hormone concentration following thyrotropin-releasing hormone injection in patients with acromegaly or gigantism. J Clin Endocrinol Metab 1972;35:97–100.
29. Grinspoon S, Clemmons D, Swearingen B, Klibanski A. Serum insulin-like growth factor-binding protein-3 levels in the diagnosis of acromegaly. J Clin Endocrinol Metab 1995;80:927–932.
30. Ezzat S, Ren S, Braunstein GD, Melmed S. Octreotide stimulates insulin-like growth factor binding protein-1 (IGFBP-1) levels in acromegaly. J Clin Endocrinol Metab 1991;73:441–443.
31. Acromegaly therapy consensus development panel. Consensus statement: benefits versus risks of medical therapy for acromegaly. Am J Med 1994;97:468–473.
32. Sano T, Asa SL, Kovacs K. Growth hormone-releasing hormone-producing tumors: clinical, biochemical, and morphological manifestations. Endocr Rev 1988;9:357–373.
33. Frohman LA. Ectopic hormone production by tumors. Clinical Neuroendocrine Perspectives 1984;3:201–224.
34. Bates AS, Van't Hoff W, Jones JM, Clayton RN. An audit of outcome of treatment in acromegaly. Q J Med 1993;86:293–299.
35. Ross DA, Wilson CB. Results of transsphenoidal microsurgery for growth hormone-secreting pituitary adenomas in a series of 214 patients. J Neurosurg 1988;68:854–867.
36. Fahlbusch R, Honegger J, Buchfelder M. Surgical management of acromegaly. Endocrinol Metab Clin North Am 1992;21:669–692.
37. Tindall GT, Oyesiku NM, Watts NB, Clark RV, Christy JH, Adams DA. Transsphenoidal adenomectomy for growth hormone-secreting pituitary adenomas in acromegaly: outcome analysis and determinants of failure. J Neurosurg 1993;78:205–215.
38. Zervas NT. Multicenter surgical results in acromegaly. In: Ludecke DK, Tolis G, eds. Growth Hormone, Growth Factors, and Acromegaly. Raven, Press New York, 1987, p. 253.
39. Melmed S, Ho K, Thorner M, Klibanski A, Reichlin S. Recent advances in pathogenesis, diagnosis and management of acromegaly. J Clin Endocrinol Metab 1995;80:3395–3402.
40. Faglia G, Arosio M, Bazzoni N. Ectopic acromegaly. Endocrinol Metab Clin North Am 1992;21:575–595.
41. Eastman RC, Gorden P, Glatstein E, Roth J. Radiation therapy of acromegaly. Endocrinol Metab Clin North Am 1992;21:693–712.
42. Eastman RC, Gorden P, Roth J. Conventional supervoltage irradiation is an effective treatment for acromegaly. J Clin Endocrinol Metab 1979;48:931–940.
43. Gorden P, Glatstein E, Oldfield E, Roth J. Conventional supervoltage radiation in the treatment of acromegaly. In: Robbins RJ, Melmed S, eds. Acromegaly. A Century of Scientific and Clinical Progress. Plenum, New York, 1987, pp. 211–228.
44. Dowsett RJ, Fowble B, Sergott RC, Savino PJ, Bosley TM, Snyder PJ, Gennarelli TA. Results of radiotherapy in the treatment of acromegaly: lack of ophthalmologic complications. Int J Radiat Oncol Biol Phys 1990;19:453–459.
45. Brada M, Ford D, Ashley S, Bliss JM, Crowley S, Mason M, Rajan B, Traish D. Risk of second brain tumour after conservative surgery and radiotherapy for pituitary adenoma. B M J 1992;304:1343–1346.
46. Tsang RW, Laperriere NJ, Simpson WJ, Brierley J, Panzarella T, Smyth HS. Glioma arising after radiation therapy for pituitary adenoma. Cancer 1993;72:2227–2233.
47. Reubi JC, Landolt AM. High density of somatostatin receptors in pituitary tumors from acromegalic patients. J Clin Endocrinol Metab 1984;59:1148–1151.
48. Reubi JC, Landolt AM. The growth hormone responses to octreotide in acromegaly correlate with adenoma somatostatin receptor status. J Clin Endocrinol Metab 1989;68:844–850.
49. Ur E, Mather SJ, Bomanji J, Ellison D, Britton KE, Grossman AB, Wass JAH, Besser GM. Pituitary imaging using a labelled somatostatin analogue in acromegaly. Clin Endocrinol 1992;36:147–150.
50. Greenman Y, Melmed S. Heterogeneous expression of two somatostatin receptor subtypes in pituitary tumors. J Clin Endocrinol Metab 1994;78:398–403.
51. Greenman Y, Melmed S. Expression of three somatostatin receptor subtypes in pituitary adenomas: evidence for preferential SSTR5 expression in the mammosomatotroph lineage. J Clin Endocrinol Metab 1994;79:724–729.

52. Ezzat S, Snyder PJ, Young WF, Boyajy LD, Newman C, Klibanski A, Molitch ME, Boyd AE, Sheeler L, Cook DM, Malarkey WB, Jackson I, Lee Vance M, Thorner MO, Barkan A, Frohman LA, Melmed S. Octreotide treatment of acromegaly: a randomized, multicenter study. Ann Intern Med 1992;117:711–718.
53. Flogstad AK, Halse J, Haldorsen T, Lancranjan I, Marbach P, Bruns C, Jervell J. Sandostatin LAR in acromegalic patients: a dose-range study. J Clin Endocrinol Metab 1995;80:3601–3607.
54. Newman CB, Melmed S, Snyder PJ, Young WF, Boyajy LD, Levy R, Stewart WN, Klibanski A, Molitch ME, Gagel RF, Boyd AE, Sheeler L, Cook D, Malarkey WB, Jackson IMD, Lee Vance M, Thorner MO, Ho PJ, Jaffe CA, Frohman LA, Kleinberg DL. Safety and efficacy of long term octreotide therapy of acromegaly: results of a multicenter trial in 103 patients—a clinical research center study. J Clin Endocrinol Metab 1995;80:2768–2775.
55. Grunstein RR, Ho KY, Sullivan CE. Effect of octreotide, a somatostatin analog, on sleep apnea in patients with acromegaly. Ann Intern Med 1994;121:478–483.
56. Lim MJ, Barkan AL, Buda AJ. Rapid reduction of left ventricular hypertrophy in acromegaly after suppression of growth hormone hypersecretion. Ann Intern Med 1992;117:719–726.
57. von Werder K, Losa M, Muller OA, Schweiberer L, Fahlbusch R, del Poso E. Treatment of metastasing GRH-producing tumor with a long-acting somatostatin analogue. Lancet 1984;2:282–283.
58. Jaffe CA, Barkan AL. Treatment of acromegaly with dopamine agonists. Endocrinol Metab Clin North Am 1992;21:713–735.
59. Lamberts SWJ, Zweens M, Verschoor L, del Pozo E. A comparison among the growth hormone-lowering effects in acromegaly of the somatostatin analog SMS 201–995, bromocrptine, and the combination of both drugs. J Clin Endocrinol Metab 1986;63:16–20.
60. Chen WY, Chen N, Yun J, Wagner TE, Kopchick JJ. In vitro and in vivo syudies of antagonistic effects of human growth hormone analogs. J Biol Chem 1994;269:15,892–15,897.
61. Shimon I, Melmed S. Growth hormone- and GHRH-producing tumors. In: Arnold A, ed. Endocrine Neoplasms; Cancer Treatment and Research Series. Kluwer, Norwell, MA. 1997; in press.

8 ACTH

Normal Physiology

Richard I. Dorin, MD
and Lawrence M. Crapo, MD, PhD

Contents

INTRODUCTION

The hypothalamic-pituitary-adrenal (HPA) axis as depicted in Fig. 1 regulates the secretion of cortisol from the adrenal glands and, by doing so, helps preserve the body's homeostatic integrity under basal and stress conditions. It is striking that the structural and functional determinants regulating the HPA axis are strongly conserved across mammalian species. Thus, this unique system has served the adaptation to physiologic and psychologic stress over a broad sweep of evolutionary time. The HPA axis evolved under very primitive conditions of mammalian and human life when stresses such as salt and water depletion, infection, hemorrhage, and lack of food occurred more frequently than in modern life. Nevertheless, the critical role of the HPA axis in promoting survival from these unpredictable and intermittent episodes of illness and stress is underscored by the brief life expectancy of subjects with adrenal insufficiency prior to the availability of exogenous glucocorticoid replacement therapy *(1)*.

Adrenocorticotrophic hormone (ACTH) resides at the center of the HPA axis. It is a 39-amino acid peptide that is produced by enzymatic cleavage of a larger precursor peptide, called pro-opiomelanocortin (POMC). In humans, the corticotroph cell of the anterior pituitary is the primary source of circulating ACTH. Secretion of ACTH from the corticotrophs is pulsatile and demonstrates diurnal variation.

From: *Contemporary Endocrinology, Vol. 3: Diseases of the Pituitary: Diagnosis and Treatment*
Edited by M. E. Wierman Humana Press Inc., Totowa, NJ

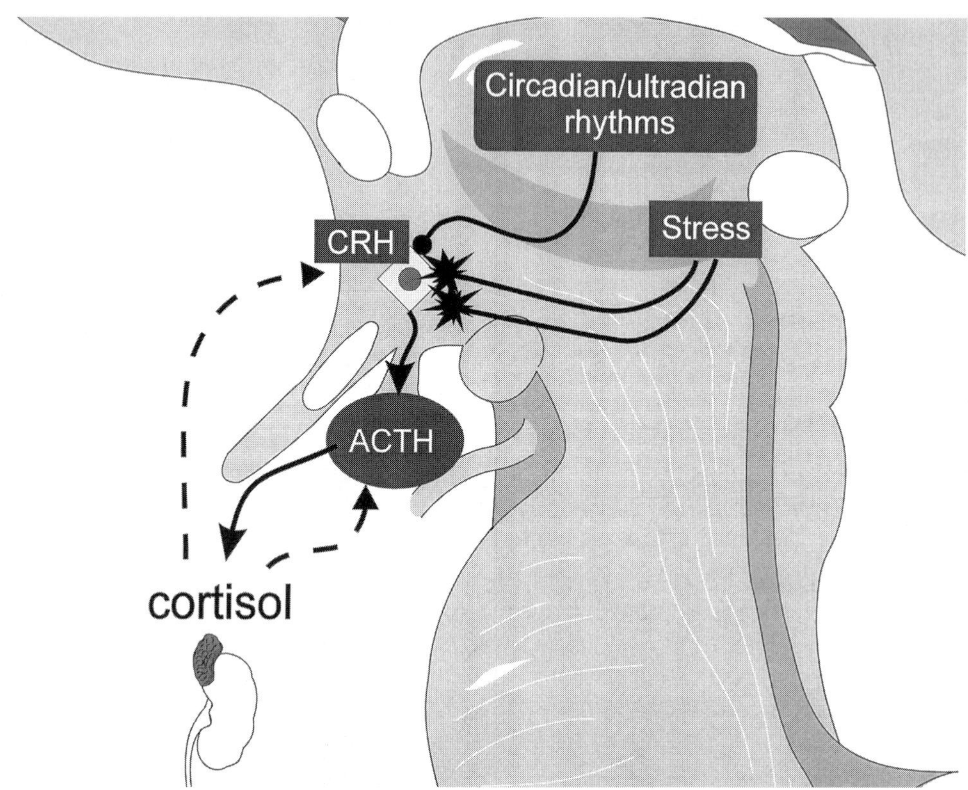

Fig. 1. Overview of the HPA axis. The key regulatory components of the HPA axis include the central nervous system, which generates signals mediating circadian and ultradian rhythms and the HPA response to stress. CNS afferents are integrated at the level of the hypothalamic CRH-producing neuron, which in turn projects to the median eminence and secretes CRH directly into the pituitary portal circulation. CRH (and other ACTH-secretagogs) act directly on the ACTH-producing corticotroph cell of the anterior pituitary, which stimulates the adrenal cortex to produce and secrete corticosteroids, including cortisol, which participates in negative feedback regulation of the HPA axis. Positive regulation is indicated by solid line, and inhibitory regulation (negative feedback) is indicated by the broken line.

The central nervous system (CNS) governs pituitary ACTH secretion through the release of hypothalamic factors that reach the pituitary portal circulation and regulate ACTH synthesis and secretion. Secretion of ACTH is stimulated by corticotropin releasing hormone (CRH), arginine vasopressin (AVP), and other neuropeptides; it is suppressed by peripheral feedback of cortisol from the adrenals. Central factors mediate the ACTH response to stress and activation of ACTH secretion following corticosteroid removal. Central regulatory factors also determine the circadian variation and the ultradian rhythm of ACTH secretion associated with periodic (approx q 40 min) secretory bursts of ACTH and cortisol. As in the case of other pituitary hormones, the pulsatile release of ACTH is believed to correspond to hypothalamic activation resulting in synchronous release of CRH and/or other ACTH secretagogs *(2)*.

In the periphery, on the systemic side of the blood–brain barrier, there are two components of the HPA axis, the pituitary and the adrenals. The ACTH from the pituitary stimulates a rapid rise in adrenal cortisol secretion within 5–10 min. Cortisol in turn exerts feedback suppression of ACTH secretion through pituitary as well as suprapituitary effects. In the pituitary, cortisol interacts with intracellular glucocorticoid receptors of the corticotroph cell to directly inhibit POMC mRNA synthesis and secretion of ACTH. Unbound cortisol also passes freely across the blood–brain barrier and acts at multiple CNS sites, including the hypothalamus and hippocampus, to inhibit synthesis and secretion of hypothalamic CRH, AVP, and other ACTH secretagogs.

The HPA axis plays a vital role in the maintenance and defense of homeostatic equilibrium. Under nonstressed conditions, the maintenance of circadian and ultradian rhythms of ACTH and cortisol secretion serves important physiological and permissive functions, as illustrated by the clinical impact of chronic hypocortisolism associated with the syndrome of ACTH deficiency (secondary adrenal insufficiency). During stress, CRH and AVP producing neurons in the hypothalamus receive and integrate neural and humoral inputs from a variety of organ systems, including the CNS, peripheral nervous system (PNS), and cardiovascular and immune systems. The central activation of ACTH leads in turn to elevated systemic levels of cortisol, which plays a critical role in the successful adaptation to stress. The mechanism by which ACTH secretion is maintained in spite of feedback by high circulating levels of cortisol is uncertain, but probably reflects a balance in which central activation dominates over peripheral feedback inhibition.

Across the span of evolutionary time, a highly conserved hormonal system, the HPA axis, has been forged to defend homeostatic equilibrium in higher organisms. The centerpiece of the system is ACTH, and this chapter focuses on the normal physiology of this fascinating hormone.

ACTH SYNTHESIS AND SECRETION

Cell of Origin

ACTH is synthesized from the precursor peptide, pro-opiomelanocortin (POMC), within specialized corticotroph cells that are distributed primarily throughout the central region (median wedge) of the anterior pituitary gland. The corticotrophs can be easily distinguished from other cells by antibody staining against ACTH and other POMC-derived peptides, such as beta-lipotropin. Ultrastructural features of the corticotroph include neurosecretory granules and a well-developed endoplasmic reticulum and Golgi apparatus. Pituitary ACTH producing corticotroph cells can be identified in man by the eighth week of gestation. During fetal life, the corticotroph is sensitive to hormonal regulation, including stimulation by CRH and feedback inhibition by corticosteroids.

Pro-Opiomelanocortin (POMC) Gene Expression

The principal synthetic product of the human corticotroph cell is POMC, which is encoded by a single gene composed of three exons *(3)* and located on chromosome 2p23 (*see* Fig. 2). Regulation of POMC gene transcription is the first step at which POMC gene expression and ACTH biosynthesis are controlled, and is an important component of the hormonal regulation of ACTH production. Accordingly, the 5′-

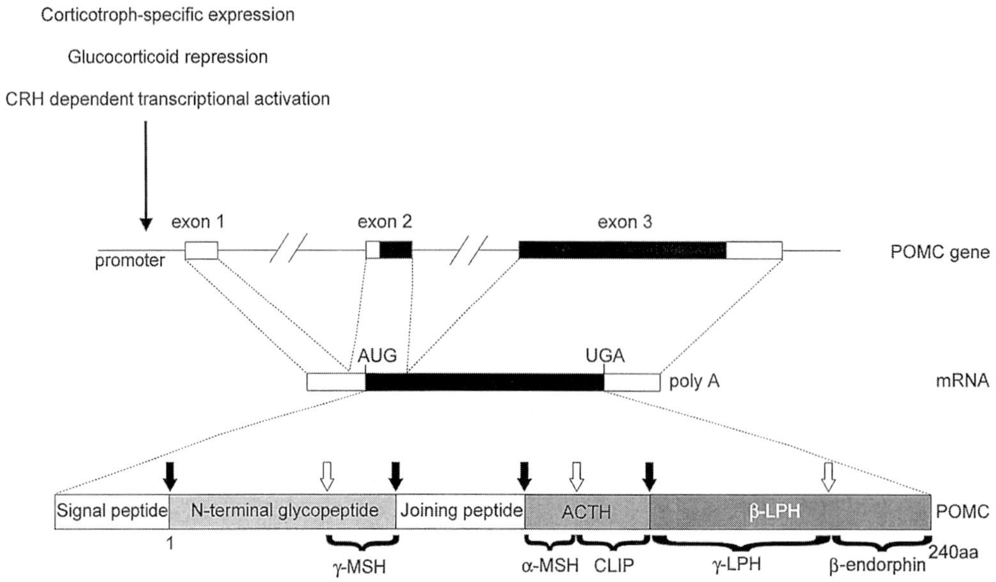

Fig. 2. Structure of the ACTH precursor gene and peptide, proopiomelanocortin (POMC). The structure of the POMC gene (upper panel) includes 5′-regulatory sequences, which confer corticotroph-specific expression, glucocorticoid-dependent repression, and transcriptional activation by CRH. Intron splicing yields the mature POMC mRNA, which includes untranslated (open fill) and translated regions (solid fill). The POMC peptide (lower panel) is cleaved at dibasic amino acids in a tissue-specific manner. POMC cleavage characteristic of the anterior pituitary (solid arrows) yield ACTH ACTH and β-LPH. Additional dibasic cleavage sites (open arrows) utilized in other tissues, such as brain and neurointermediate lobe of the pituitary, yield additional peptide products, including α-MSH, γ-LPH, and β-endorphin (lower brackets). Adapted with permission from ref. *112*.

regulatory sequences upstream of the POMC transcription start site are conserved across species and confer developmental, tissue specific, and hormonal regulation of gene transcription in transgenic animals and in vitro models *(4,5)*. Regulatory sequences contained within the first 500 bp of the POMC promoter confer corticotroph-specific expression, transcriptional activation by CRH, and repression by corticosteroids (*see* Fig. 2).

POMC Peptide and Posttranslational Processing

The primary translation product of POMC mRNA is a 266-amino acid precursor peptide that contains a secretory leader sequence and multiple potential dibasic cleavage sites. Posttranslation processing of the POMC precursor, including enzymatic cleavage, glycosylation, acetylation, phorphorylation, and amidation, can give rise to a number of peptides having distinct biological activities *(6)*. As shown in Fig. 2, these include opioid peptides (β-endorphin), melanotropic peptides (alpha-, beta-, and gamma-MSH), and corticotrophic peptides (ACTH). Posttranslational processing of POMC varies according to the site of expression *(7)*. In humans, for example, POMC is expressed in the anterior pituitary and cleaved to yield ACTH and β-lipotropin. In other mammals, POMC is also expressed in the intermediate lobe of the pituitary, where it is cleaved to produce beta-endorphin and α-MSH. However, the neurointermediate lobe is not well developed in humans and, except during fetal development and in certain forms of Cushing's disease, does not appear to contribute to circulating levels of POMC-derived peptides in normal physiology.

POMC is also expressed and synthesized in a number of extrapituitary sites, including the gonad, leukocytes, and neuroendocrine cells of the lung, gut, and adrenal medulla. In many of these extrapituitary sites, POMC transcription is initiated at a site in exon 3, and the cognate protein therefore lacks a signal peptide. This observation suggests that POMC products, including ACTH and β-endorphin, are synthesized but not secreted in these tissues *(8,9)*. In addition, POMC is expressed in the CNS, notably the arcuate nucleus of the hypothalamus, where it is processed to yield β-endorphin, which functions as an opioidergic neurotransmitter. With the exception of ectopic production of ACTH from neuroendocrine tumors, the corticotroph cell of the anterior pituitary is the sole source of physiologically significant levels of circulating ACTH in humans. Accordingly, conditions that result in corticotroph cell destruction, such as hypophysectomy, hemorrhage, and autoimmune injury, are associated with very low or undetectable systemic levels of ACTH and complete secondary adrenal insufficiency.

Signal Transduction Pathways Regulating ACTH Synthesis and Secretion

In addition to POMC, corticotrophs produce a variety of other proteins that influence ACTH synthesis and secretion. These include specific peptidase enzymes involved in tissue-specific processing of POMC *(10)*, and cell surface and intracellular proteins that participate in regulation of POMC gene expression and ACTH secretion. The corticotroph cell expresses specific cell surface receptors for both CRH and AVP *(11,12)*, and a variety of membrane-associated G proteins that participate in distinct signal transduction pathways of CRH, AVP, and other ACTH secretagogues. CRH appears to influence ACTH synthesis and secretion primarily through activation of adenylate cyclase and phosphorylation events mediated through the cAMP-dependent protein kinase A (PKA) pathway *(13)*. AVP stimulates membrane phopholipase C activity, resulting in phosphoinositol turnover, in tracellular Ca^{2+} release, and protein kinase C (PKC) activation *(14)*. The synergistic ACTH response to CRH and AVP *(15,16)* reflects the distinct as well as overlapping signal transduction pathways by which these peptides influence ACTH synthesis and secretion *(17)*.

In addition, corticotroph cells express intracellular receptors, most notably the classical type II glucocorticoid receptor, with a high affinity for dexamethasone and other glucocorticoid compounds, such as prednisone and cortisol. Ligand-activated glucocorticoid receptor binds directly to the 5′-regulatory domain of the POMC gene to suppress gene transcription *(5,18)*. The direct corticosteroid suppression of pituitary ACTH secretion is also mediated through the type II glucocorticoid receptor, but may involve additional mechanisms, as yet unclarified, that are distinct and more rapid in onset than negative regulatory effects on ACTH biosynthesis *(19,20)*.

ACTH Secretion

In vitro studies suggest that the corticotroph cell secretes ACTH through two distinct pathways, termed constitutive and secretory (or "granular"), that appear to cor-

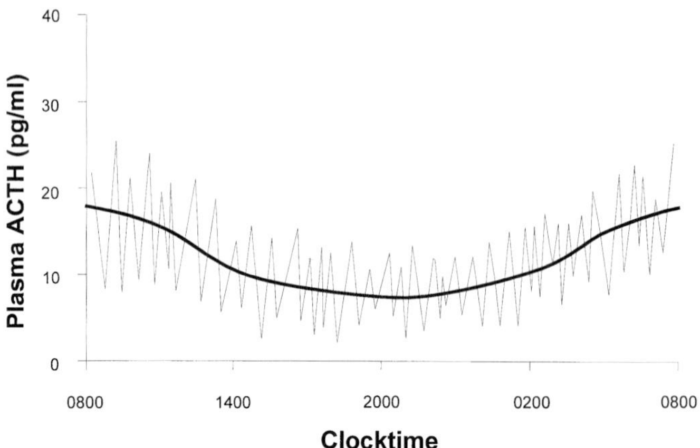

Fig. 3. Schematic representation of frequently sampled plasma ACTH levels in healthy (unstressed) human subjects, illustrating circadian periodicity and ultradian pulsatility of the HPA axis. ACTH (and cortisol) levels are lowest between 8 PM and midnight, with increased HPA activity beginning before awakening. Ultradian pulses (having periodicity of less than 24 h) occur throughout the 24 h cycles at approximately 90-min intervals.

respond to continuous and pulsatile components of ACTH secretion in humans *(21,22)*. The ACTH secretory pulse occurs in response to central stimulation, and can be reproduced by administration of exogenous CRH or exposure to stressful stimuli such as insulin-mediated hypoglycemia *(23,24)*. These stimuli entrain the ACTH pulse by activating the coordinated fusion of neurosecretory granules with the extracellular membrane through a mechanism that appears to involve changes in intracellular calcium concentration *(25)*. The resulting quantal release of stored hormone into the systemic circulation produces transient increments in plasma ACTH concentrations, and corresponding changes in serum cortisol. Nonpulsatile ACTH secretion is less clearly understood, but appears to be related to a continuous, low level "leak" of newly synthesized ACTH to the extracellular compartment through a transport mechanism that is independent of neurosecretory granules *(21)*.

Circadian and Ultradian Rhythms of ACTH Secretion

When plasma ACTH is measured at frequent intervals in humans, characteristic patterns of ACTH secretory activity, corresponding to circadian and ultradian rhythms, are observed *(22,26)*. Circadian rhythm refers to a regular pattern of hormone secretion that occurs over the 24-h diurnal cycle, whereas ultradian rhythm refers to periodicity of ACTH secretory activity over a shorter interval. Like many other endocrine rhythms, the rhythm of ACTH and cortisol secretion is closely linked to light–dark and sleep-activity cycles *(27)*. As illustrated in Fig. 3, activation of the HPA axis typically begins about 4:00 AM and reaches a peak around 8:00 AM. The ACTH and cortisol levels gradually diminish, and the HPA axis becomes relatively quiescent between 8:00 PM and 2:00 AM.

The circadian pattern of ACTH secretion is centrally mediated, and is organized by a CNS "clock" that is localized to the suprachiasmatic nucleus (SCN). This pattern of ACTH (and cortisol) secretion is maintained in subjects who are blind or removed from visual cues with a periodicity of about 25 h. However, in normal individuals, the clock is "set" or entrained by visual cues and the light–dark cycle. Since CRH-deficient mice with a deleted CRH gene lose their diurnal variation of corticosterone secretion, it appears that the presence of CRH is a necessary condition for the maintenance of the ACTH diurnal cycle *(28)*. However, it is also likely that factors other than CRH play an important role in generating the diurnal ACTH rhythm, since circadian variation is maintained during continuous CRH infusion in human subjects with suppression of endogenous HPA activity *(29)*.

An ultradian rhythm of periodic ACTH secretory bursts, with a frequency of about 40 bursts/24-h period, has been identified using pulse detection and deconvolution algorithms *(22,26)*. Thus, as shown in Fig. 3, the normal profile of ACTH and cortisol secretion reflects both the frequency of ACTH pulses and the amount of ACTH secreted per pulse. The amplitude and mass/burst of the ACTH pulse is influenced by stimulus intensity (for example, concentration of CRH), which is believed to reflect incremental recruitment of ACTH secretory granules and corresponding release of ACTH. The circadian variation in ACTH secretion is related to changes in ACTH pulse amplitude, but not frequency *(26)*. Similarly, stress stimuli, such as insulin-mediated hypoglycemia, are associated with an increase in ACTH pulse amplitude *(24)*. Corticosteroids act through a direct pituitary effect to decrease the amplitude of endogenous or stimulated ACTH pulses *(30)*.

Maintenance Functions of HPA Activity

The circadian and ultradian rhythms of the HPA axis serve important physiologic functions even in the absence of stress. The normal, daily, episodic secretion of ACTH and cortisol obviously maintains a variety of permissive endocrine and metabolic functions. When ACTH is absent, resulting in secondary adrenal insufficiency, the loss of these permissive functions contributes to the syndrome of chronic adrenal insufficiency, characterized by nausea, anorexia, weight loss, fatigue, and occasional hypoglycemia. Daily activation of the HPA axis is also important in maintaining the integrity of adrenal cortical function. In the absence of adequate daily ACTH secretion, the enzymes responsible for adrenal steroidogenesis are downregulated, adrenal weight falls, and cortisol secretory capacity is decreased. Thus, the ability to mount an adequate cortisol response to life-threatening stress is critically dependent on the normal, daily maintenance functions of the HPA axis.

CENTRAL REGULATION OF THE HPA AXIS

Hypothalamic-Pituitary Portal ACTH Secretagogs

The CNS regulates four critical variables influencing ACTH secretion:

1. Diurnal variation in ACTH pulse amplitude;
2. Amplitude and frequency of ultradian ACTH pulses;
3. Activation of pulsatile ACTH secretion in response to stress; and
4. Central HPA activation in response to corticosteroid removal.

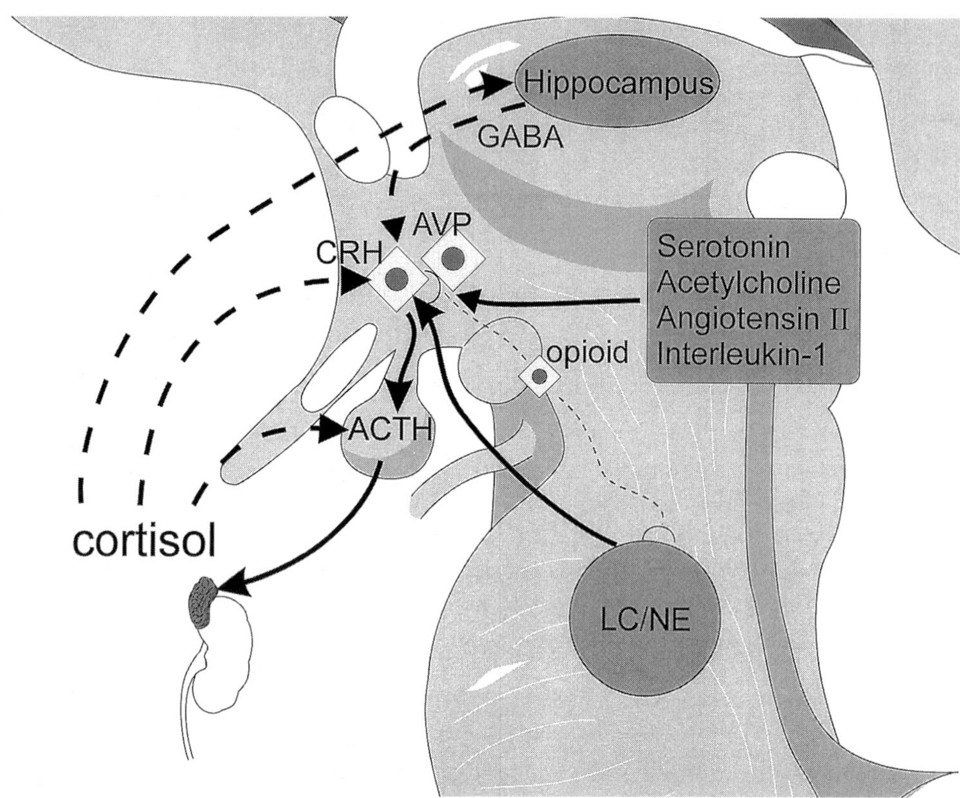

Fig. 4. Schematic representation of neuroendocrine regulation of the HPA axis. A variety of central nervous system structures and neurotransmitters project to the hypothalamus to provide stimulatory (solid lines) or inhibitory (broken lines) regulation of CRH synthesis and secretion. CNS noradrenergic afferents from the locus coeruleus (LC/NE) also stimulate CRH synthesis and release. Other ACTH secretagogs, such as AVP, regulate ACTH secretion and modify the response to CRH by direct release into the hypophyseal portal circulation. Negative feedback by cortisol (broken lines) is mediated at multiple sites that express cortisol responsive (type I and type II) corticosteroid receptors, including pituitary, hypothalamus, and hippocampus.

As indicated in Fig. 4, a variety of CNS structures, neuronal networks, and neurotransmitter systems indirectly influence ACTH secretion. These regulatory influences are integrated at the level of the hypothalamus and ultimately expressed through release of specific effector molecules, termed ACTH secretagogs, that act directly on the corticotroph cell to stimulate ACTH secretion. These ACTH secretagogs are synthesized in the hypothalamus and reach the pituitary via direct release into a specialized circulatory conduit, the pituitary portal vessels. Thus, ACTH secretagogs must fulfill several criteria, including:

1. Hypothalamic expression and synthesis;
2. Secretion into the pituitary portal circulation at physiologically active concentrations;
3. The presence of specific corticotroph cell receptors for the putative secretagog; and
4. Pituitary ACTH releasing activity in vitro and in vivo.

Having fulfilled such criteria, the physiologic significance of ACTH secretagogs has been experimentally addressed by assessing the effect of functional ablation employing immunoneutralization and/or gene knockout methodologies on the ACTH and corticosteroid response to centrally mediated stimuli.

Both CRH and AVP meet all criteria for physiologically important ACTH secretagogues *(31)*. Originally isolated in 1981 from ovine hypothalami by virtue of in vitro ACTH releasing activity in primary pituitary cultures *(32)*, CRH is clearly the dominant hypothalamic peptide mediating stimulation of ACTH production and secretion. AVP also activates ACTH secretion independently and through synergistic interactions with CRH *(17)*. A variety of other compounds, including CCK, NPY, catecholamines, interleukin-1, angiotensin II, and leukemic inhibitory factor (LIF), also appear to have a minor role in the central regulation of ACTH secretion *(33)*. It seems likely that the role of many of these secretagogs may be to modulate the effect of CRH, but at present their physiological significance is uncertain.

Animal Models of CRH Deficiency

The primacy of CRH in central regulation of ACTH secretion is emphasized by the severe defiiciency of ACTH and corticosteroid observed in the murine model of CRH deficiency using gene knockout methods *(34,35)*. In CRH-deficient mice, the lack of corticosterone (the principal rodent glucocorticoid) during development leads to deficient fetal surfactant production and death of the animals from neonatal respiratory distress syndrome. However, these mice can be rescued antenatally by administration of dexamethasone and then survive into adulthood without any further administration of exogenous glucocorticoids *(35)*.

In adult CRH-deficient mice, basal ACTH and corticosterone levels are markedly below normal, suggesting that no other ACTH secretagogs, including AVP, are able to compensate for the lack of CRH in spite of markedly diminished glucocorticoid feedback. In addition, CRH-deficient mice lack the normal circadian pattern of ACTH and corticosteroid secretion, and exhibit a blunted, but not absent, ACTH response to stress *(28)*. Thus, it appears that compounds other than CRH can mediate some degree of ACTH responsiveness to centrally acting stress stimuli. Interestingly, there is a marked difference in both basal and stress-induced ACTH and corticosterone secretion between male and female mice lacking CRH, with consistently higher ACTH and corticosterone levels noted in female knockout mice. Thus, there exists sexual dimorphism in the HPA axis, which is amplified when CRH is absent *(28)*. These knockout mice demonstrate a normal ACTH response to CRH, and their anterior pituitary glands show normal histology and POMC levels, suggesting that CRH is not necessary for the development and maintenance of corticotroph function *(28)*. However, this normal ACTH response to exogenous CRH occurs at a very low level of circulating corticosterone in CRH-deficient mice; this response may actually be decreased relative to CRH-intact mice at comparable levels of corticosterone. These findings in the CRH knockout mouse model indicate CRH plays a critical role, either active or permissive, in all components of the central regulation of ACTH secretion, including response to stress, corticosteroid removal, and circadian variation.

Hypothalamic CRH-Producing Neurons

Parvocellular neurons that synthesize and secrete CRH are located in the paraventlicular nucleus (PVN) of the hypothalamus *(36)*. These CRH neurons play a primary role in the central regulation of ACTH secretion. They project axons to capillaries in the median eminence, thereby providing a mechanism for direct secretion of CRH into the hypothalamic-pituitary portal system.

As with other hypothalamic releasing hormones, CRH is found in portal blood at physiologically active concentrations (10^{-9}–$10^{-10}M$) and is rapidly diluted in the systemic circulation *(37,38)*. Since peripheral or petrosal sinus plasma levels of CRH do not clearly reflect pituitary portal concentrations of CRH, hypothalamic CRH secretion in humans can only be indirectly assessed through measurement of ACTH secretion.

In addition to hypothalamic CRH producing neurons, CRH is expressed in neurons located in other CNS sites, including the cerebral cortex and amygdala *(39)*. Functional CRH receptors are also widely distributed in extrahypothalamic sites of the CNS *(40)* so that injection of CRH into the cerebral ventricles results in a variety of physiologic effects, such as anxiety, arousal, and conflict avoidance *(41–43)*. These extrahypothalamic sites of CRH expression do not project to the median eminence and therefore play no direct role in pituitary ACTH secretion, but they may mediate central effects of stress other than activation of the HPA axis *(44)*.

CRH Synthesis and Secretion

CRH is expressed from a single-copy gene with a highly conserved structure of two exons and one intron that is localized on chromosome 8q13 in humans. As in the case of POMC, gene transcription is an important component of physiologic regulation of CRH, and sequences within the 5′-regulatory region of the CRH gene confer developmental and tissue-specific expression *(45–47)* as well as activation in response to increased intracellular cAMP and neuronal depolarization believed to participate in the transcriptional activation of CRH in response to stress *(48–50)*. The CRH is transcribed from two distinct promoter sites, yielding mRNA species that differ in the 5′-untranslated region but produce the same pre-pro CRH peptide *(45,51)*. The functional significance of differential transcription initiation sites is uncertain, but may be related to differences in CRH mRNA stability or transcriptional regulation *(52,53)*. The 5′-regulatory sequences of the CRH gene also influence transcriptional repression by corticosteroids *(54–56)*, although the CRH promoter lacks a consensus glucocorticoid response element and the precise site and mechanism of corticosteroid-dependent repression remains uncertain. The functional importance of these 5′-regulatory sequences is emphasized by the remarkable degree of sequence conservation across species, with > 90% homology between human and mouse genes *(57)*, as illustrated in Fig. 5. This degree of nucleotide conservation indicates that transcriptional determinants of CRH expression confer an important survival advantage and that mechanisms of regulation are similar across phylogenetic lines. CRH is a 41-amino acid peptide that is cleaved from the carboxyl terminus of a larger 170-amino acid precursor called pre-proCRH. The CRH peptide is modified during post-translational processing by amidation of the C-terminal glycine, a step required for biological activity of CRH.

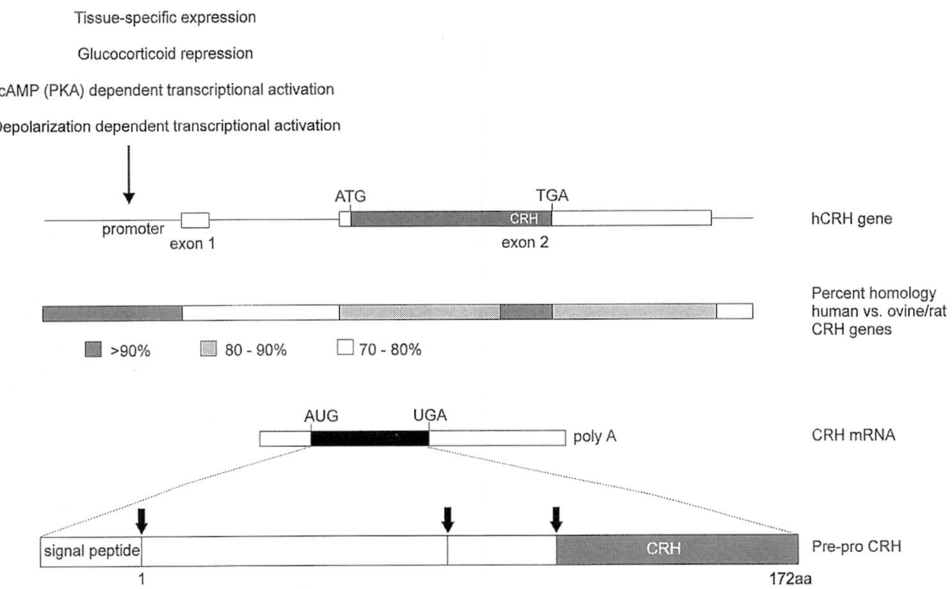

Fig. 5. Structure of the human CRH gene (upper panel) with 5′-regulatory sequence of the CRH promoter and translated regions (solid fill). Percent homology between the human CRH gene and the ovine and rat. CRH genes (middle panel) demonstrates a high degree of conservation (>90%) for 5′-regulatory and CRH coding regions. The CRH mRNA and CRH prepropeptide are indicated in the lower panel, with dibasic cleavage sites indicated by solid arrows. Adapted with permission from ref. *113*.

Regulation of CRH Secretion

As illustrated in Fig. 4, a variety of different afferent neurons project from the CNS and PNS to the region of the hypothalamus that contains the CRH neurons. Noradrenergic fibers originating in the locus ceruleus, for example, appear to activate CRH secretion and synthesis. This may account for the attenuation of ACTH secretion by clonidine, a drug that depletes central noradrenergic activity *(58)*. Serotonergic and cholinergic pathways also lead to the stimulation of ACTH secretion, and interleukin-1 activates ACTH release through central mechanisms involving CRH secretion.

In addition to these positive regulatory pathways, there are negative opioidergic pathways that suppress CRH and ACTH secretion. Consequently, an opioid receptor blocker, such as naloxone, causes a transient stimulation of ACTH secretion mediated through release of endogenous CRH *(59)*. It is presently unclear whether endogenous opioids, and their inhibition by naloxone, act directly on CRH neurons in the hypothalamus or indirectly through effects on other regulatory pathways *(60)*, such as noradrenergic afferents originating in the locus coeruleus (*see* Fig. 4).

Source and Significance of AVP

AVP is synthesized in both parvocellular and magnocellular divisions of the PVN, and both sources contribute to pituitary portal AVP concentrations. Whereas magnocellular neurons secrete AVP principally into the systemic circulation, they also contribute to pituitary portal AVP levels through anastomotic connections. AVP is coexpressed with CRH in parvocellular neurons of the PVN *(61,62)*. Thus, whereas AVP is a considerably less potent stimulus for ACTH secretion than CRH, the synergistic effect of AVP with CRH is significant under conditions in which both secretagogues are coordinately released *(63,64)*.

Administration of CRH in Humans

A variety of clinically useful maneuvers can be employed to stimulate ACTH secretion. Intravenous infusion of CRH is associated with a rapid rise in plasma ACTH and serum cortisol, with a maximal response occurring 15–30 min after CRH administration *(23)*. Both human and ovine CRH compounds have been used in this setting *(65)*. Human CRH (hCRH) has a shorter half-life and duration of action, owing to the presence of a serum CRH binding protein (CRH-BP), which attenuates the biological action of the hormone *(66,67)*. Ovine CRH (oCRH) by contrast, does not bind CRH-BP and therefore has a more extended duration of action. Accordingly, the greater magnitude of the ACTH response to oCRH confers improved diagnostic sensitivity and specificity relative to hCRH in defined clinical situations *(68)*. A dose of 100 μg or 1 μg/kg of ovine or human CRH has been typically used in human studies. Higher doses produce a greater ACTH response, but are associated with increased incidence of side effects, such as flushing, dyspnea, chest tightness, and hypotension. At present, neither ovine nor human CRH is commercially available for clinical application.

Considerable heterogeneity in the ACTH response to standardized doses of iv CRH is observed in healthy human subjects *(23,69)*. Several variables influence the magnitude of the ACTH response, including inhibitory effects of endogenous cortisol secretion. However, marked heterogeneity is also observed when endogenous cortisol secretion is blocked with metyrapone, indicating that other factors influence corticotroph responsiveness *(70,71)*. A positive correlation between the unstimulated (basal) ACTH level and the stimulated response to exogenous CRH has also been observed *(72)*. Factors determining these individual differences in the set point for pituitary response, hormone biosynthesis and secretion, and feedback inhibition are incompletely understood.

When iv CRH is given as a continuous infusion or repeated serial boluses, there is a sustained ACTH response with consequent hypercortisolism, suggesting that desensitization of the corticotroph to CRH is not a characteristic feature of the HPA axis *(73–75)*. This contrasts sharply with the gonadotroph axis, in which continuous infusion of GnRH results in downregulation and suppression of gonadotroph function with diminished LH and FSH secretion. The robust responsiveness of the corticotroph to repeated or continuous CRH stimulation supports the idea that clinical conditions associated with increased CRH from either a central source, as may occur during depression, or from tumors producing ectopic CRH, can result in chronic HPA axis activation with excessive cortisol secretion. These observations, as well as transgenic models in which the CRH gene is overexpressed *(76)*, demonstrate that chronic hypersecretion of CRH can stimulate an otherwise normal corticotroph-adrenal axis to produce sustained hypercortisolism.

PERIPHERAL REGULATION OF THE HPA AXIS

Pituitary Effects on the HPA Axis

The dominant regulatory effect of ACTH is the stimulation of adrenal corticosteroid synthesis and secretion. ACTH acts through high affinity receptors localized in the surface membrane of adrenal cortex cells, which are coupled to the generation of intracellular cyclic AMP. The daily morning surge of ACTH helps maintain adrenal steroidogenesis by regulating the transcription of a variety of p450 enzymes *(77)*. In addition, ACTH stimulates secretion of cortisol and other adrenocortical steroids, including aldosterone, 17-hydroxy-progesterone, and adrenal androgens.

Cortisol Synthesis and Secretion

Cortisol secretion occurs rapidly within 5–10 min of ACTH stimulation. Analysis of spontaneous ACTH and cortisol secretory dynamics in humans confirms that cortisol pulses closely follow ACTH pulses *(22)*. The dose–response curve of ACTH and cortisol is linear within the physiologic range of ACTH so that, during CRH testing, subjects having a higher ACTH response will also demonstrate an increased level of cortisol secretion *(23)*. However, the dose–response curve flattens out at supraphysiologic concentrations of ACTH such as those achieved during the standard 250 μg cortrosyn (ACTH 1–24) stimulation test.

Prior exposure to ACTH has an important influence on the adrenal cortisol response to ACTH. For example, when ACTH is deficient, there is downregulation of adrenal steroidogenic enzymes and adrenal cortical atrophy, which results in a blunted cortisol response to a defined dose of exogenous ACTH. By contrast, when ACTH is chronically excessive, as in ACTH-dependent Cushing's syndrome, then the adrenal cortex hypertrophies and a given dose of ACTH produces a greater than normal rise in serum cortisol.

Short-Loop Feedback of ACTH Secretion

Since the pituitary gland is situated on the systemic side of the blood–brain barrier, it is conceivable that ACTH, or other POMC-derived peptides such as β-lipotropin, act through a direct systemic feedback loop to modulate pituitary ACTH secretion. However, available evidence does not support the existence of such a feedback mechanism *(22,78)*. By the same token, the observation that retrograde flow from pituitary to hypothalamus may occur in the hypophyseal vessels suggests a mechanism by which ACTH might directly influence the secretion of CRH. Available data on this issue is contradictory and does not clearly support the presence of a negative regulatory effect of pituitary ACTH, or other POMC-derived peptides, on HPA function. Accordingly, our feedback schemes, outlined in Fig. 1, emphasize the positive regulation of CRH on ACTH and of ACTH on cortisol, whereas cortisol itself is the dominant negative regulatory agent in the HPA axis.

Feedback Inhibition by Cortisol

Feedback regulation of ACTH secretion by glucocorticoids is most clearly demonstrated at the level of the pituitary. Thus, exogenous CRH stimulation of ACTH is blunted by infusion of hydrocortisone or dexamethasone and increased by removal of cortisol feedback either by surgical adrenalectomy or by administration of metyrapone, an inhibitor of adrenal steroidogenesis *(71)*. In vitro studies of ACTH producing corticotroph cells indicate that glucocorticoids act through a homogenous type II glucocorticoid receptor population to inhibit POMC gene transcription as well as ACTH secretion *(18)*.

By contrast, assessment of glucocorticoid CNS feedback has been less amenable to analysis, owing to the difficulty in culturing neuronal cells and the inability to accurately measure portal blood concentrations of CRH and other ACTH secretagogs. Nevertheless, central feedback regulation is clearly important in mediating suppression of HPA axis activity. The primary role of the CNS in glucocorticoid feedback inhibition is most clearly illustrated by the suppression of the HPA axis in humans following termination of chronic hypercortisolism *(29)*. Such subjects demonstrate a normal ACTH response to an iv infusion of CRH, indicating that central, rather than pituitary, factors limit the recovery of the HPA axis from chronic glucocorticoid suppression. Whether or not this long-term suppression is mediated through direct inhibition of CRH secretion by hypothalamic CRH neurons or through intermediate effects on afferent pathways regulating CRH is at present uncertain. However, these clinical data provide compelling evidence that long-term suppression of the HPA axis following chronic glucocorticoid excess is mediated through central mechanisms and can be reversed by infusion of CRH.

Glucocorticoid receptors that mediate central feedback regulation involve distinct populations of receptor subtypes that are distributed in a broad spatial and cellular array in the CNS *(79,80)*. Classical (type II) glucocorticoid receptors are expressed in a variety of neuronal and glial cells, including the hypothalamic CRH producing neurons *(81)*. Available evidence suggests that glucocorticoids can act directly at the CRH producing neuron to inhibit CRH secretion as well as gene transcription *(54,82)*. The latter conclusion is supported by in vitro studies demonstrating that the CRH promoter is negatively regulated by glucocorticoids in a variety of cell lines *(55,56)*.

In addition to those direct effects on the CRH producing neurons located in the PVN, corticosteroids appear to inhibit ACTH secretion by indirect effects that are mediated through other CNS sites, most notably the hippocampus. In addition to type II glucocorticoid receptors, the hippocampus expresses the type I (mineralocorticoid or corticosterone preferring) receptor, which has a high affinity for cortisol *(83,84)*. In animal studies, ligand occupancy of hippocampal corticosteroid receptors has been associated with suppression of basal ACTH and cortisol secretion, as well as attenuation of stress-induced HPA axis activation *(85,86)*. Conversely, when hippocampal receptors are decreased with aging or chronic stress, then there is decreased sensitivity to glucocorticoid feedback inhibition with augmented ACTH secretion *(87)*. Although the importance of hippocampal feedback regulation by glucocorticoids is well established in animal models, its relevance in humans remains uncertain *(88)*. The age-associated changes in HPA axis function and the age-dependent increase in HPA abnormalities associated with depression in humans may reflect a decline in hippocampal glucocorticoid receptors *(89)*.

STRESS AND THE HPA AXIS

Stress implies an action being exerted on an object. These two components, action and object, both need to be defined in order to specify what stress means. Mechanical stress is a load or force of such magnitude that it produces strain in the object on which it is exerted. Physiological or psychological stress, on the other hand, is a stimulus of sufficient magnitude such that it disturbs the homeostatic equilibrium of an organism. The organism in its basal state is placed under a strain by the perturbation. The fact that the activation of the HPA represents a final common pathway in response to diverse forms of stress emphasizes the critical role of the HPA axis in the maintenance of homeostasis.

Stress can be detected by various defense systems in the body, such as the CNS, PNS (peripheral nervous system), vascular system, and immune system, that activate systematic changes throughout the body. These include increased arousal, tolerance to pain, and changes in the immune, cardiovascular, endocrine, and nervous systems. Thus, central activation of the HPA axis is but one component of the adaptation to stress that includes release of catecholamines, cytokines, neuropeptides, and other modulators of homeostasis, whose pattern will depend on the nature of the stress experienced. However, CRH, ACTH, and cortisol may be the most consistent participants in the preservation of the body's homeostatic equilibrium. Accordingly, stress can be defined operationally by the centrally mediated increase in ACTH secretion above the normal background of circadian and ultradian ACTH release.

The range of stressful stimuli that activate ACTH secretion is quite broad and includes such diverse conditions as pain, infection, hemorrhage, trauma, fright, hypoxia, exercise, depression, hypoglycemia, and mental and osmotic stress. These various forms of stress influence ACTH secretion through distinct neuronal pathways that may differ with respect to magnitude of ACTH response, sensitivity to corticosteroid inhibition, and array of hypothalamic ACTH secretagogs released into the portal circulation *(90)*. The acute or chronic nature of specific stresses may also influence the HPA response *(91)*.

An important feature of the stress reaction is that activation of the HPA axis will override feedback suppression by cortisol. Thus, when stress is present in sufficient magnitude, CRH and ACTH will continue to be produced in the face of very high levels of plasma cortisol. The molecular basis for this resistance to corticosteroid repression of ACTH secretion is uncertain, but is probably mediated at the level of the CNS rather than pituitary *(92)*. In view of observations that persistent hypersecretion of CRH can provoke an otherwise normal HPA axis into a state of hypercortisolism, it is likely that activation of CRH during stress will override the feedback suppression of elevated cortisol levels.

CLINICAL EVALUATION OF CORTICOTROPH FUNCTION

Measurement of ACTH

Modern approaches to the measurement of plasma ACTH levels include radioimmunoassay (RIA) and immunometric assay (IMA) methodologies. Single antibody RIA methods may have significant crossreactivity with other POMC-derived peptides; depending on the specific antibody reagents, IMA methods may provide improved specificity for the intact ACTH(1–39) peptide. Current assays can detect plasma ACTH with a sensitivity of 0.2–5 pg/mL with inter-assay and intra-assay coefficients of variation both < 10%.

For routine testing, ACTH levels are typically measured during peak hours of hypothalamic-pituitary-adrenal (HPA) axis activity between 6:00 and 9:00 AM. Subjects should be in a nonstressed state during the time of plasma collection since stress or illness can elevate the ACTH concentration. Handling of blood samples and separation of plasma requires special attention. ACTH may adhere to glass surfaces, requiring collection of EDTA plasma samples in plastic or siliconized glass containers. ACTH may be unstable in whole blood at room temperature due to degradation by proteases. Thus, whole blood samples are ideally transported on ice and plasma should be separated from cells as quickly as possible. ACTH is relatively stable in plasma stored at −20 to −70°C.

Normal Variation in ACTH Secretion

Even in the absence of stressful stimuli or intrinsic disorders of the HPA axis, there is still considerable normal variation in ACTH secretion patterns. Thus, the time of peak and nadir HPA axis activity may vary considerably between different individuals and within the same individual on different days. Gender differences in ACTH secretion exist, with a trend to lower ACTH levels in menstruating women, and lower mean plasma ACTH levels in women taking oral contraceptives. Gender differences in ultradian patterns of ACTH, but not cortisol, secretion have been observed, with greater pulse frequency, amplitude, and integrated 24-h ACTH secretion in males compared to females *(93)*.

Age may also have an impact on HPA axis function. Animal studies suggest that normal aging is associated with decreased HPA axis activity and altered central feedback regulation by glucocorticoids. However, it has been difficult to establish age-associated changes in HPA axis activity in humans.

Pregnancy is associated with increased plasma levels of ACTH, an increase in urine-free cortisol excretion, and a subnormal ACTH response to exogenous CRH *(94,95)*. All of these changes may be mediated by placentally derived CRH, progesterone, or other factors *(96)*.

Evaluation of the Integrity of ACTH Secretion

As described above, normal ACTH secretory dynamics involve both basal and pulsatile ACTH secretion subject to circadian rhythms, activation in response to stress, and inhibition by glucocorticoids. As might be expected, no single test can approximate these diverse components of normal ACTH secretory dynamics. Most clinically applied tests have focused on decreased ACTH secretory capacity or excessive ACTH secretion as it relates to the two principal disorders of adrenal function: adrenal insufficiency and cortisol excess (Cushing's syndrome).

Importance of Ambient Cortisol Concentrations

At all times it is important to remember that, like many other pituitary hormones, plasma ACTH concentrations must be evaluated within the context of its target gland hormone level, in this case cortisol originating from the adrenal gland. So what is considered a "normal" plasma ACTH level will depend on the simultaneous plasma cortisol level. Thus, even if plasma ACTH concentrations could be measured throughout the day, it would be impossible to establish a diagnosis of excessive or impaired ACTH secretion without understanding the context of antecedent and concurrent cortisol concentrations. For example, the loss of cortisol feedback inhibition in primary adrenal insufficiency (Addison's disease) is associated with increased ACTH concentrations and augmented ACTH response to CRH or stressful stimuli. Conversely, the finding of normal ACTH concentrations in the presence of hypercortisolism and Cushing's syndrome is inappropriate in the context of chronic cortisol excess. Finally, excess CRH secretion, as occurs in stress or depression, can produce ACTH-dependent hypercortisolism without implying any intrinsic abnormality of the pituitary or adrenal glands.

Cortisol as a Surrogate for ACTH

Pulsatile secretion of ACTH is rapidly followed by secretion of cortisol; consequently, ACTH and cortisol are closely correlated over the physiologic range of plasma ACTH concentrations *(97)*. Since sample collection and assay methods for serum cortisol are simpler than for plasma ACTH, cortisol is often used as a surrogate endpoint for ACTH. There is also some inherent gain in the pituitary-adrenal axis, such that serum cortisol demonstrates a more sensitive and robust response than ACTH following administration of exogenous CRH *(23)*. In the clinical context, integrated tests of the HPA axis that include adrenal function are also useful in establishing the normality of the axis.

Limited Value of Random Hormone Levels

Because of the normal variation and pulsatility of ACTH secretion, a random plasma ACTH concentration is difficult to interpret. As emphasized above, an ACTH level by itself cannot be used to establish a diagnosis of adrenal insufficiency or excess. However, once adrenal function has been established by other means, plasma ACTH concentration may be useful in differential diagnosis. In adrenal insufficiency, a clearly elevated ACTH level is supportive of primary rather than secondary hypoadrenalism. In Cushing's syndrome, an elevated or inappropriately normal plasma ACTH level is consistent with ACTH-dependent hypercortisolism. Extremely high levels of ACTH are often, but not always, associated with the syndrome of ectopic ACTH secretion.

Time of Day as a Variable

The informative value of ACTH (or cortisol) levels can be enhanced by taking advantage of the normal circadian variation in HPA axis activity. Since the HPA axis is usually active in the early morning, a low ACTH or cortisol value obtained at 8:00 A.M. may result from impaired secretory reserve. Conversely, activity of the HPA axis diminishes during the late afternoon and evening. Thus, elevated evening ACTH or cortisol levels, associated with loss of normal diurnal variation, is suggestive of Cushing's syndrome *(98)*.

By the same token, results of dynamic tests of ACTH secretion are influenced by the time of day. ACTH response to CRH administered in the morning, for example, may be diminished relative to the same test in the late afternoon or evening. This may be related to background ACTH secretory activity, producing elevations of baseline relative to stimulated ACTH levels, or to the inhibitory effect of cortisol secretion *(23)*.

DYNAMIC TESTS OF ACTH SECRETION

Adrenal Component of HPA Function (the Short ACTH Stimulation Test)

It is not intuitively obvious why the level of cortisol produced in response to acute administration of exogenous ACTH should provide a reflection of endogenous ACTH secretory capacity. The informative value of this test stems from the chronic trophic effects of ACTH on biosynthetic and secretory capacity of the adrenal cortex. Thus, in chronic ACTH excess, adrenal weight is increased and the cortisol response to ACTH is augmented. Conversely, in chronic ACTH deficiency, the cortisol response to exogenous ACTH is blunted. Therefore, the acute adrenal response to ACTH is a reflection of the antecedent milieu of ACTH secretion that correlates well with more sophisticated tests of the HPA axis, such as the insulin tolerance test. Adrenal atrophy and decreased secretory capacity associated with ACTH deficiency is dynamic in time. Since there is no intrinsic abnormality in the adrenal gland itself, the decreased secretory capacity associated with ACTH deficiency can be reversed by continuous ACTH administration over several days.

The short cortrosyn (ACTH 1–24) stimulation test is typically performed by determination of baseline serum cortisol concentration, im or iv administration of cosyntropin at a dose of 250 μg, and determination of serum cortisol 30–60 min later. An increase in plasma cortisol above 20 μg/dL usually reflects normal adrenal and ACTH secretory reserve, although the accuracy of the test is limited in some circumstances. For simplicity, in outpatient settings we prefer giving 250 μg of ACTH(1–24) by im injection followed by a single plasma cortisol determination 45 min later. In addition, the ACTH levels produced by 250 μg of ACTH (1–24) are well above physiologic, and may overcome mild forms of secondary adrenal insufficiency. Recent studies suggest that the sensitivity of the test may be improved by employing more physiologic doses in the range of 1–5 μg of cosyntropin *(99,100)*.

Pituitary Component of HPA Function (Exogenous CRH and AVP Administration)

Both CRH and AVP act on the corticotroph, and therefore exogenous administration of these ACTH secretagogs directly stimulate pituitary ACTH secretion. The direct action of CRH on the pituitary corticotroph supports an application of the CRH stimulation test in primary pituitary disorders, including ACTH deficiency and excess associated with hypopituitarism and Cushing's disease (corticotroph adenoma), respectively *(101)*. However, the clinical utility of the CRH test to distinguish normal from abnormal ACTH response has been limited by several factors. These include the significant degree of normal variability in ACTH response to CRH and the modulatory effect of endogenous cortisol secretion on CRH-stimulated ACTH secretion. In addition, the maintenance of normal ACTH response to exogenous CRH under conditions of chronic CRH excess or deficiency limit the value of the CRH test. These factors also limit the distinction between hypercortisolemic conditions associated with corticotroph adenoma (Cushing's disease) and hypothalamic hypercortisolism (pseudo-Cushing's syndrome) associated with psychiatric disorders, such as depression *(102,103)*. Whereas most tumors associated with ectopic ACTH secretion do not respond, several exceptions have been reported, thus limiting the usefulness of CRH testing in ACTH-dependent Cushing's syndrome *(104,105)*.

Accordingly, the main clinical utility of exogenous CRH administration has been realized in conjunction with other HPA investigations. Thus, administration of CRH during petrosal sinus sampling improves the sensitivity and specificity of that procedure in distinguishing pituitary from peripheral sources of ACTH secretion *(106)*. Similarly, use of CRH in conjunction with the dexamethasone suppression test improves the discrimination between hypothalamic hypercortisolism (pseudo-Cushing's syndrome) and corticotroph adenoma *(107,108)*.

AVP has been also used alone or in combination with CRH to stimulate ACTH secretion. The ACTH responses to AVP generally parallel those produced by CRH, and the two stimuli together produce a synergistic ACTH response.

Central Component of HPA Function (Insulin-Induced Hypoglycemia, Metyrapone, and Naloxone)

The insulin tolerance test (ITT) has also been used to activate ACTH and cortisol secretion. Typically, insulin is administered as an iv bolus at a dose of 0.1–0.15 U/kg, with the aim of achieving blood glucose levels of 30–40 mg/dL and mildly symptomatic hypoglycemia. A plasma cortisol level greater than 20 µg/dL following hypoglycemia is considered a normal response. By producing a physiological stress, the ITT acts through central mechanisms, involving release of CRH and other ACTH secretagogs. This property is advantageous in two respects. First, a normal cortisol response to insulin-induced hypoglycemia implies that central, pituitary, and adrenal components of the HPA axis are all intact and that the HPA axis will activate normally in the event of other stress, such as surgery. Second, by involving central activation of CRH, the ITT may be useful in identifying clinical conditions associated with central dysregulation of HPA axis function. For example, CRH is appropriately suppressed by chronic hypercortisolism associated with a corticotroph adenoma (Cushing's disease), resulting in a blunted ACTH and cortisol response to hypoglycemia *(98)*.

The clinical utility of the ITT is limited by several important factors. These include the cost of multiple assays and physician time in performing the test. Moreover, hypoglycemia is a real stress and may be associated with side effects, such as angina, seizure, or CNS ischemia; in patients with compensated adrenal insufficiency, the ITT may produce frank acute adrenal crisis. In addition, the diagnostic accuracy of the test is limited. This is owing in part to individual variability in the degree of hypoglycemia produced by insulin as well as differences in the glycemic threshold for activation of the HPA axis. In addition, since hypoglycemia activates other stress-responsive systems, such as sympathetic and adrenal medullary catecholamine secretion, it may stimulate ACTH secretion through mechanisms that are independent of CRH. These factors limit the diagnostic sensitivity and specificity of the ITT in evaluation of adrenal disorders. Endogenous pyrogen has been used in a similar manner to simulate stress, although side effects limit the practicality of this method.

The metyrapone test activates ACTH secretion by removing feedback inhibition mediated by endogenous cortisol secretion. Metyrapone acts at the adrenal cortex to block cortisol synthesis primarily by inhibition of the 11-β–hydroxylase enzyme. Like the ITT, the response to metyrapone is believed to involve central as well as pituitary components of the HPA axis. The normal response to metyrapone administration is an increase in the ACTH level, which leads to increased secretion of corticosteroid precursors that build up behind the metyrapone block, especially 11-deoxycortisol (compound S). Interpretation of this test also requires documentation of the effectiveness of metyrapone in blocking cortisol biosynthesis, which can be accomplished by simultaneous serum cortisol determination.

Administration of the opiate antagonist naloxone also stimulates the release of ACTH and cortisol in animals and humans. Although the mechanism underlying this effect is not certain, CRH producing neurons in the hypothalamus appear to be under tonic inhibitory control by endogenous opioids, and the reversal of this effect by naloxone leads to central activation of HPA axis secretory activity *(59,109)*. In normal subjects, naloxone produces a rise in ACTH and cortisol comparable to that produced by CRH stimulation *(30)*. The commercial availability and safety of naloxone offer advantages relative to CRH and ITT, respectively. Because of its central site of action, naloxone may provide an integrated assessment of HPA axis function comparable to the ITT. Preliminary studies suggest that the ACTH response to naloxone is blunted in pituitary Cushing's disease, but exaggerated in conditions associated with hypothalamic hypercortisolism, e.g., pseudo-Cushing's syndrome seen with depression *(110,111)*. Additional data will be necessary to evaluate the role of naloxone in the clinical evaluation of secondary adrenal insufficiency and cortisol excess states.

SUMMARY AND CONCLUSION

The HPA axis is vitally important in the maintenance of homeostasis and senses as a key defense system against stressful perturbation. The hormones CRH, ACTH, and cortisol form an interdependent triad that are responsible for HPA axis integrity. Several of these hormones, their precursors, and their transcriptional units are highly conserved over the sweep of evolutionary time, suggesting that the structures are extremely important in homeostatic regulation.

The central hormone of the HPA axis is ACTH. It originates from a larger precursor peptide POMC through selective enzymatic processing, and is secreted in discrete pulses whose amplitude and frequency result in circadian and ultradian rhythms. ACTH secretion is stimulated by secretagogues introduced into the pituitary portal circulation and is supressed by cortisol feedback inhibition.

CRH is the dominant ACTH secretagog, but AVP and other neuropeptides play a minor role in ACTH secretion. In animal models of CRH deficiency using gene knockout methods, ACTH levels are extremely low, the normal circadian pattern is absent, and there is a blunted ACTH response to stress, emphasizing the dominant role of CRH relative to AVP and other secretagogs in maintaining the integrity of the HPA. The CRH secretion from hypothalamic neurons is regulated by the CNS and PNS, as well as by cortisol feedback inhibition. These interactions are complicated and involve noradrenergic, serotonergic, cholinergic, and opioidergic pathways that have stimulatory and inhibitory effects on CRH neurons and other ACTH secretagogues.

In summary, the HPA axis is a marvelously and complexly coordinated entity. The axis has been assembled from ancestral scraps of interesting molecules, conserved in structure, and entrained into a flexible and dynamic system for the defense of the body's homeostatic integrity.

REFERENCES

1. Kendall EC. Cortisone. Charles Scribner's Sons, New York, 1971.
2. Williams CL, Nishihara M, Thalabard JC, Grosser PM, Hotchkiss J. Knobil E. Corticotropin-releasing factor and gonadotropin-releasing hormone pulse generator activity in the rhesus monkey. Electrophysiological studies. Neuroendocrinology 1990;52:133–137.
3. Takahashi H. Hakamata Y. Watanabe Y. Kikuno R. Miyata T. Numa S. Complete nucleotide sequence of the human corticotropin-β-lipotropin precursor gene. Nucleic Acids Res 1983;11:6847–6858.
4. Hammer GD, Fairchild-Huntress V, Low MJ. Pituitary-specific and hormonally regulated gene expression directed by the rat proopiomelanocortin promoter in transgenic mice. Mol Endocrinol 1990;4:1689–1997.
5. Therrien M, Drouin J. Molecular determinants for cell specificity and glucocorticoid repression of the proopiomelanocortin gene. Ann NY Acad Sci 1993;680:663–671.
6. Eipper BA, Mains RE. Structure and biosynthesis of proadrenocorticotropin/endorphin and related peptides. Endocr Rev 1980;1:1–27.
7. Smith AI, Funder JW. Proopiornelanocortin processing in the pituitary, central nervous system and periperhal tissues. Endocr Rev 1988;9:159–179.
8. Lacaze MT, De Keyzer Y. Luton JP, Kahn A, Bertagna X. Characterization of proopiomelanocortin transcripts in human nonpituitary tissues. Proc Natl Acad Sci USA 1987;84:7261–7265.
9. Clark AJ, Lavender PM, Coates P. Johnson MR, Rees LH. In vitro and in vivo analysis of the processing and fate of the peptide products of the short proopiomelanocortin mRNA. Mol Endocrinol 1990;4:1737–1743.
10. Benjannet S. Rondeau N. Day R. Chretien M, Seidah NG. PC1 and PC2 and proprotein convertases capable of cleaving proopiomelanocortin at distinct pairs of basic residues. Proc Natl Acad Sci USA 1991;88:3564–3568.
11. Potter E, Sutton S. Donaldson C, et al. Distribution of corticotropin-releasing factor receptor mRNA expression in the rat brain and pituitary. Proc Natl Acad Sci USA 1994;91:8777–8781.
12. Baertschi AJ, Friedli M. A novel type of vasopressin receptor on anterior pituitary corticotrophs. Endocrinology 1985;116:499–502.
13. Reisine T. Rougon G. Barbet J. Affolter HU. Corticotropin-releasing factor-induced adrenocorticotropin hormone release and synthesis is blocked by incorporation of the inhibitor of cyclic AMP-dependent protein kinase into anterior pituitary tumor cells by liposomes. Proc Natl Acad Sci USA 1985;82:8261–8265.
14. Carvallo P. Aguilera G. Protein kinase C mediates the effect of vasopressin in pituitary corticotrophs. Mol Endocrinol 1989;3:1035–1943.
15. Lamberts SWJ, Verleun T. Oosterom R. et al. Corticotropin releasing factor and vasopressin exert a synergistic effect on adrenocorticotropin release in man. J Clin Endocrinol Metab 1984;58:298–305.
16. DeBold CR, Sheldon WR, DeCherney GS, et al. Arginine vasopressin potentiates adrenocorticopin release induced by ovine corticotropin-releasing factor. J Clin Invest 1984;75:533–538.
17. Abou-Samra AB, Hanvood JP, Manganiello VC, Catt KJ, Aguilera G. Phosbol 12-myristate 13-acetate and vasopressin potentiate the effect of corticotropin-releasing factor on cyclic AMP production in rat anterior pituitary cells. J Biol Chem 1987;262:1129–1136.
18. Ebenvine JH, Roberts JL. Glucocorticoid regulation of pro-opiomelanocortin gene transcription in the rat pituitary. J Biol Chem 1984;259:2166–2170.
19. Keller-Wood ME, Dallman MF. Corticosteroid inhibition of ACTH secretion. Endo Rev 1984;5:1–24.

20. Dayanithi G. Antoni FA. Rapid as well as delayed inhibitory effects of glucocorticoid hormones on pituitary adrenocorticotropic hormone release are mediated by type II glucocorticoid receptors and require newly synthesized messenger ribonucleic acid as well as protein. Endocrinology 1989;125:308–313.
21. Gumbiner B. Kelly RB. Two distinct intracellular pathways transport secretory and membrane glycoproteins to the surface of pituitary tumor cells. 1982; Cell 58:51–59.
22. Iranmanesh A, Lizarralde G. Short D, Veldhuis JD. Intensive venous sampling paradigms disclose high frequency adrenocorticotropin release episodes in normal men. J Clin Endocrinol Metab 1990;71:1276–1283.
23. Orth DN. Corticotropin-releasing hormone in humans. Endo Rev 1992;13:164–191.
24. Iranmanesh A, Lizarralde G. Veldhuis JD. Coordinate activation of the corticotropic axis by insulin-induced hypoglycemia: simultaneous estimates of beta-endorphin, adrenocorticotropin and cortisol secretion and disappearance in normal men. Acta Endocrinol 1992;128:521–528.
25. Childs CV. Structure-function correlates in the corticotropes of the anterior pituitary. Front Neuroendocrinol 1992;13:271–317.
26. Veldhuis JD, Iranmanesh A, Johnson ML, Lizarralde G. Amplitude, but not frequency, modulation of adrenocorticotropin secretory bursts gives rise to the nyctohemeral rhythm of the corticotropic axis in man. J C'lin Endocrinol Metab 1990;71:452–463.
27. Veldhuis JD, Iranmanesh A, Johnson ML, Lizarralde G. Twenty-four-hour rhythms in plasma concentrations of adenohypophyseal hormones are generated by distinct amplitude and/or frequency modulation of underlying pituitary secretory bursts. J Clin Endocrinol Metab 1990;71:1616–1623.
28. Muglia L, Jacobson L, Luedke C, Majzoub JA. Regulation of the hypothalamic-pituitary-adrenal axis in corticotropin-releasing hormone deficient mice. 77th Annual Meeting of the Endocrine Society, Washington, DC, June 1995.
29. Gomez MT, Magiakou MA, Mastorakos G. Chrousos GP. The pituitary corticotroph is not the rate limiting step in the postoperative recovery of the hypothalamic-pituitary-adrenal axis in patients with Cushing syndrome. J Clin Endocrinol Metab 1993;77:173–177.
30. Dorin RI, Ferries LM, Roberts B, Qualls CR, Veldhuis JD, Lisansky EJ. Assessment of stimulated and spontaneous adrenocorticotropin secretory dynamics identifies distinct components of cortisol feedback inhibition in healthy humans. J Clin Endocrinol Metab 1996;81:3883–3891.
31. Antoni FA. Hypothalamic control of adrenocorticotropin secretion: advances since the discovery of 41-residue corticotropin-releasing factor. Endo Rev 1986;7:351–378.
32. Vale W. Spiess J. Rivier C, Rivier J. Characterization of a 41-residue ovine hypothalamic peptide that stimulates secretion of corticotropin and beta-endorphin. Science 1981;213:1394–1397.
33. Akita S. Webster J. Ren SG. et al. Human and murine pituitary expression of leukemia inhibitory factor: novel intrapituitary regulation of adrenocorticotropin hormone synthesis and secretion. J Clin Invest 1995;95:1288–1298.
34. Muglia LJ, Jenkins NA, Gilbert DJ, Copeland NG, Majzoub JA. Expression of the mouse corticotropin-releasing hormone gene in vivo and targeted inactivation in embryonic stem cells. J Clin Invest 1994;93:2066–2072.
35. Muglia L, Jacobson L, Dikkes P. Majzoub JA. Corticotropin-releasing hormone deficiency reveals major fetal but not adult glucocorticoid need. Nature 1995;373:427–432.
36. Sawchenko PE, Imaki T. Potter E, Kovacs K, Imaki J. Vale W. The functional neuroanatomy of corticotropin-releasing factor. Ciba Found Symp 1993;172:5–29.
37. Rivier CL, Plotsky PM. Mediation by corticotropin releasing factor (CRF) of adenohypophysial hormone secretion. Ann Rev Physiol 1986;48:475–494.
38. Plotsky PM, Vale W. Hemorrhage-induced secretion of corticotropin-releasing factor-like immunoreactivity into the rat hypophysial portal circulation and its inhibition by glucocorticoids. Endocrinology 1984;114:164–169.
39. Swanson LW, Sawchenko PE, Rivier J. Vale WW. Organization of ovine corticotropin-releasing factor immunoreactive cells and filbers in the rat brain: an immunohistochemical study. Neuroendoclinology 1983;36:165–186.
40. Potter E, Sutton S. Donaldson C, et al. The distribution of CRF receptor mRNA expression in the rat brain and pituitary. 76th Annual Meeting of the Endocrine Society Anaheim, CA, 1994.

41. Tazi A, Dantzer R. Le Moal M, Rivier J. Vale W. Koob GF. Corticotropin-releasing factor antagonist blocks stress-induced fighting in rats. Regul Pept 1987;18:37–42.
42. Sutton RE, Koob GF, Le Moal M, Rivier J. Vale W. Corticotropin releasing factor produces behavioural activation in rats. Nature 1982;297:331–3.
43. Cole BJ, Cador M, Stinus L, et al. Central administration of a CRF antagonist blocks the development of stress-induced behavioral sensiitization. Brain Res 1990;512:343–346.
44. Chrousos GP, Gold PW. The concepts of stress and stress system disorders. Overview of physical and behavioral homeostasis. JAMA. 1992;267:1244–1252.
45. Vamvakopoulos NC, Chrousos GP. Hormonal regulation of human corticotropin-releasing hormone gene expression: implications for the stress response and immune/inflammatory reaction. Endocr Rev 1994; 15:409–420.
46. Keegan CE, Karolyi IJ, Knapp LT, Bourbonais FJ, Camper SA, Seasholtz AF. Expression of corticotropin-releasing hormone transgenes in neurons of adult and developing mice. Mol Cell Neurosci 1994;5:505–514.
47. Mugele K, Kugler H. Spiess J. Immortalization of a fetal rat brain cell line that expresses corticotropin-releasing factor mRNA. DNA Cell Biol 1993;12:119–126.
48. Dorin RI, Takahashi H. Nakai Y. Fukata J. Naitoh Y. Imura H. Regulation of human corticotropin-releasing hormone gene expression by 3′,5′-cyclic adenosine monophosphate in a transformed mouse corticotroph cell line. Mol Endocrinol 1989;3:1537–1544.
49. Seasholtz AF, Thompson RC, Douglass JO. Identification of a cyclic adenosine monophosphate-responsive element in the rat corticotropin-releasing hormone gene. Mol Endocrinol 1988;2:1311–1319.
50. Guardiola-Diaz HM, Boswell C, Seasholtz AF. The cAMP-responsive element in the corticotropin-releasing hormone gene mediates transcriptional regulation by depolarization. J Biol Chem 1994;269:14784–14791.
51. Robinson BG, D'Angio LA,Jr., Pasieka KB, Majzoub JA. Preprocorticotropin releasing hormone: cDNA sequence and in vitro processing. Mol Cell Endocrinol 1989;61:175–180.
52. Dorin RI, Zlock DW, Kilpatrick K. Transcriptional regulation of human corticotropin releasing factor gene expression by cyclic adenosine 3′,5′-monophosphate: differential effects at proximal and distal promoter elements. Mol Cell Endocrinol 1993;96:99–111.
53. Vamvakopoulos NC, Chrousos GP. Regulated activity of the distal promoter-like element of the human corticotropin-releasing hormone gene and secondary structural features of its corresponding transcripts. Mol Cell Endocrinol 1993;94:73–78.
54. Herman JP, Schafer MK, Thompson RC, Watson SJ. Rapid regulation of corticotropin-releasing hormone gene transcription in vivo. Mol Endocrinol 1992;6:1061–1069.
55. Van LP, Spengler DH, Holsboer F. Glucocorticoid repression of 3′,5′-cyclic-adenosine monophosphate-dependent human corticotropin-releasing-hormone gene promoter activity in a transfected mouse anterior pituitary cell line. Endocrinology 1990;127:1412–1418.
56. Majzoub JA, Emanuel R. Adler G. MDartinez C, Robinson B. Wittert G. Second messenger regulation of mRNA for corticotropin-releasing factor. Ciba Found Symp 1993;172:30–43.
57. Vamvakopoulos NC, Karl M, Mayol V, et al. Structural analysis of the regulatory region of the human corticotropin releasing hormone gene. FEBS Lett 1990;267: 1–5.
58. Jackson RV, Grice JE, Jackson AJ, Hockings GI. Naloxone-induced ACTH release in man is inhibited by clonidine. Clin Exp Pharm Physiol 1990;17:179–184.
59. Estienne M, Kesner J. Arb B. Kraeling R. Rampacek G. On the site of action of naloxone: stimulated cortisol secretion in gilts. Life Sci 1988;43:161–166.
60. Koh T. Nakai Y. Kinoshita F. Tsujii S. Tsukada T. Imura H. Evidence for noradrenergic involvement in naloxone-induced stimulation of luteinizing hormone release in prepubertal female rats. Eur J Pharm 1983;89:275–278.
61. Kiss JZ, Mezey E, Skirboll L. Corticotropin-releasing factor-immunoreactive neurons of the paraventricular nucleus become vasopressin positive after adrenalectomy. Proc Natl Acad Sci USA 1984;81:1854–1858.
62. Wolfson B. Manning RW, Davis LG, Arentzen R. Baldino F, Jr. Co-localization of corticotropin releasing factor and vasopressin mRNA in neurones after adrenalectomy. Nature 1985;315:59–61.

63. Whitnall MH, Mezey E, Gainer H. Co-localization of corticotropin-releasing factor and vasopressin in median eminence neurosecretory vesicles. Nature 1985;317:248–250.
64. Raff H. Interactions between neurohypophysial hormones and the ACTH-adrenocortical axis. Ann NY Acad Sci 1993;689:411–425.
65. Hermus AR, Pieters GF, Pesman GJ, et al. Differential effects of ovine and human corticotrophin-releasing factor in human subjects. Clin Endocrinol 1984;21:589–595.
66. Schurmeyer TH, Schulte HM, Avgerinos PC, et al. Pharmacology of ovine and human CRH. Horm Metab Res Suppl 1987;16:24–30.
67. Behan DP, Potter E, Sutton S. Fischer W. Lowry PJ, Vale WW. Corticotropin-releasing factor-binding protein: a putative peripheral and central modulatory of the CRF family of neuropeptides. Ann NY Acad Sci 1993;697:1–8.
68. Nieman LK, Cutler GB,Jr., Oldrleld EH, Loriaux DL, Chrousos GP. The ovine corticotropin-releasing hormone (CRH) stimulation test is superior to the human CRH stimulation test for the diagnosis of Cushing's disease. J Clin Endocrinol Metab 1989;69:165–169.
69. Gold PW, Kling MA, Whitfield HJ, et al. The clinical implications of corticotropin-releasing hormone. Adv Expt Med Biol 1988;245:507–519.
70. DeBold C, Orth DN, DeCherney GS, et al. Cortdicotropin-releasing hormone: stimulation of ACTH secretion in normal man. Horm Metab Res Suppl 1987;16:8–16.
71. DeBold CR, Jackson RV, Kamilaris TC, et al. Effects of ovine corticotropin-releasing hormone on adrenocorticotropin secretion in the absence of glucocorticoid feedback inhibition in man J Clin Endocrinol Metab 1989;68:431–437.
72. Hermus AR, Pieters GF, Smals AG, Benraad TJ, Klolppenborg PW. Plasma adrenocorticotropin, cortisol, and aldosterone responses to corticotropin-releasing factor: modulatory effect of basal cortisol levels. J Clin Endocrinol Metab 1984;58:187–191.
73. Avgerinos PC, Schurmeyer TH, Gold PW, et al. Pulsatile administration of human corticotropin-releasing hormone in patients with secondary adrenal insufficiency: restoration of the normal cortisol secretory pattern. J Clin Endocrinol Metab 1986;62:816–821.
74. Schulte HM, Chrousos GP, Gold PW, et al. Continuous administration of synthetic ovine corticotropin- releasing factor in man. Physiological and pathophysiological implications. J Clin Invest 1985;75:1781–1785.
75. Ur E, Capstick C, McLoughlin L, Checkley S. Besser GM, Grossman A. Continuous administration of human corticotropin-releasing hormone in the absence of glucocorticoid feedback in man. Neuroendocrinology 1995;61:191–197.
76. Stenzel-Poore MP, Cameron VA, Vaughan J. Sawchenko PE, Vale W. Development of Cushing's syndrome in corticotropin-releasing factor transgenic mice. Endocrinology 1992;130:3378–3386.
77. Keeney DS, Waterman MR. Regulation of steroid hydroxylase gene expression: importance to physiology and disease. Pharm Ther 1993;58:301–317.
78. Raff H. Findling JW, Wong J. Short loop adrenocorticotropin feedback after ACTH 1–24 injection in man is an artifact of the immunoradiometric assay. J Clin Endocrinol Metab 1989;69:678–680.
79. Whitfield HJ, Jr., Brady LS, Smith MS, Mamalaki E, Fox RJ, Herkenham M. Optimization of cRNA probe in situ hybrdidization methodology for localization of glucocorticoid receptor mRNA in rat brain: a detailed protocol. Cell Mol Neurobiol 1990;10:145–157.
80. Arriza JL, Simerly RB, Swanson LW, Evans RM. The neuronal mineralocorticoid receptor as a mediator of glucocorticoid response. Neuron 1988;1:887–900.
81. Covenas M, deLeon M, Cintra A, Bjelke B. Gustafsson J-A, Fuxe K. Coexistence of c-Fos and glucocorticoid immunoreactivities in the CRF immunoreactive neurons of the paraventricular hypothalamic nucleus of the rat after acute immobilization stress. Neurosci Lett 1993;149:149–152.
82. Kovacs KJ, Mezey E. Dexamethasone inhibits corticotropin-releasing factor gene expression in the rat paraventricular nucleus. Neuroendocrinology 1987;46:365–368.
83. Meaney MJ, Sapolsky RM, McEwen BS. The development of the glucocorticoid receptor system in the rat limbic brain. II. An autoradiographic study. Brain Research 1985;350:165–168.
84. Herman JP, Patel PD, Akil H. Watson SJ. Localization and regulation of glucocorticoid and mineralocorticoid receptor messenger RNAs in the hippocampal formation of the rat. Mol Endocrinol 1989;3:1886–1894.
85. Herman JP, Schafer MK, Young EA, et al. Eviclence for hippocampal regulation of neuroendocrine neurons of the hypothalamo-pituitary-adrenocortical axis. J Neurosci 1989;9:3072–3082.

86. Sapolsky RM, Meaney MJ, McEwen BS. The development of the glucocorticoid receptor system in the rat limbic brain. III. Negative-feedback regulation. Brain Research 1985;350:169–173.
87. Sapolsky RM, Krey LC, McEwen BS. Glucocorticoid-sensitive hippocampal neurons are involved in terminating the adrenocortical stress response. Pro Natl Acad Sci USA 1984;81:6174–6177.
88. Seeman TE, Robbins RJ. Aging and hypothalamic-pituitary-adrenal response to challenge in humans. Endocr Rev 1994;15:233–260.
89. Sapolsky RM, Krey LC, McEwen BS. The neuroendocrinology of stress and aging: the glucocorticoid cascade hypothesis. Endo Rev 1986;7:284–301.
90. Imaki T. Nahan JL, Rivier C, Sawchenko PE, Vale W. 1991 Differential regulation of corticotropin-releasing factor mRNA in rat brain regions by glucocorticoids and stress. J Neurosci 11:585-599.
91. Aguilera G. Regulation of pituitary ACTH secretion during chronic stress. Front Neuroendocrinol 1994;15:321–350.
92. Imaki T. Xiao-Quan W. Shibasaki T. et al. Stress-induced activation of neuronal activity and corticotropin-releasing factor gene expression in the paraventricular nucleus is modulated by glucocorticoids in rats. J Clin Invest 1995;96:231–238.
93. Horrocks PM, Jones AF, Ratcliffe WA, et al. Patterns of ACTH and cortisol pulsatility over twenty-four hours in normal males and females. Clin Endocrinol 1990;32:127–134.
94. Carr BR, Parker CR, Madden J. MacDonald PC, Porter JC. Maternal adrenocorticotropin and cortisol relationships throughout human pregnancy. American J Obstet Gynecol 1981;139:416–422.
95. Schulte HM, Weisner D, Allolio B. The corticotrophin releasing hormone test in late pregnancy: lack of adrenocorticotrophin and cortisol response. Clin Endocrinol 1990;33:99–106.
96. Allolio B. Hoffmann J. Linton EA, Winkelmann W. Eusche M, Schulte HM. Diurnal salivary cortisol patterns during pregnancy and after delivery: relationship to plasma corticotrophin-releasing-hormone. Clin Endocrinol 1990;33:279–289.
97. Iranmanesh A, Lizarralde G. Johnson ML, Veldhuis JD. Circadian, ultradian, and episodic release of beta-endorphin in men, and its temporal coupling with cortisol. J Clin Endocrinol Metab 1989;68:1019–1026.
98. Crapo L. Cushing's syndrome: a review of diagnostic tests. Metabolism 1979;28:955–977.
99. Tordjman K, Jaffe A, Grazas N. Apter C, Stern N. The role of the low dose (1 microgram) adren-corticotropin test in the evaluation of patients with pituitary disease. J Clin Endocrinol Metab 1995;80:1301–1305.
100. Broide J. Soferman R. Kivity S. et al. Low-dose adrenocorticotropin test reveals impaired adrenal function in patients taking inhaled corticosteroids. J Clin Endocrinol Metab 1995;80:1243–1246.
101. Chrousos GP, Schuermeyer TH, Doppman J. et al. NIH conference. Clinical applications of corticotropin-releasing factor. Ann Intern Med 1985;102:344–358.
102. Gold PW, Goodwin FK, Chrousos GP. Clinical and biochemical manifestations of depression. Relation to the neurobiology of stress New Engl J Med 1988;319:413–420.
103. Gold PW, Loriaux L, Roy A, et al. Responses to corticotropin-releasing hormone in the hypercor tisolism of depression and Cushing's disease. New Engl J Med 1986;314:1329–1335.
104. Kaye TB, Crapo L. The Cushing syndrome: an update on diagnostic tests. Annals of Internal Medicine 1990;112:434–444
105. Suda T. Kondo M, Totani R. et al. Ectopic adrenocorticotropin syndrome caused by lung cancer that responded to corticotropin-releasing hormone. J Clin Endocrinol Metab 1986;63:1047–1051.
106. Oldfield EH, Doppman JL, Nieman LK, et al. Petrosal sinus sampling with and without corticotropin-releasing hormone for the differential diagnosis of Cushing's syndrome. New Engl J Med 1991;325:897–905.
107. Yanovski JA, Cutler GB,Jr., Chrousos GP, Nieman LK. Corticotropin-releasing hormone stimulation following low-dose dexamethasone administration. A new test to distinguish Cushing's syndrome from pseudo-Cushing's states. JAMA 1993;269:2232–2238.
108. Heuser I, Yassouridis A, Holsboer F. The combined dexamethasone/CRH test: a refined laboratory test for psychiatric disorders. J Psych Res 1994;28:341–356.
109. Hockings GI, Grice JE, Walters MM, Crosbie GV, Torpy DJ, Jackson RV. A synergistic adrenocorticotropin response to naloxone and vasopressin in normal humans: evidence that naloxone stimulates endogenous corticotropin-releasing hormone. Neuroendocrinology 1995;61:198–206.

110. Gaitan D, Loosen PT, Burns D, Edkhator N. Orth DN. Plasma ACTH response to naloxone in major depressive disorder (MDD), chronic alcoholism (ALC), Cushing's disease (CD) and normal subjects (NL). 75th Annual Meeting of the Endocrine Society, June 1993, Las Vegas, NV.
111. Hockings GI, Grice JE, Ward WK, Walter MM, Jensen GR, Jackson RV. Hypersensitivity of the hypothalamic-pituitary-adrenal axis to naloxone in post-traumatic stress disorder. Biol Psychiatry 1993;33:585–593.
112. Holm IA, Majzoub JA. Adrenocorticotropin. In: Melmed S, ed. The Pituitary. Blackwell Scientific, Cambridge, MA, 1995, pp. 45–97.
113. Thompson RC, Seasholtz AF, Herbert E. Rat corticotropin-releasing hormone gene: sequence and tissue distribution. Mol. Endocrinol. 1987;1:333–370.

9

Cushing Syndrome

Differential Diagnosis and Treatment

Maria Alexandra Magiakou, MD,
George Mastorakos, MD,
and George P. Chrousos, MD

CONTENTS

ETIOLOGY

Harvey Cushing first described the homonymous syndrome in 1912 *(1)*. Cushing syndrome, which results from prolonged exposure of the organism to high levels of glucocorticoids, represents a subcategory of hypercortisolism (Table 1).

The cause of Cushing syndrome can be exogenous, resulting from the administration of glucocorticoids or ACTH, or endogenous, secondary to increased secretion of cortisol, ACTH or CRH *(2)*. Exogenous administration of glucocorticoids, mostly iatrogenic or rarely factitious (self-induced), accounts for the majority of cases of ACTH-independent Cushing syndrome, because supraphysiologic doses of glucocorticoids are frequently prescribed for a wide range of nonendocrine diseases *(3)*. The incidence of endogenous Cushing syndrome is two to five new cases per million of population per year with a female to male preponderance of 9:1; approximately 10% of these cases occur in children and adolescents. The classification of endogenous Cushing syndrome and rate of occurrence for ages >7 yr, are summarized in Table 2.

Spontaneous (endogenous) Cushing syndrome can result from ACTH excess (ACTH-dependent), which can arise from the pituitary gland or ectopic ACTH

From: *Contemporary Endocrinology, Vol. 3: Diseases of the Pituitary: Diagnosis and Treatment*
Edited by M. E. Wierman Humana Press Inc., Totowa, NJ

Table 1
Classification of Hypercortisolism

Physiologic States
Stress
Pregnancy
Chronic strenuous exercise
Pathophysiologic States
Cushing syndrome
Endogenous
Exogenous
Psychiatric states
Melancholic depression (Pseudocushing syndrome)
Chronic active alcoholism (Pseudocushing syndrome)
Anorexia nervosa
Obsessive-compulsive disorder
Panic anxiety
Narcotic withdrawal
Metabolic syndrome X
Complicated diabetes mellitus
Primary cortisol (glucocorticoid) resistance

Modified from Kamilaris and Chrousos *(2)*.

Table 2
Classification of Endogenous Cushing Syndrome and Rate of Occurrence (Ages > 7 yr)

Classification	*Occurrence*
ACTH-Dependent	85%
Pituitary (disease)	80%
Ectopic ACTH	20%
Ectopic CRH	Rare
ACTH-Independent	15%
Adrenal adenoma	30%
Adrenal carcinoma	70%
Micronodular adrenal disease	Rare
Massive macronodular adrenal disease	Rare
Glucocorticoid hypersensitivity syndrome	Rare
"Transitional States"	Rare
Other Autonomous Adrenal Hyperfunctioning	
McCune-Albright syndrome, ACTH hypersensitivity	Rare
Feeding-induced	Rare

Modified from Kamilaris and Chrousos *(2)*.

or CRH secreting tumors, or from autonomous secretion of cortisol (ACTH-independent) by a cortisol secreting adrenal tumor(s), "micronodular" dysplastic adrenals (primary pigmented nodular adrenocortical disease, PPNAD), "massively macronodular" adrenals (massive macronodular adrenal disease, MMAD), or other autonomous adrenal processes *(4–8)*. ACTH-dependent Cushing syndrome, which accounts for approximately 85% of endogenous cases, is caused by pituitary ACTH secretion (microadenomas, macroadenomas, corticotroph hyperplasia) in 80% of cases and ectopic ACTH secretion in 20%. Pituitary ACTH secretion has been traditionally called "Cushing disease." A very small number of patients with ACTH-dependent Cushing syndrome might have tumors secreting CRH *(9,10)*. Also, a very small number of patients with chronic Cushing disease go on to develop adrenal macroadenomas autonomously secreting cortisol *(11)*. This has been called a "transitional state."

In children younger than 7 yr, ACTH-independent causes—primarily adrenal carcinoma—are more frequently seen than ACTH-dependent ones *(2,4)*. The incidence of adrenal carcinomas is higher in patients younger than 10 yr, or between 40 and 50 yr. There is female predominance, although there is a higher incidence of nonfunctional tumors in males.

The molecular pathophysiology of ACTH secreting tumors, either in the pituitary or ectopically, remains elusive. Although abnormalities of the G proteins are not frequent, approximately 50% of these tumors carry mutations of the *p53* tumor-suppressor gene *(12)*. Adrenal adenomas or carcinomas are monoclonal in origin. Abnormalities of the p53 gene or of the inhibitory subunit of G proteins and overexpression of insulin-like growth factors were identified in a subset of these neoplasms and might be implicated in their pathogenesis *(13)*. PPNAD is a hereditary autosomal dominant disorder usually manifesting in childhood or young adulthood *(5)*. It can be associated with cardiac myxomas and multiple spotty pigmentations of the skin and mucosae, a triad referred to as Carney's complex. Other endocrine and nonendocrine abnormalities may be present in this disorder, whose genetic locus was recently mapped on chromosome region 2p16.

CLINICAL PRESENTATION

Table 3 summarizes the clinical features of Cushing syndrome in patients of all ages. Cushing syndrome is a multisystem disorder; the clinical changes are due to glucocorticoid excess combined to mineralocorticoid and/or adrenal androgen excess.

One of the earliest signs in almost all patients with Cushing syndrome is obesity, which is mostly truncal, and is characterized by facial rounding (moon facies) and plethora (Fig. 1). The typical clinical presentation in adults includes emotional and sleep disturbances, muscle weakness and fatigue, hirsutism, and typical purple skin striae. Hypertension, carbohydrate intolerance or diabetes, amenorrhea, loss of libido, easy bruising, or spontaneous fractures of ribs and vertebrae may be encountered. Although all patients may exhibit some of these features at the time of diagnosis, few, if any, will have all of them. Pictures of the patient taken over a period of years are particularly helpful in the clinical evaluation *(2,4)*. The clinical manifestations of the syndrome in children are different from those in adults *(14)*. Weight gain and growth retardation are the prevailing signs (Fig. 2), and pubertal advance or delay may be present. The bone age may be appropriate for the chronological age, delayed, or advanced, depending on the relative elevation and effects of glucocorticoids and adrenal androgens. Mental changes (including emotional lability, irritability, or depression), muscle weakness, and sleep disturbances are rare in comparison to adults with Cushing syndrome.

Table 3
Clinical Presentation in Cushing Syndrome (all ages)

Symptoms/signs	*Frequency, %*
Obesity or weight gain (>115% IBW[a])	80
Thin skin	80
Moon facies	75
Hypertension	75
Purple skin striae	65
Hirsutism	65
Abnormal glucose tolerance	55
Impotence	55
Menstrual disorders (usually amenorrhea)	60
Plethora	60
Proximal muscle weakness	50
Truncal obesity	50
Acne	45
Bruising	45
Mental changes	45
Osteoporosis	40
Edema of lower extremities	30
Hyperpigmentation	20
Hypokalemic alkalosis	15
Diabetes	15

[a]IBW, ideal body wt.

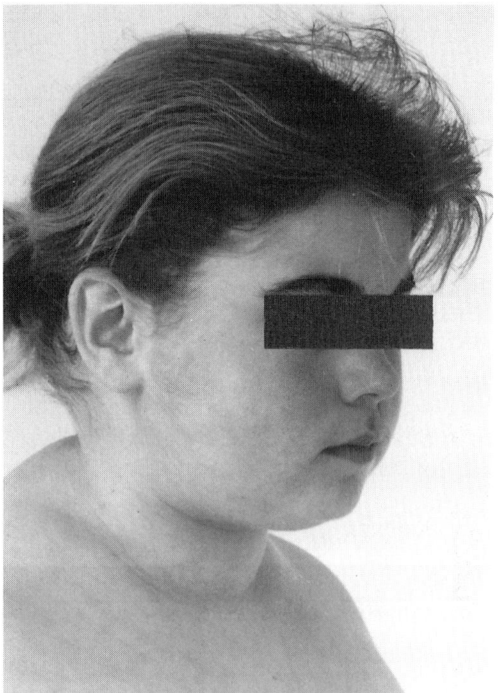
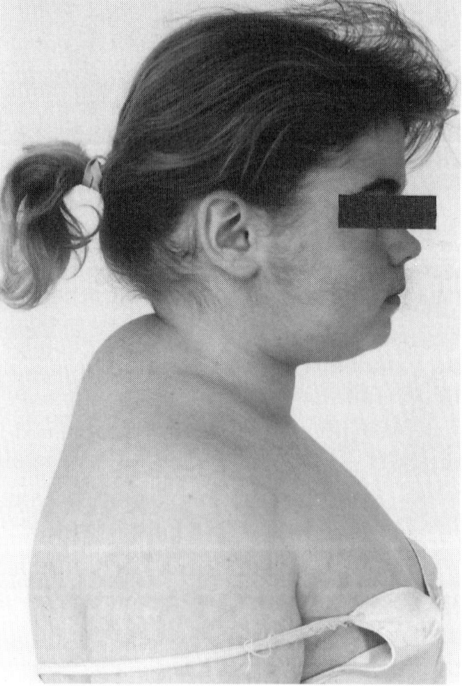

Fig. 1. Close-up of a 15-yr-old girl with Cushing disease. Note the facial rounding, the facial hirsutism, and the filling-in of the supraclavicular fossae.

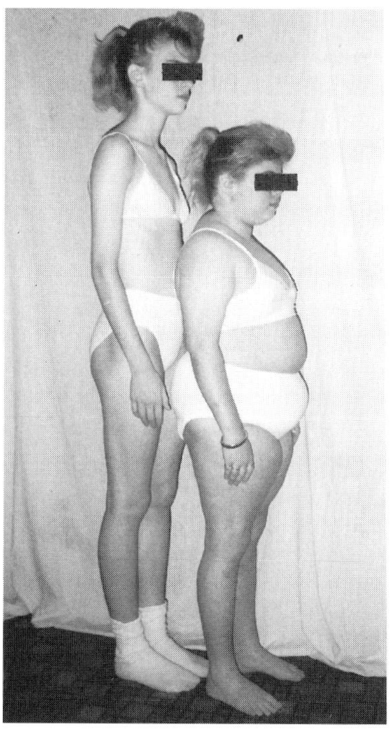
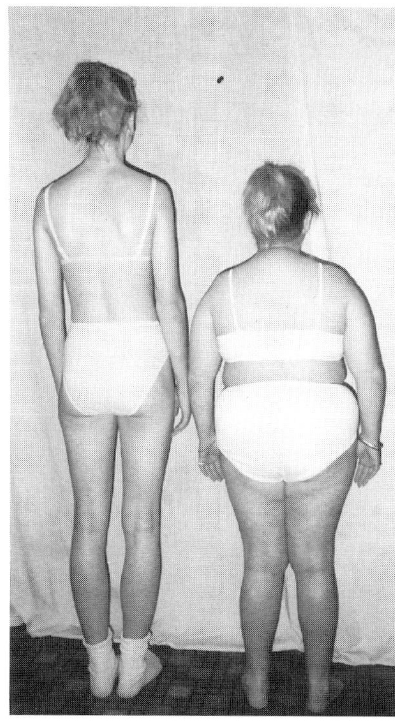

Fig. 2. Characteristic growth retardation and obesity in a 15-yr-old patient with Cushing disease in comparison to her healthy identical twin sister.

Generally, rapidly progressing, very severe Cushing syndrome points toward the ectopic ACTH syndrome. Severe hypertension with hypokalemic alkalosis and/or hyperpigmentation are also frequently due to an ectopic ACTH-secreting tumor *(4)*. Rapid and severe virilization is frequently due to adrenocortical carcinoma *(15,16)*. Patients with adrenocortical carcinomas may be asymptomatic, or may present with abdominal pain or fullness, symptoms and signs of Cushing syndrome (30%), virilization (20%), combined symptoms of Cushing syndrome and virilization (30%), feminization (10%), or hyperaldosteronism (5–10%).

DIAGNOSIS OF CUSHING SYNDROME

In addition to the history and clinical evaluation, the laboratory evaluation of a patient with cushingoid appearance is necessary to establish the diagnosis of hypercortisolism.

Diagnosis of Hypercortisolim

The first step is the biochemical documentation of endogenous hypercortisolism, which can usually be accomplished by outpatient tests. These include measurement of 24-h urinary free cortisol excretion (corrected for body surface area) and/or the determination of 24-h urinary 17-hydroxysteroid excretion (corrected per gram of excreted creatinine), as well as performance of the single dose dexamethasone suppression test.

The determination of 24-h urinary free cortisol excretion is an excellent first-line test for documentation of endogenous Cushing syndrome *(17)*. Values consistently in excess of 300 μg/d are virtually diagnostic of Cushing syndrome. Assuming correct collection, there are very few false-negative results. False-positive results, however, may be obtained in several non-Cushing hypercortisolemic states (Table 1), but these states rarely show urinary free cortisol levels higher than 300 μg/d. Urinary free cortisol remains constant throughout life when adjusted for square meter of body surface area, thus obviating establishing age-specific normal values in children or obese subjects. Normal values are < 70 $mg/m^2/d$ *(18)*.

Urinary 24-h 17-hydroxysteroid excretion corrected for the urinary creatinine excretion gives an indirect measure of the rate of cortisol secretion and, thus, it also can be used for the establishment of hypercortisolism. These compounds include all cortisol metabolites with a 17-dihydroxyacetone side chain and, thus, give an indirect measure of the rate of cortisol secretion. Correction is required, however, for urine creatinine excretion because size and adiposity influence its daily production. Normal values are 2–7 mg/g creatinine/d. On occasion, there is discrepancy between the urinary free cortisol excretion value, which is normal or slightly elevated, and the value of 17-hydroxysteroid excretion, which is clearly elevated and more compatible with the Cushing manifestations of the patient. This is due to deviations in the activity of cortisol metabolizing enzymes, and in such instances the urinary 17-hydroxysteroids corrected per gram creatinine should be employed as the index of hypercortisolism *(19)*.

The overnight 1 mg (in children 15 μg/kg body weight) dexamethasone suppression test is a useful screening procedure for hypercortisolism. It is simple and has a low incidence of false normal suppression (< 3%). The same test, however, has a high incidence of false-positive results (approximately 20–30%). A plasma cortisol level > 5 mg/dL suggests hypercortisolism *(20,21)*.

Cushing syndrome is generally excluded if the response to a single-dose dexamethasone suppression test and the 24-h urinary free cortisol or 17-hydroxysteroid excretion tests are normal, although one should keep in mind that periodic and intermittent cortisol hypersecretion occurs in approximately 5–10% of patients with Cushing syndrome of any etiology, and may confuse the picture.

Isolated plasma ACTH and cortisol determinations are of limited value since both hormones are secreted episodically and in a circadian fashion in normals, and their secretion is influenced by physical or emotional stress. Five consecutive morning and five evening plasma samples should be drawn for determination of diurnal levels of cortisol *(22)*. The averages of the morning and evening values are used for the evaluation of the circadian rhythmicity of plasma cortisol values. Over 80% of patients with Cushing syndrome have equally elevated mean morning and evening values and, thus, no circadian rhythm. Also, frequently, patients with Cushing syndrome have single or several plasma ACTH and cortisol measurements in the normal range.

If the diagnosis of Cushing syndrome is in doubt because of a discrepancy between the urinary free cortisol and the 17-hydroxysteroid excretion value, frequent plasma sampling over 24 h for measurement of cortisol concentrations may be of help. One should take into account the concentrations of cortisol-binding globulin (CBG), however, and, if available, should obtain measurements of plasma free cortisol or salivary cortisol concentrations.

Hypercortisolemic States of Unusual Laboratory Behavior

Periodic Cushing Syndrome

"Periodic," "cyclic," or "episodic" hormonogenesis, which accounts for 5–10% of cases with Cushing syndrome, has been described in patients with Cushing disease, the ectopic ACTH syndrome (bronchial carcinoids were involved in half of the reported cases), and benign or malignant adrenal tumors or micronodular adrenal disease. Biochemically, patients with periodic hormonogenesis may have paradoxically "normal" responses to dexamethasone and poor responsiveness to metyrapone. Discrepancies between the clinical picture and the biochemical pattern are typical *(23)*. Thus, patients with clinical stigmata of Cushing's syndrome may have consistently normal 24-h urinary free cortisol excretion and normal responses to dexamethasone. In such patients, several weekly 24-h urinary free cortisol determinations for a period of 3–6 mo may be necessary to establish the diagnosis.

Cushing Syndrome in Pregnancy

In normal pregnancy, a small progressive rise in plasma ACTH, and a two- to threefold increase in plasma total and free cortisol occur. Urinary free cortisol is also elevated above normal, especially between the 34th and 40th week of gestation (90–350 mg/d). In the later part of pregnancy, immunoreactive CRH of placental origin is detected in plasma, with levels reaching up to 10,000 pg/mL. Because plasma cortisol is poorly suppressed in response to dexamethasone in normal pregnancy, the diagnosis of mild or early Cushing syndrome may be difficult to ascertain *(24)*. Transient pregnancy-related and -limited Cushing syndrome has been described. Its etiology is unknown; however, deficiency of CRH-binding protein might explain its pregnancy-limited expression.

Primary Cortisol Resistance

Biologically confirmed hypercortisolism without Cushing syndrome stigmata has been found in several families or individual patients with primary glucocorticoid resistance *(25,26)*. Patients with this rare syndrome have an apparent end-organ insensitivity to cortisol owing to molecular defects of the glucocorticoid receptor. They may be totally asymptomatic or may present with hyperandrogenism (acne, hirsutism, menstrual irregularities, precocious puberty) or with signs of mineralocorticoid excess (hypertension, hypokalemic alkalosis), as a result of hyperfunctioning adrenal cortices, and increased secretion of steroids with androgen and mineralocorticoid activity *(27)*. In such patients, the dexamethasone suppression tests show suboptimal suppressibility, however the circadian rhythmicity and stress responsiveness of ACTH and cortisol are normal, albeit with high basal levels.

Chronic Disease

Hyperthyroidism, liver disease, and renal failure may cause confusion in the interpretation of adrenal tests. Hyperthyroidism causes elevations of plasma cortisol-binding globulin (CBG) and increased secretion and metabolism of cortisol. Although plasma cortisol levels and urinary cortisol metabolites may be elevated in hyperthyroidism, urinary free cortisol values are generally within the upper normal range. In patients with liver disease, a blunting of circadian periodicity of cortisol has been described, along with a concomitant decrease in the clearance of corticosteroids. In patients with severe renal failure (creatinine clearance <15 mL/min/1.73 m^2), the urinary values of free cortisol and 17-hydroxysteroids may be falsely low *(2)*.

Drugs

Urinary free cortisol excretion may be elevated in patients receiving drugs such as phenytoin, phenobarbital, and primidone. These drugs accelerate the metabolism of dexamethasone and may cause nonsuppression in a dexamethasone suppression test owing to the lower plasma dexamethasone levels achieved *(28)*. Delayed clearance of dexamethasone owing to idiosyncratic factors, on the other hand, may give spurious cortical suppression in patients with Cushing syndrome *(29,30)*. Hydrocortisone suppression tests have been developed for patients with idiosyncratic changes in the metabolism of dexamethasone, and for patients receiving drugs that accelerate the metabolism of this synthetic steroid *(31)*. Concurrent measurement of plasma dexamethasone concentrations can help in defining changes in the absorption or metabolic clearance of dexamethasone.

DIFFERENTIAL DIAGNOSIS

Distinguishing Mild Cushing Syndrome From Pseudocushing States

Differentiating pseudocushing from Cushing syndrome is sometimes very difficult *(32–34)*. The clinical and biochemical presentation of mild hypercortisolism in Cushing syndrome is often indistinguishable from that seen in pseudocushing states, such as depression or chronic active alcoholism (Table 1). A hyperactive or hyperresponsive hypothalamic CRH neuron is central to the hypercortisolism of pseudocushing states in the context of a hypothalamic-pituitary-adrenal (HPA) axis that is otherwise appropriately, albeit not fully, restrained by negative cortisol feedback *(33)*. In contrast, the hypercortisolism of Cushing syndrome feeds back negatively and completely suppresses hypothalamic CRH secretion. These concepts are the basis of the tests employed in the differential diagnosis of mild hypercortisolism.

Levels of UFCs up to 100% above upper normal range are usually compatible with pseudocushing or mild Cushing syndrome. Most patients with Cushing syndrome (80–90%) show inadequate suppression to low dose dexamethasone (0.5 mg every 6 h for 2 d) and do not respond to insulin-induced hypoglycemia (in contrast to the normal responses of depressed and other pseudocushing state patients). In addition, most patients with Cushing disease (85%) have a normal or exaggerated ACTH response to CRH, whereas most patients with depression (75%) show a blunted response. The diagnostic accuracy of these three tests, considered individually or in combination in the differential diagnosis of mild hypercortisolism, however, does not exceed 80%.

A combined dexamethasone suppression (0.5 mg every 6 h for 2 d) test with an oCRH stimulation test was recently developed to optimize the latter's efficacy in distinguishing between pseudocushing states and Cushing disease *(35)*. In the former, the pituitary corticotroph is appropriately restrained by glucocorticoid feedback and does not respond to CRH, whereas in the latter, the corticotroph tumor is generally resistant to this dose of dexamethasone and responds to CRH. Thus, the dexamethasone-CRH test achieves nearly 100% specificity, sensitivity, and diagnostic accuracy. This test should be reserved, however, for borderline or mildly hypercortisolemic patients who have already shown failure to suppress with 1 mg of overnight dexamethasone, and who the clinician suspects as having Cushing disease. The criterion used for the diagnosis of Cushing disease is a cortisol level of >38 nmol/L 15 min after the CRH injection *(35)*.

Although both pseudocushing and Cushing syndrome patients respond clinically to antidepressant therapy, UFC improves usually only in the former. Moreover, the natural course of disease is different; the former is usually self-limited, whereas the latter is progressively deteriorating.

Determining Cushing Syndrome Causes

Once the diagnosis of endogenous Cushing syndrome has been established, testing should be undertaken to clarify the specific cause. The tests include: those that examine the biochemistry of the HPA axis (baseline hormone determinations and dynamic endocrine testing), several imaging techniques used mainly to examine the size and shape of the pituitary and adrenal glands or to detect and evaluate tumors, and catheterization studies to localize ACTH-secreting tumors in the pituitary vs a peripheral site *(2,4)*.

Baseline Hormone Determinations

The first category includes measurements of plasma ACTH, CRH, POMC, DHEAS, and/or other adrenal androgen concentrations.

When a reliable and sensitive ACTH assay is available *(36)*, determination of plasma ACTH simultaneously with plasma cortisol provides useful information about the etiology of Cushing syndrome, as it would distinguish ACTH-dependent from non-ACTH-dependent Cushing syndrome. Thus, adrenal cortisol secreting tumors and micro- and macronodular adrenal disease are associated with suppressed levels of plasma ACTH, whereas Cushing disease and the ectopic ACTH syndrome are associated with normal or elevated plasma ACTH concentrations. The magnitude of elevation of plasma ACTH may have differential diagnostic value, since often, patients with the ectopic ACTH syndrome have greater plasma ACTH levels than those with Cushing disease *(2,4)*.

There are also reliable assays available for determination of plasma POMC, CRH, DHEAS, and other adrenal androgens, which may be of help with several differential diagnostic problems. Thus, plasma POMC is elevated in the ectopic ACTH syndrome *(37)*, CRH in the ectopic CRH syndrome *(9,10,38)*, whereas adrenal androgens are high in adrenal cancer and suppressed in benign, cortisol secreting adrenal adenomas *(27)*.

Sometimes, in the diagnosis of ectopic ACTH secretion, special tests are required. When, e.g., medullary carcinoma of the thyroid is suspected, basal or post calcium or pentagastrin plasma calcitonin should be determined. In the case of a pheochromocytoma secreting ACTH, plasma and urinary catecholamines or urinary VMA and metanephrines should be measured. When an abdominal carcinoid secreting serotonin is suspected, urinary 5-HIAA should also be determined.

Endocrine Dynamic Testing of the HPA Axis

It is essential that dynamic testing of the HPA axis is performed while the patient is hypercortisolemic. This state should always be documented at the time of testing to avoid mistakes. For that purpose, all adrenal blocking agents should be discontinued for at least 6 wk prior to testing. The major tests in the differential diagnosis of Cushing syndrome and results expected according to diagnosis are shown in Table 4.

Liddle Dexamethasone Suppression Test. The standard high-dose dexamethasone test as described by Liddle is an established, reliable procedure for differentiating Cushing disease from the ectopic ACTH syndrome *(39)*. In patients with Cushing disease, the abnormal corticotrophs are sensitive to glucocorticoid inhibition only at high doses of dexamethasone (2.0 mg every 6 h for 2 d). More than 65% of patients with Cushing disease demonstrate a decrease in urinary 17-hydroxysteroid or urinary free cortisol excretion to values respectively < 50 and 90% of the baseline values on d 6 of the test, whereas < 10% of patients with the ectopic ACTH syndrome or ACTH-independent Cushing syndrome respond in this manner *(14,40)*.

It should be mentioned that nonsuppression at the low dose of the standard dexamethasone suppression test might be owing to a technical error (inaccurate urinary collection, error in dexamethasone uptake, laboratory errors), to increased metabolism of dexamethasone (idiosyncratic, drugs), to stress and/or pseudocushing states, or to the syndrome of glucocorticoid resistance. On the other hand, normal suppression at the low dose in Cushing syndrome might be owing to incomplete urinary collection, decreased clearance of dexamethasone, periodic hormonogenesis or increased pituitary sensitivity to dexamethasone. Moreover, failure of patients with Cushing disease to suppress at the high dose of the standard dexamethasone suppression test might again be a result of technical error, increased metabolism of dexamethasone or decreased pituitary sensitivity to dexamethasone. Furthermore, suppression of nonpituitary Cushing syndrome patients at the high dexamethasone dose might either mean dexamethasone-suppressible ectopic ACTH syndrome or dexamethasone-suppressible adrenocortical carcinoma. Paradoxical responses to dexamethasone point toward either micronodular adrenal disease or ectopic ACTH secreting tumors.

Overnight 8-mg Dexamethasone Suppression Test. A proposed modification of the Liddle dexamethasone suppression test is administration of 8 mg dexamethasone orally at midnight as a single dose, and measurement of plasma cortisol concentrations in the following morning. Its advantages are outpatient administration and the avoidance of errors owing to incomplete urine collections. The diagnostic accuracy of this test may be similar to that of the standard Liddle test *(41,42)*.

Metyrapone Stimulation Test. The standard metyrapone test is relatively simple but not as reliable as the dexamethasone suppression test. It is rapidly becoming obsolete but remains an option in cases in which all other tests mentioned here have failed to provide an unequivocal diagnosis. Eighty percent of patients with Cushing disease have normal or increased responses to metyrapone (> 5% on d 2 or 3 of the test), whereas most patients with the ectopic ACTH syndrome fail to respond in this manner *(43)*.

Corticotropin Releasing Hormone Stimulation (CRH) Test. The ovine (o) CRH test is of equal or greater value than the standard dexamethasone suppression test in differentiating between Cushing disease and ectopic ACTH secretion *(44–46)*. Eighty percent of patients with Cushing disease respond to oCRH with increases in plasma levels of ACTH and cortisol, whereas >95% of patients with ectopic ACTH production do not. The (o)CRH test is rapidly superseding the classic tests of dexamethasone suppression and metyrapone stimulation because it is simple, brief, reliable, cost-effective, and can be performed on an outpatient basis. However, the existing pitfalls concerning this test should be mentioned. About 5% of patients with ectopic ACTH tumors respond, whereas 15–20% of patients with Cushing disease do not respond to oCRH. Also, this test is useful only when the patient is hypercortisolemic. Thus patients with periodic or mild Cushing syndrome, or on medical therapy, may respond, regardless of etiology, when the patient is not hypercortisolemic at the time of testing.

The diagnostic power of the Liddle dexamethasone suppression test and the oCRH test is enhanced when both tests are employed. Negative results from both tests rule out the diagnosis of Cushing disease with a diagnostic accuracy of more than 98% *(45)*.

Imaging Evaluation

Imaging techniques can help clarify the etiology of hypercortisolism. These include computed tomographic (CT) scanning and magnetic resonance imaging (MRI) of the pituitary gland, and CT scan, MRI, and ultrasound imaging of the adrenal glands. Computed tomographic and MRI scans of the chest and abdomen are also employed when tumors secreting ectopic ACTH are suspected.

Pituitary. Over 95% of pituitary ACTH secreting tumors are microadenomas with a diameter <7 mm. Plain sella radiographs and sella tomography are normal in the majority of patients, with <5% having a large enough tumor (macroadenoma) to cause changes in the sella turcica, including sellar enlargement or erosion of the floor. Less than 30% can be seen by CT of the sella *(47)*.

The most appropriate initial procedure to detect pituitary ACTH secreting tumors is an MRI scan of the pituitary. The availability of thin-section, high-resolution MRI scanners and the image enhancer gadolinium now permit recognition of approximately 50% of pituitary tumors secreting ACTH *(14,48,49)*.

Adrenals. Imaging by CT or MRI of the adrenal glands is useful in the distinction between Cushing disease and a cortisol secreting adrenal adenoma or carcinoma. The adrenal CT or MRI scans of the adrenals in patients with Cushing disease demonstrate bilateral cortical hyperplasia, diffuse or nodular, including bilateral enlargement of the adrenal glands with thickening or nodularity and a relatively normal overall glandular configuration in approximately 60% of the patients *(50,51)*. Most adrenocortical carcinomas, on the other hand, are quite large in patients with Cushing syndrome and, hence, are easily detectable by CT or MRI. Although adrenocortical adenomas are usually smaller (< 5 cm in diameter) than carcinomas, most can also be demonstrated by CT or MRI. Generally, since most adrenal adenomas causing hypercortisolism are > 2 cm in diameter, they can be easily detected because of the excess retroperitoneal periadrenal fat present in Cushing syndrome. Although it may be functionally atrophic, the contralateral gland usually appears normal. Furthermore, adrenocortical adenomas show no enhancement at the T2 relaxation time of the MRI, whereas adrenocortical carcinomas do *(52)*. In patients with micronodular adrenal disease, the adrenal CT shows bilateral or unilateral nodularity with normal size glands in about 60% of patients, and is grossly normal in the other 40% *(5,14)*.

The widespread use of abdominal CT or MRI scan has led to increasing discovery of incidental adrenal masses, the majority of which are nonfunctioning adenomas ("incidentalomas"), and this should be taken into account. "Incidentalomas" are rare in children and their frequency increases with age, after the age of 40 yr.

Ultrasonography provides another noninvasive means for imaging of adrenal lesions, but its sensitivity and accuracy are less than those of the CT or MRI scans. Ultrasound has been useful in thin patients who have little fat to outline structures on CT or MRI. However, considerable technical and diagnostic skill is required for this technique *(2,4)*.

The iodocholesterol scan is rarely necessary in the evaluation of patients with Cushing syndrome, since this scanning procedure has been largely superceded by CT or MRI scans, which are simpler and faster and involve less radiation. The iodocholesterol scan, however, may on occasion have some advantages over CT or MRI scans. ACTH-dependent macronodules in Cushing disease or chronic ectopic ACTH secretion and cortisol-secreting adrenal adenomas concentrate iodocholesterol and, hence, image. Bilateral, symmetrical (adrenocortical hyperplasia), or asymmetrical (macronodular adrenal hyperplasia) adrenal visualization occurs as a result of ACTH-secreting pituitary or ectopic tumors, whereas unilateral visualization is present in unilateral ACTH-independent adrenal macroadenomas. Cortisol secreting adrenocortical carcinomas, on the other hand, do not image because they are very inefficient in taking up and incorporating cholesterol. The iodocholesterol scan is also useful to localize ectopic adrenal tissue or an adrenal remnant that is causing recurrent hypercortisolism after bilateral adrenalectomy. In this instance, it should be kept in mind that, frequently, 2 d after administration of iodocholesterol may not be sufficient time to allow for visualization of adrenal tissue. Rather, 3–7 d may be necessary before the tissue is visualized *(53,54)*.

Ectopic Tumors. A chest X-ray should be performed routinely and CT and/or MRI of the chest and/or abdomen should be obtained when tumors secreting ACTH ectopically are suspected, since over half of tumors responsible for the ectopic ACTH syndrome are located in the thorax, and 25–30% of ectopic ACTH secreting tumors are occult at the time of the initial evaluation. The location and kind of tumors causing the ectopic ACTH syndrome are depicted in Table 4. Corticotropin-producing thymic carcinoids and pheochromocytomas are generally apparent on CT at initial presentation *(55,56)*. Patients with negative CT findings should undergo MRI of the chest and abdomen using T2-weighted and STIR sequences in which carcinoid tumors demonstrate high signal intensity *(57)*. There are still a significant number of small ectopic tumors, most frequently bronchial carcinoids, that elude CT and MRI detection *(58)*. In these cases, 3- to 6-mo follow-up examinations with MRI of the chest are indicated. In some cases, a body scan following injection of the radiolabeled somatostatin analog, octreotide, might be helpful in detecting occult carcinoids.

Catheterization Studies

The differential diagnosis of Cushing disease from the ectopic ACTH syndrome can be quite difficult, since both entities can have similar clinical and laboratory features. In addition, half of pituitary microadenomas and up to 30% of ectopic ACTH secreting tumors may be radiologically occult. Simultaneous bilateral inferior petrosal venous sinus (BIPSS) and peripheral vein catheterization for measurement of plasma ACTH concentrations before and after oCRH stimulation is one of the most specific tests available to localize the source of ACTH production (Fig. 3) *(59–61)*.

Venous blood from the anterior pituitary drains into the cavernous sinus and subsequently into the inferior petrosal sinuses. Two separate catheters are led into each inferior petrosal sinus via the ipsilateral femoral vein. The location of the catheters is

Table 4
Results of Diagnostic Testing in Cushing's Syndrome and Pseudocushing's States

Disorder	*CRH test*	*Dexamethasone and CRH test*	*Liddle test (Urinary 17-OHS)*	*Metapyrone tests (Urinary 17-OHS)*	*CT or MRI*	*BIPSS*
Corticotropin-Dependent Cushing's Syndrome						
Pituitary	Corticotropin ↑ Cortisol ↑	Corticotropin ↑ Cortisol ↑	Low dose – High Dose ↓	↑	Pituitary ± Adrenal ↑ (macronodules)	Gradient lateralization
Ectopic corticotropin	Corticotropin – Cortisol –	Corticotropin – Cortisol –	Low dose – High dose –	–	Pituitary – Adrenal ↑ (macronodules)	No gradient
Ectopic CRH	High plasma CRH	?	Low dose – High dose ±	? (±)[a]	Pituitary – Adrenal ↑	Gradient[a]
Corticotropin-Independent Cushing's Syndrome						
Adrenal adenoma	Corticotropin ↓ Cortisol –	Corticotropin ↓ Cortisol –	Low dose – High dose –	–	+	Corticotropin ↓
Adrenal carcinoma	Corticoptropin ↓ Cortisol –	Corticotropin ↓ Cortisol –	Low dose – Low dose –	–	+	Corticotropin ↓
Micronodular adrenal disease	Corticotropin ↓ Cortisol –	Corticotropin ↓ Cortisol –	Low dose – High dose – Paradoxical ±	–	±	Corticotropin ↓
Massive macronodular adrenal disease	Corticotropin ↓ Cortisol –		Low dose – High dose –			
Pseudocushing's States						
Depression	Corticotropin blunted Cortisol ↑	Corticotropin ↓ Cortisol ↓	Low dose ± ↓ High dose ↓	↑	?	Nondiagnostic

[a]These results are theoretically expected.
↑, elevation or enlargement; ↓, suppression; +, positive test; –, negative test or no change; ±, positive or negative.
CT, computed tomography; MRI, magnetic resonance imaging; OHS, hydroxysteroid.
(Modified from ref. *2* with permission.)

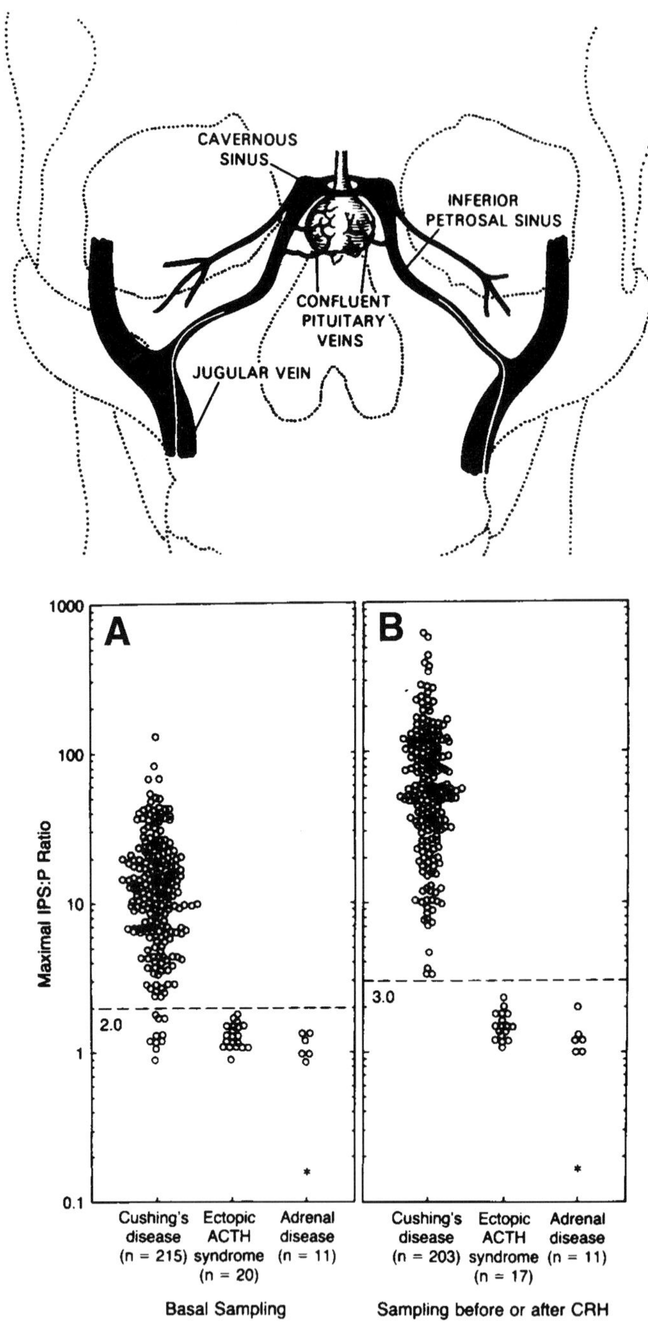

Fig. 3. Results of bilateral inferior petrosal sinus sampling (modified from refs. *60* and *61* and with permission).

confirmed radiologically by injection of radio-opaque solution. Samples for measurement of plasma ACTH are collected simultaneously from each inferior petrosal sinus and a peripheral vein both before and 3, 5, and 10 min after injection of 1 μg/kg oCRH. Generally, patients with the ectopic ACTH syndrome have no ACTH concentration gradient between either inferior petrosal sinus and the peripheral sample before or after oCRH. On the other hand, an increased baseline or stimulated gradient (>2 and >3, respectively) of plasma ACTH between any or both of the inferior petrosal sinuses and the peripheral sample is highly suggestive of Cushing disease. Basal gradients distinguish 95% of patients with Cushing disease from those with ectopic. Stimulated gradients separate up to 98% *(14)*. In addition to distinguishing between Cushing disease and ectopic ACTH secretion, BIPSS provides information about the side of the pituitary in which the adenoma resides. The predictive value of lateralization in unoperated patients is approximately 75–80%. Thus, if a microadenoma cannot be identified at surgery, the only data on which the surgeon can base the decision to perform hemihypophysectomy are the results of bilateral inferior petrosal sinus sampling (BIPSS). The usefulness of BIPSS in distinguishing patients with previous transsphenoidal surgery from patients with ectopic ACTH secretion is as high as in unoperated patients. The value of this test in lateralizing an adenoma in patients with previous transsphenoidal surgery, however, is less than that in unoperated patients *(59–61)*. The overall diagnostic value of the BIPSS depends on its being performed while the patient is hypercortisolemic at the time of the study, and this should be always assured prior to performing the test.

BIPSS is technically difficult and, like all invasive procedures, can never be completely risk-free even in the most experienced hands *(62)*. It should be reserved only for patients with classic Cushing disease symptoms and negative or equivocal MRI findings of the pituitary, and patients with positive pituitary MRI findings but equivocal suppression and stimulation test results. In the former group, BIPSS unequivocally distinguishes ACTH secreting pituitary adenomas from pituitary stimulating lung and thymic carcinoid tumors, and provides lateralization data of potential value to the surgeon. In the latter group, BIPSS will exclude the possibility of a pituitary inciden taloma, which can be visualized on MRI in as many as 10% of young women.

In the case of search for an occult ectopic tumor secreting ACTH, thymic vein sampling for measurement of ACTH concentrations can be of help in localizing the tumor to the thorax, but not necessarily the thymus *(63)*. Presence of a concentration gradient is compatible with a thymic or lung carcinoid tumor.

Proposed Algorithm

We recommend the following diagnostic scheme in patients with Cushing syndrome. First, the presence of hypercortisolism should be established by demonstrating increased urinary cortisol or 17-hydroxysteroid excretion on several occasions. Second, plasma ACTH should be measured and a CRH test performed to distinguish between ACTH-dependent and ACTH-independent Cushing syndrome, and pituitary MRI scans should be obtained in all patients with the former type of disorder. In the case of a positive CRH test and an unequivocally positive pituitary MRI scan, the diagnosis of Cushing disease is made, and transsphenoidal surgery is indicated. If the pituitary MRI scan is negative or equivocal, BIPSS should be performed. Patients with CRH test results that suggest ectopic ACTH secretion and negative pituitary MRI scans should also undergo BIPSS and chest and abdominal CT or MRI scans. If an ectopic ACTH secreting tumor is identified, it should be excised. If basal plasma ACTH values suggest ACTH-independent Cushing syndrome, CT or MRI scanning of the adrenal glands should be performed, to establish the diagnosis of primary adrenal disease.

TREATMENT OF CUSHING SYNDROME

Therapy is indicated in all patients with clinical signs and laboratory confirmation of Cushing syndrome. The treatment of choice depends on the specific cause of the hypercortisolism, which must be established unequivocally. Optimal treatment is the correction of hypercortisolism without permanent dependence on hormone replacement.

Cushing Disease

Currently, four therapeutic modalities are available for the treatment of pituitary ACTH secreting tumors: transsphenoidal removal of the adenoma, pituitary irradiation with concomitant therapy with the adrenolytic agent mitotane (o,p′-DDD [Lysodren]), therapy with mitotane or steroidogenic enzyme inhibitors (aminoglutethimide [Cytadren], metyrapone, trilostane, ketoconazole [Nizoral]), and bilateral adrenalectomy *(2,4,64)*.

TRANSSPHENOIDAL SURGERY

Transsphenoidal adenomectomy is the treatment of choice for most cases of Cushing syndrome caused by pituitary microadenomas *(65–67)*. If preoperatively the presence of a pituitary microadenoma can be demonstrated by imaging techniques or BIPSS, transsphenoidal selective resection of the adenoma is indicated. In most specialized centers the success rate of first transsphenoidal surgery exceeds 90%. If BIPSS has lateralized the microadenoma and the surgeon cannot identify it at surgery, 75–80% of patients can be cured by ipsilateral hemihypophysectomy. Successful surgery leads to cure of hypercortisolism with no need for permanent glucocorticoid replacement. A small percentage of patients (approximately 5%) suffer recurrences, however.

Treatment failures are most common in patients with pituitary macroadenomas. The success rate of repeat transsphenoidal surgery is considerably lower in patients with recurrent Cushing disease after a previously successful operation, or in patients with a previously failed transsphenoidal operation, than in unoperated patients *(68)*.

Transient diabetes insipidus and, less frequently, inappropriate antidiuretic hormone secretion may occur during the early weeks following surgery. Central and primary hypothyroidism (autoimmune), growth hormone deficiency, hypogonadism and permanent hypocortisolism may occur. Permanent diabetes insipidus, hemorrage, cerebrospinal fluid rhinorrhea, injury of internal carotid, cranial nerve palsy and meningitis are uncommon complications but may occur more frequently in patients with repeated transsphenoidal surgery. The perioperative mortality rate of transsphenoidal surgery is probably < 1%, but lower than that of bilateral adrenalectomy (approximately 3%).

Success after transsphenoidal surgery is defined as a drop in serum cortisol or urinary free cortisol to an undetectable level in the immediate postoperative period. Also, an oCRH stimulation test has been used in the postoperative evaluation of patients cured of Cushing disease by selective microadenomectomy or hemipituitectomy. At the early postoperative period, these patients are hypocortisolemic with subnormal ACTH responses to CRH, presumably on the basis of suppression of hypothalamic CRH neurons, because of long-standing hypercortisolism. Normal cortisol levels and a normal response to CRH at this time may identify a subgroup of patients at risk for suboptimal resection and recurrence of the disease *(69)*.

After a successful transsphenoidal operation in Cushing disease, a period of adrenal insufficiency ensues in most of patients cured, during which glucocorticoids must be replaced. This abnormality of the HPA axis can last as long as 1 yr or longer, or, rarely, it can be permanent *(70)*. The rate limiting step in the recovery of the HPA axis during this postoperative period is not the corticotrope, but the defect probably resides in the hypothalamic CRH neuron and/or its higher regulatory inputs *(71)*. Intraoperatively, and during the first two postoperative days, 100 mg/m^2/d of hydrocortisone or its equivalent is given iv. Once the patient has recovered from the surgical procedure, oral replacement doses of hydrocortisone, 20–30 mg (12–15 mg/m^2) per day, are started. Patients often complain of weakness, lack of energy, and irritability at these doses. This is a sign of successful surgery and the symptoms could be alleviated with pharmacologic doses of glucocorticoids. The replacement dose of hydrocortisone is maintained for 3 mo and adrenocortical function is evaluated at that time with a rapid Cortrosyn test (250 μg ACTH 1–24 iv bolus, with plasma cortisol measured at 0, 30, and 60 min). If the test is normal (cortisol >18 and >20 μg/dL at 30 and 60 min, respectively), glucocorticoid replacement is discontinued. If the response is subnormal, the patient is reevaluated at 3 mo intervals. Approximately 70–80% of the patients will have a normal test at 6 mo postoperatively. Patients should be given extra glucocorticoids during stress (twice replacement for minor stress, such as febrile illness or dental surgery, and 8–10 times replacement for major stress, such as major trauma or surgery).

Combined Pituitary X-Irradiation and Mitotane Therapy

This is a reasonable alternative treatment after failure of transsphenoidal surgery, presence of cavernous sinus wall invasion by the tumor, or as the first line of treatment in patients judged unsuitable for surgery. The recommended dosage of pituitary irradiation is 4500–5000 rad total. High voltage, conventional X-radiation is given in 180- to 200-rad fractions over a period of 6 wk. This treatment alone cures only 10–15%, but markedly improves another 25–30% of untreated adult patients (better responses in adults under 40 yr of age) and presumably up to 80% of children younger than 18 yr. Biochemical and clinical amelioration occurs with preservation of pituitary and adrenal function, but is delayed by several months (6–18 mo). Full effect can take years to occur. Heavy particle beam irradiation and Bragg peak proton irradiation therapy appear to be equally effective to conventional irradiation; however, the prevalence of postradiation panhypopituitarism is higher with the former techniques.

Progressive anterior hypopituitarism, including growth hormone deficiency, hypothyroidism, and hypogonadism, occurs in > 40% of patients. These complications may occur several years after radiotherapy.

Usually, concommittantly with and following pituitary radiation, drug therapy (mitotane) is given at low doses, ranging from 1–4 g/d. Combined pituitary radiation and mitotane improves the success rate of either modality given alone curing approximately two-thirds of the patients *(72,73)*.

PHARMACOTHERAPY

Drug therapy alone is rarely used to treat Cushing disease except temporarily, prior to definitive treatment. Mitotane (Lysodren) is the only available pharmacologic agent that both inhibits biosynthesis of corticosteroids (inhibits 11-β hydroxylase and cholesterol side-chain cleavage enzymes) and destroys adrenocortical cells secreting cortisol, thus producing a long-lasting effect. Therapy with mitotane alone can be successful in 30–40% of patients with Cushing disease. Addition of aminoglutethimide, up to 1 g/d orally in four divided doses, or metyrapone, up to 1 g/d in four divided doses, can improve the success rate. During treatment, the urinary free cortisol excretion should be monitored and the dose of mitotane titrated to maintain urinary free cortisol excretion in the normal range. If adrenal insufficiency is suspected, oral hydrocortisone should be added.

Although mitotane is a selective inhibitor of the *reticularis* and *fasciculata* zones of the adrenal cortex, it may on occasion affect the *zona glomerulosa* leading to hypoaldosteronism that requires replacement with oral fludrocortisone (Florinef) 50–300 μg/d. Because mitotane induces liver mono-oxygenases (cytochrome P450 enzymes) that metabolize steroids and other drugs, an adequate dose of hydrocortisone and fludrocortisone may be higher than expected. Measuring urinary 17-hydroxysteroid excretion does not provide a reliable index of adrenal suppression by the drug, since an early fall in the urinary excretion of this metabolite occurs independently of the effect of the drug on cortisol secretion. This phenomenon is a result of mitotane-induced enhancement of liver 6-hydroxylase activity that results in diverting cortisol metabolism to 6-alpha-hydroxylated metabolites that are not detected by the Porter-Silber reaction *(4,74)*.

Adrenal enzyme inhibitors—aminoglutethimide, metyrapone, trilostane, and ketoconazole—have been used alone or in combination with mitotane or each other to control some of the symptoms and metabolic abnormalities associated with the hypercortisolemia in Cushing disease. Combinations are recommended because they usually prevent "breakthroughs" that occur when the drugs are used alone. In addition, one can employ moderate doses with fewer side-effects from each agent *(4,74)*.

Aminoglutethimide (Cytadren) acts in the first step of steroid biosynthesis, where it blocks the conversion of cholesterol to pregnenolone in the adrenal cortex. As a result, the synthesis of cortisol, aldosterone, and androgens is inhibited. The drug has been used in children at doses ranging of 0.5–2 g/d. Aminoglutethimide alone is only transiently effective, since the inhibitory effect of the drug on cortisol biosynthesis is overcome by increasing plasma concentrations of ACTH *(4,74)*.

Metyrapone (Metopirone), an 11-beta hydroxylase inhibitor, blocks the final step of cortisol biosynthesis by preventing the conversion of 11-deoxycortisol to cortisol. Treatment with metyrapone alone (250 mg twice daily to 1 g divided four times daily) or in combination with mitotane or aminoglutethimide can result in biochemical and clinical remission in patients with Cushing disease. Combination of metyrapone and aminoglutethimide should lead to increased therapeutic effectiveness with decreased individual drug doses and fewer side-effects *(4,74)*.

Trilostane (Modrastane), which until recently was an investigational drug, inhibits the conversion of pregnenolone to progesterone, another critical step in cortisol biosynthesis. Trilostane at doses of 200–1000 mg/d has similar side-effects to those observed with aminoglutethimide *(4,74)*.

Ketoconazole (Nizoral), an imidazole containing antifungal agent, is an excellent adrenal steroidogenesis inhibitor, that affects multiple enzymes. This drug can be given at doses ranging from 600–1200 mg/d in three or more divided doses. A gradual increase of the dosage over 7–10 d starting with 200 mg/d is recommended. Amelioration of clinical and metabolic manifestations of hypercortisolism can be seen within 4–6 wk of treatment. Etomidate, an imidazole containing anesthetic agent, also inhibits cortisol secretion in a manner similar to that of ketoconazole *(75)*.

BILATERAL ADRENALECTOMY

The indications for adrenal surgery for Cushing disease have been altered radically by the success and low morbidity of transsphenoidal surgery. Bilateral adrenalectomy could be considered for patients who have failed selective pituitary adenomectomy or hemihypophysectomy. When performed properly, it leads to cure of hypercortisolism. The major disadvantages of bilateral adrenalectomy are that the individual is committed to lifelong daily cortisol and fludrocortisone replacements; that it fails to attack the cause underlying the hypersecretion of ACTH; and that relapses, although uncommon, can occur as a result of growth of adrenal rest tissue or an adrenal remnant. In addition, perioperative mortality is approximately three times higher than that of transsphenoidal surgery, although it can be minimized by careful perioperative preparation.

Also, Nelson syndrome, i.e., large pituitary macroadenomas secreting great amounts of ACTH and β-lipotropin resulting in skin hyperpigmentation, may occur in approximately 10–15% of patients with Cushing disease treated with bilateral adrenalectomy. Clinically apparent Nelson syndrome may occur months or years after bilateral adrenalectomy. These ACTH-secreting macroadenomas may be locally invasive and extend above the diaphragma sellae, causing visual field defects. Rarely, they can metastasize locally in the brain and distant hepatic metastatic nodules have been reported. Treatment for such ACTH secreting macroadenomas is usually difficult and includes transsphenoidal surgery followed by 5000 rad of conventional pituitary X-radiation *(76)*.

Ectopic ACTH Syndrome

The treatment of choice for ectopic ACTH secretion is surgical and directed toward complete excision of the tumor, if it is resectable and its location known. If there is evidence of invasion of adjacent lymph nodes, local radiation may be recommended after surgery. If surgical cure is impossible, blockade of steroidogenesis is indicated, and combination chemotherapy or radiation therapy may be administered. With bronchial carcinoids, which are by far the most common tumors producing the ectopic ACTH syndrome, lung lobectomy may be sufficient for cure. Carcinoids, however, should not be considered benign. They may be extremely slow growing but have the potential for both local invasion and distant metastases.

In approximately 30% of all cases with ectopic ACTH secretion, tumors cannot be found despite severe hypercortisolism. These patients should be medically controlled as suggested above, in order to correct the symptoms and should have periodic imaging evaluations to localize the source of ACTH. RU486, a glucocorticoid receptor antagonist at doses of 5–20 mg/kg/d may also be employed. The most common side effects of this drug include gynecomastia, skin rash, and hypothyroidism *(77)*.

Medical control of hypercortisolism may allow eventual detection of an occult tumor and spare the patient from adrenalectomy. Repeat searches for the tumor should be undertaken every 6–12 mo. If by 2 yr the tumor has escaped detection, or, if medical control is not possible, a bilateral adrenalectomy should be considered. This procedure may need to be done earlier in developing children in whom ketoconazole and other medications may interfere with growth and pubertal progression. Periodic evaluation must continue in the case of an occult tumor, until the tumor is found and removed *(74)*.

Primary Adrenal Disease

The therapeutic approach to ACTH-independent Cushing syndrome is also surgical. Unilateral or bilateral adrenalectomy is the recommended therapy, depending on whether one or both adrenals are affected. The cure rate of benign adenomas and micronodular disease should be 100%.

Adrenocortical carcinomas are implicated in 0.2% of cancer deaths. The tumor is characterized as stage I when it is <5 cm in diameter and confined to the adrenal gland, as stage II when it is >5cm in diameter also confined to the adrenal gland, as stage III when there is involvement of local lymph nodes or local capsular invasion, and as stage IV when there is involvement of local organs or distant metastases. They usually require surgical excision followed by chemotherapy, and have a poor prognosis with practically a 100% rate of either local recurrence or distant metastases. Less than 30% of patients who undergo surgery survive for 5 yr.

In all cases, adrenalectomy may be performed by either the abdominal approach or via posterior flank incision. The latter is associated with fewer complications and lower mortality *(74)*.

Medical control of hypercortisolism as suggested above with Cushing disease or ectopic ACTH secretion is indicated in cases in which surgical treatment is not an option at the time of the decision. Use of mitotane for adrenal carcinomas at very high doses up to 12 g/d may leads to partial response in 15–20% of the patients, but does not increase the length of survival.

CONCLUSIONS

The diagnosis of Cushing syndrome requires the demonstration of hypercortisolism, best achieved by 24-h urinary free cortisol excretion determinations. In borderline or confusing cases, a combined dexamethasone oCRH test may be helpful in ruling out pseudocushing states. Distinction between ACTH-dependent and ACTH-independent Cushing syndrome is made on the basis of basal and oCRH-stimulated plasma ACTH determinations and adrenal CT. In the majority of cases of ACTH-dependent Cushing syndrome, differential diagnosis is achieved by the oCRH test and a pituitary MRI with gadolinium. If no discrete lesion is present or if the oCRH test is equivocal, BIPSS with oCRH administration is necessary to distinguish between a pituitary and an ectopic source. Once the source is identified, surgery is the treatment of choice for all forms of Cushing syndrome. In cases of Cushing disease, in which transsphenoidal surgery fails, or in which the disease recurs, repeat transsphenoidal surgery and radiation therapy in association with mitotane treatment are reasonable alternatives. Bilateral adrenalectomy effectively cures hypercortisolism if resection of the ACTH secreting tumor is unsuccessful and radiation or medical therapy fails.

REFERENCES

1. Cushing H. The Pituitary Body and Its Disorders. Lippincott, Philadelphia, PA, 1912, pp. 219.
2. Tsigos C., Kamilaris T, Chrousos GP. Adrenal diseases. In: Moore WT, Eastman R, eds. Diagnostic Endocrinology. B.C. Decker, Toronto, 1996, pp. 123–156.
3. Magiakou MA, Chrousos GP. Corticosteroid therapy, nonendocrine disease and corticosteroid withdrawal. In: Bardin CW, ed. Current Therapy in Endocrinology and Metabolism. 5th ed., Mosby, New York, 1994, pp. 120–124.
4. Magiakou MA, Chrousos GP. Diagnosis and treatment of Cushing disease In: Imura H, ed. The Pituitary Gland. 2nd ed., Raven, New York, 1994, pp. 391–508.
5. Doppman JL, Travis WD, Nieman L, Miller DL, Chrousos GP, Gomez GT, Cutler GB Jr, Loriaux DL, Norton JA. Cushing syndrome due to primary pigmented nodular adrenocortical disease: findings at CT and MR imaging. Radiology 189; 172:415–420.
6. Doppman JL, Nieman LK, Travis WD, Miller DL, Cutler GB Jr, Chrousos GP, Norton JA. CT and MR imaging of massive macronodular adrenocortical disease: a rare cause of autonomous primary adrenal hypercortisolism. J Comput Assist Tomogr 1991; 15:773–779.
7. Lacroix A, Bolte E, Tremblay J, Dupre J, Poitras P, Fournier H, Garon J, Garrel D, Bayard F, Taillefer R. Gastric inhibitory polypeptide-dependent cortisol hypersecretion—a new cause of Cushing's syndrome. N Engl J Med 1992; 327:974–980.
8. Danon M, Robboy SL, Kim S, Scully R, Crawford JD. Cushing syndrome, sexual precocity, and polyostotic fibrous dysplasia (Albright syndrome) in infancy. J Pediatr 1975; 87:917–921.
9. Carey RM, Varma SK, Drake CR Jr, Thorner MO, Kovacs K, Rivier J, Vale W. Ectopic secretion of corticotropin-releasing factor as a cause of Cushing's syndrome. N Engl J Med 1984; 311:13–20.
10. Auchus RJ, Mastorakos G, Friedman TC, Chrousos GP. Corticotropin-releasing hormone production by a small cell carcinoma in a patient with ACTH-dependent Cushing syndrome. J Endocrinol Invest 1994; 17:447–452.
11. Malchoff CD, Rosa J, DeBold CR, Kozol RA, Ramsby GR, Page DL, Malchoff DM, Orth DN. Adrenocorticotropin-independent bilateral macronodular adrenal hyperplasia: an unusual cause of Cushing's syndrome. J Clin Endocrinol Metab 1989; 68:855–860.
12. Buckley N, Bates AS, Broome JC, Strange RC, Perrett CW, Burke CW, Clayton RN. P53 protein accumulates in Cushing's adenomas and invasive non-functional adenomas. J Clin Endocrinol Metab 1994; 79:1518–1521.
13. Tsigos C, Chrousos GP. Clinical presentation, diagnosis and treatment of Cushing's syndrome in Current opinion in Endocrinology and Diabetes, Current Science, Philadelphia, 1995; p.1–11.
14. Magiakou MA, Mastorakos G, Oldfield EH, Gomez MT, Doppman JL, Cutler GB Jr, Nieman LK, Chrousos GP. Cushing syndrome in children and adolescents: Presentation, Diagnosis and Therapy. N Engl J Med 1994; 331:629–636.
15. Plotz CM, Knowlton AL, Ragan C. The natural history of Cushing's syndrome. Am J Med 1952; 13:597–614.
16. Soffer LJ, Iannaccone A, Gabrilove JL. Cushing's syndrome: a study of fifty patients. Am J Med 1961; 30:129–146.
17. Murphy BEP. Clinical evaluation of urinary cortisol determinations by competitive protein-binding radioassay. J Clin Endocrinol Metab 1968; 28:343–348.
18. Gomez MT, Malozowski S, Winterer J, and Chrousos GP. Urinary free cortisol values in normal children and adolescents. J Pediatrics 1968; 118:256–258.
19. Schoneschofer M, Weber B, Oelkers W, Nahoul K, Mantero F. Measurement of urinary free 20 alphadihydrocortisol in biochemical diagnosis of chronic corticoidism. Clin Chem 1986; 32:808–810.
20. Connolly CK, Gore MBR, Stanley N, Wills MR. Single-dose dexamethasone suppression in normal subjects and hospital patients. Brit Med J 1968; 2:665–667.
21. Pavlatos FC, Smilo RP, Forsham PH. A rapid screening test for Cushing's syndrome. J Amer Med Assoc 193:720–723.
22. Kao M, Voina S, Nichols A, Horton R. Parallel radioimmunoassay for plasma cortisol and 11-deoxycortisol. Clin Chem 1965; 1975; 21:1644–1647.
23. Brown RD, Van Loon GR, Orth DN, Liddle GW. Cushing's disease with periodic hormonogenesis: one explanation for paradoxical response to dexamethasone. J Clin Endocrinol Metab 1973; 36:445–451.
24. Buescher MA, McClamrock HD, Adashi EY. Cushing syndrome in pregnancy. Obstet Gynecol 1992; 79:130–137.

25. Chrousos GP, Vingerhoeds A, Brandon D, Eil C, Pugeat M, DeVroede M, Loriaux DL, Lipsett MB. Primary cortisol resistance in man: a glucocorticoid receptor-mediated disease. J Clin Invest 1982; 69:1261–1269.
26. Chrousos GP, Detera-Wadleigh SD, Karl M. Syndromes of glucocorticoid resistance. Ann Intern Med 1993; 119:1113–1124.
27. Mastorakos G, Chrousos GP. Adrenal androgens In: Reproductive Endocrinology, Surgery, and Technology. Adashi EY, Rock JA, Rosenwaks Z, eds. Lippincott-Raven, New York 1996; 1539–1553.
28. Jubiz W, Meikle AW, Levinson RA, Mizutani S, West CD, Tyler FH. Effect of diphenylhydantoin on the metabolism of dexamethasone. N Engl J Med 1970; 283:11–14.
29. Caro JF, Meikle AW, Check JH, Cohen SN. "Normal suppression" to dexamethasone in Cushing's disease: an expression of decreased metabolic clearance for dexamethasone. J Clin Endocrinol Metab 1978; 47:667–670.
30. Meikle AW, Lagerquist LG, Tyler FH. Apparently normal pituitary-adrenal suppressibility in Cushing's syndrome: dexamethasone metabolism and plasma levels. J Lab Clin Med 1975; 86:472–478.
31. Carey RM. Suppression of ACTH by cortisol in dexamethasone-non-suppressible Cushing's disease. N Engl J Med 1980; 302:275–279.
32. Sachar EJ. Twenty-four-hour cortisol secretory patterns in depressed and manic patients. Prog Brain Res 1975; 42:81–91.
33. Gold PW, Loriaux DL, Roy A, Kling MA, Calabrese JR, Kellner CH, Nieman LK, Post RM, Pickar D, Gallucci W. Responses to corticotropin-releasing hormone in the hypercortisolism of depression and Cushing's disease: pathophysiology and diagnostic implications. N Engl J Med 1986; 314:1329–1335.
34. Lamberts SWJ, Klijn JGM, deJong FH, Birkenhager JC. Hormone secretion in alcohol-induced pseudo-Cushing's syndrome. Differential diagnosis with Cushing's disease. J Am Med Assoc 1979; 242:1640–1643.
35. Yanovski JA, Cutler GB Jr, Chrousos GP, Nieman LK. Corticotropin-Releasing Hormone stimulation following low-dose dexamethasone administration: a new test to distinguish Cushing's syndrome from pseudo-Cushing's states. JAMA 1993; 269:17:2232–2238.
36. Orth DN. Adrenocorticotropic hormone (ACTH). In Jaffe PM, Behram HR (eds) Methods of Hormone Radioimmunoassay. Academic, New York 1978; 245–284.
37. White A, Stewart MF, Farrell WE, Crosby SR, Lavender PM, Twentyman PR, Rees LH, Clark AJ. Proopiomelanocortin gene expression and peptide secretion in human small-cell lung cancer cell lines. J Mol Endocrinol 1989; 3:1:65–70.
38. Schteingart DE, Lloyd RV, Akil H, Chandler WF, Ibarra-Perez G, Rosen SG, Ogletree R. Cushing's syndrome secondary to ectopic corticotropin-releasing hormone-adrenocorticotropin secretion. J Clin Endocrinol Metab 1986; 63:770–775.
39. Liddle GW. Tests of pituitary-adrenal suppressibility in the diagnosis of Cushing's syndrome. J Clin Endocrinol Metab 1960; 20:1539–61.
40. Flack MR, Oldfield EH, Cutler GB Jr, Zweig MH, Malley JD, Chrousos GP, Loriaux DL, Nieman LK. The use of urine free cortisol in the high dose dexamethasone suppression test for the differential diagnosis of Cushing's syndrome. Ann Int Med 1992; 116:211–217.
41. Tyrrell JB, Findling JW, Aron DC, Fitzgerald PA, Forsham PH. An overnight high-dose dexamethasone suppression test for rapid differential diagnosis of Cushing's syndrome. Ann Intern Med 1986; 104:180–186.
42. Dichek HL, Nieman LK, Oldfield EH, Pass HI, Malley JD, Cutler GB Jr. A comparison of the standard high dose dexamethasone suppression test and the overnight 8-mg dexamethasone suppression test for the differential diagnosis of the adrenocorticotropin-dependent Cushing's syndrome. J Clin Endocrinol Metab 1994; 78:418–422.
43. de Lange WE, Sluiter WJ, Pratt JJ, Doorenbos H. Plasma 11-deoxycortisol, androstenedione, testosterone and ACTH in comparison with the urinary excretion of tetrahydro-11-deoxycortisol as indices of the pituitary-adrenal response to oral metyrapone. Acta Endocrinol 1980; 93:488–494.
44. Chrousos GP, Schulte HM, Oldfield EH, Gold PW, Cutler GB Jr, Loriaux DL. The corticotropin releasing factor stimulation test: an aid in the evaluation of patients with Cushing's syndrome. N Engl J Med 1984; 310:622–626.
45. Nieman LK, Chrousos GP, Oldfield EH, Avgerinos PC, Cutler GB Jr, Loriaux DL. The ovine CRH test and the dexamethasone suppression test in the differential diagnosis of Cushing's syndrome. Ann Intern Med 1986; 105:862–867.

46. Nieman LK, Cutler GB Jr, Oldfield EH, Loriaux DL, and Chrousos GP. The ovine corticotropin-releasing hormone stimulation test is superior to the human corticotropin-releasing hormone stimulation test for the diagnosis of Cushing's disease. J Clin Endocrinol Metab 1989; 69:165–170.
47. Saris SC, Patronas NJ, Doppman JL, Loriaux DL, Cutler GB Jr, Nieman LK, Chrousos, GP, Oldfield EH. Pituitary CT scanning in Cushing's syndrome. Radiology 1986; 162:775–777.
48. Dwyer AJ, Frank JA, Doppman JL, Oldfield EH, Hickey AM, Cutler GB Jr, Loriaux DL, Schiable TF. Gadolinium DTPA enhanced magnetic resonance imaging of pituitary adenomas in patients with Cushing's disease: initial experience. Radiology 1987; 163:421–426.
49. Doppman JL, Frank JA, Dwyer AJ, Oldfield EH, Miller DL, Nieman LK, Chrousos GP, Cutler GB Jr, Loriaux DL. Gadolinium DPTA enhanced MR imaging of ACTH-secreting microadenomas of the pituitary gland. J Comp Assist Tom 1988; 12:728–735.
50. Aron DC, Findling JW, Fitzgerald PA, Brooks RM, Fisher FE, Forsham PH, Tyrrell JB. Pituitary ACTH dependency of nodular adrenal hyperplasia in Cushing's syndrome-report of 2 cases and review of the literature. Am J Med 1981; 71:302–306.
51. Doppman Jl, Miller DL, Dwyer AJ, Loughlin T, Nieman LK, Cutler GB Jr, Chrousos GP, Oldfield EH, Loriaux DL. Macronodular adrenal hyperplasia in Cushing's disease. Radiology 1988; 166:347–352.
52. Flack MR, Chrousos GP. Neoplasms of the adrenal cortex in Holland JF, Frei III E, Bast Jr. RC, Kufe DW, Morton DL, Weichselbaum RR, eds. Cancer Medicine, third ed, Lea and Febiger, PA, p. 1147–1152.
53. Sarkar SD, Cohen EL, Beierwaltes WH, Ice RD, Cooper R, Gold EN. A new superior adrenal imaging agent, 131I-6β-iodomethyl-19-norcholesterol (NP-59): evaluation in humans. J Clin Endocrinol Metab 1977; 45:353–362.
54. Herwig KR, Schteingart DE. Successful removal of adrenal remnant localized by I-19-iodocholesterol. J Urol 1984; 111:713–714.
55. Doppman JL, Nieman LK, Miller DL, Pass HI, Chung R, Cutler GB Jr, Schauf M, Chrousos GP, Norton JA, Zirrsman HA, Oldfield EH, Loriaux DL. Ectopic adrenocorticotropic hormone syndrome: localization studies in 28 patients. Radiology 1989; 172:115–124.
56. Leinung MC, Young WF Jr, Whitaker MD, Scheithauer BW, Tvastek VF, Kvols LK. Diagnosis of corticotropin-producing bronchial carcinoid tumors causing Cushing's syndrome. Mayo Clin Proc 1990; 65:1314–1321.
57. Doppman JL, Pass HI, Nieman LK, Findling TW, Dwyer AJ, Fenerstein IM, Ling A, Travis WD, Cutler GB Jr, Chrousos GP, Loriaux DL. Detection of ACTH-producing bronchial carcinoid tumors: MR imaging versus CT. Am J Radiol 1991; 156:39–43.
58. Limper AH, Carpenter PC, Scheithauser B, Staats BA. The Cushing syndrome induced by bronchial carcinoid tumors. Ann Intern Med 1992; 117:209–214.
59. Miller DL, Doppman JL. Petrosal sinus sampling; technique and rationale. Radiology 1991; 178:37–47.
60. Oldfield EH, Chrousos GP, Schulte HM, Loriaux DL, Schaaf M, Doppman JL. Preoperative lateralization of ACTH secreting pituitary microadenomas by bilateral and simultaneous inferior petrosal sinus sampling. N Engl J Med 1985; 312:100–103.
61. Oldfield EH, Doppman J, Nieman LK, Chrousos GP, Miller DL, Katz DA, Cutler GB Jr, Loriaux DL. Petrosal sinus sampling with and without corticotropin releasing hormone in patients with Cushing's syndrome. N Engl J Med 1991; 325:897–905.
62. Miller DL, Doppman JL, Peterman SB, Nieman LK, Oldfield EH, Chang R. Neurologic complications of petrosal sinus sampling. Radiology 1992; 185:143–147.
63. Doppman JL, Pass HI, Nieman LK, Miller DL, Chang R, Cutler GB Jr, Chrousos GP, Jaffe GS, Norton JA. Corticotropin-secreting carcinoid tumors of the thymus: diagnostic unreliability of thymic venous sampling. Radiology 1992; 184:71–74.
64. Loriaux DL, Cutler GB Jr. Diseases of the adrenal glands. In: Kohler PO, ed. Clinical Endocrinology. Wiley, New York, 1986, pp. 167–238.
65. Tyrrell JB, Brooks RM, Fitzgerald PA, Cofoid PB, Forsham PH, Wilson CB. Cushing's disease. Selective transsphenoidal resection of pituitary microadenomas. N Engl J Med 1978; 298:753–758.
66. Salassa RM, Laws ER Jr, Carpenter PC, Northcutt RC. Transsphenoidal removal of pituitary microadenoma in Cushing's disease. Mayo Clin Proc 1978; 53:24–28.
67. Malpalam TJ, Tyrrell JB, Wilson CB. Transsphenoidal microsurgery for Cushing disease: a report of 216 cases. Ann Intern Med 1989; 109:487–493.
68. Friedman RB, Oldfield EH, Nieman LK, Chrousos GP, Doppman JL, Cutler GB Jr, Loriaux DL. Repeat transsphenoidal surgery in Cushing's disease. J Neurosurg 1989; 71:520–527.

69. Avgerinos PC, Chrousos GP, Nieman LK, Oldfield EH, Loriaux DL, Cutler GB. The corticotropin releasing hormone test in the postoperative evaluation of patients with Cushing's syndrome. J Clin Endocrinol Metab 1987; 65:906–913.
70. Doherty GM, Nieman LK, Cutler GB Jr, Chrousos GP, Norton JA. Time to recovery of the hypothalamic-pituitary-adrenal axis after curative resection of adrenal tumors in patients with Cushing's syndrome. Surgery 1990; 108:1085–1090.
71. Gomez MT, Magiakou MA, Mastorakos G, Chrousos GP. The pituitary corticotroph is not the rate limiting step in the postoperative recovery of the hypothalamic-pituitary-adrenal axis in patients with Cushing syndrome. J Clin Endocrinol Metab 1992; 77:173–177.
72. Schteingart DE, Tsao HS, Taylor CI, McKenzie A, Victoria R, Therrien BA. Sustained remission of Cushing's disease with mitotane and pituitary irradiation. Ann Intern Med 1980; 92:613–619.
73. Jennings AS, Liddle GW, Orth DN. Results of treating childhood Cushing's disease with pituitary irradiation. N Engl J Med 1977; 297:957–962.
74. Gomez MT, Chrousos GP. Cushing's syndrome. In: Bardin W, ed. Current Therapy in Endocrinology and Metabolism, 4th ed. BC Decker, Toronto, pp. 134–137.
75. Tabarin A, Navarranne A, Guerin J, Corcuff JB, Parneix M, Roger P. Use of ketokonazole in the treatment of Cushing's disease and ectopic ACTH syndrome. Clin Endocrinol (Oxf) 1991; 34:63–69.
76. Moore TJ, Dluhy RG, Williams GH, Cain JP. Nelson's syndrome: frequency, prognosis, and effect of prior pituitary irradiation. Ann Intern Med 1976; 85:731–734.
77. Laue L, Kawai S, IJdelsman R. Glucocorticoid antagonists: pharmacological attributes of the prototype antiglucocorticoid RU 486. In: Lichtenstein LM, Claman H, Oronsky A, Schleimer RP, eds. Antiinflammatory Steroid Action: Basic and Clinical Aspects. New York: Academic, New York, 1989, pp. 643–649.

10 Gonadotropins
Normal Physiology

François P. Pralong, MD,
and William F. Crowley, Jr., MD

CONTENTS

INTRODUCTION

The gonadotropins, luteinizing hormone (LH) and follicle stimulating hormone (FSH), are dimeric pituitary glycoprotein hormones controlling gonadal steroidogenesis and gametogenesis. Their biosynthesis and secretion is tightly regulated by counterbalancing positive inputs from the hypothalamus (GnRH) and negative feedback from the gonads (steroid and peptide hormones). The differential secretion of FSH vs LH can also be achieved by local factors produced within the pituitary gland itself (activin, inhibin, and follistatin). Integration of these different signals by the gonadotrope results in the coordinate secretion of LH and FSH, ultimately promoting sexual maturation and normal reproductive function. Therefore, gonadotropins play a central role in reproductive biology.

CHEMISTRY

Gonadotropins belong to a family of glycoprotein hormones that include pituitary thyroid stimulating hormone (TSH) and placental chorionic gonadotropin (CG). All four are heterodimers constituted of two noncovalently linked subunits called α and β. Whereas the α-subunit is common to all glycoproteins, each β-subunit is hormone-specific and unique *(1,2)*. The hormones LH, FSH, TSH, and CG are known under the generic name of glycoproteins, because their subunits are glycosylated at specific residues *(3)*.

From: *Contemporary Endocrinology, Vol. 3: Diseases of the Pituitary: Diagnosis and Treatment*
Edited by M. E. Wierman Humana Press Inc., Totowa, NJ

These α- and β-subunits are encoded by different genes located on separate chromosomes and heterodimerization is an essential feature of glycoproteins as uncombined subunits have no known biological activity. Once association between an α- and a β-subunit occurs, the resulting dimers confer hormonal bioactivity, the differences in primary amino acid sequences between the various β-subunits imparting its unique biological specificity.

α-Subunit

In the human, a single gene located on chromosome 6 *(4,5)* encodes for a 24-amino acid leader peptide followed by the 94-amino acid mature common α-subunit. This gene is expressed in the anterior pituitary gland as well as in the placenta. The most striking feature of the mature α-subunit is the presence of 10 highly conserved cystine residues, oxidized to form five disulfide bonds that are crucial to the tertiary "cystine knot" structure of the mature protein *(1)* and hence to dimerization and ligand-receptor interaction. Aside from these cystines, the mature α-subunit also bears two asparagine-linked oligosaccharides at residues 56 and 83 *(3)* that play an important role for the biological activity of the molecule.

β-Subunits

The human LHβ-subunit is encoded by a member of a cluster of eight different genes *(6)* located on chromosome 19, which also comprise the gene coding for the CGβ-subunit *(7)*. It is believed that these genes have evolved by duplication *(8)*, and that most represent either pseudogenes or are expressed at very low levels. The LHβ-subunit is expressed in the pituitary, whereas the related CGβ-subunit is expressed mainly in the placenta of human and primates. The CG gene, however, may also be expressed at low levels in several endocrine and nonendocrine tissues, including the pituitary *(9)*. The protein encoded by the LHβ gene consists of a leader peptide of 24 amino acids, followed by the 121-amino acid mature LHβ-subunit *(1)*. The human FSHβ-subunit also consists of a leader peptide of 19 amino acids followed by a mature peptide of 111 amino acids *(10)*. It is encoded by a single gene located on chromosome 11 *(11)* and, as expected, is expressed only in the anterior pituitary.

Regardless of differences in their primary amino acid sequences, the four different human β-subunits share two important structural features. Like the α-subunit, they all bear a highly conserved backbone of 12 cystine residues that oxidize to form six disulfide bonds *(1)*, and they contain either one (LHβ) or two (FSHβ) glycosylation sites *(3)*.

Functional Role of Glycosylation

The assembly of gonadotropin hormone subunits into heterodimers and their glycosylation occurs cotranslationally in the rough endoplasmic reticulum during subunit biosynthesis. Following these early steps, further specific processing of the Asn-linked oligosaccharides (i.e., terminal sulfation or sialylation) occurs in the Golgi apparatus. These newly synthesized gonadotropins are then directed to the regulated secretion pathway, where they are stored in secretory granules, and released following GnRH binding to its receptor. It has been postulated that differences in glycosylation pattern between LH and FSH may represent the signal that differentially segregates both hormones to different secretory granules, which, in turn, is a prerequisite for their differential secretion from the gonadotrope (for a complete review on glycosylation of gonadotropins, *see* ref. *3*). The α-subunit is synthesized in considerable excess of both LH- and FSH β-subunits by the gonadotrope and is costored and cosecreted with the dimeric hormones in its free or uncombined form following pulsatile GnRH stimulation *(12)*.

The functional importance of these posttranslational modifications of gonadotropins has long been recognized: Oligosaccharides are important determinants of hormone half-lives as well as their bioactivity *(13)*. The clearance of these gonadotropin hormones is a complex phenomenon involving liver metabolism as well as renal excretion and the subset of predominantly sulfated oligosaccharides has a shorter plasma half-life than those with sialylated oligosaccharides *(14,15)*. Therefore, the significantly higher content of sialic acid in human FSH probably accounts in part for the longer circulating half-life of FSH compared to LH. In the human, the half-life of LH has been reported to range from 10 to 50 min *(16,17)*, whereas values of 1–4 h are generally accepted for FSH *(18,19)*.

Glycosylation of gonadotropin subunits is not mandatory for their heterodimerization, or binding of the mature hormone to its cognate receptor *(20)*. However, deglycosylated hormones display little or no ability to stimulate cAMP production in target cells (in fact, they can act as antagonists), demonstrating the important functional role of oligosaccharides in determining bioactivity *(20,21)*. Studies conducted with gonadotropins bearing deglycosylated α- or β-subunits have demonstrated that the β-subunit determines binding specificity, whereas the α-subunit is probably most important in initiating signal transduction *(21,22)*.

A remarkable feature of the Asn-linked oligosaccharides is that neither their sialylation nor their sulfation patterns are fixed for a given hormone. Consequently, several isomeric forms of LH and FSH *(23)* can coexist in the serum of a given individual and these variations in the carbohydrate moieties are thought to constitute a "fine-tuning" mechanisms for the control of gonadal activity. For example, shifts toward more biologically active isoforms of circulating gonadotropins occur at specific phases of the human menstrual cycle *(24)* or at the onset of puberty *(25)*.

Structural Biology of Gonadotropins

The heterodimeric structure and the presence of extensive disulfide bonding within each subunit are the most remarkable features of gonadotropins. These features result in extensive protein folding and therefore multiple noncontiguous segments of the primary amino acid sequence contribute to receptor binding and activation (for review, *see* ref. *26*). The recent elucidation of the tridimensional structure of the human CG by crystallography has demonstrated that the noncovalent association of the two subunits depends on a unique "seat-belt" arrangement provided by a single disulfide pairing between the highly conserved cystine residues within each subunit *(27)*. These results confirmed the biological importance of several regions of the α- and β-subunit that contribute to receptor binding *(26)* by allowing to correlate the functional significance of specific residues and their localization on the surface. Moreover, this study *(27)* disclosed the surprising fact that structurally, human CG belongs to the superfamily of the cystine-knot growth factors, together with nerve growth factor (NGF), transforming growth factor -β (TGF-β), and platelet-derived growth factor-β (PDGF-β). It is fully expected that the tridimensional structure of LH and FSH (whose sequence homologies with hCG are 90 and 50%, respectively) will be essentially similar to that of the CGβ.

PHYSIOLOGY

During the early research on the hypothalamic control of gonadotropin secretion, it had been postulated that there would be two distinctly different hypothalamic hypophysiotropic factors regulating LH and FSH. Although 25 yr have passed since the isolation of the decapeptide LH-RH by Schally and his colleagues (now referred to as GnRH by virtue of the absence of an FSH-RH) *(28)*, a second gonadotropic factor has yet to be found. Even though there is some evidence for its existence *(29)*, most investigators now believe that all situations in which LH and FSH are secreted differentially can probably be explained via a differential modulation of GnRH actions by the sex steroid milieu, the secretion of inhibin which affects selectively FSH *(30–34)*, or by autocrine/paracrine interactions between inhibin, activin *(35–37)*, and the activin-binding protein follistatin *(38,39)* at the pituitary level. In this debated context, the fascinating finding that pituitary expression of inhibin/activin/follistatin is regulated by GnRH *(40,41)* could eventually provide the missing link between GnRH and the differential control of FSH. Further characterization of these interactions is currently the object of very intense research.

Physiologic Importance of Pulsatile Mode of GnRH Stimulation

The hallmark of the hypothalamic secretion of GnRH is the pulsatile characteristic of its release into the hypophyseal portal blood, resulting in episodic stimulation of the gonadotrope. In the late 1970s, the seminal work of Knobil and colleagues demonstrated the absolute requirement for such a pulsatile stimulus to sustain physiologic gonadotrope function *(42)*. Using castrate monkeys bearing hypothalamic lesions rendering them hypogonadotropic, these authors were able to restore normal gonadotropin secretion with pulsatile GnRH administration, whereas continuous infusion of the peptide was completely ineffective (Fig. 1).

Following its secretion into the hypophyseal portal blood, GnRH then binds to a high-affinity receptor expressed exclusively by the pituitary gonadotrope (a G protein-coupled receptor), triggering a cascade of intracellular events (recently reviewed in ref. *43*). Phospholipase C is activated, and the resultant hydrolysis of inositol phosphates and increase in intracellular calcium stimulates the release of mature LH and FSH from their secretory granules. Further phosphorylation of protein kinase C then leads to stimulation of gonadotropin biosynthesis via as-yet-unknown second messengers. Gonadotropins are then cosecreted in an episodic manner from the gonadotrope with each gonadotropin pulse being preceded by a GnRH pulse and each GnRH pulse followed by a LH pulse *(44,45)*. In the human, the study of gonadotropin secretion by frequent (i.e., q10') blood sampling can therefore be used to infer the antecedent activity of the human hypothalamic GnRH pulse generator. The study of normal subjects, combined or not with the use of GnRH-deficient men and women in whom the pattern of GnRH replacement can be controlled, has provided critical information on the control of the gonadotrope by hypothalamic and/or gonadal factors in the human *(46,47)*. The frequency of blood sampling and the serum half-life of the hormones measured are two crucial de-

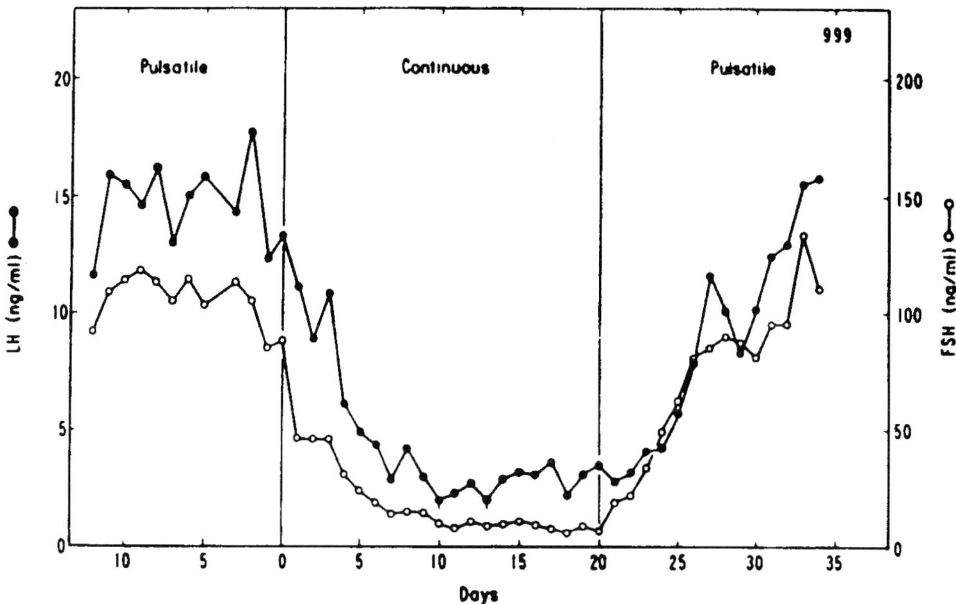

Fig. 1. Suppression of plasma LH and FSH concentrations after initiation, on d 0, of a continuous GnRH infusion (1 µg/min) in an ovariectomized rhesus monkey with a radio frequency lesion in the hypothalamus; gonadotropin secretion had been reestablished by the intermittent (pulsatile) administration of the decapeptide (1 µg/min for 6 min once per hour). The inhibition of gonadotropin secretion was reversed after reinstitution of the intermittent mode of GnRH stimulation on d 20 (reproduced from ref. *42* with permission).

terminants of the level of precision achieved with such studies. Luteinizing hormone sampled every 10 min has been more valuable than FSH, which is cleared much more slowly from the circulation *(18,19)* with a pituitary expression that is modulated by autocrine-paracrine factors other than GnRH *(35–39)*. The common α-subunit is also released from the gonadotrope in its uncombined form in response to GnRH stimulation and its pulsatile secretion in the human parallels that of LH in most physiological situations *(12,48)*. Because of its shorter half-life of about 15 min, it represents a particularly useful marker of gonadotrope activation in conditions in which GnRH is secreted at high frequencies (i.e., during the preovulatory LH surge and in castrate models).

In addition to its importance in maintaining gonadotrope function, the pattern of pulsatile GnRH secretion encodes considerable information from the hypothalamus to the gonadotrope *(49,50)*. A pulsatile stimulus can generally be characterized by its magnitude (i.e., amplitude), the average rate of its occurrence (i.e., frequency), its variability around this mean frequency (i.e., its interpulse interval), and its contour (i.e., dose–duration characteristics). Studies in various animal and human models of GnRH deficiency have demonstrated that each of these characteristics may modulate gonadotrope function independently *(41,47,51–55)*. The importance of this phenomenon becomes immediately apparent when remembering that a single hypothalamic factor (GnRH) regulates the differential synthesis and secretion of two different gonadotrope products (LH and FSH).

The human menstrual cycle may well represent a physiological circumstance during which such mechanisms come into play. During the human luteal phase, the frequency of hypothalamic GnRH secretion decreases significantly under the influence of progesterone secretion from the corpus luteum *(56)*. Following this period of slow frequency, FSH is secreted preferentially when GnRH stimulation increases again during the luteal-follicular transition *(57)*. As it turns out, decreasing the frequency of GnRH stimulation in a rat model of GnRH-deficiency results in a differential increase in FSH biosynthesis as measured by gene transcription *(55)*. Therefore, it may well be that the slow luteal phase frequency of GnRH pulses acts to prepare for the differential gonadotropin release at the luteal-follicular transition by building up relatively more intracellular stores of mature FSH. Changing frequency of GnRH secretion thus translates to both changes in secretion as well as gene activation indicating the fundamental importance of this mode of signaling.

Conversely, when the frequency of exogenous GnRH stimulation is increased in GnRH-deficient men, mean LH and FSH secretion increases initially but then decreases at the highest frequencies used *(58)*. This decrease is most compatible with homologous desensitization of the gonadotrope. Again, the menstrual cycle provides a situation in which this observation may be physiologically relevant. In sheep, very high levels of GnRH persist in the hypothalamo-hypophyseal portal blood several hours after the termination of the LH surge *(59)*, and the mechanisms responsible for the termination of the LH surge in the face of continuing GnRH stimulation are far from being fully elucidated *(60)*. Therefore, the observation that high GnRH frequencies can induce pituitary desensitization *(58)* is at least consistent with the hypothesis that this may constitute a mechanism for the hypothalamus to terminate the LH surge.

Ontogeny of Gonadotropin Secretion

Gonadotropins are first detectable in the peripheral blood of the human fetus by approximately wk 12–14 of gestation *(61)*. Their biosynthesis at this earliest stage of development appears to be at least partially dependent on GnRH as evidenced by the absence of LH and FSH β-subunits within the pituitary glands of anencephalic infants lacking a hypothalamus *(61)* and the ability for GnRH to induce LH synthesis and secretion in fetal human pituitary cells in vitro *(62)*. In female fetuses, levels of LH and FSH increase steadily thereafter throughout the gestation, whereas, in males, they tend to decrease during the third trimester *(61)*. This sexual dimorphism has been at least partially ascribed to differences in the relative sensitivity of the developing hypothalamus and pituitary to male and female gonadal steroid feedback. In primates, testosterone is a potent inhibitor of gonadotropin secretion early in fetal life *(63)* and the developing testes secrete very high levels of testosterone in response to maternal hCG, which binds to the LH receptor. In addition, both subunits of inhibin appear in the human testis during the second trimester of gestation *(64)*. In sharp contrast, the fetal ovary does not seem to express FSH receptors until the ninth month of gestation *(65)*, and the appearance of inhibin subunits in the ovary lags well behind the testis *(64)*. Taken together, these differences may well explain the higher levels of gonadotropins, particularly FSH, measured in the female fetus *(61)*.

Pulsatile gonadotropin secretion in early infancy persists at adult levels up to 12 wk after birth with a similar sexual dimorphism in the pattern of LH and FSH secretion *(66)* observed *in utero (61)*. It thereafter vanishes during childhood years, although low amplitude pulses of LH and FSH have been observed in children as early as 5 yr old *(67)*. This observation suggests that the mechanism(s) responsible for this quiescence of childhood resides in the hypothalamus, and not in the pituitary, which can respond (after priming) to exogenous GnRH stimulation. Many hypotheses have been formulated to explain both the low levels of secretion of gonadotropins during childhood and the subsequent awakening of the whole hypothalamo-pituitary-gonadal axis that heralds clinical puberty (reviewed in refs. *68,69*) but the definitive answer to these questions has not yet been provided.

Whatever the mechanism(s) implicated, reactivation of the hypothalamic GnRH pulse generator at the time of puberty results in progressive increases in the amplitude and frequency of gonadotropin pulses. Classically, this pulsatile secretion is initially entrained by sleep and then occurs during the daytime as puberty progresses *(70)*. As mentioned earlier, this increased LH and FSH secretion may also be accompanied by an altered ratio of bioactive over immunoactive hormone *(71)*. These dynamic changes concur to elicit gonadal development, resulting in testis enlargement and sperm production in boys, whereas the ovary begins its cyclic folliculogenesis in girls. Increasing levels of gonadal steroids trigger the development of secondary sexual characteristics in both sexes. At the same time, and probably in conjunction with gonadal peptides, sex steroids begin to modulate gonadotropin secretion dynamically via classical endocrine feedback mechanisms. It is interesting to note that the same sexual dimorphism that exists in gonadotropin secretion *in utero* is present during infancy, with girls secreting significantly more FSH than LH, whereas in boys this is not present *(66)*.

In women, menstrual cycles become irregular during the fourth decade of life. FSH levels can begin to rise at a time when LH secretion is still in the premenopausal range *(72)*, indicating declining ovarian function. This selective rise in gonadotropin secretion continues as the ovary is failing, reflecting the waning negative feedback effects of both steroid and nonsteroid gonadal products. The effects of aging in men are certainly not as dramatic; however, some data suggest that there are age associated changes in the pituitary-gonadal function of elderly men *(73,74)*.

BIOLOGICAL FUNCTIONS

The target organs of LH and FSH are the gonads. In the ovary, LH induces ovulation of the mature follicle and stimulates estrogen production by promoting synthesis of the requisite androgen precursors in theca cells. These androgens then diffuse into neighboring granulosa cells, where they are aromatized into estrogens under the control of FSH. Finally, LH helps to sustain luteinization of the ruptured Graaffian follicle, which then forms a corpus luteum during the second half of the ovulatory cycle by stimulating progesterone synthesis. In the testis, the primary role of LH is to stimulate testosterone biosynthesis by Leydig cells, whereas FSH is responsible for initiation of spermatogenesis. Whether or not FSH is required for maintenance of spermatogenesis in the adult remains an open question.

The FSH in the ovary is responsible for the development of a mature follicle that will eventually ovulate in response to the rapidly increasing LH levels that occur at the midcycle gonadotropin surge. Interestingly, at the same time that FSH promotes the final development of the dominant follicle that will ovulate, it also seems to initiate the recruitment of the next generation of follicles that will grow during the following cycles. As stated above, FSH also participates in estrogen production by stimulating aromatization of androgens in granulosa cells. In the testis, FSH has classically been regarded as a key factor in the development of seminiferous tubules and the initiation of puberty. This belief has recently been challenged by the demonstration that mice in which the FSHβ gene has been knocked out exhibit normal spermatogenesis and fertility *(75)*. It is, however, not clear at this time whether this will prove true in humans, since marked differences in the spermatogenic process exist between humans and other mammals.

Gonadotropin Hormone Receptors

It has been long recognized that gonadotropins stimulate cAMP production in their target cells *(76)*, therefore suggesting that their receptor would be a member of the G protein-coupled family of receptors. The cloning of the receptors for LH in 1989 *(77,78)*, and FSH shortly thereafter *(79)*, confirmed this hypothesis. Binding of either LH or FSH to their cognate receptor stimulates the adenylate cyclase-cAMP pathway (for a review, *see* ref. *80*). It has also been demonstrated that the effects of LH can be mediated by several other intracellular second messenger systems including the phospholipase A_2, C, and D pathways. In addition, it appears that steroidogenesis can be modulated by several other factors present locally within the gonads, including GnRH itself, GHRH, CRH, and TGFα *(80)*.

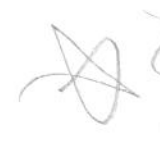

Both the LH and the FSH receptor consist of a large extracellular N-terminus domain, followed by both the classical seven transmembrane domain of α-helices and a small intracytoplasmic C-terminus domain characteristic of this family of receptors (Fig. 2). In contrast to other family members, their extracellular domain is significantly larger than usual, comprising as many as 341 residues for the LH-CG receptor. It contains several leucine repeats which may be very important for ligand-receptor interactions *(78)*. Moreover, most G protein-coupled receptors share the striking feature of being encoded by intronless genes, whereas the genes for the LH and FSH receptors contain 11 and 10 exons, respectively *(81,82)*. It is therefore believed that these receptors have evolved by recombination between a gene encoding for a leucine-rich ligand-binding protein and an intronless gene encoding for a G protein-coupled receptor.

The largest of these exons (11 for the LHR and 10 for the FSHR) encodes for the entire transmembrane and intracellular domains of the protein, whereas the other exons encode for various segments of the extracellular domain (Fig. 3). Interestingly, alternatively spliced transcripts of the LH receptor gene that lack the transmembrane domain have been identified intracellularly *(77)*. This alternative splicing may have some physiological importance because such proteins, if secreted, could act as antagonists of gonadotropin actions by binding circulating hormones with high affinity. To date, however, all available evidence suggests that transcripts lacking the transmembrane domain remain trapped within the cells *(83)*.

In the initial report on the LH receptor, its expression seemed to be confined to the gonads *(78)*. This finding was somewhat expected, given that the known biological ac-

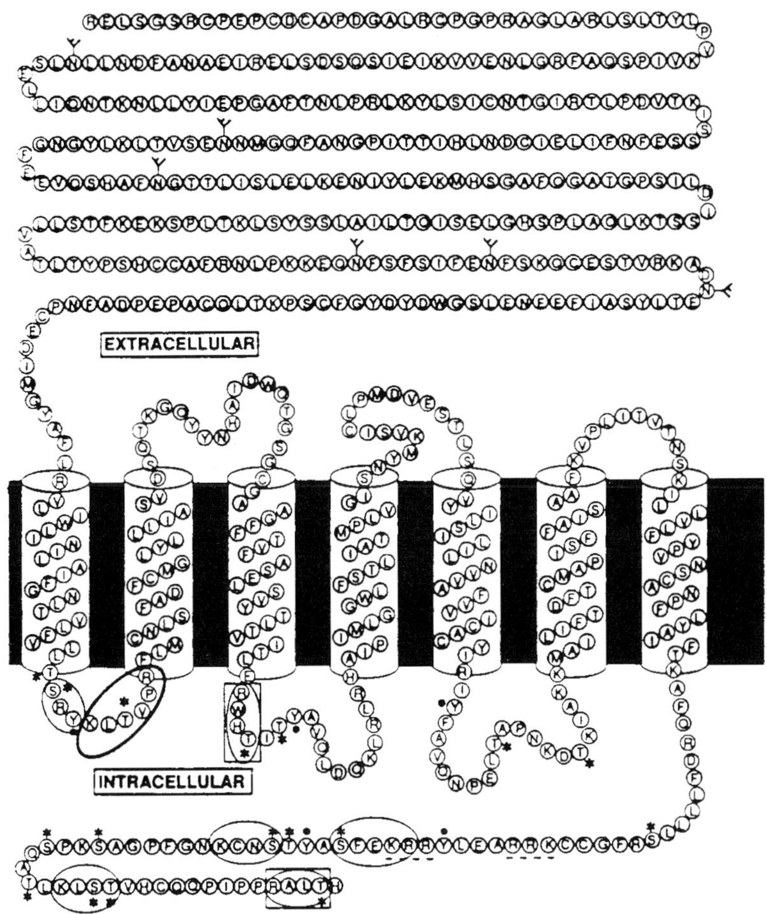

Fig. 2. Amino acid sequence, orientation, and proposed topology of the rat LH/CG receptor in the plasma membrane. Potential sites for N-linked glycosylation are shown by the branch-like structures. The sequences underlined with dashes in the cytoplasmic tail mark two clusters of basic amino acids which might represent potential tryptic cleavage sites. Potential intracellular sites for phosphorylation are denoted by asterisks or dark dots. The rectangles denote weak consensus sequences for cAMP-dependent phosphorylation. The ovals and heavy ovals denote weak and strong consensus sequences for C kinase-catalyzed phosphorylation, respectively (reproduced from ref. *83* with permission).

tivity of gonadotropins is limited to these target organs. Recent data have, however, demonstrated the presence of the LH/CG-receptor in the rat hypothalamus *(84)* and further work using the mouse GnRH neuronal cell line GT 1-7 *(85)* confirmed that the LH receptor is expressed and functional in these cells *(86)*. These recent observations therefore corroborate the hypothesis that gonadotropins feedback on hypothalamic GnRH neurons via a short loop feedback mechanism *(87,88)*. However, the dramatic increase in gonadotropin secretion observed after castration in most species suggests that this effect is probably physiologically less important.

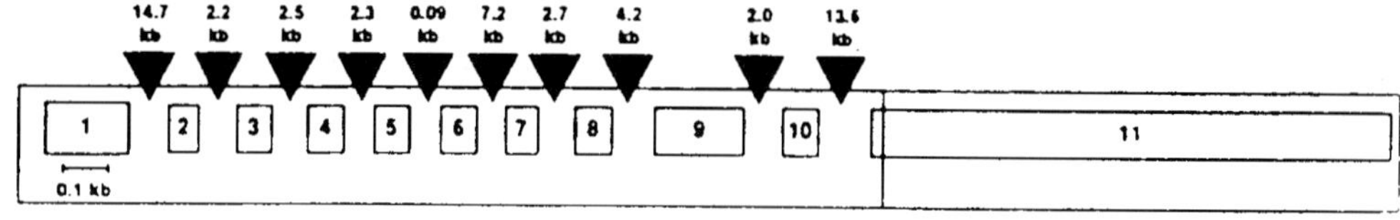

Fig. 3. Genomic organization of the rat LH/CG receptor. Exons and introns are represented by the open rectangles and shaded triangles, respectively. The size of the different introns is indicated on the top of each triangle. The exons are drawn to scale indicated under exon 1. The first 10 exons encode for the majority of the extracellular domain. Exon 11 encodes for a small portion of the extracellular domain, all the transmembrane region, and the entire C-terminal cytoplasmic tail (reproduced from ref. *83* with permission).

FEEDBACK CONTROL OF GONADOTROPIN SECRETION

Modulation Sex Steroid Hormones

In women, estrogens can exert a dual feedback effect upon gonadotropin secretion. A clear demonstration of the negative feedback effects of estrogens in normal women is provided by the elevation in LH and FSH levels observed after the menopause *(72)* and their decrease following estrogen replacement after castration *(89)*. During the normal menstrual cycle, the feedback effects exerted by estrogens will eventually shift from negative to positive towards the late follicular phase, triggering the midcycle surge of LH and FSH secretion. The mechanism of this positive feedback effect is not well understood. The dose and perhaps pattern of exposure to estradiol may be responsible for this shift from negative to positive. Studies performed in normal and GnRH-deficient subjects *(90–92)* indicate that, whereas estrogens modulate gonadotropin secretion mainly at the pituitary level, there is also ample evidence suggesting the implication of hypothalamic GnRH in the generation of the midcycle LH surge in women, i.e., positive feedback *(93,94)*.

The principal effect of progesterone is to decrease the frequency of gonadotropin pulses *(56)* and it is therefore believed to act primarily at the hypothalamic level. This feature is most evident in normal human physiology by the slowing of gonadotropin pulse frequency observed during the luteal phase while progesterone levels are rising. Because hypothalamic GnRH neurons do not express sex steroid receptors *(95)*, these central effects of estrogen and progesterone are likely to be mediated by afferent nerve terminals; it has been hypothesized that opioidergic pathways from the brainstem and other hypothalamic neurons play an important role in this mediation. Finally, an additional pituitary effect of progesterone cannot be excluded at the present time.

Testosterone and its aromatized derivative estradiol are the two steroid hormones that exert negative feedback effects on gonadotropin secretion in the male *(96,97)*. Tandem studies conducted in normal and in GnRH-deficient men have elucidated the respective sites of action of these effects in the human male *(90–92)*. Gonadotropin secretion following infusions of testosterone or estradiol in normal men were compared with GnRH-deficient men in whom the dose and frequency of exogenous GnRH replacement were kept constant. In normal men, gonadal steroids can modulate the function of the gonadotrope either by directly inhibiting LH or FSH secretion from the pituitary, and/or by inhibiting GnRH secretion from the hypothalamus. In GnRH-deficient men in whom the exogenous GnRH replacement regimen is kept constant, any effect of changing gonadal steroid levels on gonadotropin secretion must thus directly reflect a pituitary site of action.

Comparisons made between both human models demonstrated that testosterone, unlike estradiol, has a dual site of action (Fig. 4). It decreases the frequency of gonadotropin pulses in normal men, therefore demonstrating a hypothalamic site of action. However, it also decreases mean LH levels secreted in response to GnRH in GnRH-deficient men, which represents evidence of an additional pituitary site of action *(91)*. The effects of estradiol were identical in both models, demonstrating that estrogens act primarily at the pituitary level *(90)*. The most striking finding of these studies was the demonstration that some feedback effects of testosterone are mediated via its aromatization to estradiol. The administration of testolactone, a potent inhibitor of aromatization, permitted some insight into the mechanism of this feedback. The hypothalamic effects appear to be mediated directly by androgens (i.e., independent of aromatization), whereas both testosterone itself and estradiol can directly suppress gonadotropin secretion from the pituitary *(90,91)*.

Gonadal Peptide Hormone Modulation

Although the existence of the gonadal protein, inhibin, was demonstrated in 1932 *(98)*, 50 yr were to elapse before the eventual isolation and cloning of its α- and β-subunits *(99)*. Inhibins are now divided into two different subtypes, inhibin A and inhibin B, according to the subtype of their β-subunit (β_A and β_B). One important biological role of inhibin is to inhibit FSH biosynthesis and secretion by the gonadotrope selectively (for review, *see* ref. *100*), and it also probably plays an important autocrine/paracrine role in the gonads. Although the first RIAs for circulating inhibin were developed almost 10 yr ago *(101)*, their initial lack of specificity for dimeric inhibin *(102)* has made it difficult to firmly elucidate its role in the human reproduction with precision. For example, the initial assay whose specificity was only for the α-subunit, failed to establish a correlation between inhibin and FSH in normal and infertile men *(103)*. The recent development of dimer-specific immunoradiometric assays *(104)* has enabled characterization of circulating levels of dimeric inhibin in the human more accurately *(105)*. These studies demonstrated that 32-kDa dimeric inhibin-A is surprisingly not a major endocrine regulator of FSH in the human male. However, very recent data have demonstrated that there is convincing evidence in the human male to suggest that inhibin-B circulates in levels compatible with its function as an endocrine signal of gonadal origin, potentially stimulated by gonadotropins. In the female, inhibin A is secreted by dominant follicles and corpora lutea as indicated by its high circulating levels during the late follicular and luteal phase (Fig. 5). Inhibin B levels appear to be elevated only in the late luteal and early follicular phase of the cycle i.e., quite different and reciprocal in pattern of inhibin-A during the cycle. Overall, the physiology of inhibin in the human has yet to be defined precisely. These more sensitive and specific assays will certainly help determine the role played in the endocrine regulation of FSH in the human by the different subtypes of inhibin as well as its higher molecular weight precursors, which are bioactive and circulate in μg/mL quantities in the human.

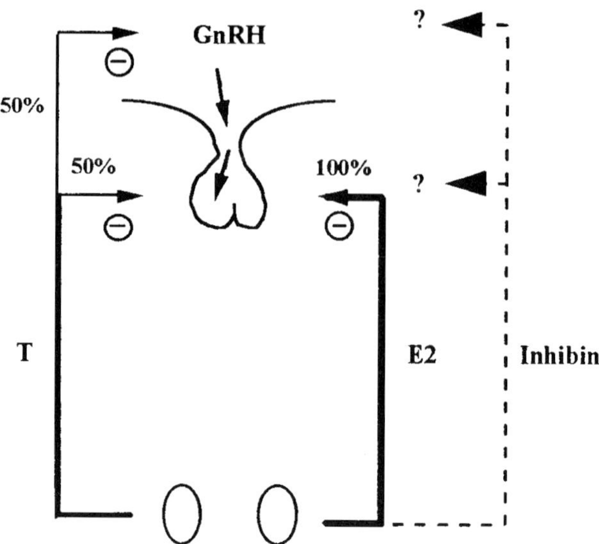

Fig. 4. Summary of the relative sites of action of sex steroids on the hypothalamo-pituitary axis. The effects of testosterone, schematized on the left, are both mediated by the pituitary and the hypothalamus, whereas those of estradiol (right arrow) are mainly mediated at the pituitary level. The exact site of action and physiologic role played by dimeric inhibin in the human remain to be fully elucidated.

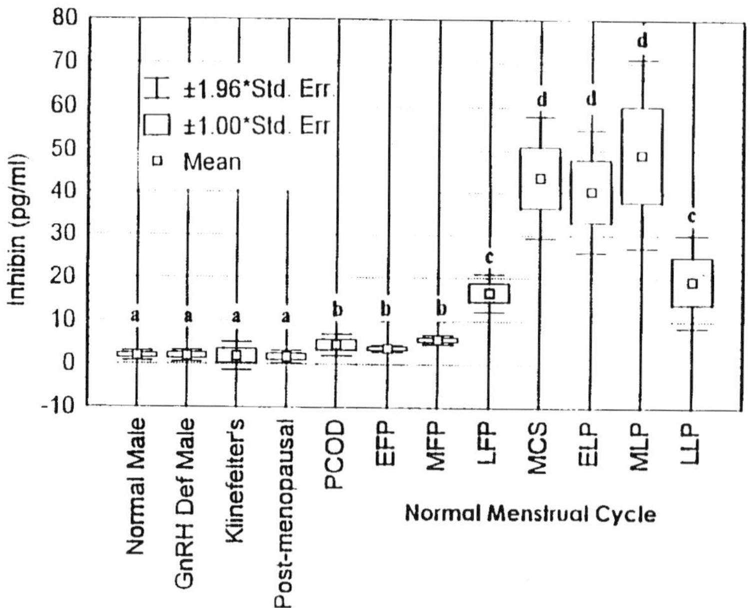

Fig. 5. Mean dimeric inhibin-A levels in serum from several fertile and infertile groups of men and women. Groups with different letter symbols have significantly different means ($p < 0.05$) (reproduced from ref. *105* with permission).

CONCLUSION

The control of pituitary gonadotropin secretion in the human is very tightly modulated by factors of hypothalamic, pituitary, and gonadal origin. The "fine tuning" existing between such factors with often opposite effects on the gonadotrope results in the regulation of gonadal steroidogenesis and gametogenesis. Recent years have witnessed significant advances in the field of gonadotropin physiology such as the cloning of their receptors and the elucidation of their crystal structure. This, in turn, will lead to the design of better agonists and antagonists of gonadotropins. As our basic understanding of human physiology grows, the potential clinical applications of such new tools for treatment of reproductive disorders as well as for the investigation of newer contraceptive agents will certainly blossom.

REFERENCES

1. Pierce JG, Parsons TF. Glycoprotein hormones: structure and function. Ann Rev Biochem 1981, 50:465–495.
2. Gharib SD, Wierman ME, Shupnik MA, Chin WW. Molecular biology of the pituitary gonadotropins. Endocrine Rev 1990; 11:177–199.
3. Baenziger JU, Green ED. Pituitary glycoprotein hormone oligosaccharides: structure, synthesis and function of the asparagine-linked oligosaccharides on lutropin, follitropin and thyrotropin. Biochem Biophys Acta 1988; 947:287–306.
4. Naylor SL, Chin WW, Goodman HM, Lalley PA, Grzeschik KH, Sakaguchi AY. Chromosome assignment of genes encoding the alpha and beta subunits of glycoprotein hormones in man and mouse. Som Cell Genetics 1983; 9:757–770.
5. Fiddes JC, Goodman HM. Isolation, cloning and sequence analysis of the cDNA for the a-subunit of human chorionic gonadotropin. Nature 1979; 281:351–356.
6. Boorstein WR, Vamvakopoulos NC, Fiddes JC. Human chorionic gonadotropin b-subunit is encoded by at least eight genes arranged in tandem and inverted pairs. Nature 1982; 300:419–422.
7. Julier C, Weil D, Couillin P, et al. The beta chorionic gonadotropin-beta luteinizing gene cluster maps to human chromosome 19. Human Genetics 1984; 67:174–177.
8. Talmadge K, Boorstein WR, Fiddes JC. The human genome contains seven genes for the beta-subunit of chorionic gonadotropin but only one gene for the beta-subunit of luteinizing hormone. DNA 1983; 2:281–289.
9. Sawitzke AL, Griffin J, Odel WD. Purified preparations of human luteinizing hormone are contaminated with small amounts of chorionic gonadotropin-like material. J Clin Endocrinol Metab 1991; 72:841–846.
10. Jameson JL, Becker CB, Lindell CM, Habener JF. Human follicle-stimulating hormone b-subunit gene encodes multiple messenger ribonucleic acids. Mol Endocrinol 1988; 2:806–815.
11. Watkins PC, Eddy R, Beck AK, et al. DNA sequence and regional assignment of the human follicle-stimulating hormone beta-subunit gene to the short arm of human chromosome 11. DNA 1987; 6:205–212.
12. Whitcomb RW, O'Dea LS, Finkelstein JS, Heavern DM, Crowley WF, Jr. Utility of free alpha-subunit as an alternative neuroendocrine marker of gonadotropin-releasing hormone (GnRH) stimulation of the gonadotroph in the human: evidence from normal and GnRH-deficient men. J Clin Endocrinol Metab 1990; 70:1654–1661.
13. Morell AG, Gregoriadis G, Scheinberg IH, Hickman J, Ashwell G. The role of sialic acid in determining the survival of glycoproteins in the circulation. J Biol Chem 1971; 246:1461–1467.
14. Fiete D, Srivastava V, Hindsgaul O, Baenziger JU. A hepatic reticuloendothelial cell receptor specific for SO_4-4GalNAcb1,4GlcNAcb1,2Mana that mediates rapid clearance of lutropin. Cell 1991; 67:1103–1110.
15. Baenziger JU, Kumar S, Brodbeck RM, Smith PL, Beranek MC. Circulatory half-life but not interaction with the lutropin/chorionic gonadotropin receptor is modulated by sulfation of bovine lutropin oligosaccharides. Proc Natl Acad Sci USA 1992; 89:334–338.

16. Veldhuis JD, Johnson ML. *In Vivo* dynamics of luteinizing hormone secretion and clearance in man: assessment by deconvolution mechanics. J Clin Endocrinol Metab. 1988; 66:1291–1300.
17. Yen SSC, Llerena O, Little B, Pearson OH. Disappearance rates of endogenous luteinizing hormone and dhorionic gonadotropin in man. J Clin Endocrinol Metab. 1968; 28:1763–1767.
18. Urban RJ, Padmanabhan V, Beitins I, Veldhuis JD. Metabolic clearance of human follicle-stimulating hormone assessed by radioimmunoassay, immunoradiometric assay, and *in Vitro* Sertoli cell bioassay. J Clin Endocrinol Metab 1991; 73:818–823.
19. Yen SSC, Llerena LA, Pearson OH, Littell AS. Disappearance rates of endogenous follicle-stimulating hormone in serum following surgical hypophysectomy in man. J Clin Endocrinol. 1970; 30:325–329.
20. Matzuk MM, Boime I. Mutagenesis and gene transfer define site-specific roles of the gonadotropin oligosacharides. Biol Repro. 1989; 40:48–53.
21. Sairam MR, Bhargavi GN. A role for the glycosylation of the alpha-subunit in the transduction of biological signal in glycoprotein hormones. Science 1985; 229:65–67.
22. Keutmann HT, McIlroy PJ, Bergert ER, Ryan RJ. Chemically deglycosylated human chorionic gonadotropin subunits: characterization and biological properties. Biochemistry 1983; 22:3067–3072.
23. Stanton PG, Pozvek G, Burgon PG, Robertson DM, Hearn MTW. Isolation and characterization of human LH isoforms. J Endocrinol 1993; 138:529–543.
24. Strollo F, Harlin J, Hernandez-Montes H, Robertson DM, Zaidi AA, Diczfalusy E. Qualitative and quantitative differences in the isoelectrofocusing profile of biologically active lutropin in the blood of normally menstruating and post-menopausal women. Acta Endocrinol 1981; 97:166–175.
25. Lucky AW, Rich BH, Rosenfield RL, Fang VS, Roche-Bender N. LH bioactivity increases more than immunoreactivity during puberty. J Ped 1980; 97:205–513.
26. Keutmann HT. Receptor-binding regions in human glycoprotein hormones. Mol Cell Endocrinol 1992; 86:C1–C6.
27. Lapthorn AJ, Harris DC, Littlejohn A et al. Crystal structure of human chorionic gonadotropin. Nature 1994; 369:455–461.
28. Matsuo H, Baba Y, Nair RM, Arimura A, Schally AV. Structure of the porcine LH- and FSH-releasing hormone. I. The proposed amino acid sequence. Biochem Biophys Res Commun 1971; 43:1334–1339.
29. McCann SM, Mizunuma H, Samson WK. Differential hypothalamic control of FSH secretion: a review. Psychoneuroendocrinol 1983; 8:299–308.
30. Carroll RS, Corrigan AZ, Gharib SD, Vale W, Chin WW. Inhibin, activin, and follistatin: regulation of follicle-stimulating hormone messenger ribonucleic acid levels. Mol Endocrinol 1989; 3:1969–1976.
31. Rivier C, Rivier J, Vale W. Inhibin-mediated feedback control of follicle-stimulating hormone secretion in the female rat. Science 1986; 234:205–208.
32. Majumdar SS, Mikuma N, Ishwad PC et al. Replacement with recombinant human inhibin immediately after orchidectomy in the hypophysiotropically clamped male rhesus monkey (Macaca mulatta) maintains follicle-stimulating hormone (FSH) secretion and FSH beta messenger ribonucleic acid levels at precastration values. Endocrinology 1995; 136:1969–1977.
33. Christensen RB, Forage RG, Steiner RA, Bremner WJ. Effects of castration and recombinant human inhibin administration on circulating levels of inhibin and gonadotropins in adult male monkeys. J Andrology 1994; 15:5–31.
34. DePaolo LV, Shimonaka M, Schwall RH, Ling N. In vivo comparison of the follicle-stimulating hormone-suppressing activity of follistatin and inhibin in ovariectomized rats. Endocrinology 1991; 128:668–674.
35. Meunier H, Rivier C, Evans RM, Vale W. Gonadal and extragonadal expression of inhibin alpha, beta-A, and beta-B subunits in various tissues predicts diverse functions. Proc Natl Acad Sci 1988; 85:247–251.
36. Weiss J, Harris PE, Halvorson LM, Crowley WF, Jr., Jameson JL. Dynamic regulation of follicle-stimulating hormone-beta messenger ribonucleic acid levels by activin and gonadotropin-releasing hormone in perifused rat pituitary cells. Endocrinology 1992; 131:1403–1408.
37. Roberts V, Meunier H, Vaughan J, et al. Production and regulation of inhibin subunits in pituitary gonadotropes. Endocrinology 1989; 124:552–554.
38. Kaiser UB, Lee BL, Carroll RS, Unabia G, Chin WW, Childs GV. Follistatin gene expression in the pituitary: localization in gonadotropes and folliculostellate cells in diestrous rats. Endocrinology 1992; 130:3048–3056.
39. Kogawa K, Nakamura T, Sugino K, Takio K, Titani K, Sugino H. Activin-binding protein is present in the pituitary. Endocrinology 1991; 128:1434–1440.

40. Halvorson LM, Weiss J, Bauer-Dantoin AC, Jameson JL. Dynamic regulation of pituitary follistatin messenger ribonucleic acids during the rat estrous cycle. Endocrinology 1994; 134:1247–1253.
41. Kirk SE, Dalkin AC, Yasin M, Haisenleder DJ, Marshall JC. Gonadotropin-releasing hormone pulse frequency regulates expression of pituitary follistatin messenger ribonucleic acid: a mechanism for differential gonadotrope function. Endocrinology 1994; 135:876–880.
42. Belchetz PE, Plant TM, Nakai Y, Keogh EJ, Knobil E. Hypophysial responses to continuous and intermittent delivery of hypopthalamic gonadotropin-releasing hormone. Science 1978; 202:631–633.
43. Stojilkovic SS, Reinhart J, Catt KJ. Gonadotropin-releasing hormone receptors: structure and signal transduction pathways. Endocrine Rev 1994; 15:462–499.
44. Levine JE, Pau KY, Ramirez VD, Jackson GL. Simultaneous measurement of luteinizing hormone-releasing hormone and luteinizing hormone release in unanesthetized, ovariectomized sheep. Endocrinology 1982; 111:.
45. Clarke IJ, Cummins JT. The temporal relationship between gonadotropin releasing hormone (GnRH) and luteinizing hormone (LH) secretion in ovariectomized ewes. Endocrinology 1982; 111:1737–1739.
46. Marshall JC, Dalkin AC, Haisenleder DJ, Paul SJ, Ortolano GA, Kelch RP. Gonadotropin-releasing hormone pulses: regulators of gonadotropin synthesis and ovulatory cycles. [Review]. Rec Prog Horm Res 1991; 47:155–187.
47. Crowley WF, Jr., Whitcomb RW, Jameson JL, Weiss J, Finkelstein JS, O'Dea LS. Neuroendocrine control of human reproduction in the male. [Review]. Rec Prog Horm Res 1991; 47:27–62.
48. Winters SJ, Troen P. Pulsatile secretion of immunoreactive alpha-subunit in man. J Clin Endocrinol Metab 1985; 60:344–348.
49. Marshall JC, Kelch RP. Gonadotropin-releasing hormone: role of pulsatile secretion in the regulation of reproduction. N Engl J Med 1986; 315:1459–1468.
50. Knobil E. Patterns of hormonal signals and hormone action. N Engl J Med 1981; 305:1582, 1583.
51. Handelsman DJ, Boylan LM. Pharmacodynamics of gonadotropin-releasing hormone (GnRH). II. Pattern of GnRH delivery alters pituitary luteinizing hormone secretion in women. J Clin Endocrinol Metab 1988; 67:175–179.
52. Gross KM, Matsumoto AM, Bremner WJ. Differential control of luteinizing hormone and follicle-stimulating hormone secretion by luteinizing hormone-releasing hormone pulse frequency in man. J Clin Endocrinol Metab 1987; 64:675–680.
53. Gross KM, Matsumoto AM, Berger RE, Bremner WJ. Increased frequency of pulsatile luteinizing hormone-releasing hormone administration selectively decreases follicle-stimulating hormone levels in men with idiopathic azoospermia. Fert. Sterility 1986; 45:392–396.
54. Wildt L, Hausler A, Marshall G, et al. Frequency and amplitude of gonadotropin-releasing hormone stimulation and gonadotropin secretion in the rhesus monkey. Endocrinology 1981; 109:376–385.
55. Haisenleder DJ, Dalkin AC, Ortolano GA, Marshall JC, Shupnik MA. A pulsatile gonadotropin-releasing hormone stimulus is required to increase transcription of the gonadotropin subunit genes: evidence for differential regulation of transcription by pulse frequency in vivo. Endocrinology 1991; 128:509–517.
56. Nippoldt TB, Reame NE, Kelch RP, Marshall JC. The roles of estradiol and progesterone in decreasing luteinizing hormone pulse frequency in the luteal phase of the menstrual cycle. J Clin Endocrinol Metab 1989; 69:67–76.
57. Hall JE, Schoenfeld DA, Martin KA, Crowley WF, Jr. Hypothalamic gonadotropin-releasing hormone secretion and follicle-stimulating hormone dynamics during the luteal-follicular transition. J Clin Endocrinol Metab 1992; 74:600–607.
58. Spratt DI, Finkelstein JS, Butler JP, Badger TM, Crowley WF, Jr. Effects of increasing the frequency of low doses of gonadotropin-releasing hormone (GnRH) on gonadotropin secretion in GnRH-deficient men. J Clin Endocrinol Metab 1987; 64:1179–1186.
59. Moenter SM, Caraty A, Locatelli A, Karsch FJ. Pattern of gonadotropin-releasing hormone (GnRH) secretion leading up to ovulation in the ewe: existence of a preovulatory GnRH surge. Endocrinology 1991; 129:1175–1182.
60. Caraty A, Antoine C, Delaleu B, et al. Nature and bioactivity of gonadotropin-releasing hormone (GnRH) secreted during the GnRH surge. Endocrinology 1995; 136:3452–3460.
61. Kaplan SL, Grumbach MM. The ontogenesis of human foetal hormones. II. Luteinizing hormone (LH) and follicle stimulating hormone (FSH). Acta Endocrinol 1976; 81:808–829.
62. Castillo RH, matteri RL, Dumesic DA. Luteinizing hormone synthesis in cultured fetal human pituitary cells exposed to gonadotropin-releasing hormone. J Clin Endocrinol Metab. 1992; 75:318–322.

63. Resko JA, Ellinwood WE. Negative feedback regulation of gonadotropin secretion by androgens in fetal rhesus macaques. Biol Repro 1985; 33:346–352.
64. Rabinovici J, Goldsmith PC, Roberts VJ, Vaughan J, Vale W, Jaffe RB. Localization and secretion of inhibin/activin subunits in the human and. J Clin Endocrinol Metab 1991; 73:1141–1149.
65. Rannikki AS, Zhang FP, Huhtaniemi IT. Ontogeny of follicle-stimulating hormone receptor gene expression in the rat testis and ovary. Mol Cell Endocrinol 1995; 107:199–208.
66. Waldhauser F, Weissenbacher G, Frisch H, Pollak A. Pulsatile secretion of gonadotropins in early infancy. Eur J Pediatr 1981; 137:71–74.
67. Jakacki RI, Kelch RP, Sauder SE, Lloyd JS, Hopwood NJ, Marshall JC. Pulsatile secretion of luteinizing hormone in children. J Clin Endocrinol Metab 1982; 55:453–458.
68. Terasawa E. Control of luteinizing hormone-releasing hormone pulse generation in nonhuman primates. [Review]. Cell Molecular Neurobiol 1995; 15:141–164.
69. Bourguignon JP, Gerard A, Alvarez GML, Franchimont P. Control of pulsatile secretion of gonadotrophin releasing hormone from hypothalamic explants. [Review]. Human Reprod 1993; 2:18–22.
70. Boyar R, Finkelstein J, Roffwarg H, Kapen S, Weitzman E, Hellman L. Synchronization of augmented luteinizing hormone secretion with sleep during puberty. N Engl J Med 1972; 287:582–586.
71. Lucky AW, Rich BH, Rosenfield RL, Fang WS, Roche-Bender N. LH bioactivity increases more than immunoreactivity during puberty. J Ped 1980; 97:205–213.
72. Sherman BM, Korenman SG. Hormonal characteristics of the human menstrual cycle throughout reproductive life. J Clin Inv 1975; 55:699–706.
73. Zumoff B, Strain GW, Kream J, et al. Age variation of the 24-hour mean plasma concentrations of androgens, and gonadotropins in normal adult men. J Clin Endocrinol Metab 1982; 54:534–538.
74. Veldhuis JD, Urban RJ, Lizarralde G, Johnson ML, Iranmesh A. Attenuation of luteinizing hormone secretory burst amplitude as a proximate basis for the hypoandrogenism of healthy aging in men. J Clin Endocrinol Metab 1992; 75:707–713.
75. Dong J, Nishimori K, Kumar TR, Wang Y, Lu N, Guo Q, Matzuk MM. Transgenic mouse models to study folliculogenesis. Abstract. Int Symp on Life Cycle of the Ovarian Follicle 1995; Ft Lauderdale.
76. Sutherland EW, Robinson GA. Role of cyclic 3'-5'AMP in response to catecholamines and other hormones. Pharmacol. Rev 1966; 18:145–161.
77. Loosfelt H, Misrahi M, Atger M, et al. Cloning and sequencing of porcine LH-hCG receptor cDNA: variants lacking transmembrane domain. Science 1989; 245:525–528.
78. McFarland KC, Sprengel R, Phillips HS, et al. Lutropin-choriogonadotropin receptor: an unusual member of the G protein-coupled receptor family. Science 1989; 245:494–499.
79. Sprengel L, Braun T, Nikolics K, Segaloff DL, Seeburg PH. The testicular receptor for follicle stimulating hormone: structure and functional expression of cloned cDNA. Mol Endocrinol 1990; 4:525–530.
80. Leung PCK, Steele GL. Intracellular signaling in the gonads. Endocrine Rev 1992; 13:476–498.
81. Tsai-Morris CH, Buczko E, Wang W, Xie XZ, Dufau ML. Structural organization of the rat luteinizing hormone (LH) receptor gene. J Biol Chem 1991; 266:11355–11359.
82. Heckert LL, Daley IJ, Griswold MD. Structural organization of the follicle-stimulating hormone receptor gene. Mol Endocrinol 1992; 6:70–80.
83. Segaloff DL, Ascoli M. The lutropin/choriogonadotropin receptor . . . 4 years later. Endocrine Rev 1993; 14:324–347.
84. Lei ZM, Rao CV, Kornyei JL, Licht P, Hiatt ES. Novel expression of human chorionic gonadotropin/luteinizing hormone receptor gene in brain. Endocrinology 1993; 132:2262–2270.
85. Mellon PL, Windle JJ, Goldsmith PC, Padula CA, Roberts JL, Weiner RI. Immortalization of hypothalamic GnRH neurons by genetically targeted tumorigenesis. Neuron 1990; 5:1–10.
86. Lei ZM, Rao CV. Novel presence of luteinizing hormone/human chorionic gonadotropin (hCG) receptors and the down-regulating action of hCG on gonadotropin-releasing hormone gene expression in immortalized hypothalamic GT1-7 neurons. Mol Endocrinol 1994; 8:1111–1121.
87. Melrose PA. In vitro evidence for short-loop gonadotropin feedback on gonadotropin-releasing hormone neurons harvested from adult male rats. Endocrinology 1987; 121:200–204.
88. Padmanabhan V, Evans NP, Dahl GE, McFadden KL, Mauger DT, Karsch FJ. Evidence for short or ultrashort loop negative feedback of gonadotropin-releasing hormone secretion. Neuroendocrinology 1995; 62:248–258.
89. Geola FL, Frumar AM, Tataryn IV, et al. Biological effects of various doses of conjugated equine estrogens in postmenopausal women. J Clin Endocrinol Metab 1980; 51:620–625.

90. Finkelstein JS, O'Dea LS, Whitcomb RW, Crowley WF, Jr. Sex steroid control of gonadotropin secretion in the human male. II. Effects of estradiol administration in normal and gonadotropin-releasing hormone-deficient men. J Clin Endocrinol Metab 1991; 73:621–628.
91. Finkelstein JS, Whitcomb RW, O'Dea LS, Longcope C, Schoenfeld DA, Crowley WF, Jr. Sex steroid control of gonadotropin secretion in the human male. I. Effects of testosterone administration in normal and gonadotropin-releasing hormone-deficient men. J Clin Endocrinol Metab 1991; 73:609–620.
92. Bagatell CJ, Dahl KD, Bremner WJ. The direct pituitary effect of testosterone to inhibit gonadotropin secretion in men is partially mediated by aromatization to estradiol. J Andrology 1994; 15:15–21.
93. Moenter SM, Caraty A, Locatelli A, Karsch FJ. Pattern of gonadotropin-releasing hormone (GnRH) secretion leading up to ovulation in the ewe: existence of a preovulatory GnRH surge. Endocrinology 1991; 129:1175–1182.
94. Kolp LA, Pavlou SN, Urban RJ, Rivier JC, Vale WW, Veldhuis JD. Abrogation by a potent gonadotropin-releasing hormone antagonist of the estrogen/progesterone-stimulated surge-like release of luteinizing hormone and follicle-stimulating hormone in postmenopausal women. J Clin Endocrinol Metab 1992; 75:993–997.
95. Shivers BD, Harlan RE, Morrell JI, Pfaff DW. Absence of estradiol concentration in cell nuclei of LHRH-immunoreactive neurones. Nature 1983; 304:345–347.
96. Winters SJ, Janick JJ, Loriaux DL, Sherins RJ. Studies on the role of sex steroids in the feedback control of gonadotropin concentrations in men. II. Use of the estrogen antagonist, clomiphen citrate. J Clin Endocrinol Metab 1979; 48:222–227.
97. Sherins RJ, Loriaux DL. Studies on the role of sex steroids in the feedback control of FSH concentrations in men. J Clin Endocrinol Metab 1973; 36:886–893.
98. McCullagh DR. Dual endocrine activity of testes. Science 1932; 76:19.
99. Mason AJ, Hayflick JS, Ling N, et al. Complementary DNA sequences of ovarian follicular fluid inhibin show precursor structure and homology with transforming growth factor-beta. Nature 1985; 318:659–663.
100. Vale W, Rivier C, Hsueh A. Chemical and biological characterization of the inhibin family of protein hormones. Rec Prog Horm Res 1988; 44:1–34.
101. McLachlan RI, Robertson DM, Burger HG, de KDM. The radioimmunoassay of bovine and human follicular fluid and serum inhibin. Mol Cell Endocrinol 1986; 46:175–185.
102. Schneyer AL, Mason AJ, Burton LE, Ziegner JR, Crowley WF, Jr. Immunoreactive inhibin alpha-subunit in human serum: implications for radioimmunoassay. J Clin Endocrinol Metab 1990; 70:1208–1212.
103. DeKretser DM, McLachlan RI, Robertson DM, Burger HG. Serum inhibin levels in normal men and men with testicular disorders. J Clin Endocrinol Metab 1989; 70:1414–1419.
104. Groome N, O'Brien M. Immunoassays for inhibin and its subunits: further applications of the synthetic peptide approach. J Immunol Methods 1993; 165:167–176.
105. Lambert-Messerlian GM, Hall JE, Sluss PM, et al. Relatively low levels of dimeric inhibin circulate in men and women with polycystic ovarian syndrome using a specific two-site enzyme-linked immunosorbent assay. J Clin Endocrinol Metab 1994; 79:45–50.

11 Gonadotropin Deficiency

Differential Diagnosis and Treatment

Corrine K. Welt, MD, *and Janet E. Hall,* MD

CONTENTS

Gonadotropin deficiency is the manifestation of a heterogeneous group of disorders affecting the hypothalamic-pituitary-gonadal axis. Abnormal patterns of gonadotroph stimulation, deficiency of gonadotropin production, inappropriate feedback loops, and genetic defects resulting in abnormal gonadotropin structure encompass the variety of pathophysiologic mechanisms underlying gonadotropin deficiency (Table 1). Despite diverse etiologies, the resulting clinical characteristics are shared among the disorders. It is only through understanding the underlying mechanisms that accurate diagnoses can be made and appropriate treatment administered.

CLINICAL CHARACTERISTICS OF GONADOTROPIN DEFICIENCY

Gonadotropin deficiency manifests itself clinically as hypogonadism. The time of onset of gonadotropin deficiency, whether occurring before or after the onset of puberty, determines the clinical presentation, which is further modified by the severity of the defect.

Primary gonadotropin deficiency is characterized by the absence of puberty by age 14 in boys and age 13 in girls. Males typically present with a small phallus (<3–5 cm) and testes (<5 mL), the absence of scrotal pigment and rugae, azospermia, a prepubertal pattern of hair growth, decreased muscle mass and increased subcutaneous fat,

From: *Contemporary Endocrinology, Vol. 3: Diseases of the Pituitary: Diagnosis and Treatment*
Edited by M. E. Wierman Humana Press Inc., Totowa, NJ

Table 1
Classification of Gonadotropin Deficiency

- Abnormalities in GnRH Stimulation
  - Tumors and destructive/infiltrative disorders of the hypothalamus
    - Tumors (craniopharyngiomas, germinomas, gliomas, meningiomas, endodermal sinus tumors, chordomas, metastases, teratomas)
    - Other space occupying lesions (aneurysms, arachnoid cysts, dermoid and epidermoid cysts, Rathke's cleft cysts)
    - Cranial irradiation
    - Infiltrative disorders (Langerhan's histiocytosis, tuberculosis, sarcoidosis)
  - Isolated GnRH deficiency
    - Idiopathic hypogonadotropic hypogonadism
    - Kallmann's syndrome
    - Fertile eunuch
  - Congenital syndromes
    - Prader-Willi syndrome
    - Bardet-Biedl syndrome
    - Moebius syndrome
    - Familial cerebellar ataxia
    - X-linked congenital adrenal hypoplasia
  - Functional hypothalamic dysfunction
    - Anorexia nervosa and bulimia nervosa
    - Excessive exercise, weight loss, and fasting
    - Physical and psychological stress
    - Acute and chronic illness, burn injury, and head trauma
  - Hyperprolactinemia
  - Cushing's syndrome and exogenous steroid use
  - Miscellaneous disorders of hypothalamic function
    - Alcohol use
    - Aging
- Intrapituitary Abnormalities
  - Pituitary tumors
  - Destructive disorders
    - Hemochromatosis
    - Lymphocytic hypophysitis
    - Granulomatous hypophysitis
    - Adenohypophyseal necrosis
    - Empty sella syndrome
  - Abnormalities of gonadotropin structure
    - Isolated FSH deficiency
    - Immunologically anomalous LH
    - Biologically inactive LH
- Abnormal Feedback
  - Estradiol excess (Leydig cell tumors, feminizing adrenal tumors, choriocarcinomas)
  - Obesity
  - Anabolic steroid use

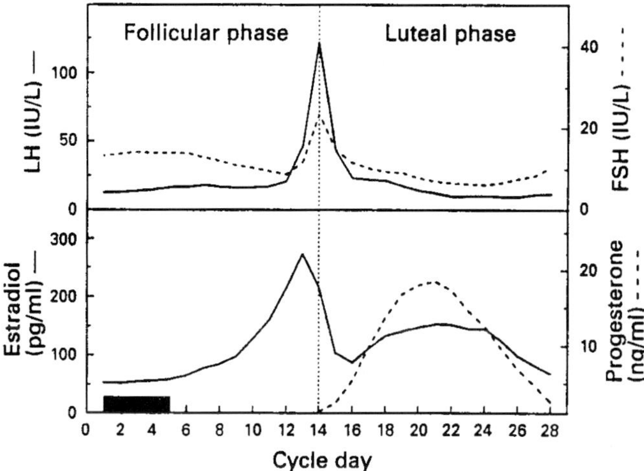

Fig. 1. Dynamic changes in mean LH, FSH, estradiol, and progesterone levels throughout the normal menstrual cycle based on daily blood samples in over 100 normal cycles. Menses is indicated by the solid box. The dotted line indicates ovulation.

eunuchoidal skeletal proportions (upper/lower body ratio <1 with an arm span 6 cm > standing height), and a high-pitched voice. In females, gonadotropin deficiency is manifested by primary amenorrhea, the absence of thelarche and hip development, and absence of cervical mucous with a nonestrogenized vaginal mucosa. Both sexes manifest delayed bone age. Even in cases of primary gonadotropin deficiency, adrenarche which is regulated independently of gonadarche, occurs normally. Thus, axillary and pubic hair growth are present, although development of these characteristics is augmented by androgens in boys and estrogens in girls.

The clinical manifestations of secondary gonadotropin deficiency depend on their relative severity. Males may experience impotence, decreased libido, decreased ejaculate volume with oligo or azoospermia and infertility, and loss of facial, axillary, chest, and pubic hair. Females generally present with secondary amenorrhea or irregular menses, but may also present with infertility or loss of libido. The hypogonadism that results from gonadotropin deficiency results in decreased bone density for both sexes.

Regulation of Gonadotropin Secretion

Gonadotropins are released in a pulsatile manner, in response to hypothalamic GnRH secretion. Pulsatile stimulation of the gonadotrophs by GnRH is critical, as constant stimulation results in desensitization and abolition of gonadotropin secretion *(1)*. The response of LH and FSH to GnRH stimulation is not identical, however, as reflected by differential changes of the two hormones during the menstrual cycle (Fig. 1) and the differential response of LH and FSH to GnRH receptor blockade *(2–4)*. Evidence suggests that these differences are owing, in part, to differential sensitivity of the secretory products of the gonadotroph to both GnRH stimulation and estradiol negative feedback. However, there are other recently discovered peptides that selectively mediate FSH biosynthesis and secretion as discussed in Chapter 10 and are likely to play important endocrine and/or paracrine roles in the human. Pituitary activin increases FSH biosynthesis and secretion *(5)*, whereas follistatin, which is found in the pituitary, the gonad as well as other organs, inhibits FSH through inactivation of activin *(6–8)*. Gonadal secretion of specific inhibins that inhibit FSH synthesis and secretion may function in an endocrine mode in the female (inhibin A and/or inhibin B) and in the male (inhibin B). In addition, there is some evidence that favors a separate FSH-releasing hormone *(9)*.

NORMAL GONADOTROPIN SECRETION

The pattern of gonadotropin secretion varies across developmental stages (*see* Chapter 10), across each reproductive cycle in the female, and in both males and females in direct response to GnRH stimulation. The response to GnRH stimulation is more marked for LH, whereas the changes in FSH within a day are much less apparent due to the relatively longer half-life of FSH. Knowledge of the variation in gonadotropin pulsatility in both men and women is an important framework upon which to build an understanding of pathophysiology.

Gonadotropin Secretion in Normal Men

In adult males, mean gonadotropin levels and the frequency and amplitude of LH pulses show considerable variation over a 24-h period within and between individuals (Fig. 2). This variability was demonstrated in a study of 20 healthy males with normal sexual function, testosterone levels, and semen analyses, and in whom gonadotropins were sampled every 10 min *(10)*. This study revealed a variation in mean LH levels of 4.7–18.4 IU/L with a diurnal variation characterized by greater nighttime LH secretion. The mean LH pulse amplitude varied between 4.5 ± 0.8 and 16.3 ± 2.5 IU/L, whereas the frequency of pulsatile episodes of LH varied from 6–19 pulses over 24 h. Mean FSH levels varied between 3.3 and 15.7 IU/L, with pulses only rarely detected. Resulting testosterone levels, measured at 6-h intervals, ranged from 105–1316 ng/dL, with testosterone values dipping below the normal range during the day in some subjects. A diurnal variation in testosterone has also been demonstrated in many studies *(11,12)*, although not seen here, with higher levels in the morning compared to the evening. The variability in normal gonadotropin and testosterone levels throughout the day both within and between individuals emphasizes the need to exercise caution in interpreting single LH and testosterone values in males. FSH, owing to its longer half-life, is much less variable.

Gonadotropin Secretion in Normal Women

In adult females, considerable variation in GnRH pulse frequency has been demonstrated across the menstrual cycle *(13–17)* (Fig. 3). The early follicular phase is characterized by pulses of LH that occur every 90 min and a unique slowing of pulsatile secretion during the nighttime hours *(13,18–19)*, which has now been shown to be specifically related to sleep rather than time of day and is more pronounced with deeper sleep *(20)*. Pulses of FSH may be seen in the very early follicular phase when FSH levels are at their highest in the cycle *(21)*, with the exception of the midcycle surge. In the midfollicular phase, LH pulse amplitude decreases, and LH pulse frequency increases to every 60 min, whereas in the late follicular phase, the amplitude again increases and

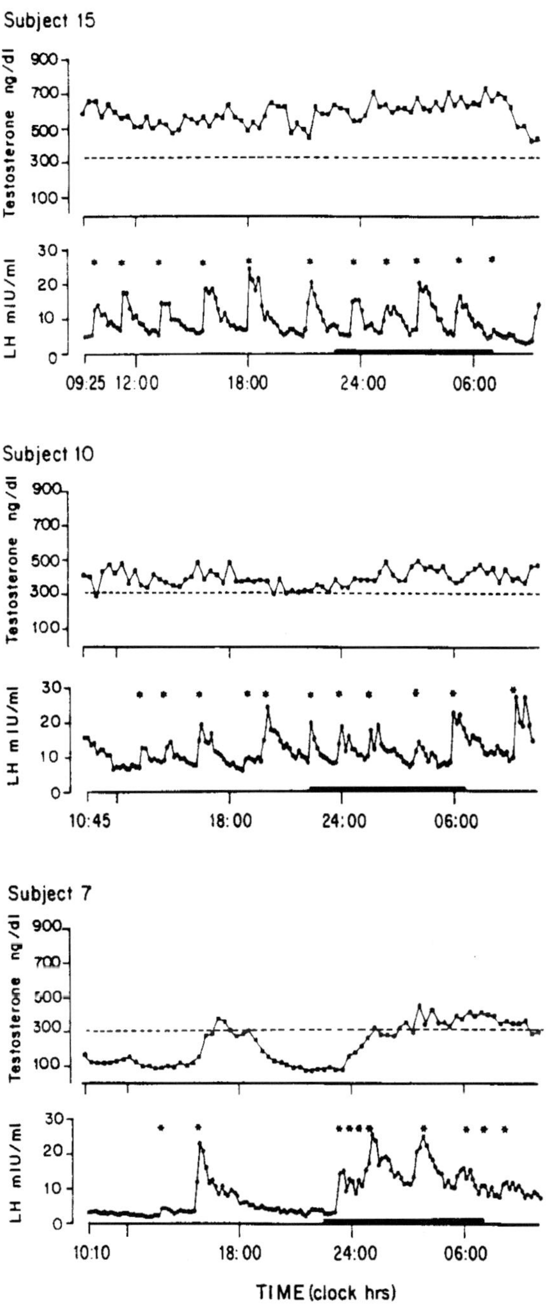

Fig. 2. Serum luteinizing hormone concentration determined at 10-min intervals and testosterone (T) concentration determined at 20-min intervals in three subjects. The dotted line indicates the lower of normal range T concentrations. Note that serum T concentrations were sometimes determined to be below the normal range in these men with normal reproductive function. The bar at the bottom of the bottom of each panel indicates nighttime hours. The LH pulsations are indicated by an asterisk. Reproduced from ref. *10* with permission.

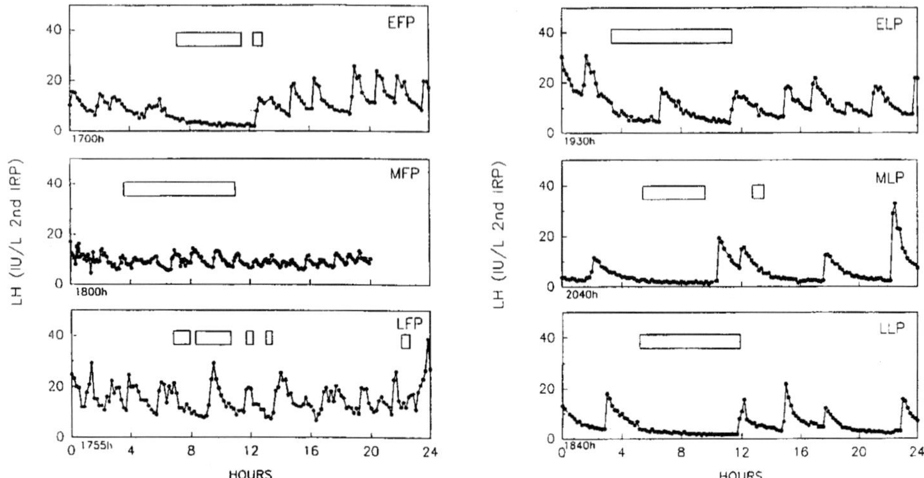

Fig. 3. Representative studies showing the pattern of pulsatile LH secretion in normal women in the early follicular phase (EFP), midfollicular phase (MFP), late follicular phase (LFP), early luteal phase (ELP), midluteal phase (MLP), and late luteal phase (LLP). Sleep is indicated by the bars. Reproduced from ref. *13* with permission.

the frequency remains approximately every 60 min. FSH levels fall progressively from the mid through the late follicular phase, and pulses of FSH are not apparent.

Mean LH levels and the amplitude of LH pulses increase sevenfold from the late follicular phase to the midportion of the midcycle gonadotropin surge, falling rapidly as the surge terminates. The frequency of LH pulses does not increase from the late follicular phase through the midportion of the gonadotropin surge, but a decrease in frequency is apparent as the surge terminates. FSH may also be pulsatile during the midcycle gonadotropin surge and FSH levels rise to a brief peak, coincident with the peak of LH. The failure of GnRH pulse frequency to increase and the apparent decrease in the overall amount of GnRH secreted during the surge *(22)* argue strongly that, in the human, the positive feedback that generates the midcycle surge is almost exclusively mediated at the level of the pituitary gonadotroph, although several lines of evidence indicate that there is an absolute requirement for GnRH.

The luteal phase is characterized by a progressive decrease in the frequency of pulsatile LH secretion from approximately every 100 min in the early luteal phase, to approximately every 216 min in the late luteal phase. The decrease in pulse frequency is associated with a dramatic increase in LH pulse amplitude. In addition, the LH pulses are associated with dramatic excursions in progesterone *(23)* and estradiol *(24)*, as FSH levels reach their nadir. The luteal-follicular transition is marked by a dramatic increase in LH pulse frequency and mean FSH, both of which occur prior to the onset of menses. Whereas release from the negative feedback of estradiol *(25)* and possibly also inhibin A *(26,27)* contributes to the selective rise of FSH during the transition, we have recently demonstrated that the increasing frequency of pulsatile GnRH stimulation contributes significantly to the rate of rise of FSH at this critical time *(28)*.

GONADOTROPIN DEFICIENCY: ABNORMALITIES IN GNRH STIMULATION

Tumors and Destructive/Infiltrative Disorders of the Hypothalamus

Structural lesions in the hypothalamus interfere with the normal pattern of GnRH secretion through compression or destruction of critical areas of the median eminence of the hypothalamus and result in hypogonadotropic hypogonadism. In general, these disorders result in multiple abnormalities in secretion of anterior and/or posterior pituitary hormones and may also present with headache. Craniopharyngiomas are the most common of these abnormalities, usually presenting with growth retardation, visual impairment, or headache. Other tumors and space occupying lesions with a predilection for midline CNS structures such as the hypothalamus include germinomas, gliomas, meningiomas, endodermal sinus tumors, Rathke's cleft cysts, as well as rare aneurysms, arachnoid cysts, chordomas, metastatic tumors, dermoid and epidermoid cysts, and teratomas *(29)*. Langerhans histiocytosis and infiltrative disorders of the hypothalamus such as sarcoidosis and tuberculosis generally manifest with diabetes insipidus and typically exhibit systemic signs in addition to evidence of pituitary dysfunction *(29)*.

The hypothalamic effects of cranial irradiation are an important cause of pituitary dysfunction including gonadotropin deficiency. The hypothalamus is significantly more radiosensitive than is the pituitary and the degree of residual dysfunction depends on the dose and type of radiation employed and the age at which the patient is subjected to radiation, with younger patients showing increased endocrine susceptibility *(30–33)*. In addition, there appears to be a hierarchy of susceptibility to disruption of normal hypothalamic-pituitary function, with the GH axis being extremely sensitive to the effects of radiation, the ACTH axis generally the least sensitive, and the thyroid and reproductive axes having intermediate susceptibility. After cranial irradiation, the incidence of menstrual irregularities secondary to hypothalalmic or pituitary dysfunction may be as high as 70%, with hormonal evaluation indicating the presence of hypogonadotropic hypogonadism *(33)*. Dysfunction of the reproductive axis in these patients may, therefore, result from abnormalities in hypothalamic GnRH secretion, whether directly or secondary to hyperprolactinemia, or from an abnormality at the level of the pituitary.

Isolated GnRH Deficiency

Idiopathic hypogonadotropic hypogonadism (IHH) is characterized by an isolated deficiency of GnRH secretion in the absence of a structural CNS lesion *(34)*. Although IHH is found in both males and females, there is a marked male predominance. The complete absence of pulsatile LH secretion combined with the ability of a pulsatile regimen of exogenous GnRH to completely reverse the gonadotropin abnormality has localized the defect in this disorder to the hypothalamus.

Anosmia occurs in conjunction with IHH in approximately 30–50% of cases *(34,35)*, and its pattern of inheritance was first reported by Kallmann in 1944 *(36)*. It is now recognized that other abnormalities may be present in association with GnRH deficiency and anosmia, including midline cranial defects (i.e., cleft lip and palate), deafness, color blindness, gaze-evoked nystagmus, cerebellar ataxia, synkinesia, mental retardation, unilateral renal agenesis, and pes excavatum. Autosomal dominant, autosomal recessive and X-linked modes of inheritance have been described, indicating genetic heterogeneity *(37,38)*. A fivefold excess of affected males to females is seen; however, the X-linked mode of inheritance appears to be the least common mode of inheritance *(35)*.

Despite abnormalities in the GnRH gene on chromosome 8 which characterize the hypogonadotropic (hpg) mouse, an animal model of GnRH deficiency, studies in males and females with isolated GnRH deficiency have indicated no such abnormalities in the GnRH gene, to date *(39,40)*. A genetic abnormality has, however, been identified in patients with the X-linked form of Kallmann's syndrome. Recent studies using deletion mapping in patients with an apparent X-linked inheritance in association with X-linked ichthyosis and other contiguous gene syndromes, localized the KAL gene to the short arm of the X chromosome (Xp22.3) *(41,42)*. Subsequent descriptions of Kallmann's patients with small deletions or single-base mutations within the KAL gene confirmed the gene location *(43,44)*. Domain A of the predicted protein product contains a sequence typically coding for a four-disulfide core, shared by proteins including protease inhibitors and neurophysins, whereas domains B and C contain typical sequences coding for fibronectin type III repeats, also found in neural cell adhesion molecules and tyrosine phosphatases *(41)*. The homology with proteins involved in neural development and migration *(45)* suggests that in these patients, GnRH deficiency results from a migration arrest of GnRH neurons on their path to the hypothalamus *(46)*.

Idiopathic hypogonadotropic hypogonadism including Kallmann's syndrome is characterized clinically by failure to progress through puberty in both men and women. Occasionally, individuals present with hypogonadotropic hypogonadism in the setting of already complete sexual maturation, representing an acquired form of GnRH deficiency. An additional variant of IHH in men is the "fertile eunuch" syndrome, in which patients have sufficient GnRH induced gonadotropin secretion to achieve the high intratesticular testosterone levels required for spermatogenesis, yet inadequate testosterone levels for complete virilization.

Congenital Syndromes

Other congenital syndromes share the association of hypogonadotropic hypogonadism and neurological disorders. In patients with Prader-Willi syndrome, characterized by neonatal hypotonia, obesity, short stature, and mental retardation, hypogonadism is thought to result from hypothalamic dysfunction *(47)*. A small deletion on the paternal chromosome 15 is often present. Bardet-Biedl syndrome, an autosomal recessive disorder, combines retinal dystrophy, polydactyly, mental retardation, renal anomalies, obesity, and hypogonadism. The hypogonadism is most commonly due to primary gonadal failure, although hypogonadotropic hypogonadism has also been reported *(48)*. Moebius syndrome is characterized by oculofacial paralysis, seizures, mental retardation, and in some cases, hypogonadotropic hypogonadism. In the hypogonadotropic hypogonadism described in association with familial cerebellar ataxia, the reported site of the abnormality, hypothalamus *(49)* or pituitary *(50)*, has yet to be determined.

It is also unclear whether the hypogonadotropic hypogonadism associated with X-linked congenital adrenal hypoplasia is hypothalamic *(51)* or pituitary *(52)* in origin.

The recent discovery that mutations in the gene DAX-1 are responsible for the syndrome should help elucidate the etiology of the hypogonadism *(53,54)*.

Functional Hypothalamic Dysfunction

In the majority of women in whom low levels of gonadotropins accompany hypoestrogenism, a structural neuroanatomical lesion cannot be found. The diagnosis given to this group of patients who comprise two-thirds to three-quarters of all patients presenting with amenorrhea, is "hypothalamic amenorrhea" *(55)*. Hypothalamic amenorrhea has been associated with exercise, with nutritional deprivation, with abnormal eating behaviors, and with specific stressors such as moving away from home. However, in many cases, no proximate cause can be identified. A syndrome of hypothalamic dysfunction has also been described in men, but it appears that more severe stressors are required before reproductive dysfunction occurs.

In this disorder, LH levels are normal to low as are FSH levels. In addition, FSH may be higher than LH. The pattern of pulsatile secretion of LH in patients with secondary amenorrhea in the absence of a history of excessive exercise, weight reduction, or stress has been compared to that in normal women in the early follicular phase, i.e., matched for ambient sex steroid levels. These studies revealed an underlying spectrum of defects of pulsatile LH, and thus, GnRH secretion, which presumably accounts for the clinical spectrum encountered in such patients *(56–58)* (Fig. 4). The most severe form of this abnormality is characterized by a complete lack of GnRH-induced gonadotropin secretion, whereas other abnormalities such as low amplitude, slow frequency, and nighttime augmentation of secretion all appear to provide inadequate GnRH secretion to sustain the gonadotropin pattern required for orderly folliculogenesis and ovulation *(56)*. Occasional patients exhibit a pattern of LH secretion that is normal in terms of both frequency and amplitude of GnRH secretion *(56)*. It is unclear why this pattern is not associated with normal folliculogenesis although recent studies would suggest that the absence of cyclic regulation of GnRH pulse frequency may result in relatively tonic FSH secretion which is inadequate to promote follicular recruitment.

These abnormalities in pulsatile LH secretion are seen in a wide variety of disorders of hypothalamic GnRH secretion in both females and males. Apulsatile patterns are seen in patients with IHH and Kallmann's syndrome and in patients with anorexia nervosa *(59)*. Nighttime augmentation has also been described in males and females recovering from anorexia nervosa as well as in normal puberty *(59,60)* (Fig. 5). Slow frequency and/or low amplitude LH pulse patterns have been found in patients whose amenorrhea is associated with excessive exercise *(61)*, weight loss, and bulimia nervosa *(62)*. In males as well as females, decreased LH pulse frequency is seen in cases of burn injury *(63)*, and decreased LH pulse amplitude has been documented in acute head injury *(64)*. Stress, acute or chronic illness *(65,66)*, and protein calorie malnutrition also result in hypogonadism associated with low levels of gonadotropins.

Attempts have been made to separate the effects of exercise, energy expenditure, and weight loss on changes in hypothalamic function. Exercise itself, with or without weight loss, has been shown to disrupt menstrual cyclicity *(67,68)*. It appears that it is an energy imbalance (dietary energy intake – exercise energy expenditure) that results in initial dysfunction of the GnRH pulse generator as manifested by decreased LH pulse frequency *(69,70)*. In highly conditioned male marathon runners *(71)* and in fasting nor-

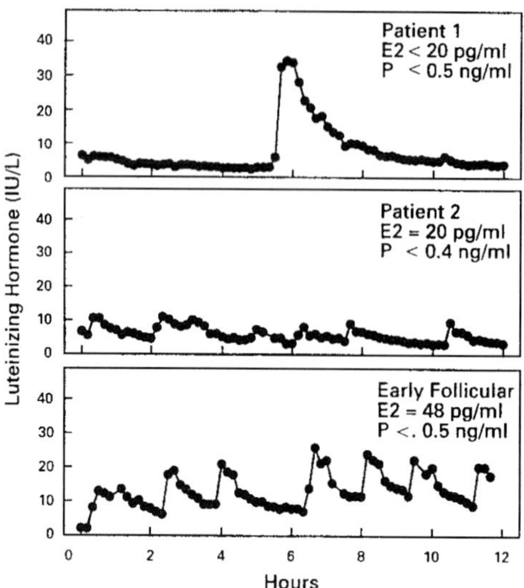

Fig. 4. Three representative patterns of pulsatile LH secretion, estradiol (E2) and progesterone (P) levels in women with hypothalamic amenorrhea compared with the pulse pattern, E2 and P levels seen in normal women in the early follicular phase (lower panel). Low frequency (upper panel) and low amplitude (middle panel) LH pulsations are demonstrated. Reproduced from ref. *58a* with permission.

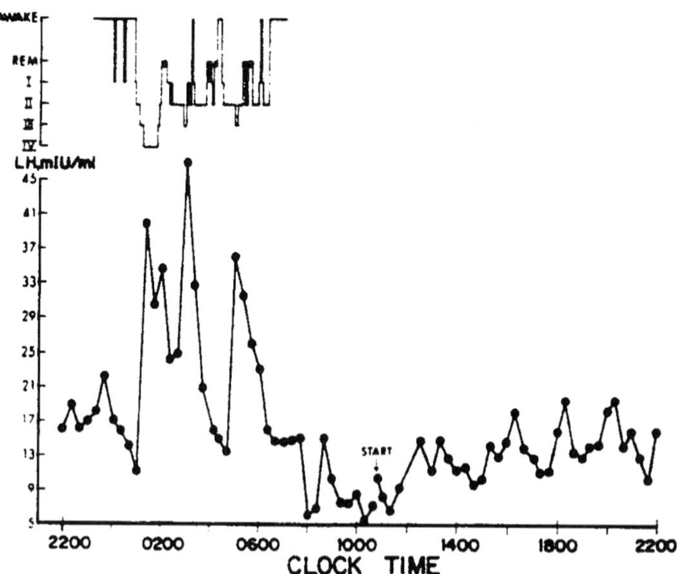

Fig. 5. Plasma LH concentration measured every 20 min for 24 h in a patient with anorexia nervosa and primary amenorrhea. The study demonstrates nighttime augmentation of LH pulsation which is also seen in normal puberty. Reproduced from ref. *59* with permission.

mal males *(72,73)*, a decrease in LH pulse frequency and amplitude has also been described. However, in the male, it is only in cases of severe stress, such as prolonged exercise associated with weight loss and sleep deprivation *(74)* that testosterone falls into the hypogonadal range.

It is likely that abnormalities of the GnRH pulse generator in these disorders are secondary to abnormal regulation of one or more neurotransmitters. Numerous studies have attempted to delineate the role of putative neurotransmitter abnormalities in the pathogenesis of hypothalamic amenorrhea. For example, endorphins and dopamine are inhibitory to GnRH secretion. Blockade of opioids with naloxone *(58,75)* and of dopamine with metoclopramide *(75,76)* both increase LH pulse frequency in a subset of patients with hypothalamic amenorrhea. Melatonin, which is known to regulate reproductive activity in seasonal breeding animals, was found to be increased in patients with hypothalamic amenorrhea in two studies *(77,78)*.

The elevated cortisol levels seen in anorexia nervosa *(79)*, hypothalamic amenorrhea *(80)*, and amenorrheic runners *(81)*, suggest a role for the hypothalamic-pituitary-adrenal axis in hypothalamic dysfunction. In women with hypothalamic amenorrhea *(82)* and in highly trained male runners *(83)*, elevated basal ACTH and cortisol levels, and blunted ACTH and cortisol responses to CRH, suggest chronic activation of this axis. In animals, intraventricular injection of CRH decreased GnRH *(84)* and LH secretion *(85,86)*, whereas a CRH antagonist reversed the effect of stress on inhibition of LH secretion *(87)*. Human studies using short-term CRH infusions have also shown a decrease in basal plasma gonadotropin levels, but no effect on GnRH-induced gonadotropin secretion *(88)*. There may also be a direct hypothalamic effect of cortisol (*see* section on Cushing's Syndrome and Exogenous Steroid Use). Taken together, the evidence points to a role for CRH in the pathogenesis of hypothalamic dysfunction.

Hyperprolactinemia

Although hyperprolactinemia results in hypogonadotropic hypogonadism, it is rare that the mass effect of a pituitary tumor is the cause of gonadotropin deficiency. Hyperprolactinemia most commonly results from pituitary microadenomas or stalk compression, and produces a picture similar to that of hypothalamic amenorrhea. In women, prolactin elevation is associated with low to normal mean LH levels *(89)*. LH secretion has varied from a pattern of slow frequency pulses of increased amplitude *(90)* to completely absent pulsatile secretion *(89)* whereas the secretory capacity of the pituitary as assessed by the response to exogenous GnRH is preserved *(91)*, and normal ovulation can be induced with exogenous pulsatile GnRH *(92)*.

The mechanism of GnRH inhibition in hyperprolactinemia is controversial. Hyperprolactinemia appears to induce increased dopamine turnover in the hypothalamus, resulting in inhibition of GnRH, and therefore LH secretion *(93)*. Dopamine's inhibitory control on prolactin is lost, however, consistent with decreased lactotroph receptor number or affinity *(94)*, or altered dopamine metabolism *(93)*. Alternatively, naloxone infusion in hyperprolactinemic patients results in a rise in LH and FSH levels and return of normal LH pulsatility, suggesting that inhibition of GnRH secretion may be owing to increased endogenous opiate tone *(95)*.

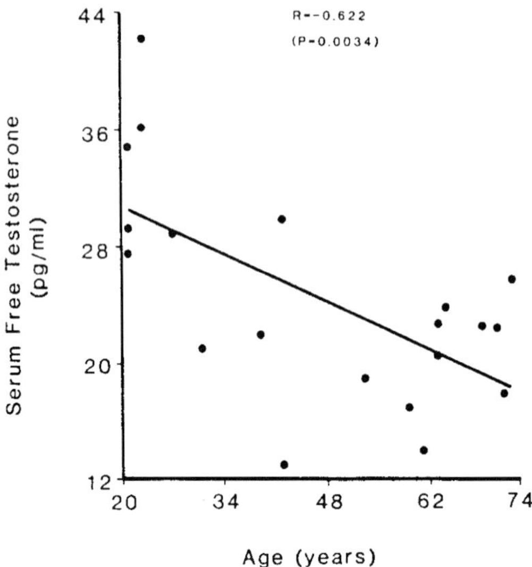

Fig. 6. Relationship of age and serum free testosterone concentrations in 22 healthy men ages 21–73. Increasing age was associated with a significant decrease in serum free testosterone concentration. Reproduced from ref. *108* with permission.

Cushing's Syndrome and Exogenous Steroid Use

Disturbance of menstrual cyclicity in women, even in the absence of hyperandrogenism, and sexual dysfunction in men are common complaints in patients with Cushing's syndrome, regardless of the etiology. In males, the hypogonadism is characterized by low testosterone levels in the setting of suppressed LH *(96)*. Similar endocrine abnormalities have been described with exogenous glucocorticoid therapy *(97)*. After 1 mo of hydrocortisone administration, LH pulse frequency in the early follicular phase of normally cycling women was significantly decreased *(98)*. A similar decrease seen with long-term hydrocortisone administration in orchiectomized monkeys was reversed with pulsatile GnRH administration *(99)*, suggesting a hypothalamic site of action. Increased CRH may also result in gonadotropin deficiency, as discussed above.

Miscellaneous Disorders of Hypothalamic Function

Alcohol exerts its effects at all levels of the hypothalamic-pituitary-gonadal axis. A direct toxic effect of alcohol on the testicular Leydig cells has been demonstrated in the male rat *(100)*. Few studies on the effects of alcohol have been performed in females, but moderate to heavy alcohol intake does result in anovulation in a subset of women *(101)*. Despite the presence of low testosterone in men and estradiol in women, gonadotropin levels are often low to normal, suggesting hypothalamic or pituitary dysfunction also plays a role. Indirect evidence for an inhibitory effect of alcohol on the hypothalamus comes from a study of generally healthy alcoholic men, in which LH and FSH pulse amplitude was elevated 3 d after withdrawal of alcohol and returned toward normal after 5 wk *(102)*. In addition to the direct effects of alcohol, chronic malnutrition and weight loss may also contribute to hypothalamic and pituitary dysfunction in alcoholic patients.

Aging is associated with a decline in normal sperm motility and morphology *(103)* as well as Leydig cell number *(104)* and function *(105)* in the male. Despite a slight elevation of gonadotropins, testosterone and free testosterone levels are decreased when compared to levels in young controls *(106)* (Fig. 6). Further, a decrease in LH secretory burst amplitude *(107,108)* suggests that central mechanisms may contribute to decreasing testosterone levels with age. Despite the benefits of testosterone therapy, including improved energy, sense of well-being, and increased lean body mass, testosterone replacement in the normal elderly male remains controversial owing to potential adverse effects on lipids and risk of progression of an occult prostate cancer.

GONADOTROPIN DEFICIENCY: INTRAPITUITARY ABNORMALITIES

Pituitary Tumors

Most pituitary tumors cause gonadotropin deficiency as a result of mass compression of normal gonadotrophs. Further damage to gonadotrophs occurs as a result of surgery, whereas irradiation is less likely to result in direct pituitary dysfunction than in hypogonadotropism secondary to abnormal hypothalamic stimulation *(33)*. In cases of ACTH secreting tumors and prolactinomas, gonadotropin deficiency is also more likely to result from hypothalamic dysfunction.

Nonfunctioning pituitary adenomas represent a unique group of tumors resulting in hypogonadotropic hypogonadism. Despite the in vitro synthesis and secretion of glycoprotein hormones and/or free α- and β-subunits detected in a majority of these tumors, in vivo hormone production is less common *(109)*. In fact, 96% of patients with nonfunctioning adenomas present with hypogonadism, frequently associated with inappropriately normal or low gonadotropin levels suggestive of central hypogonadism *(110,111)*. In addition to central hypogonadism due to tumor mass effect, gonadotropin deficiency may result from mild hyperprolactinemia and its effect on GnRH secretion as noted above. In addition, secretion of bioinactive gonadotropin subunits rather than intact and bioactive gonadotropin heterodimers will result in inadequate gonadotropin stimulation of the gonads *(109)*. Surgical removal of the tumor with a decrease in the mass effect has been shown to restore gonadotroph function in 32% of patients studied *(110)*.

Destructive Disorders of the Pituitary

Hypogonadism is a known complication of hemochromatosis in males. Although primary hypogonadism has been reported *(112)*, hypogonadotropic hypogonadism is the most common finding. Iron deposition in the pituitary gonadotrophs, and failure of pulsatile GnRH therapy to restore testosterone and LH pulsatility *(113)*, localize the defect to the pituitary gland. The hypogonadism may be reversible by phlebotomy if performed at an early age *(112,114)*.

Lymphocytic hypophysitis most commonly presents with headache and visual field deficits or pituitary dysfunction in women in the third trimester of pregnancy or in the postpartum period, although it has also been described in postmenopausal females and rarely in males *(115)*. The diagnosis is often made on biopsy by the characteristic lymphocytic infiltrate of the anterior pituitary. Gonadotropin deficiency occurs as a late consequence of the lymphocytic infiltrate *(115)*, in contrast to pituitary adenomas in which gonadotropin function is often lost early. An autoimmune etiology is suggested by the coincidental occurrence of other autoimmune disease and the predominance in women, although specifity *(116)* of the antipituitary antibody appears to be poor and the predictive value is unknown. Improvement in pituitary function has been documented with decompressive surgery and with steroids *(117)*, but spontaneous recovery has also been reported *(118)*.

Granulomatous hypophysitis is distinguished pathologically from lymphocytic hypophysitis by the presence of histiocytes and multinucleated giant cells perhaps due to a foreign-body type reaction *(119)*. Typically, pituitary insufficiency is the presenting feature and it appears to affect both genders equally *(119)*. Systemic granulomatous disease, such as tuberculosis or sarcoid, must be ruled out.

Adenohypophyseal necrosis generally occurs following a delivery complicated by hemorrhage and hypotension, in which case it is also known as Sheehan's syndrome *(120)*. This disorder may result in single or multiple hormone deficiencies, including gonadotropin deficiency. The syndrome is often heralded by inability to breast feed postpartum. In addition to its presentation during the postpartum period, adenohypophyseal necrosis may also occur spontaneously in diabetics *(121,122)*. Spontaneous antepartum pituitary necrosis has been reported in diabetic females suggesting that the combination of pregnancy and diabetes increases the risk of this disorder *(122,123)*.

The empty sella syndrome, a benign condition probably caused by elevated intracranial pressure remodelling the sellar anatomy through an incompetent sellar diaphragm *(124)*, most commonly presents without endocrine dysfunction. In those patients with abnormalities, however, isolated hypogonadism (6%) and hyperprolactinemia (4%) are the most common findings *(125)*.

Abnormalities of Gonadotropin Structure

Selective abnormalities in gonadotropin structure and function have been described for both LH and FSH, and provide insight into the normal function of the two gonadotropin hormones. Isolated FSH deficiency is a reported, albeit rare cause of infertility in males *(126,127)* and females *(128)*. Analysis of the gene coding the FSHβ-subunit in one woman presenting with primary amenorrhea, infertility, and isolated FSH deficiency revealed homozygosity for a frameshift deletion in exon 3, which resulted in a premature termination codon. The location of the deletion predicts a β-subunit that has lost the regions important for binding the α-subunit and the FSH receptor. Administration of exogenous FSH resulted in ovulation and pregnancy in the proband *(128)*.

Selective LH deficiency, owing to an immunologically anomalous form of LH, has been described. In this anomalous form of LH, two point mutations in the LH β gene cause amino acid substitutions, one of which introduces an extra glycosylation site into the protein. The resultant LH is not detected in a two-site immunometric assay using a specific MAb to the LH α/β dimer, but is detectable with other antibody combinations and in in vitro bioassay. The LH variant has an increased in vitro bioactivity and a decreased in vivo half life. The variant LH, detectable in 28% of the Finnish population, causes no abnormality in GnRH pulse patterns and no clinical evidence of infertility in homozygotes *(129)*. The same mutation has been described in Japanese subjects

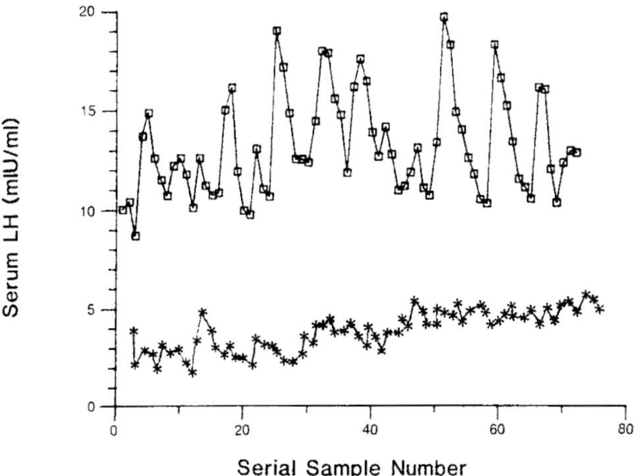

Fig. 7. Serum immunoactive LH concentration measured every 20 min for 24 h before surgery, indicated by the asterisks, and 2 wk after surgery, indicated by the open squares. Note the increased concentrations and amplitudes of LH pulses observed 2 wk after removal of the estrogen-secreting adrenal tumor. Reproduced from ref. *134* with permission.

suffering from infertility *(130)*, although the relationship of this LH variant and infertility may be coincidental *(129)*.

Secretion of biologically inactive LH has also been described *(131)*. The homozygous form is characterized clinically by failure of spontaneous puberty and infertility. These findings are associated with low testosterone, elevated but bioinactive LH levels, and a normal testosterone response to exogenous LH. The heterozygous form in males results in impaired fertility, low testosterone levels, and normal to elevated LH levels. Female heterozygotes appear to have normal sexual development and fertility. The molecular defect in this disorder has been identified as a single base mutation in the LHβ gene, resulting in the substitution of an arginine for a glutamine at amino acid 54, and inability of LH to bind to the LH receptor *(131)*.

GONADOTROPIN DYSFUNCTION: ABNORMAL FEEDBACK

Estradiol exerts negative feedback at the pituitary level in both males *(132)* and females. Thus, any condition of estradiol excess might be expected to result in gonadotropin deficiency and hypogonadism. Direct production of estradiol and/or estrone by Leydig cell tumors *(133)* and feminizing adrenal tumors *(134)*, as well as indirect increases in estradiol and estrone associated with hCG secreting choriocarcinomas *(135)*, are examples of such conditions. Decreased immunoactive and bioactive LH and decreased LH pulse amplitude associated with a feminizing adrenal tumor increased significantly upon surgical removal *(134)* (Fig. 7), attesting to the negative feedback of estradiol and/or estrone.

In obesity, serum testosterone levels are low *(136)*, whereas estradiol and estrone levels are elevated *(137)*. In fact, free testosterone, SHBG and total testosterone decrease in proportion to the degree of obesity *(138)*. In addition, LH pulse amplitude is decreased suggesting that gonadotropin deficiency is the consequence of hypogonadotropism *(139)*, perhaps due to increased estradiol and estrone feedback. Obese patients with obstructive sleep apnea may also have hypothalamic dysfunction on this basis *(140)*.

Anabolic steroid use also results in hypogonadotropic hypogonadism through negative feedback at both the pituitary and hypothalamus and mediated partially through the aromatization of androgens to estrogens *(141)*. The hypogonadal state in these individuals is characterized by impaired spermatogenesis and decreased testosterone *(142)* and may last for months after drugs are discontinued *(143)*.

GONADOTROPIN DYSFUNCTION: DIAGNOSIS

A careful and directed clinical history can provide many clues to the underlying cause of the patient's disorder. Specific questions should focus on the developmental history, including history of cryptorchidism, pattern of growth and pubertal development, as well as parental height, family history of pubertal delay, infertility, and anosmia. The menstrual history is important in women and should include age and weight at menarche, regularity and duration of menstrual interval and flow, the presence or absence of symptoms associated with ovulation, date of the last menstrual period, and history of pregnancy. The history of sexual function in males should include an assessment of libido, frequency of intercourse, erectile function including presence or absence of morning erections, ejaculate volume, and fertility history. Relevant localizing symptoms for both sexes include anorectic behaviors or attitudes, exercise patterns, medications, drug and alcohol use, galactorrhea and breast development, headache or visual disturbances, significant weight changes, symptoms of other endocrine dysfunction, systemic illness, head trauma, and depression.

Physical examination should include measurement of height, weight, and arm span, and a careful examination for the presence of secondary sexual characteristics, visual field defects, galactorrhea and gynecomastia, and signs of anorexia nervosa, such as lanugo hair or carotenemia. A careful genitourinary examination for penile size, hypospadias, scrotal rugae, testicular masses, and testicular size in men, and size of the ovaries and uterus along with estrogenization of the vaginal mucosa in women, is also important.

Establishment of hypogonadotropic hypogonadism will be the initial step in the diagnosis in patients presenting as above. The LH measurements should be used with caution in the diagnosis of hypogonadotropic hypogonadism because of their pulsatile nature, but can be used to determine whether values are within the normal or low range. The FSH, because of its longer half-life, is much less variable and is critical in ruling out primary gonadal dysfunction. Testosterone levels in males should also be interpreted with a view to normal variability, and several measurements may be required at differing times over several days for accuracy. Administration of medroxyprogesterone acetate in females (10 mg for 5 d) provides an assessment of overall estrogen status. A prolactin level should be measured in all patients presenting with hypogonadism, whereas full anterior pituitary testing should be performed in patients with mass lesions, head trauma, and idiopathic hypogonadotropic hypogonadism.

The role of GnRH testing in the differential diagnosis of hypogonadotropic hypogonadism continues to be controversial. In differentiating pituitary from hypothalamic causes, single bolus GnRH testing is not generally useful. There are, in fact, many patients with GnRH deficiency and normal pituitary function who do not respond to bolus GnRH but require repetitive dosing before LH and FSH release can be documented. In some instances, a full 7 d of pulsatile administration of GnRH with periodic sampling for LH following GnRH administration may be helpful in ensuring the presence of normal gonadotroph function. A full 12- or 24-h sampling study to document a lack of pulsatile LH secretion is performed in a research setting, but clinical use is limited by cost and availability.

In patients with an elevated prolactin level or primary hypogonadotropic hypogonadism and in situations in which a functional cause is not apparent by history, cranial imaging is also warranted. Although a cranial CT or MRI can be used to rule out the presence of mass lesions, the increased resolution of the pituitary region by the MRI makes it the current diagnostic choice. Measurement of bone density is suggested if it will help the physician or the patient determine a course of treatment.

GONADOTROPIN DYSFUNCTION: TREATMENT

The treatment of gonadotropin deficiency depends on the underlying diagnosis, the age of the patient, and the goals of therapy. When the underlying disorder is reversible, as in cases of weight loss or excessive exercise, or when the underlying pathology is remediable, the primary treatment course should be undertaken. In other situations, treatment with sex steroid, exogenous gonadotropins, or GnRH replacement will be directed by the patient's needs.

Pubertal Treatment

In the prepubertal patient with gonadotropin deficiency, testosterone or estradiol therapy should be started at a low dose and gradually increased to adult doses with development of secondary sexual characteristics. In females, institution of therapy with 5 μg ethinyl estradiol or 0.3 mg conjugated estrogen daily is followed by cyclic therapy with a progestagen after 6 mo. In males, 50 100 mg testosterone enanthate or cypionate im can be dosed monthly. HCG treatment, 200–500 IU 2–3 times per week, administered im or sc, is another option in males as treatment results in some testicular enlargement in addition to normalization of testosterone levels.

Treatment if Fertility Is not Desired

In adult males, treatment of hypogonadism is required for maintenance of secondary sexual characteristics and sexual performance, libido, maintenance of muscle mass, and preservation of bone mass. Males with low testosterone levels often present because of sexual dysfunction and desire immediate treatment. Testosterone replacement can be administered in the form of testosterone cypionate or enanthate in doses of 200–300 mg im every 3 wk or can be given as a transdermal preparation, with the dose titered to the trough level of testosterone drawn immediately prior to the administration of the next dose.

Estrogen replacement should be seriously considered after 6 mo of amenorrhea in women to prevent bone loss, a serious complication in women with hypoestrogenism from any cause. An oral contraceptive agent is often a convenient form of estrogen in women who do not desire pregnancy. Replacement with conjugated estrogens 0.625 mg, in conjunction with a cyclic or continuous progesterone regimen for endometrial protection, is also adequate to spare bone mass, but cannot be relied on to provide contraception.

Treatment if Fertility Is Desired

In cases in which fertility is desired, therapy with exogenous gonadotropins or pulsatile GnRH is necessary for folliculogenesis and spermatogenesis. Exogenous gonadotropin therapy is the only option in patients with a nonfunctioning pituitary. Current treatment includes the use of hCG, which binds and activates the gonadal LH receptor and is particularly useful owing to its relatively long half-life, and human menopausal urinary gonadotropins (hMG) which include both FSH and LH. Pergonal and Metrodin (a more purified preparation of FSH), are traditional preparations. Recombinant human gonadotropins are currently being developed for this use and may eventually replace the traditional sources of exogenous gonadotropins.

In males, treatment with exogenous gonadotropin therapy is individualized, beginning with hCG 500–1000 IU im or sc 3 times per week and titrating to normal testosterone levels. Doses of hMG at 37.5–150 IU im 3 times per week is added if significant testicular growth has not occurred, and the dose is titrated to sperm count. A subset of males with testicular volumes of > 4 mL may respond to hCG alone *(144)*, and once initiated, it may be possible maintain spermatogenesis with hCG alone.

Treatment with GnRH may also be an option for men with hypogonadotropic hypogonadism who desire fertility. Successful treatment will depend on the ability of the pituitary to respond to a physiologic pattern of exogenous pulsatile GnRH, which can be administered sc. Importantly, several days of pituitary priming with pulsatile GnRH may be required to determine the ability of the pituitary to respond to GnRH and a negative GnRH stimulation test prior to pituitary priming may provide misleading information. For treatment, a pulse frequency of every 2 h, based on normative data *(10)*, and a dose ranging from 25–600 ng/kg per bolus has been successful *(145)* (Fig. 8). The individual GnRH dose correlates negatively with testicular size and positively with body weight. Semen analysis is performed when the testis volume reaches 8 mL. GnRH has several advantages over gonadotropin therapy including lower testosterone and estradiol levels and therefore less gynecomastia, a more pronounced rise in testicular volume, and possibly, more rapid achievement of spermatogenesis *(146)*. To date, pulsatile GnRH is FDA approved for treatment of GnRH deficiency in the female only.

In females desiring fertility, ovulation induction may be achieved with estrogen antagonists, exogenous gonadotropins, or pulsatile GnRH. Although the use of estrogen antagonists, such as clomiphene citrate, is the easiest route for ovulation induction, it may be unsuccessful in patients with low estrogen states such as functional amenorrhea. In addition, its use requires intact pituitary function. However, a therapeutic trial is warranted in the appropriate patients due to the convenience and relatively low risk associated with this form of therapy.

Exogenous gonadotropin therapy is the treatment of choice for women with no pituitary function. A typical starting dose of hMG is 150 IU. Frequent ultrasound monitoring, daily estradiol levels, and dose adjustment are necessary to avoid ovarian

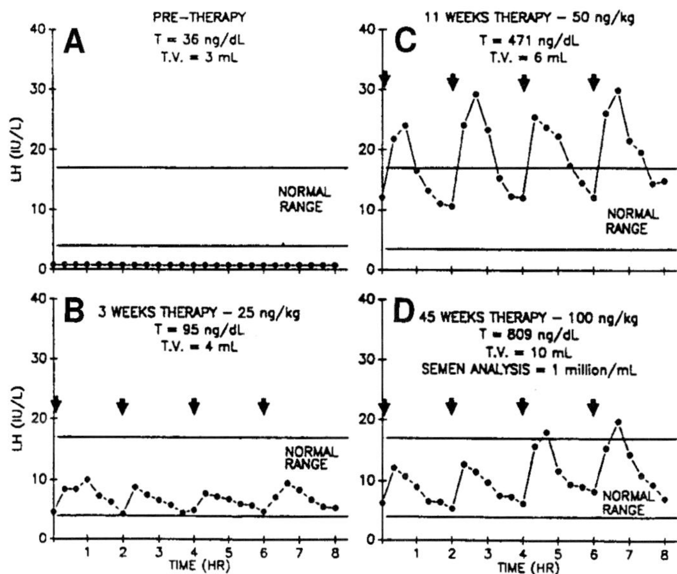

Fig. 8. Response of a representative 25-yr-old man with isolated GnRH deficiency to pulsatile GnRH. **(A)** Pretherapy admission demonstrates low serum testosterone level (T), infantile testes volume (TV), and a complete absence of LH pulsation. **(B)** After 3 wk of pulsatile GnRH at 2-h intervals (arrows) at a dose of 25 ng/kg, a pulsatile LH pattern has been established, but T levels remain in the prepubertal range. **(C)** After 11 wk of therapy, at a dose of 50 ng/kg, the serum T is normal, the TV has doubled, and LH pulses are above the normal range. **(D)** At 45 wk of therapy, LH levels are within the normal range, TV has increased to 10 ml and sperm are now present in the ejaculate. Reproduced from ref. *145* with permission.

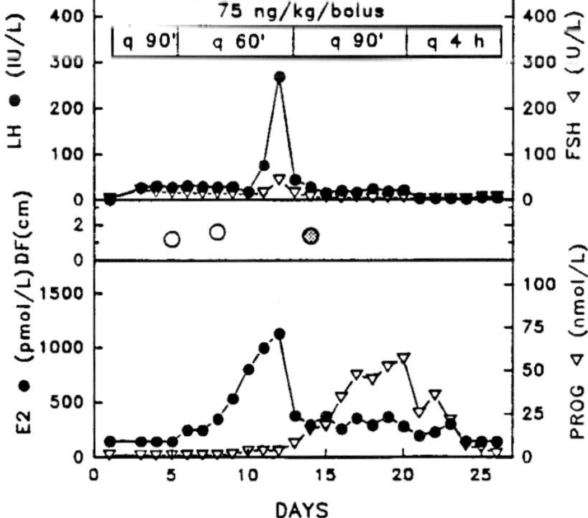

Fig. 9. Daily hormonal results in a representative cycle of pulsatile GnRH therapy, indicating normal gondotropin and sex steroid dynamics. The size of the dominant follicle is presented in the middle panel. The shaded circle represents the presence of intrafollicular echoes. GnRH puse frequency is indicated in the boxes. Reproduced from ref. *149* with permission.

hyperstimulation and multiple gestations. Intravenous pulsatile GnRH confers an advantage over gonadotropins because of its ability to mimic normal menstrual cycle dynamics, and thus result in single follicle ovulation. Treatment of patients with hypothalamic amenorrhea using pulsatile GnRH at a dose of 75 ng/kg and a pulse frequency mimicking the normal female menstrual cycle *(56,147)* resulted in similar rates of ovulation and conception when compared to treatment with exogenous gonadotropins *(148)*. Importantly, the cumulative rate of conception was higher in the GnRH treatment group and the rate of multiple folliculogenesis, higher order multiple gestations, and cycle cancellation was lower *(148)*. Thus, pulsatile GnRH therapy is the treatment of choice in infertility resulting from disordered GnRH secretion. In addition, pulsatile GnRH can be used successfully in patients with GnRH deficiency secondary to treatment of cranial tumors *(149)* (Fig. 9). In many of these patients, hypothalamic dysfunction appears to contribute substantially to gonadotropin deficiency and hypogonadism.

REFERENCES

1. Belchetz PE, Plant TM, Nakai Y, et al. Hypophysial responses to continuous and intermittent delivery of hypothalamic gonadotropin-releasing hormone. Science 1978; 202:631–633.
2. Hall JE, Brodie TD, Badger TM, et al. Evidence of differential control of FSH and LH secretion by gonadotropin-releasing hormone (GnRH) from the use of a GnRH antagonist. J Clin Endocrinol Metab 1988; 67:524–531.
3. Hall JE, Whitcomb RW, Rivier JE, et al. Differential regulation of luteinizing hormone, follicle-stimulating hormone, and free α-subunit secretion from the gonadotrope by gonadotropin-releasing hormone (GnRH): evidence from the use of two GnRH antagonists. J Clin Endocrinol Metab 1990; 70:328–335.
4. Pavlou SN, Debold CR, Island DP, et al. Single subcutaneous doses of a luteinizing hormone-releasing hormone antagonist suppress serum gonadotropin and testosterone levels in normal men. J Clin Endocrinol Metab 1986; 63:303–308.
5. DePaolo LV, Bicsak TA, Erickson GF, Shimisaki S, Ling N. Follistatin and activin: a potential intrinsic regulatory system within diverse tissues. Proc Soc Exp Med 1991; 198:500–512.
6. Sugino K, Kurosawa N, Nakamura T, et al. Molecular heterogeneity of follistatin, an activin-binding protein. J Biol Chem 1992; 68:15,579–15,587.
7. Nakamura T, Takio K, Eto Y, Shibai H, Titani K, Sugino H. Activin-binding protein from rat ovary is follistatin. Science 1990; 247:836–838.
8. Schneyer A, Rzucidlo DA, Sluss PM, Crowley WF Jr. Characterization of unique binding kinetics of follistatin and activin or inhibin in serum. Endocrinology 1994; 135:667–674.
9. Lumpkin MD, Moltz JH, Yu WH, et al. Purification of FSH-releasing hormone: its dissimilarity from LHRH of mammalian, avian, and piscian origin. Brain Res Bull 1987; 18:175–178.
10. Spratt DI, O'Dea LSL, Schoenfeld D, et al. Neuroendocrine-gonadal axis in men: frequent sampling of LH, FSH, and testosterone. Am J Physiol 1988; 254:E658–E666.
11. Okamoto MC, Setaish K, Nadagawa Y, Hriuchi K, Moriya K, Itoh S. Diurnal variations in the levels of plasma and urinary androgens. J Clin Endocrinol Metab 1971; 32:846–851.
12. Faiman C, Winter JSD. Diurnal cycles in plasma FSH, testosterone and cortisol in men. J Clin Endocrinol Metab 1971; 33:186–192.
13. Filicori M, Santoro N, Merriam GR, Crowley Jr WF. Characterization of the physiological pattern of episodic gonadotropin secretion throughout the human menstrual cycle. J Clin Endocrinol Metab 1986; 62:1136–1144.
14. Backstrom CT, McNeilly AS, Leask RM, Baird DT. Pulsatile secretion of LH, FSH, prolactin, oestradiol and progesterone in the human menstrual cycle. Clin Endocrinol (Oxf) 1982; 17:29–42.
15. Reame N, Sauder SE, Kelch RP, Marshall JC. Pulsatile gonadotropin secretion during the human menstrual cycle: evidence for altered frequency of gonadotropin-releasing hormone secretion. J Clin Endocrinol Metab 1984; 59:328–337.

16. Yen SSC, Tsai CC, Naftolin F, Vandenberg G, Ajabor L. Pulsatile patterns of gonadotropin release in subjects with and without ovarian function. J Clin Endocrinol Metab 1972; 34:671–675.
17. Evans WS, Sollenberger MJ, Booth Jr RA, et al. Contemporary aspects of discrete peak-detection algorithms. II. The paradigm of the luteinizing hormone pulse signal in women. Endocr Rev 1992; 13:81–104.
18. Soules MR, Steiner RA, Cohen NL, Bremner WJ, Clifton DK. Nocturnal slowing of pulsatile luteinizing hormone secretion in women during the follicular phase of the menstrual cycle. J Clin Endocrinol Metab 1985; 61:43–49.
19. Rossmanith WG, Boscher S, Kern W, Fehm HL. Impact of sleep on the circadian excursions in the pituitary gonadotropin responsiveness of early follicular phase in women. J Clin Endocrinol Metab 1993; 76:330–336.
20. Hall JE, Richardson GS, Sullivan JP, Kaplowitz L, Welsh DK. Nocturnal slowing of GnRH secretion in the early follicular phase is specifically related to slow wave sleep: evidence from sleep reversal studies. Endocrine Soc 74th Annual Program and Abstracts. 1992; 873:270 (abstract).
21. Ross GT, Cargille CM, Lipsett MB. Pituitary and gonadal hormones in women during spontaneous and induced ovulatory cycles. Recent Prog Horm Res 1970; 26:1–62.
22. Hall JE, Taylor AE, Martin KA, Rivier J, Schoenfeld DA, Crowley Jr WF. Decreased release of gonadotropin-releasing hormone during the preovulatory midcycle luteinizing hormone surge in normal women. Proc Natl Acad Sci 1994; 91:6894–6898.
23. Filicori M, Butler JP, Crowley Jr WF. 1984 Neuroendocrine regulation of the corpus luteum in the human. J Clin Invest 1984; 73:1638–1647.
24. Rossmanith WG, Laughlin GA, Mortola JF, Johnson ML, Veldhuis JD, Yen SSC. Pulsatile cosecretion of estradiol and progesterone by the midluteal phase corpus luteum: temporal link to luteinizing hormone pulses. J Clin Endocrinol Metab 1990; 70:990–995.
25. LeNestour E, Marraoui J, Lahlou N, Roger M, de Ziegler D, Bouchard Ph. Role of estradiol in the rise in follicle-stimulating hormone levels during the luteal-follicular transition. J Clin Endocrinol Metab 1993; 77:439–442.
26. McLachlan RE, Robertson DM, Healy DL, Burger HG, deKretser DM. Circulating immunoreactive inhibin levels during the normal human menstrual cycle. J Clin Endocrinol Metab 1987; 65:954–961.
27. Roseff SH, Bangah ML, Kettel LM, et al. Dynamic changes in circulating inhibin levels during the luteal-follicular transition of the human menstrual cycle. J Clin Endocrinol Metab 1989; 69:1033–1039.
28. Welt CK, Martin KA, Smith JA, Taylor AE, Crowley Jr WF, Hall JE. GnRH pulse frequency: a key determinant of the luteal-follicular rise in FSH. 10th Int Cong of Endocrin 1996; 397:854 (abstract).
29. Post KD, McCormick PC, Bello JA. Differential diagnosis of pituitary tumors. Endocrinol Metab Clin North Am 1987; 16:609–645.
30. Samaan NA, Bakdash MM, Caderao JB, Cangir A, Jesse Jr RH, Ballantyne AJ. Hypopituitarism after external irradiation. Ann Intern Med 1975; 83:771–777.
31. Shalet SM, Morris-Jones PH, Beardwell CG, Pearson D. Pituitary function after treatment of intracranial tumours in children. Lancet 1975; 2:104–107.
32. Lam KSL, Tse VKC, Wang C, Yeung RTT, Ho JHC. Effects of cranial irradiation on hypothalamic-pituitary function-a 5-year longitudinal study in patients with nasopharyngeal carcinoma. Q J Med 1991; 78:165–176.
33. Constine LS, Woolf PD, Cann D, et al. Hypothalamic-pituitary dysfunction after radiation for brain tumors. N Engl J Med 1993; 328:87–94.
34. Christensen RB, Matsumoto AM, Bremner WJ. Idiopathic hypogonadotropic hypogonadism with anosmia (Kallmann's syndrome). Endocrinologist 1992; 2:332–340.
35. Waldstreicher J, Seminara SB, Jameson JL, et al. The genetic and clinical heterogeneity of gonadotropin-releasing hormone deficiency in the human. 1996; 81:4388–4395.
36. Kallmann F, Schoenfeld WA, Barrera SE. The genetic aspects of primary eunuchoidism. Am J Mental Defic 1944; 48:203–236.
37. Santen RJ, Paulsen CA. Hypogonadotropic eunuchoidism. I. Clinical study of the mode of inheritance. J Clin Endrinol Metab 1973; 36:47–54.
38. White BJ, Rogol AD, Brown KS, et al. The syndrome of anosmia with hypogonadotropic hypogonadism: a genetic study of 18 families and a review. Am J Med Genetics 1983; 15:417–435.
39. Weiss J, Adams E, Whitcomb RW, et al. Normal sequence of the gonadotropin-releasing hormone gene in patients with idiopathic hypogonadotropic hypogonadism. Biol Reprod 1991; 45:743–747.

40. Weiss J, Crowley WF, Jameson JL. Structure of the GnRH gene in patients with idiopathic hypogonadotropic hypogonadism. J Clin Endocrinol Metab 1989; 69:299–303.
41. Franco B, Guioli S, Pragliola A, et al. A gene deleted in Kallmann's syndrome shares homology with neural cell adhesion and axonal path-finding molecules. Nature 1991; 353:529–536.
42. Legouis R, Hardelin J-P, Levilliers J, et al. The candidate gene for the X-linked Kallmann syndrome encodes a protein related to adhesion molecules. Cell 1991; 67:423–435.
43. Bick D, Franco B, Sherins RJ, et al. Intragenic deletion of the *KALIG-1* gene in Kallmann's syndrome. N Engl J Med 1992; 326:1752–1777.
44. Hardelin J-P, Levilliers J, del Castillo I, et al. X chromosome-linked Kallmann syndrome: stop mutations validate the candidate gene. Proc Natl Acad Sci USA 1992; 2:311–314.
45. Rugarli EI, Ballabio A. Kallmann syndrome: from genetics to neurobiology. JAMA 1993; 270:2713–2716.
46. Schwanzel-Fukada M, Bick M, Pfaff DW. Luteinizing hormone-releasing hormone (LHRH)-expressing cells do not migrate normally in an inherited hypogonadal (Kallmann) syndrome. Mol Brain Res 1989; 6:311–326.
47. Bray GA, Dahms WT, Swerdloff RS, Fiser RH, Atkinson RL, Carrel RE. The Prader-Willi Syndrome: a study of 40 patients and a review of the literature. Medicine 1983; 62:59–80.
48. Green JS, Parfrey PS, Harnett JD, et al. The cardinal manifestations of Bardet-Biedl syndrome, a form of Laurence-Moon-Biedl syndrome. N Engl J Med 1989; 321:1002–1009.
49. Berciano J, Amando JA, Freijanes J, Rebollo M, Vaquero A. Familial cerebellar ataxia and hypogonadotropic hypogonadism: evidence for hypothalamic LHRH deficiency. J Neurol Neurosurg Psychiatry 1982; 45:747–751.
50. Abs R, Van Vleymen E, Parizel PM, Van Acker K, Martin M, Martin J. Congenital cerebellar hypoplasia and hypogonadotropic hypogonadism. J Neurol Sciences 1990; 98:259–265.
51. Kruse K, Sippell WG, Schnakenburg KV. Hypogonadism in congenital adrenal hypoplasia: evidence for a hypothalamic origin. J Clin Endocrinol Metab 1984; 58:12–17.
52. Kikuchi K, Kaji M, Momoi T, et al. Failure to induce puberty in a man with X-linked congenital adrenal hypoplasia and hypogonadotropic hypogonadism by pulsatile administration of low dose gonadotropin-releasing hormone. Acta Endocrinol 1987; 114:153–160.
53. Zanaria E, Muscatelli F, Bardoni B, et al. An unusual member of the nuclear hormone receptor superfamily responsible for X-linked adrenal hypoplasia congenita. Nature 1994; 372:635–641.
54. Muscatelli F, Strom TM, Walker AP, et al. Mutations in the DAX-1 gene give rise to both X-linked adrenal hypoplasia congenita and hypogonadotropic hypogonadism. Nature 1994; 372:672–676.
55. Albright F, Halstead J. Studies on ovarian dysfunction. II. The application of the "hormonal measuring sticks" to the sorting out and to the treatment of the various types of amenorrhea. N Engl J Med 1935; 212:250–257.
56. Santoro N, Filicori M, Crowley Jr WF. Hypogonadotropic disorders in men and women: diagnosis and therapy with pulsatile gonadotropin-releasing hormone. Endocr Rev 1986; 7:11–23.
57. Reame NE, Sauder SE, Case GS, et al. Pulsatile gonadotropin secretion in women with hypothalamic amenorrhea: evidence that reduced frequency of gonadotropin-releasing hormone secretion is the mechanism of persistent anovulation. J Clin Endocrinol Metab 1985; 61:851–858.
58. Khoury SA, Reame NE, Kelch RP, Marshall JC. Diurnal patterns of pulsatile luteinizing hormone secretion in hypothalamic amenorrhea: reproducibility and responses to opiate blockage and an (α2-adrenergic agonist. J Clin Endocrinol Metab 1987; 64:755–762.
58a. Crowley Jr WF, Filicori M, Spratt DE, Santoro NF. The physiology of gonadotropin-releasing hormone (GnRH) secretion in men and women. Recent Prog Horm Res 1985; 41:473–531.
59. Boyar RM, Katz J, Finkelstein JW, et al. Anorexia nervosa: immaturity of the 24-hour luteinizing hormone secretory pattern. N Engl J Med 1974; 291:861–865.
60. Pirke KM, Fichter MM, Lund R, Doerr P. Twenty-four hour sleep-wake pattern of plasma LH in patients with anorexia nervosa. Acta Endocrinol 1979; 92:193–204.
61. Loucks AB, Mortola JF, Girton L, Yen SSC. Alterations in the hypothalamic-pituitary-ovarian and the hypothalamic-pituitary-adrenal axes in athletic women. J Clin Endocrinol Metab 1989; 68:402–411.
62. Schweiger U, Pirke J, Laessle RG, Fichter MM. Gonadotropin secretion in bulimia nervosa. J Clin Endocrinol Metab 1992; 7:112–117.
63. Semple CC, Robertson WR, Mitchell R, et al. Mechanisms leading to hypogonadism in men with burns injuries. Br Med J 1987; 295:403–407.

64. Clarke JDA, Raggatt PR, Edwards OM. Abnormalities of the hypothalamo-pituitary-gonadal axis after head injury. Clin Endocrinol 1992; 36:481–485.
65. Woolf PD, Hamill RW, McDonald JV, Lee LA, Kelly M. Transient hypogonadotropic hypogonadism caused by critical illness. J Clin Endocrinol Metab 1985; 60:444–450.
66. Spratt DI, Bigos ST, Beitins I, Cox P, Longcope C, Orav J. Both hyper- and hypogonadotropic hypogonadism occur transiently in acute illness: bio- and immunoactive gonadotropins. J Clin Endocrinol Metab 1992; 75:1562–1570.
67. Bullen BA, Skrinar GS, Beitins IZ, von Mering G, Turnbull BA, McArthur JW. Induction of menstrual disorders by strenuous exercise in untrained women. N Engl J Med 1985; 312:1349–1353.
68. Warren MP. The effects of exercise on pubertal progression and reproductive function in girls. J Clin Endocrinol Metab 1980; 51:1150–1157.
69. Loucks AB, Heath EM. Dietary restriction reduces luteinizing hormone (LH) pulse frequency during waking hours and increases LH pulse amplitude during sleep in young menstruating women. J Clin Endocrinol Metab 1994; 78:910–915.
70. Loucks AB, Brown R, King K, Thuma JR, Verdun M. A combined regimen of moderate dietary restriction and exercise training alters luteinizing hormone pulsatility in regularly menstruating, young women. Proc 77th Ann Meeting Endo Soc 1995; P3-360 (Abstract).
71. MacConnie SE, Barkan A, Lampman RM, Schork MA, Beitins IZ. Decreased hypothalamic gonadotropin-releasing hormone secretion in male marathon runners. N Engl J Med 1986; 315:411–417.
72. Cameron JL, Weltzin TE, McConaha C, Helmreich DL, Kaye WH. Slowing of pulsatile luteinizing hormone secretion in men after forty-eight hours of fasting. J Clin Endocrinol Metab 1991; 73:35–41.
73. Veldhuis JD, Iranmanesh A, Evans WS, Lizarralde G, Thorner MO, Vance ML. Amplitude suppression of the pulsatile mode of immunoradiometric luteinizing hormone release in fasting-induced hypoandrogenemia in normal men. J Clin Endocrinol Metab 1993; 76:587–593.
74. Opstad PR. Androgenic hormones during prolonged physical stress, sleep, and energy deficiency. J Clin Endocrinol Metab 1992; 74:1176–1183.
75. Martin KA, Hall JE, Santoro NF, Crowley Jr WF. Hypothalamic amenorrhea (HA): further neuroendocrine characterization. Clin Res 1990; 38:342A.
76. Berga SL, Loucks AB, Rossmanith WG, Kettel LM, Laughlin MA, Yen SSC. Acceleration of luteinizing hormone pulse frequency in functional hypothalamic amenorrhea by dopaminergic blockade. J Clin Endocrinol Metab 1991; 72:151–156.
77. Berga SL, Mortola JF, Yen SSC. Amplification of nocturnal melatonin secretion in women with functional hypothalamic amenorrhea. J Clin Endocrinol Metab 1988; 66:242–244.
78. Brzezinski A, Lynch HJ, Seibel MM, Deng MH, Nader TM, Wurtman RJ. The circadian rhythm of plasma melatonin during the normal menstrual cycle and in amenorrheic women. J Clin Endocrinol Metab 1988; 66:891–895.
79. Gold PW, Gwirtsman H, Avgerinos PC, et al. Abnormal hypothalamic-pituitary-adrenal function in anorexia nervosa: pathophysiologic mechanisms in underweight and weight-corrected patients. N Engl J Med 1986; 314:1335–1342.
80. Suh BY, Liu JH, Berga SL, Quigley ME, Laughlin GA, Yen SS. Hypercortisolism in patients with functional hypothalamic-amenorrhea. J Clin Endocrinol Metab 1988; 66:733–739.
81. Villaneuva AL, Schlosser C, Hopper B, Liu JH, Hoffman DI, Regar RW. Increased cortisol production in women runners. J Clin Endocrinol Metab 1986; 63:133–136.
82. Biller BMK, Federoff HJ, Koenig JI, Klibnaski A. Abnormal cortisol secretion and responses to corticotropin-releasing hormone in women with hypothalamic amenorrhea. J Clin Endocrinol Metab 1990; 70:311–317.
83. Luger A, Deuster PA, Kyle SB, et al. Acute hypothalamic-pituitary-adrenal responses to the stress of treadmill exercise: physiologic adaptations to physical training. N Engl J Med 1987; 316:1309–1315.
84. Petraglia F, Sutton S, Vale W, Plotsky P. Corticotropin-releasing factor decreases plasma luteinizing hormone levels in female rats by inhibiting gonadotropin-releasing hormone release into hypophyseal portal circulation. Endocrinology 1987; 120:1083–1088.
85. Rivier C, Vale W. Influence of corticotropin-releasing factor on reproductive functions in the rat. Endocrinol 1984; 114:914–919.
86. Rivier C, Vale W. Effect of the long-term administration of corticotropin releasing factor on the pituitary-adrenal and pituitary-gonadal axis in the male rat. J Clin Invest 1985; 75:689–694.

87. Rivier C, Rivier J, Vale W. Stress-induced inhibition of reproductive functions: role of endogenous corticotropin-releasing factor. Science 1986; 231:607–609.
88. Barbarino A, De Marinis L, Tofani A, et al. Corticotropin-releasing hormone inhibition of gonadotropin release and the effect of opioid blockade. J Clin Endocrinol Metab 1989; 68:523–528.
89. Bohnet HG, Dahlen HG, Wuttke W, Schneider HPG. Hyperprolactinemic anovulatory syndrome. J Clin Endocrinol Metab 1976; 42:132–143.
90. Sauder SE, Frager M, Case GD, Kelch RP, Marshall JC. Abnormal patterns of pulsatile luteinizing hormone secretion in women with hyperprolactinemia and amenorrhea: responses to bromocriptine. J Clin Endocrinol Metab 1984; 59:941–948.
91. Monroe SE, Levine L, Chang RJ, Keye Jr WR, Yamamoto M, Jaffe RB. Prolactin-secreting pituitary adenomas. V. Increased gonadotroph responsivity in hyperprolactinemic women with pituitary adenomas. J Clin Endocrinol Metab 1981; 52:1171–1178.
92. Caro JF, Woolf PD. Pituitary-ovarian axis responsivity to prolonged gonadotropin-releasing hormone infusion in normal and hyperprolactinemic women. J Clin Endocrinol Metab 1980; 50:999–1004.
93. Ho KY, Smythe GA, Lazarus L. Dopaminergic control of gonadotrophin secretion in normal women and in patients with pathological hyperprolactinaemia. Clin Endocrinol 1984; 20:53–63.
94. Webb CB, Thominet JL, Barowsky H, Berelowitz M, Frohman LA. Evidence for lactotroph dopamine resistance in idiopathic hyperprolactinemia. J Clin Endocrinol Metab 1983; 56:1089–1093.
95. Grossman A, Moult PJA, Gaillard RC, et al. The opioid control of LH and FSH release: effects of a met-enkephalin analogue and naloxone. Clin Endocrinol 1981; 14:41–47.
96. Luton J, Thieblot P, Valcke J, Mahoudeau JA, Bricaire H. Reversible gonadotropin deficiency in male Cushing's disease. J Clin Endocrinol Metab 1977; 45:488–495.
97. MacAdams MR, White RH, Chipps BE. Reduction of serum testosterone levels during chronic glucocorticoid therapy. Ann Int Med 1986; 104:648–651.
98. Saketos M, Sharma N, Santoro NF. Suppression of the hypothalamic-pituitary-ovarian axis in normal women by glucocorticoids. Biol Reprod 1993; 49:1270–1276.
99. Dubey AK, Plant TM. A suppression of gonadotropin secretion by cortisol in castrated male Rhesus monkeys (*Macaca mulatta*) mediated by the interruption of hypothalamic gonadotropin-releasing hormone release. Biol Reprod 1985; 33:423–431.
100. Van Thiel DH, Cobb CF, Herman GB, Perez I, Gavaler JS. An examination of various mechanisms for ethanol-induced testicular injury: studies utilizing the isolated perfused rat testes. Endocrinology 1981; 109:2009–2015.
101. Mendelson JH, Mello NK. Chronic alcohol effects on anterior pituitary and ovarian hormones in healthy women. J Pharmacol Exp Ther 1988; 245:407–412.
102. Iranmanesh A, Velhuis JD, Samojlik E, Rogol AD, Johnson ML, Lizarralde G. Alterations in the pulsatile properties of gonadotropin secretion in alcoholic men. J Androl 1988; 9:207–214.
103. Swerdloff RS, Hever D. Effects of aging on male reproductive function. In Korenman SG, ed. Endocrine Aspects of Aging. Elsevier Biomedical; New York, 1982, pp. 119–135.
104. Neaves WB, Johnson L, Porter JC, Parker CR, Petty CS. Leydig cell numbers, daily sperm production and serum gonadotropin levels in aging men. J Clin Endocrinol Metab 1984; 59:756–763.
105. Rubens R, Dhont M, Vermeulen A. Further studies on Leydig cell function in old age. J Clin Endocrinol Metab 1974; 39:40–45.
106. Korenman SG, Morley JE, Mooradian AD, et al. Secondary hypogonadism in older men: its relation to impotence. J Clin Endocrinol Metab 1990; 71:963–969.
107. Vermeulen A, Deslypere JP, Kaufman JM. Influence of antiopioids on luteinizing hormone pulsatility in aging men. J Clin Endocrinol Metab 1989; 68:68–72.
108. Veldhuis JD, Urban RJ, Lizzaralde G, Johnson ML, Iranmanesh A. Attenuation of luteinizing hormone secretory burst amplitude as a proximate basis of hypoandrogenism of healthy aging men. J Clin Endocrinol Metab 1992; 75:52–58.
109. Snyder PJ. Gonadotroph cell adenomas of the pituitary. Endocr Rev 1985; 6:552–563.
110. Arafah BM. Reversible hypopituitarism in patients with large nonfunctioning pituitary adenomas. J Clin Endocrinol Metab 1986; 62:1173–1179.
111. Katznelson L, Alexander JM, Bikkal HA, Jameson JL, Hsu DW, Klibanski A. Imbalanced follicle-stimulating hormone beta-subunit hormone biosynthesis in human pituitary adenomas. J Clin Endocrinol Metab 1992; 74:1343–1351.

112. Kelly TM, Edwards CQ, Meikle AW, Kushner JP. Hypogonadism in hemochromatosis: reversal with iron depletion. Ann Int Med 1984; 101:629–632.
113. Wang C, Tso SC, Todd D. Hypogonadotropic hypogonadism in severe β-thalassemia: effect of chelation and pulsatile gonadotropin-releasing hormone therapy. J Clin Endocrinol Metab 1989; 68:511–516.
114. Cundy T, Butler J, Bomford A, Williams R. Reversibility of hypogonadotrophic hypogonadism associated with genetic haemochromatosis. Clin Endocrinol 1993; 38:617–620.
115. Cosman F, Post KD, Holub DA, Wardlaw SL. Lymphocytic hypophysitis: report of 3 new cases and review of the literature. Medicine 1989; 68:240–256.
116. Bottazzo GF, Pouplard A, Florin-Christensen A, Doniach D. Autoantibodies to prolactin-secreting cells of human pituitary. Lancet 1975; 2:97–101.
117. Beressi N, Cohen R, Beressi J, et al. Pseudotumoral lymphocytic hypophysitis successfully treated by corticosteroid alone: first case report. Neurosurgery 1994; 35:505–508.
118. McGrail KM, Beyerl BD, Black PM, Klibanski A, Zervas NT. Lymphocytic adenohypophysitis of pregnancy with complete recovery. Neurosurgery 1987; 20:791–793.
119. Scanarini M, D'Avella D, Rotilio A, Kitromilis N, Mingrino S. Giant-cell granulomatous hypophysitis: a distinct clinicopathological entity. J Neurosurg 1989; 71:681–686.
120. Sheehan HL. Postpartum necrosis of the anterior pituitary. J Path Bact 1937; 45:189–214.
121. Brennan CF, Malone RGS, Weaver JA. Pituitary necrosis in diabetes mellitus. Lancet 1956; 2:12–16.
122. Harvey JC, de Klerk J. The Houssay phenomenon in man. Amer J Med 1955; 19:327–336.
123. Schalch DS, Burday SZ. Antepartum pituitary insufficiency in diabetes mellitus. Ann Intern Med 1971; 74:357–360.
124. Neelon FA, Goree JA, Lebovitz HE. The primary empty sella: clinical and radiographic characteristics and endocrine function. Medicine 1973; 52:73–92.
125. Brismar K, Efendic S. Pituitary function in the empty sella syndrome. Neuroendocrinology 1981; 32:70–77.
126. Al-Ansari AAK, Khalil TH, Kelani Y, Mortimer CH. Isolated follicle-stimulating hormone deficiency in men: successful long-term gonadotropin therapy. Fertil Steril 1984; 42:618–626.
127. Hargreave TB, Kyle KF, Kelly AM, England P. Releasing factor tests in men with oligozoospermia. Br J Urol 1979; 51:38–42.
128. Matthews CH, Borgato S, Beck-Peccoz P, et al. Primary amenorrhoea and infertility due to a mutation in the β-subunit of follicle-stimulating hormone. Nature Genetics 1993; 5:83–86.
129. Haavisto AM, Pettersson K, Bergendahl M, Virkamaki A, Huhtaniemi I. Occurrence and biological properties of a common genetic variant of luteinizing hormone. J Clin Endocrinol Metab 1995; 80:1257–1263.
130. Furui K, Suganuma N, Tsukahara S-I, et al. Identification of two point mutations in the gene coding luteinizing hormone (LH) β-subunit, associated with immunologically anomalous LH variants. J Clin Endocrinol Metab 1994; 78:107–113.
131. Weiss J, Axelrod L, Whitcomb RW, Harris PE, Crowley WF, Jameson JL. Hypogonadism caused by a single amino acid substitution in the β subunit of luteinizing hormone. N Engl J Med 1992; 326:179–183.
132. Finkelstein JS, O'Dea LSL, Whitcomb RW, Crowley Jr WF. Sex steroid control of gonadotropin secretion in the human male. II. Effects of estradiol administration in normal and gonadotropin-releasing hormone-deficient men. J Clin Endocrinol Metab 1991; 73:621–628.
133. Kuhn JM, Mahoudeau JA, Billaud L, et al. Evaluation of diagnostic criteria for Leydig cell tumours in adult men revealed by gynaecomastia. Clin Endocrinol 1987; 26:407–416.
134. Veldhuis JD, Sowers JR, Rogol AD, Klein FA, Miller N, Dufau ML. Pathophysiology of male hypogonadism associated with endogenous hyperestrogenism: evidence for dual defects in the gonadal axis. N Engl J Med 1985; 312:1371–1375.
135. Stepanas AB, Samaan NA, Schultz PN, Holoye PY. Endocrine studies in testicular tumor patients with and without gynecomastia: a report of 45 cases. Cancer 1978; 41:369–376.
136. Glass AR, Swerdloff RS, Bray GA, Dahms WT, Atkinson RL. Low serum testosterone and sex-hormone-binding-globulin in massively obese men. J Clin Endocrinol Metab 1977; 45:1211–1219.
137. Schneider G, Kirschner MA, Berkowitz R, Ertel NH. Increased estrogen production in obese men. J Clin Endocrinol Metab 1979; 48:633–638.
138. Zumoff B, Strain GW, Miller LK, et al. Plasma free and non-sex-hormone-binding-globulin-bound testosterone are decreased in obese men in proportion to their degree of obesity. J Clin Endocrinol Metab 1990; 71:929–931.

139. Vermeulen A, Kaufman JM, Deslypere JP, Thomas G. Attenuated luteinizing hormone (LH) pulse amplitude but normal LH pulse frequency, and its relation to plasma androgens in hypogonadism of obese men. J Clin Endocrinol Metab 1993; 76:1140–1146.
140. Santamaria JD, Prior JC, Fleetham JA. Reversible reproductive dysfunction in men with obstructive sleep apnoea. Clin Endocrinol 1988; 28:461–470.
141. Finkelstein JS, Whitcomb RW, O'Dea LSL, et al. Sex steroid control of gonadotropin secretion in the human male. I. Effects of testosterone administration in normal and gonadotropin-releasing hormone deficient men. J Clin Endocrinol Metab 1991; 73:609–620.
142. Alen M, Suominen J. Effect of androgenic and anabolic steroids on spermatogenesis in power athletes. Int J Sports Med 1984; 5:189–192.
143. Alen M, Reinila M, Vihko R. Response of serum hormones to androgen administration in power athletes. Med Sci Sports 1985; 17:354–359.
144. Burris AS, Rodbard HW, Winters SJ, Sherins RJ. Gonadotropin therapy in men with isolated hypogonadotropic hypogonadism: the response to human chorionic gonadotropin is predicted by initial testicular size. J Clin Endocrinol Metab 1988; 66:1144–1151.
145. Whitcomb RW, Crowley WF. Diagnosis and treatment of isolated gonadotropin-releasing hormone deficiency in men. J Clin Endocrinol Metab 1990; 70:3–7.
146. Schopohl J, Mehltretter G, von Zumbusch R, et al. Comparison of gonadotropin-releasing hormone and gonadotropin therapy in male patients with idiopathic hypothalamic hypogonadism. Fertil Steril 1991; 56:1143–1145.
147. Martin K, Santoro N, Hall J, Filicori M, Wierman M, Crowley Jr WF. Management of ovulatory disorders with pulsatile gonadotropin-releasing hormone. J Clin Endocrinol Metab 1990; 71:1081A–1081G.
148. Martin KA, Hall JE, Adams JM, Crowley Jr WF. Comparison of exogenous gonadotropins and pulsatile gonadotropin-releasing hormone for induction of ovulation in hypogonadotropic amenorrhea. J Clin Endocrinol Metab 1993; 77:125–129.
149. Hall JE, Martin KA, Whitney HA, Landy H, Crowley Jr WF. Potential for fertility with replacement of hypothalamic gonadotropin-releasing hormone in long term female survivors of cranial tumors. J Clin Endocrinol Metab 1994; 79:1166–1172.

12 Gonadotropin (FSH and LH) Pituitary Tumors

Differential Diagnosis and Treatment

Eun Jig Lee, MD, *and J. Larry Jameson,* MD, PhD

CONTENTS

INTRODUCTION

The majority of pituitary adenomas cause dramatic clinical manifestations as a result of hypersecretion of one or more pituitary hormones. For example, acromegaly, Cushing's disease, and amenorrhea-galactorrhea result in classic endocrine syndromes that reflect excess secretion of growth hormone (GH), adrenocorticotropin (ACTH), and prolactin (PRL), respectively. Serum determinations of these hormones are useful in the diagnosis of these pituitary tumors and as tumor markers to follow the progress of therapy. In contrast to these disorders, pituitary adenomas that secrete the gonadotropins, follicle stimulating hormone (FSH) and luteinizing hormone (LH), have traditionally been regarded as uncommon tumors and there is less experience with the clinical manifestations of these tumors. However, the application of new techniques has dramatically changed our understanding of the prevalence of gonadotropin secreting adenomas. The majority of the pituitary adenomas previously classified as nonfunctioning adenomas have been found to produce gonadotropins or their subunits *(1–12)*. Based on these and other studies, gonadotropin-secreting pituitary adenomas can now be considered to account for approximately 80% of surgically excised clinically nonfunctioning adenomas, or about 30% of all macroadenomas.

ETIOLOGY AND PATHOGENESIS

There has been much debate concerning whether pituitary tumors arise as a consequence of primary defects in pituitary cells (somatic mutations), or as a result of exces-

From: *Contemporary Endocrinology, Vol. 3: Diseases of the Pituitary: Diagnosis and Treatment*
Edited by M. E. Wierman Humana Press Inc., Totowa, NJ

sive stimulation by hypothalamic or other exogenous factors. In fact, these theories are not mutually exclusive. Chronic hormonal stimulation is well known to predispose to certain types of pituitary tumors. Typically, this circumstance gives rise to hyperplasia followed by the development of adenomas. In animal models, chronic estrogen exposure can lead to lactotrope hyperplasia and prolactinomas *(13)*, high-dose calcitonin predisposes to α-subunit secreting adenomas *(14)*, and transgenic mice that overexpress GHRH exhibit dramatic somatotroph hyperplasia followed by the development of adenomas *(15)*.

Although long-term hypogonadism occasionally results in pituitary enlargement *(16,17)*, there is no evidence that gonadotropin-secreting adenomas arise because of excessive stimulation to produce gonadotropins. Most men with gonadotropin tumors do not have evidence for gonadal dysfunction that might have caused decreased feedback inhibition *(18)*. Ovarian failure leads to menopause and persistent elevation of gonadotropins, but it is rare to develop gonadotropin secreting adenomas despite this chronic stimulus. Unlike the circumstance that occurs with chronic exposure to GHRH, excessive secretion of GnRH would be expected to desensitize gonadotropin secretion *(19)*.

The most compelling data concerning the molecular basis for the formation of gonadotropin adenomas have come from analyses of clonality *(20)*. As depicted in Fig. 1A, monoclonal tumors arise from a single progenitor cell that has acquired a growth advantage presumably because of a somatic mutation. Polyclonal tumors, on the other hand, reflect hyperplasia caused by exogenous stimulation that affects all cells equally. Recombinant DNA techniques have recently allowed the issue of pituitary tumor clonality to be addressed directly by examining whether tumor cells exhibit a uniform pattern of X-chromosome inactivation. The principle of this technique is that in females, one of the two X-chromosomes randomly undergoes inactivation according to the Lyon hypothesis. Consequently, in a monoclonal tumor, either the maternal or paternal X-chromosome should be inactivated in all cells in the tumor. In contrast, polyclonal tumors exhibit an equal distribution of inactivated X-chromosomes because they consist of cells of mixed origin. An example of clonality is shown for nonfunctioning pituitary adenomas in Fig. 1B. This group of tumors, which are essentially synonymous with gonadotropin-secreting tumors (because they were shown to be immunoreactive for gonadotropins), were found to be monoclonal using this type of analysis *(21)*. Although limited numbers of tumors have been examined in this manner, current data support the view the nonfunctioning tumors, corticotroph and somatotroph adenomas are usually monoclonal in origin *(21–24)*.

The observation that pituitary tumors are monoclonal implies the presence of a somatic mutation. Several different types of mutations have been found in pituitary tumors, although there has been relatively little progress in the case of gonadotropin secreting adenomas. For example, about one-third of somatotrope adenomas have mutations that result in activation of the Gsα-subunit *(25–27)*. These mutations cause constitutive activation of adenylyl cyclase, which is known to stimulate somatotrope cell proliferation *(28)*. The Gsα mutations appear to be restricted to somatotrope adenomas *(29)*. Mutations in other oncogenes, such as ras, Rb, and p53 are uncommon in pituitary tumors *(30–33)*. Loss of tumor suppressor genes have also been described in soma-

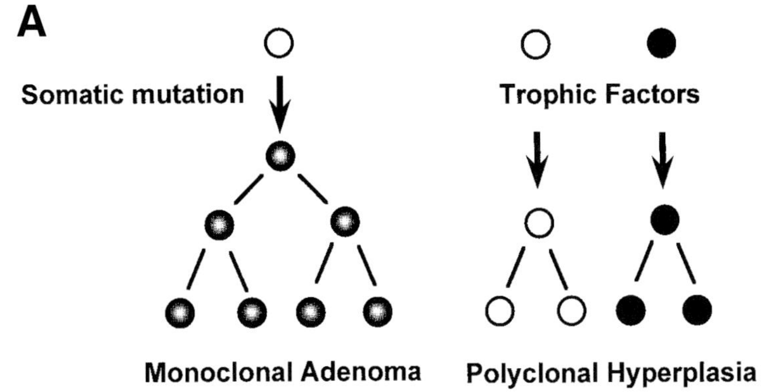

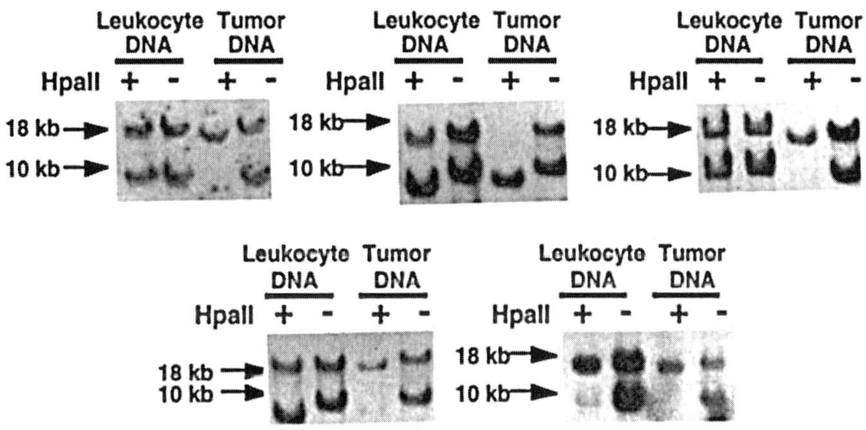

Fig. 1. Clonality of gonadotropin secreting pituitary tumors. **(A)** Schematic representation of clonality. Monoclonal tumors are depicted by expansion from a single progenitor cell after a somatic mutation. Polyclonal hyperplasia reflects equal proliferation of multiple stem cells usually in response to exogenous trophic factors or hormones. **(B)** Clonal analysis at the HPRT locus. DNA was extracted from pituitary tumor tissue, or from peripheral blood leukocytes from the same patients. DNA was digested with restriction enzymes to generate polymorphic alleles of 18 or 10 kb. Indicated lanes were also digested with *Hpa*II, a methylation-sensitive enzyme that allows discrimination of activated and inactivated X-chromosomes. After Southern blot hybridization, the presence of a single allele in the tumor specimens that were digested with *Hpa*II is consistent with monoclonality. Reproduced from ref. *21* with permission.

Table 1
Diagnostic Tests in Patients with Gonadotropin Secreting Adenomas

In Vivo Tests
Increased baseline serum hormones
FSH, LH
α, LHβ, FSHβ,
Increased hormonal response to TRH
FSH, FSHβ
LH, LHβ
MRI or CT scans showing pituitary mass
In Vitro Tests
Immunocytochemistry
Hormone secretion in cell culture
mRNA detection by *in situ* hybridization, Northern blot, or RT-PCR

totropinomas, and appear to frequently involve chromosome 11 in a region which may correspond to the MEN-1 locus *(34)*. However, similar analyses have not been performed in gonadotropin adenomas. Thus, the nature of the somatic defects in gonadotropin adenomas remain unknown, but are of great interest because this information may provide new insights into pathogenesis as well as potential strategies for therapy.

In Vitro Studies of Gonadotropin-Secreting Adenomas

Although the diagnosis of gonadotropin-producing adenomas can be difficult to establish in vivo, the tumors have been analyzed in vitro using a variety of methods (Table 1). Hormone secretion can be studied by culturing the pituitary tumor cells *(2–4,11,35)*. Although the tumor cells do not appear to divide, they continue to secrete hormone products for several weeks *(36)*. Virtually all clinically nonfunctioning tumors secrete gonadotropins in cell culture. It is notable that other pituitary hormones are not secreted, or are present at very low levels, indicating that gonadotropin secretion is unlikely to be derived from contaminating normal pituitary cells. These findings are consistent with the idea that the majority of clinically nonfunctioning tumors are of gonadotrope origin. The apparent discrepancy between the in vivo and in vitro characteristics of the gonadotropin-secreting tumors is probably explained by the quantities of hormone produced. The gonadotropin-secreting adenomas contain relatively sparse secretory granules *(37)*, and they secrete hormones inefficiently. In part, this may reflect the complex biosynthesis of the glycoprotein hormones, which require extensive glycosylation, subunit combination, and cellular trafficking. The disproportionate release of uncombined α- and β-subunits probably also reflects abnormalities in hormone biosynthesis. In comparison to the intact hormones (LH, FSH), the uncombined subunits are degraded rapidly and cleared from the circulation more quickly *(38,39)*. These features may also explain the inefficient hormone production in vivo.

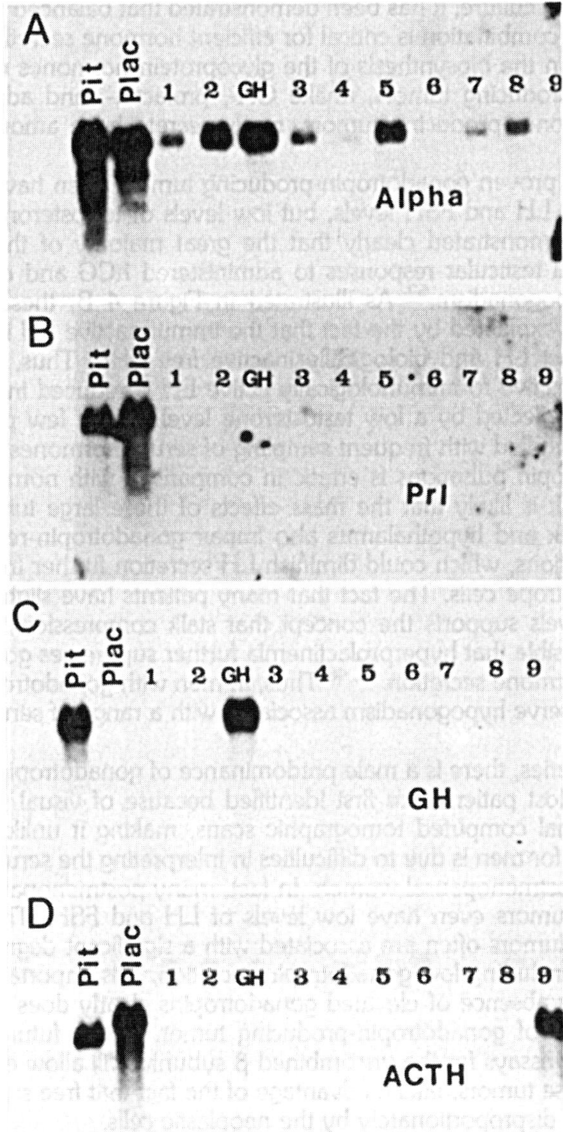

Fig. 2. Expression of gonadotropin genes in gonadotropin secreting pituitary tumors. Pituitary tumor mRNA was analyzed by Northern blot using radiolabeled probes specific for alpha, prolactin (Prl), growth hormone (GH), and adrenocorticotropin (ACTH). The same blot was rehybridized with each of the probes. Control samples in the left lanes include mRNA from normal pituitary (Pit) and placenta (Plac). The remaining lanes contain RNA from clinically nonfunctioning tumors except lane GH which contains a control specimen from a tumor known to cosecrete GH and TSH. Reproduced from ref. *4* with permission.

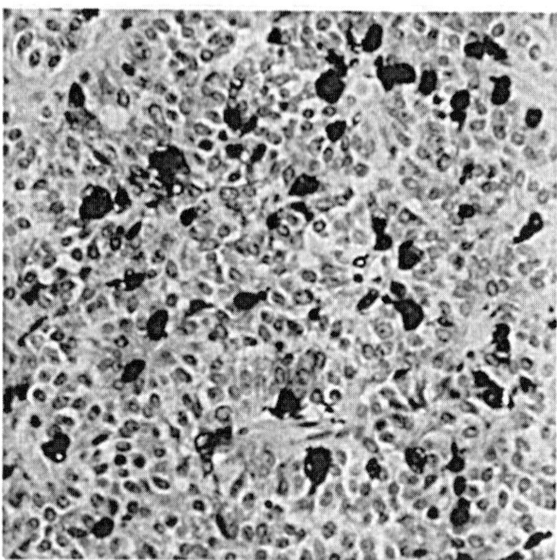

Fig. 3. Immunohistology of a gonadotropin secreting adenoma. Positive reaction for FSH is seen in a subset of cells (darkly stained). Reproduced from ref. *3* with permission.

Adenomas that are not associated with high serum levels of gonadotropins or their subunits, but with an LHβ response to TRH in vivo, secrete large amounts of intact FSH as well as LHβ in culture *(7,40,41)*. In vivo, elevation of FSH is seen much more commonly than LH *(41)*. Because FSH and LH are produced by the same cell type, one might expect more proportionate expression of the two hormones. In fact, this is seen in vitro, in which LH is secreted in large amounts even when FSH is the predominant hormone in vivo. These characteristics probably reflect differences in the mechanisms that control FSH and LH biosynthesis. FSH is highly dependent upon activin for its biosynthesis *(42,43)*, and activin is produced by gonadotropin-secreting adenomas *(44–46)*. On the other hand, LH secretion is very sensitive to the pattern of GnRH input *(19)*. Thus, tumors that are exposed to activin, but deprived of pulsatile GnRH, may tend to produce excess FSH. Overall, there is a relatively poor correlation between gonadotropin levels in vivo and hormone secretion in vitro. Nevertheless, the fact that gonadotropins are selectively secreted by the great majority of clinically nonfunctioning tumors clearly establishes the cell type of origin for these tumors.

The cloning of the human gonadotropin genes allowed studies of gene expression as a strategy for determining pituitary tumor cell type *(47)*, Northern blot analyses of extracted RNA reveals that 70–90% of clinically nonfunctioning adenomas express some combination of α-subunit, FSHβ, and LHβ mRNAs (Fig. 2) *(4,41,47,48)*. Since the initial studies using Northern blot analyses, a variety of methods have been used for mRNA studies, including reverse transcriptase-polymerase chain reaction (RT-PCR) *(45,46,49)*, and *in situ* hybridization *(50)*. Although the gene expression studies have been useful from a research perspective, they are impractical for widespread application because fresh tumor tissue is re-

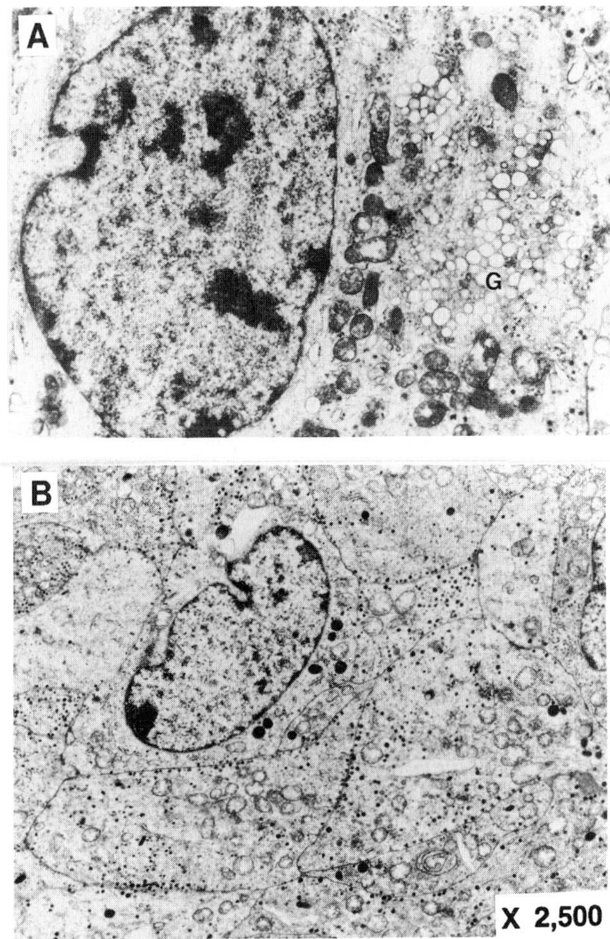

Fig. 4. Electron microscopy of gonadotropin secreting adenomas. **(A)** A gonadotrope adenoma from a female illustrating the "honeycomb" Golgi "G" and dilated endoplasmic reticulum. **(B)** Gonadotrope adenoma from a male showing sparse secretory granules.

quired to prevent mRNA degradation and the techniques for quantitative mRNA measurement remain technically sophisticated.

Immunohistology provides a practical means to establish the pathologic diagnosis of a gonadotropin producing adenoma. The fixed adenoma tissue is subjected immunocytochemical staining using specific antibodies to α, LHβ, or FSHβ *(3,10,37)*. The intensity and pattern of immunoreactivity is highly variable in different tumors, but there is positive staining for gonadotropins in approximately 70–90% of clinically nonfunctioning tumors. Commonly, one sees scattered positive cells, often clustered together (Fig. 3). The technique is most helpful when it is performed routinely as part of a panel of antibodies that are used to analyze all pituitary tumors. In this manner, there is also the possibility of detecting silent ACTH or GH tumors, as well as gonadotropin adenomas, and plurihormonal tumors.

By electron microscopy, there is additional evidence that most clinically nonfunctioning tumors arise from gonadotrope cells *(2,51)*. Interestingly, there are differences in the fine structure of gonadotropin-secreting adenomas in men and women (Fig. 4) *(52)*. Male gonadotropin-secreting adenoma cells are typically small, angular, and contain sparse small secretory granules. Their electron microscopic features are similar to that of null cell adenomas *(2)*. On the other hand, gonadotropin-secreting adenomas in women are often more highly differentiated, with abundant, dilated rough endoplasmic reticulum and Golgi sacculi (a honeycomb-like Golgi complex). The reason for the sex-related differences in cellular organelle fine structure is not understood *(10,37,52)*.

DIAGNOSIS

Clinical Features of Gonadotropin Secreting Adenomas

The previous perception that gonadotropin secreting adenomas are rare is easily understood when viewed from the context of clinical presentation. As noted, gonadotropin production from these tumors is inefficient and the detection of excess hormone levels is challenging. Unlike all other pituitary tumors, gonadotropin adenomas do not usually cause a clinical syndrome related to hormone overproduction. Rather, they typically present as clinically nonfunctioning tumors with most symptoms related to local mass effects (Table 2). In the absence of evidence for other hormone-secreting tumors, a high degree of suspicion for gonadotropin-secreting tumors can allow the diagnosis to be made in most cases.

There is a slight male predominance of gonadotropin-secreting adenomas in most series and the majority of cases occur after age 50 *(40)*. Thus, women with this type of tumor are usually postmenopausal. In this circumstance, gonadotropins are expected to be elevated and would be consistent with either menopausal elevation or production from the adenoma. As in men, many postmenopausal women with gonadotropin secreting adenomas have normal or even have low levels of LH and FSH, reflecting the common occurrence of hypopituitarism. For this reason, it is important to recognize that the absence of elevated gonadotropins does not exclude the diagnosis of gonadotropin secreting adenomas. TRH stimulations tests and assays for uncombined α- and β-subunits allow easier recognition of these adenomas (*see* below) *(53–56)*.

Case Presentation

A typical case presentation is informative because of the unusual nature of these tumors. Mr. A. N. is a 68-yr-old man who presented to his ophthalmologist because of decreased vision. After formal visual field testing, he was found to have bitemporal hemianopsia and impaired visual acuity on the left. An MRI revealed a large pituitary mass with suprasellar extension and invasion of the left cavernous sinus. He had no clinical features of Cushing's syndrome or acromegaly, and noted that his libido had declined gradually over the last 10 yr. He noted frequent headaches, particularly in the retro-orbital area. Endocrine evaluation showed normal thyroid tests, normal IGF-1, prolactin = 26 ng/mL (normal < 15 ng/mL), LH = 12 mIU/mL (normal 3–18 mIU/mL), FSH = 23 mIU/mL (normal 3–18 mIU/mL), and testosterone = 220 ng/dL (normal 300–1000 ng/dL). A TRH test for paradoxical stimulation of gonadotropins was not

Table 2
Clinical Features of Gonadotropin Secreting Adenomas

Past History
Normal pubertal development
Normal fertility
Neurological Manifestations
Headache
Visual field defects
Pituitary apoplexy
Cranial nerve palsies
Hormonal Manifestations
Hypogonadism (common)
Hypopituitarism by stalk compression
Hypogonadism, loss of libido in men
Oligoamenorrhea in women
Hypergonadotropism (rare)
Increased testosterone from ↑ LH
Testicular enlargement from ↑ FSH
Ovarian hyperstimulation from ↑ LH and FSH

performed. Transsphenoidal surgery was performed for decompression. His visual fields improved, but were not corrected entirely. Immunohistology showed scattered positive staining for α-subunit, LH, and FSH, but was negative for other pituitary hormones. It was concluded that he had a gonadotropin-secreting adenoma. The elevated basal FSH is consistent with this diagnosis as is the immunohistology. The reduced testosterone level may reflect mild hyperprolactinemia (from stalk compression), and perhaps a degree of hypopituitarism.

Mass Effects of Adenomas

Mass effects can include visual field deficits, headache, hypopituitarism, cranial nerve palsies, and pituitary apoplexy. Visual field loss due to suprasellar extension and compression of the optic chiasm is found as a presenting symptom in >70% of patients with presumed gonadotropin adenomas *(4,18,57–59)*. Headache and symptoms of hypopituitarism, particularly hypogonadism with loss of libido, are also common. Other less common neurologic presentations include palsies of cranial nerves III, IV, and VI, which result from lateral extension of the tumor into the cavernous sinus, CSF rhinorrhea, and pituitary apoplexy associated with hemorrhage and necrosis of the tumor *(60,61)*. High resolution computed tomography (CT) and magnetic resonance imaging (MRI) scans have greatly improved the diagnosis of these tumors, including increased recognition of incidental pituitary mass lesions when imaging studies are performed for unrelated indications such as head trauma.

Clinical Manifestations in Men

From first principles of hormone action, one might expect gonadotropin-secreting tumors to cause hypergonadotropic hypergonadism and excess production of sex steroids. Although such cases have been reported, they are exceedingly rare. For example, predominantly FSH-secreting adenomas in men have been associated testicular enlargement *(62)*. There have also been case reports of men with predominantly LH secreting tumors that result in increased testosterone and altered libido *(48,63)*. Gonadotropin secreting adenomas are a rare cause of precocious puberty *(64,65)*.

The most typical presentation, as in the case above, includes high normal or elevated FSH. LH levels are more variable, but are usually within the relatively broad normal range. In most cases, testosterone levels are reduced, suggesting that on average LH levels are low *(18,40,54)*.

Several explanations have been put forward to explain the hormone values in men with gonadotropin-secreting adenomas (Fig. 5). Because many men with these tumors are in older age groups, it is important to compare their gonadotropin and testosterone levels to age-matched controls, as testosterone levels decrease and gonadotropins increase with age *(66,67)*. In fact, this decline in gonadal function with age makes it even more challenging to distinguish patients with gonadotropin-secreting tumors from normals. However, age alone does not adequately explain the disproportionate secretion of FSH, nor the degree of decline in testosterone. It is also important to consider that gonadotropins are secreted in a highly pulsatile manner, and there is wide variation in pulse frequency and amplitude in normal men *(68)*. Because LH levels can vary by 10–20 mIU/mL depending on the time during a pulse when a sample is drawn, one cannot rely too heavily upon a single LH value. Secretion of FSH is also pulsatile, but the excursions are less pronounced because of its longer half-life. Patients with gonadotropin adenomas usually retain pulsatile gonadotropin secretion, although the pattern of secretion is more erratic than in normals *(48,69,70)*. It is likely that a significant component of the pulsatile gonadotropins reflects secretion from normal gonadotrope cells *(70)*. Because some degree of stalk compression is present in almost all cases (based on mildly increased prolactin), it is likely that the tumor disrupts the normal input of pulsatile GnRH and thereby decreases LH secretion from normal gonadotropes. Because many patients secrete more FSH than LH from their tumors, it is possible that a chronic imbalance in the gonadotropins leads to impaired testosterone production, but this is only conjecture at present.

Another potential explanation for the paradoxical hypogonadism involves a variety of laboratory artifacts in the measurement of immunoreactive LH. In the past, most polyclonal antibodies against LH had significant crossreactivity with the free α- and LHβ-subunits *(54,71)*. Consequently, tumors that secreted excess amounts of these bioinactive subunits had falsely high measurements for immunoreactive LH (Fig. 6). Thus, the ratio of biologically active to immunologically active LH was reduced in these patients, consistent with the low testosterone levels *(54)*. Most current measurements of LH employ immunoradiometric assays in which the crossreactivity with free subunits is negligible.

Clinical Manifestations in Women

In premenopausal women, FSH-secreting adenomas have been reported to cause ovarian hyperstimulation, leading to the development of multiple ovarian cysts and persistent elevation of serum estradiol *(72)*. However, the majority of patients do not exhibit this manifestation of hormone excess *(54)*. Rather, most women present with hypogonadotropic hypogonadism, presumably because of mass effects of the

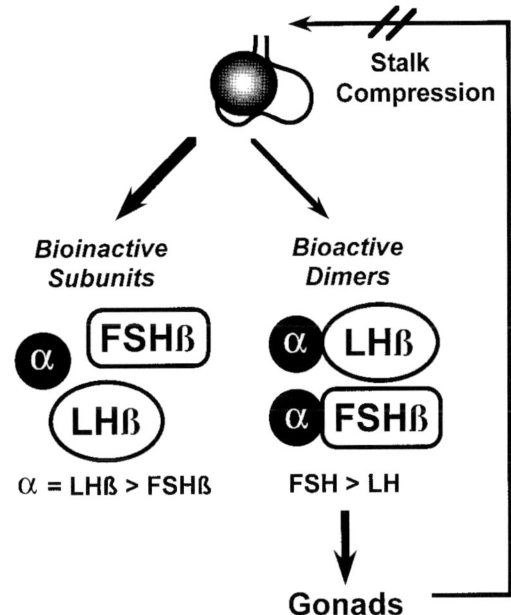

Fig. 5. Schematic illustration of gonadotropin production by gonadotropin secreting pituitary tumors. The tumors typically produce small amounts of intact, biologically active dimers, and disproportionately release bioinactive subunits. Mass effects of the tumor can also lead to impaired GnRH stimulation of normal gonadotropes and mildly elevated prolactin, both of which can cause hypogonadotropic hypogonadism. Adapted with permission from Jameson JL, Kay TWH. Glycoprotein hormone pituitary tumors. In: Advances in Endocrinology and Metabolism, E. Mazzaferri, ed. Mosby-Year Book, St. Louis, vol 2. 1991; pp. 125–147.

tumor. In premenopausal women, this can result in secondary amenorrhea *(1,41,73)*. In postmenopausal women, gonadotropin levels may not be elevated because of stalk compression.

Tests for Gonadotropin Secreting Adenomas

Because most patients present with macroadenomas and mass effects, imaging studies such as MRI or CT scan should be performed routinely in patients suspected of having gonadotropin adenomas. These scans are particularly important because of the difficulty in making the diagnosis on clinical grounds or based upon hormonal testing. In addition, the imaging studies are important for guiding the neurosurgical approach, if indicated. Visual field testing should also be performed. This should include a careful history for visual field loss, which because of compression of the optic chiasm, often involves the superior or lateral visual fields. Confrontation testing is rarely adequate for defining the borders of visual field loss. Ideally, testing should be performed by an ophthalmologist and should include evaluation for optic nerve atrophy and assessment for loss of color vision using a small red object.

Hormone testing should include basal levels of LH, FSH, and testosterone in men, and estrogen in premenopausal women (Table 2). As noted, the spectrum of go-

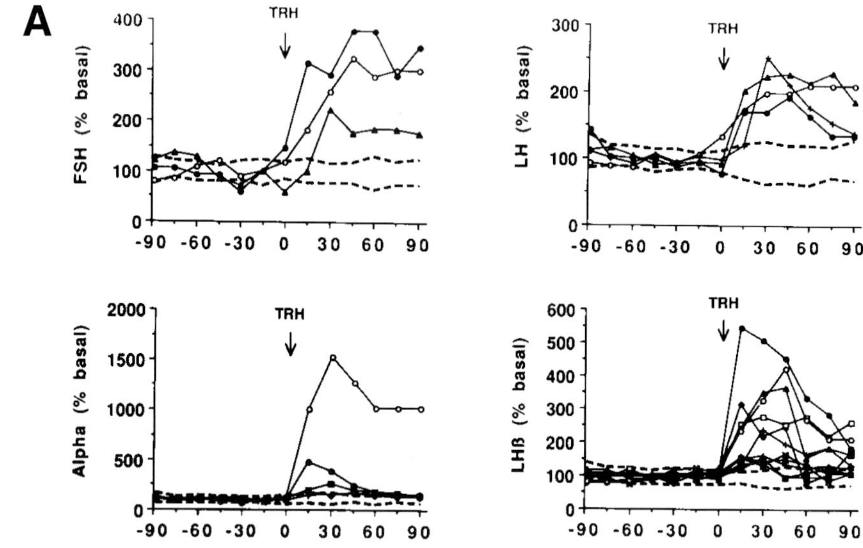

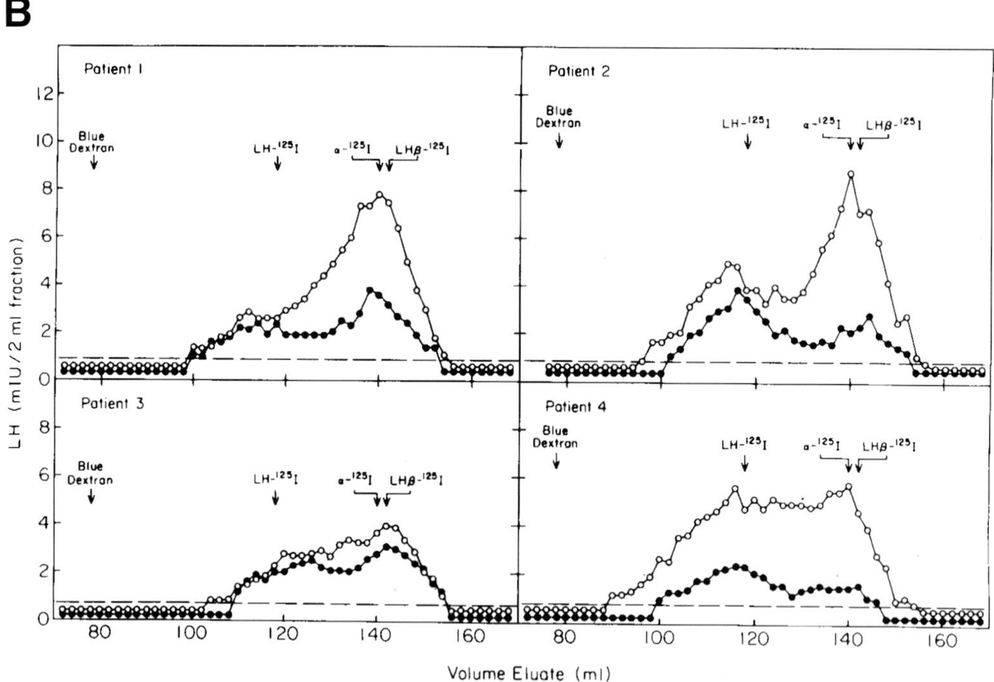

Fig. 6. TRH stimulation of gonadotropin subunits in gonadotropin secreting pituitary tumors. **(A)** In vivo responses of FSH, LH, α-subunit, and LHβ-subunit to TRH. Normal responses are indicated by dashed lines. Reproduced from ref. *55* with permission. **(B)** In vitro separation of serum LH and LHβ subunits secreted at baseline (closed circles) and after TRH stimulation (open circles). Reproduced from ref. *54* with permission.

nadotropins and sex steroids that can be seen is broad. Nevertheless, the basal levels might reveal hypergonadotropism, which can provide a tumor marker. Low levels of LH and FSH raise the possibility of hypopituitarism. Prolactin levels are of value for two reasons—first, to exclude a prolactinoma, in which case the levels are typically > 200 ng/mL; second, to evaluate the possibility of significant stalk compression, in which case the levels are typically 20–50 ng/mL. Although partial hypopituitarism is common, it is usually not necessary to perform extensive testing preoperatively. Basal thyroid function tests and a morning plasma cortisol level will usually identify patients with significant TSH or ACTH deficiency. Because pituitary function may be altered after surgery *(57)*, it is generally reasonable to reserve more extensive testing until the postoperative period. Moreover, administration of glucocorticoids during and after surgery provides adequate coverage for possible adrenal insufficiency.

Based upon other types of pituitary tumors such as Cushing's disease, one might expect that suppression testing could be useful for detecting gonadotropin producing tumors. Unfortunately, these tests have not been proven very helpful in the case of gonadotropin adenomas. Responses in normals have not been rigorously validated, and the tumors appear to vary in their responses to sex steroid administration *(65,74–76)*. However, this approach has not been evaluated extensively, especially using newer assays for gonadotropins and their subunits. GnRH stimulates gonadotropin levels in at least half of patients *(54,75,77)*, but does not reliably distinguish secretion from tumor tissue vs the normal pituitary.

The most useful hormone test for detecting gonadotropin adenomas is the TRH test *(40,53,55,56)*. Although gonadotrope cells do not normally secrete gonadotropins in response to TRH, approximately 30–70% of patients with clinically nonfunctioning pituitary adenomas secrete gonadotropins or their subunits in response to TRH stimulation. This test takes advantage of an inappropriate hormonal response and is analogous to the secretion of GH in response to TRH in patients with acromegaly. Among the responses to TRH, measurement of free LHβ appears to be most helpful. After administration of 200 μg of TRH, a 50% or greater increase in LHβ is seen in between one-third and two-thirds of patients with clinically nonfunctioning pituitary adenomas *(40,55,56,78)*. Accordingly, gonadotropin secreting pituitary adenomas can be recognized, even in postmenopausal women, by measuring the serum LHβ response to TRH, and this may also serve as a marker for residual disease *(78)*.

The composition of the TRH-responsive gonadotropins has been analyzed using gel filtration chromatography. LH immunoreactivity is typically comprised of two main peaks; one peak corresponds to intact LH and the other corresponds to the uncombined subunits, LHβ and α (Fig. 6) *(54)*. Serum FSH predominantly consists of intact FSH, although increased amounts of the uncombined FSHβ-subunit can also be identified using subunit-specific assays *(35)*.

Using immunohistochemistry 7B2 has been shown to be localized in the gonadotrope cells of the pituitary gland *(79)*, and immunoreactive 7B2 increases in response to GnRH in normal subjects *(80)*. It has been reported that some gonadotropin secreting adenomas exhibit basal elevation of plasma 7B2 and increased responses after GnRH or GnRH/TRH *(80–82)*. Thus, 7B2 may be an additional marker for gonadotropin producing pituitary adenomas, although it remains unclear whether this response distinguishes normals from patients with tumors. Similarly, chromogranin A is detected in gonadotropin secreting adenomas and is subject to regulation by GnRH. It, too, may provide an additional marker for classifying these tumors *(83–85)*.

Differential Diagnosis

Because most patients with gonadotropin secreting adenomas are identified because of mass effects of the tumor, an important first step is to exclude other types of pituitary tumors and causes of sellar masses. Usually, acromegaly and Cushing's disease can be excluded on clinical grounds. However, subtle cases may require hormonal testing to unequivocally exclude these disorders. The most important tumor to exclude is a prolactinoma. These tumors can be easily confused with gonadotropin producing pituitary tumors because prolactinomas can also result in hypogonadism. Moreover, many gonadotropin producing adenomas result in mild hyperprolactinema because of mass effects. A variety of other sellar lesions including Rathke's cleft cysts and craniopharyngiomas can usually be excluded based upon their radiographic appearance.

In the rare circumstance in which LH elevation is accompanied by increased serum testosterone, one should suspect a gonadotrope adenoma that secretes intact and bioactive LH *(48,63)*. The differential diagnosis is not extensive. An hCG-producing tumor should be excluded, particularly if the assay for LH crossreacts with hCG (which it often does). An androgen insensitivity syndrome can result in a similar pattern of hormone levels, but should be readily recognized because of incomplete virilization. Patients with androgen insensitivity are not predisposed to pituitary adenomas, and they do not have pituitary masses as in the case of LH-secreting adenomas. Supranormal FSH and LH levels that are not accompanied by elevation of serum testosterone must be distinguished from primary hypogonadism *(16,18,86)*. The majority of patients with gonadotropin-secreting adenomas have normal gonadal function based upon fertility history and testicular responses to exogenous hCG *(18)*. As noted above, the diagnosis of gonadotropin-producing tumors is even more challenging in women because of variable gonadotropin levels during the normal menstrual cycle, and elevation of gonadotropins after menopause. In young women with gonadotropin-secreting adenomas that hypersecrete gonadotropins, the LH and FSH levels might suggest premature ovarian failure. However, their estradiol levels are high rather than low. Excess secretion of LH relative to FSH is rare, but could raise the possibility of polycystic ovarian syndrome.

TREATMENT

Because gonadotropin-secreting adenomas usually come to diagnosis as result of visual or neurological symptoms, the treatment should be directed at the reducing adenoma mass and correcting visual loss (Table 3). Transsphenoidal surgery is usually the first line of treatment. Radiation therapy can be used to treat residual tumor mass or to prevent tumor recurrence after surgery. Although various pharmacologic agents such as analogs of dopamine and somatostatin, and GnRH agonists and antagonists have been used to treat gonadotropin-secreting adenomas, these treatments are not very effective in reducing tumor mass.

Table 3
Treatment of Gonadotropin Secreting Adenomas

Primary Therapy
Transsphenoidal surgery
Radiotherapy
Adjunctive Medical Therapy
Dopamine agonists
Somatostatin analogs
Gonadotropin releasing hormone antagonists

Surgery

At the time of presentation, many gonadotropin-producing tumors exhibit suprasellar or parasellar extension and local mass effects. Transsphenoidal reduction of tumor volume can allow collapse of additional tumor tissue into the sella. Vision is improved in the majority (70–80%) of patients who have abnormal visual fields due to compression of the optic chiasm *(59,87–89)*. Improvements in visual fields can often be appreciated in the early postoperative period, but it is more difficult to reverse long-standing visual loss. In a subset of patients, hypopituitarism can also be reversed by surgery, presumably owing to reduced stalk compression or pressure on the hypothalamus *(57,89)*. Transcranial and subfrontal surgery are employed less commonly because of the increased risk of serious side-effects that accompany invasion of the cranium and retraction of neural tissue.

Preoperative MRI or CT scans are important for planning surgery and are useful for predicting the outcome of surgery. Large macroadenomas, especially those with parasellar or cavernous sinus invasion, are rarely cured by surgery. Unlike patients with acromegaly or Cushing's disease, patients with gonadotropin secreting tumors do not experience adverse effects from excessive hormone secretion. Consequently, leaving small amounts of tumor tissue in inaccessible areas of the sella or parasellar regions is not as deleterious as in cases of other types of hormone-secreting pituitary tumors. For this reason, surgeons must balance the benefits of extensive tumor resection vs additional risks of complications. Recurrence rates have been reported to occur in approximately 15–25% of patients over a 4- to 8-yr period *(59,87)*. The reappearance of visual field deficit usually necessitates repeat surgery, which is associated with increased complications because of previous distortion of anatomy and scar formation *(90)*.

Many patients with gonadotropin secreting tumors have preoperative partial or complete hypopituitarism *(57,59,60)*. Significant diabetes insipidus is rare and can usually be detected from the history. Thyroid function tests can reveal secondary or tertiary hypothyroidism. It should be remembered that TSH alone is not a useful screening test in the setting of hypothalamic or pituitary disease. A low free T4 and low or normal TSH are consistent with TSH insufficiency *(91)*. Whenever possible, l-thyroxine replacement should be instituted preoperatively. However, in urgent situations, surgery can proceed safely in hypothyroid patients if adjustments are made for altered drug pharmacokinetics and perioperative care *(92)*. Most patients are covered with adequate doses of glucocorticoids during the perioperative period. If glucocorticoids are stopped after only a few days of treatment, a morning cortisol before discharge can provide an index of whether treatment should continue pending formal evaluation of the HPA axis. If the plasma cortisol is < 18 μg/dL, glucocorticoid replacement (e.g., prednisone 5 mg qAM; 2.5 mg qPM) should be continued until testing several weeks later.

Complications of transsphenoidal surgery are relatively uncommon and are increased in large tumors that extend outside of the sella *(59,60,93–95)*. In general, surgery-related mortality is on the order of 1% and serious complications including hemorrhage, CSF rhinorrhea, infection, and damage to optic and oculomotor nerves occur in approximately 5–10% of cases. Transient diabetes insipidus is relatively common and can usually be managed with aqueous vasopressin or DDAVP in conjunction with adequate fluid replacement. Although many patients will experience an improvement in pitui-tary function after surgery, an equal number will develop additional evidence of hypopituitarism *(57,59,60,88)*.

Postoperative evaluation for residual tumor, visual fields, and pituitary function is usually performed 4–8 wk after surgery. Visual fields should be formally tested by an ophthalmologist. Neuroradiological studies can be repeated to evaluate residual tumor. Although some surgeons prefer to image soon after surgery, it is advantageous to defer imaging until 3–6 mo after surgery because it can be difficult to distinguish surgical material and hemorrhage from residual tumor in earlier studies *(59)*. Subsequently, imaging can be performed at progressively longer intervals if there is no evidence of recurrence *(96)*.

For the same reason that gonadotropin tumors are difficult to diagnose based upon hormone levels, basal LH and FSH may not be of great value for detecting residual tumor tissue. Exceptions include α-subunit producing tumors, or tumors that secrete LHβ- or FSHβ-subunits in response to TRH. Reductions in hormone secretion are likely to correlate with removal of tumor *(89)*. Postoperative testing for residual pituitary function is similar to that for other types of pituitary tumors. A history of polyuria or nocturia should prompt 24-h collections for urine volume and evaluation of serum and urine osmolality. If necessary, a water deprivation test can be performed, and DDAVP can be instituted if diabetes insipidus is diagnosed. Mild diabetes insipidus can sometimes be treated with chlorpropamide as long as adequate precautions are taken to avoid hypoglycemia *(97,98)*. In the absence of contraindications, an insulin tolerance test can be used to evaluate ACTH and GH reserve. If an insulin tolerance test cannot be performed, low morning cortisol levels (when off glucocorticoid replacement) indicates the likely need for cortisol replacement. At present, there are no clear guidelines concerning growth hormone replacement in adults. As above, the evaluation of thyroid function must include a free T4 level as well as TSH. In men, if the testosterone level is low on several occasions, consideration should be given to replacement either by im injections q2–3 wk, or using a patch. In women, absent menses in conjunction with low estradiol levels should prompt consideration of estrogen/progesterone replacement to prevent osteoporosis and increased cardiovascular risk. In general, evidence for deficiency of one pituitary hormone raises the likelihood that there may be decreased reserve for others. When test results are not clear-cut, our practice is to provide hormone replacement being cautious to avoid overtreatment.

Radiation Therapy

The issue of when to use radiation treatment is controversial. Although the effects of radiation are slow, it may be appropriate as primary treatment for some patients who refuse, or cannot tolerate transsphenoidal surgery. Gamma knife radiosurgery may offer another alternative in these circumstances, but is primarily useful for small tumors that do not impinge on surrounding neural structures *(99)*. More commonly, radiation therapy is used as adjunctive treatment after surgery. Because hormone secretion is not a major issue, the primary indication for radiation is to induce further tumor regression and to prevent recurrence. Because the rate of tumor growth is usually slow, one approach is to assess the efficacy of initial surgery. If substantial tumor has been removed and the risk of recurrent mass effects is low, one could withhold radiation unless there is evidence for regrowth. On the other hand, if surgery accomplishes minimal reduction in tumor volume, radiotherapy offers a reasonably effective alternative for preventing further growth *(100)*. Conventional supervoltage radiotherapy is usually administered at a dose of about 45 Gy, divided over 20–25 doses.

The short-term side-effects of radiation therapy include fatigue and nausea, and some patients develop impaired taste or smell. Severe complications of radiation are rare, especially when the dose and field size are planned carefully *(94,100,101)*. These can include brain atrophy and necrosis, optic nerve damage, and secondary tumors *(102,103)*. Hypopituitarism is common, but it develops gradually over several years. Generally, the primary effect of radiation is on hypothalamic function, but there may be components of combined hypothalamic and pituitary deficiency. It should be emphasized that 50–80% of the patients will develop partial or panhypopituitarism after 10 yr of follow-up *(104–106)*. Therefore, it is important that these patients be evaluated for hormone deficiency at least yearly.

Medical Treatment

DOPAMINE AGONISTS

Dopamine acts via dopamine D2 receptors which have been identified in many pituitary adenomas, including glycoprotein secreting tumors *(107,108)*. Dopamine agonists, such as bromocriptine, are highly effective in the treatment of prolactinomas *(109)*. Dopamine suppresses gonadotropin secretion and reduces gonadotropin subunit mRNA accumulation in tumor tissue removed from patients with gonadotropin secreting adenomas *(110)*. In vitro studies have also shown that dopamine induces a time-dependent decrease in gonadotropin secretion from tumors maintained in long-term culture *(111)*. There are a number of case reports in which bromocriptine has been shown to lower serum gonadotropins and free α-subunit concentrations in patients with gonadotropin-secreting adenomas *(110,112–114)*. Although occasional patients respond to dopaminergic therapy *(110,112–115)*, the majority derive little benefit in terms of tumor reduction *(108)*. CV 205–502, a recently developed D2 receptor agonist, has been reported to reduce gonadotropin secretion and tumor size in some patients *(116)*. Because a subset of patients exhibit a clinically significant response to dopamine agonists, they represent a valuable adjunctive treatment in patients who are experiencing mass effects or clinical features of excess gonadotropin secretion. However, there is little justification for using these drugs in the majority of patients with gonadotropin-producing adenomas.

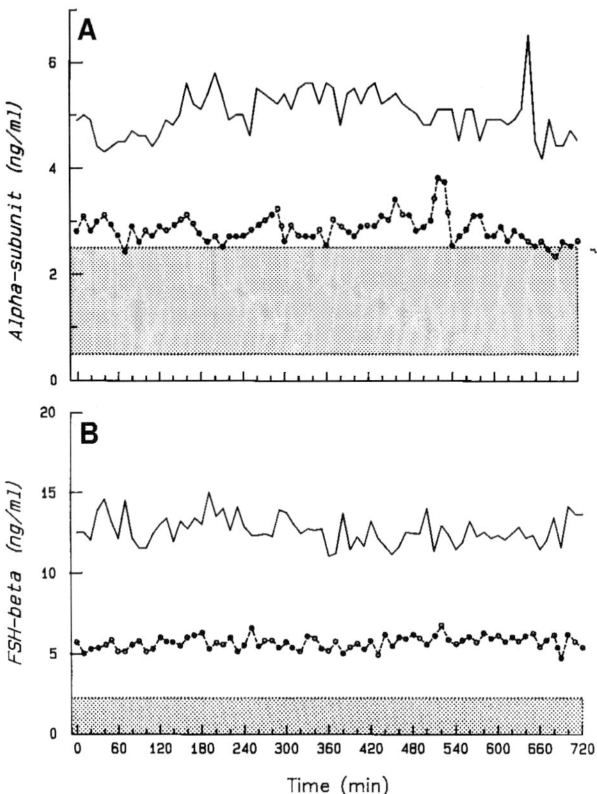

Fig. 7. Persistent agonist effects of a long acting GnRH analog in patients with gonadotropin secreting adenomas. After 4–8 wk of treatment with a long acting GnRH agonist, increased levels of alpha-subunit (panel A) and FSHβ-subunit are illustrated in two different patients. Hormone levels were determined by q10 min sampling over 12 h. Levels before treatment are shown by circles; levels after treatment are indicated by a solid line. Normal range is shown as a hatched area. Reproduced from ref. *69* with permission.

Somatostatin Analogs

Somatostatin and its analogs have been shown to have antiproliferative actions on a number of human tumors, including GH-secreting pituitary adenomas *(117–120)*. Somatostatin acts via a family of receptors which have different affinities for specific somatostatin analogs *(121–123)*. Five subtypes of somatostatin receptors have been identified *(124)*, and subtypes 2 and 5 mediate the inhibitory actions of somatostatin on GH secreting adenomas *(125)*. Somatostatin receptors have been detected in vivo in patients with clinically nonfunctioning pituitary adenomas using labeled somatostatin analogs *(126)*. Glycoprotein hormone subunit secretion is suppressed by somatostatin in a subset of adenomas studied in vitro *(127)*, suggesting that somatostatin analogs may be capable of exerting effects on gonadotropin secreting adenomas.

In a few cases, the somatostatin analog, Octreotide, has been shown to suppress LH or α-subunit secretion or to improve visual fields *(119,120,128–131)*. However, like treatment with dopamine agonists, the majority of patients with gonadotropin-secreting

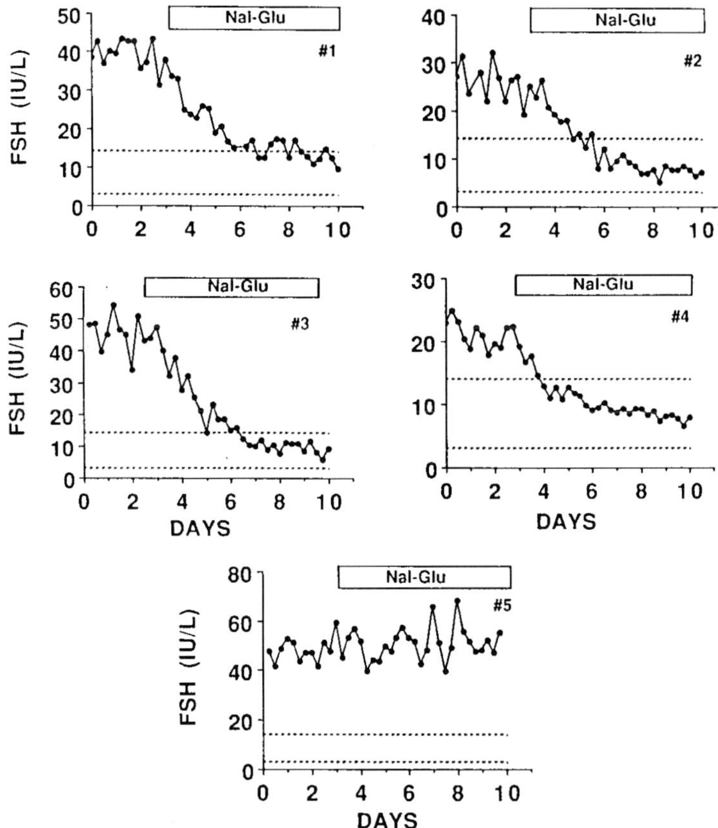

Fig. 8. Effect of a GnRH antagonist on FSH secretion in gonadotropin secreting pituitary adenomas. Short-term administration of the Nal-Glu GnRH antagonist suppressed FSH levels to normal in four of five patients. Reproduced from ref. *141* with permission.

adenomas exhibit modest responses in terms of tumor size. Nevertheless, somatostatin analogs should be considered when other forms of treatment are unsuccessful.

GnRH Agonists and Antagonists

Chronic administration of long acting GnRH agonists desensitizes GnRH receptors and decreases gonadotropin secretion from the normal gonadotrope cell *(19)*. Recent studies have confirmed expression of the GnRH receptor in pituitary tumors *(49)*. Based on the rationale that GnRH-induced desensitization might inhibit tumor growth, long acting agonists have been tried in patients with gonadotropin-secreting adenomas (Fig. 7). However, with rare exceptions, no reduction of gonadotropin secretion was observed; on the contrary, many patients exhibit an unanticipated persistent stimulatory effect on hormone secretion from the tumor *(69,132–136)*. Although there is no evidence that this treatment stimulates tumor growth, this is a theoretical concern and the absence of effective desensitization argues against their use.

Recently, a group of true GnRH antagonists have been developed. These agents act by blocking GnRH action rather than by stimulating and then desensitizing the receptor. For example, the GnRH antagonist, Nal-Glu-GnRH, produces profound and immediate hypogonadotropic hypogonadism in healthy subjects *(137–139)*. Short- and long-term administration of Nal-Glu-GnRH can reduce the secretion of FSH in patients with gonadotropin-secreting adenomas *(140–142)* (Fig. 8). However, no reduction of tumor size has been reported. Thus, GnRH antagonists can suppress excess hormone secretion, but the tumors do not appear to be particularly sensitive to GnRH deprivation.

REFERENCES

1. Beitins IZ, Lipson LG, McArthur JW. Immunoreactive luteinizing hormone, follicle stimulating hormone and their subunits in tissue culture media from normal and adenomatous, human pituitary fragments. J Clin Endocrinol Metab 1977; 45:1271–1280.
2. Asa SL, Gerrie BM, Singer W, Horvath E, Kovacs K, Smyth HS. Gonadotropin secretion in vitro by human pituitary null cell adenomas and oncocytomas. J Clin Endocrinol Metab 1986; 62:1011–1019.
3. Black PM, Hsu DW, Klibanski A, Kliman B, Jameson JL, Ridgway EC, Hedley-Whyte ET, Zervas NT. Hormone production in clinically nonfunctioning pituitary adenomas. J Neurosurg 1987; 66:244–50.
4. Jameson JL, Klibanski A, Black PM, Zervas NT, Lindell CM, Hsu DW, Ridgway EC, Habener JF. Glycoprotein hormone genes are expressed in clinically nonfunctioning pituitary adenomas. J Clin Invest 1987; 80:1472–1478.
5. Landolt AM, Heitz PU. Alpha-subunit-producing pituitary adenomas. Immunocytochemical and ultrastructural studies. Virchows Arch A Pathol Anat Histopathol 1986; 409:417–431.
6. Lipson LG, Beitins IZ, Kornblith PD, McArthur JW, Friesen HG, Kliman B, Kjellberg RN. Tissue culture studies on human pituitary tumours: radioimmunoassayable anterior pituitary hormones in the culture medium. Acta Endocrinol 1978; 88:239–249.
7. Mashiter K, Adams E, Van Noorden S. Secretion of LH, FSH, and PRL shown by cell culture and immunocytochemistry of human functionless pituitary adenomas. Clin Endocrinol 1981; 15:103–112.
8. Miura M, Matsukado Y, Kodama T, Mihara Y. Clinical and histopathological characteristics of gonadotropin-producing pituitary adenomas. J Neurosurg 1985; 62:376–382.
9. Snyder PJ. Clinically nonfunctioning pituitary adenomas. Endocrinol Metab Clin North Am 1993; 22:163–175.
10. Trouillas J, Girod C, Sassolas G, Claustrat B, Lheritier M, Dubois MP, Goutelle A. Human pituitary gonadotropic adenoma; histological, immunocytochemical, and ultrastructural and hormonal studies in eight cases. J Pathol 1981; 135:315–336.
11. Kwekkeboom DJ, de Jong FH, Lamberts SW. Gonadotropin release by clinically nonfunctioning and gonadotroph pituitary adenomas in vivo and in vitro: relation to sex and effects of thyrotropin-releasing hormone, gonadotropin-releasing hormone, and bromocriptine. J Clin Endocrinol Metab 1989; 68:1128–1135.
12. Yamada S, Asa SL, Kovacs K, Muller P, Smyth HS. Analysis of hormone secretion by clinically nonfunctioning human pituitary adenomas using the reverse hemolytic plaque assay. J Clin Endocrinol Metab 1989; 68:73–80.
13. De Nicola AF, von Lawzewitsch I, Kaplan SE, Libertun C. Biochemical and ultrastructural studies on estrogen-induced pituitary tumors in F344 rats. J Natl Cancer Inst 1978; 61:753–763.
14. Jameson JL, Weiss J, Polak JM, Childs GV, Bloom SR, Steel JH, Capen CC, Prentice DE, Fetter AW, Langloss JM. Glycoprotein hormone alpha-subunit-producing pituitary adenomas in rats treated for one year with calcitonin. Am J Pathol 1992; 140:75–84.
15. Mayo KE, Hammer RE, Swanson LW, Brinster RL, Rosenfeld MG, Evans RM. Dramatic pituitary hyperplasia in transgenic mice expressing a human growth hormone-releasing factor gene. Mol Endocrinol 1988; 2:606–612.
16. Bower BF. Pituitary enlargement secondary to untreated primary hypogonadism. Ann Intern Med 1968; 69:107–109.
17. Samaan NA, Stepanas AV, Danziger J, Trujillo J. Reactive pituitary abnormalities in patients with Klinefelter's and Turner's syndromes. Arch Intern Med 1979; 139:198–201.

18. Snyder PJ, Bigdeli H, Gardner DF, Mihailovic V, Rudenstein RS, Sterling FH, Utiger RD. Gonadal function in fifty men with untreated pituitary adenomas. J Clin Endocrinol Metab 1979; 48:309–314.
19. Crowley WF, Filicori M, Spratt DI, Santoro NF. The physiology of gonadotropin-releasing hormone (GnRH) secretion in men and women. Recent Prog Horm Res 1985; 41:473–531.
20. Johnson GL, Dhanasekaran N. The G-protein family and their interaction with receptors. Endocr Rev 1989; 10:317–331.
21. Alexander JM, Biller BM, Bikkal H, Zervas NT, Arnold A, Klibanski A. Clinically nonfunctioning pituitary tumors are monoclonal in origin. J Clin Invest 1990; 86:336–340.
22. Herman V, Fagin J, Gonsky R, Kovacs K, Melmed S. Clonal origin of pituitary adenomas. J Clin Endocrinol Metab 1990; 71:1427–1433.
23. Schulte HM, Oldfield EH, Allolio B, Katz DA, Berkman RA, Ali IU. Clonal composition of pituitary adenomas in patients with Cushing's disease: Determination by X-chromosome inactivation analysis. J Clin Endocrinol Metab 1991; 73:1302–1308.
24. Biller BMK, Alexander JM, Zervas NT, Hedley-Whyte ET, Arnold A, Klibanski A. Clonal origins of adrenocorticotropin-secreting pituitary tissue in Cushing's disease. J Clin Endocrinol Metab 1992; 75:1303–1309.
25. Landis CA, Harsh G, Lyons J, Davis RL, McCormick F, Bourne HR. Clinical characteristics of acromegalic patients whose pituitary tumors contain mutant Gs protein. J Clin Endocrinol Metab 1990; 71:1416–1420.
26. Spada A, Arosio M, Bochicchio A, Bazzoni N, Vallar L, Bassetti M, Faglia G. Clinical, biochemical, and morphological correlates in patients bearing growth hormone-secreting pituitary tumors with or without constitutively active adenylyl cyclase. J Clin Endocrinol Metab 1990; 71:1421–1426.
27. Harris PE, Alexander JM, Bikkal HA, Hsu DW, Hedley-Whyte ET, Klibanski A, Jameson JL. Glycoprotein hormone a subunit production in somatotroph adenomas with and without Gsα mutations. J Clin Endocrinol Metab 1992; 75:918–923.
28. Landis CA, Masters SB, Spada A, Pace AM, Bourne HR, Vallar L. GTPase inhibiting mutations activate the alpha chain of Gs and stimulate adenylyl cyclase in human pituitary tumours. Nature 1989; 340:692–696.
29. Lyons J, Landis CA, Harsh G, Vallar L, Grunewald K, Feichtinger H, Duh QY, Clark OH, Kawasaki E, Bourne HR, et al. Two G protein oncogenes in human endocrine tumors. Science 1990; 249:655–659.
30. Karga HJ, Alexander JM, Hedley-Whyte ET, Klibanski A, Jameson JL. Ras mutations in human pituitary tumors. J Clin Endocrinol Metab 1992; 74:914–919.
31. Cai WY, Alexander JM, Hedley-Whyte ET, Scheithauer BW, Jameson JL, Zervas NT, Klibanski A. Ras mutations in human prolactinomas and carcinomas. J Clin Endocrinol Metab 1994; 78:89–93.
32. Pei L, Melmed S, Scheithauer B, Kovacs K, Prager D. H-ras mutation in human pituitary carcinoma metastasis. J Clin Endocrinol Metab 1994; 78:842–846.
33. Jameson JL. Molecular pathogenesis of pituitary tumors: An Overview. In: Melmed S, ed. Molecular and Clinical Advances in Piuitary Disorders. Third International Pituitary Congress, Marina del Ray, 1993; pp. 15–19.
34. Thakker RV, Pook MA, Wooding C, Boscaro M, Scanarini M, Clayton RN. Association of somatotropinomas with loss of alleles on chromosome 11 and GSP mutation. J Clin Invest 1993; 91:2815–2821.
35. Snyder PJ, Bashey HM, Phillips JL, Gennarelli TA. Comparison of hormonal secretory behavior of gonadotroph cell adenomas in vivo and in culture. J Clin Endocrinol Metab 1985; 61:1061–1065.
36. Surmont DW, Winslow CL, Loizou M, White MC, Adams EF, Mashiter K. Gonadotrophin and alpha subunit secretion by human 'functionless' pituitary adenomas in cell culture: long term effects of luteinizing hormone releasing hormone and thyrotrophin releasing hormone. Clin Endocrinol (Oxf) 1983; 19:325–336.
37. Horvath E, Kovacs K. Anatomy and histology of the normal and abnormal pituitary gland. In: DeGroot LJ, ed. Endocrinology. W. B. Saunders, Philadelphia, PA, 1995, 160–177.
38. Corless CL, Matzuk MM, Ramabhadran TV, Krichevsky A, Boime I. Gonadotropin beta subunits determine the rate of assembly and the oligosaccharide processing of hormone dimer in transfected cells. J Cell Biol 1987; 104:1173–1181.
39. Matzuk MM, Kornmeier CM, Whitfield GK, Kourides IA, Boime I. The glycoprotein alpha-subunit is critical for secretion and stability of the human thyrotropin beta-subunit. Mol Endocrinol 1992; 2:95–100.
40. Snyder PJ. Gonadotroph cell adenomas of the pituitary. Endocr 1985; Rev 6:552–563.

41. Katznelson L, Alexander JM, Bikkal HA, Jameson JL, Hsu DW, Klibanski A. Imbalanced follicle-stimulating hormone beta-subunit hormone biosynthesis in human pituitary adenomas. J Clin Endocrinol Metab 1992; 74:1343–1351.
42. Weiss J, Harris PE, Halvorson LM, Crowley WF, Jr., Jameson JL. Dynamic regulation of follicle-stimulating hormone-beta messenger ribonucleic acid levels by activin and gonadotropin-releasing hormone in perifused rat pituitary cells. Endocrinology 1992; 131:1403–1408.
43. Weiss J, Crowley WF, Jr., Halvorson LM, Jameson JL. Perifusion of rat pituitary cells with gonadotropin-releasing hormone, activin, and inhibin reveals distinct effects on gonadotropin gene expression and secretion. Endocrinology 1993; 132:2307–2311.
44. Alexander JM, Jameson JL, Bikkal HA, Schwall RH, Klibanski A. The effects of activin on follicle-stimulating hormone secretion and biosynthesis in human glycoprotein hormone-producing pituitary adenomas. J Clin Endocrinol Metab 1991; 72:1261–1267.
45. Alexander JM, Swearingen B, Tindall GT, Klibanski A. Human pituitary adenomas express endogenous inhibin subunit and follistatin messenger ribonucleic acids. J Clin Endocrinol Metab 1995; 80:147–152.
46. Haddad G, Penabad JL, Bashey HM, Asa SL, Gennarelli TA, Cirullo R, Snyder PJ. Expression of activin/inhibin subunit messenger ribonucleic acids by gonadotroph adenomas. J Clin Endocrinol Metab 1994; 79:1399–1403.
47. Jameson JL, Lindell CM, Habener JF. Gonadotropin and thyrotropin alpha- and beta-subunit gene expression in normal and neoplastic tissues characterized using specific messenger ribonucleic acid hybridization probes. J Clin Endocrinol Metab 1987; 64:319–327.
48. Klibanski A, Deutsch PJ, Jameson JL, Ridgway EC, Crowley WF, Hsu DW, Habener JF, Black PM. Luteinizing hormone-secreting pituitary tumor: biosynthetic characterization and clinical studies. J Clin Endocrinol Metab 1987; 64:536–542.
49. Alexander JM, Klibanski A. Gonadotropin-releasing hormone receptor mRNA expression by human pituitary tumors in vitro. J Clin Invest 1994; 93:2332–2339.
50. Kilar F, Muhr C, Funa K. In situ hybridization histochemistry of mRNAs for hormones and chromogranins in normal pituitary tissue and pituitary adenoma. Acta Endocrinol (Copenh) 1991; 125:628–636.
51. Croue A, Beldent V, Rousselet MC, Guy G, Rohmer V, Bigorgne JC, Saint-Andre JP. Contribution of immunohistochemistry, electron microscopy, and cell culture to the characterization of nonfunctioning pituitary adenomas: a study of 40 cases. Hum Pathol 1992; 23:1332–1339.
52. Horvath E, Kovacs K. Gonadotroph adenomas of the human pituitary: sex-related fine-structural dichotomy. A histologic, immunocytochemical, and electron- microscopic study of 30 tumors. Am J Pathol 1984; 117:429–440.
53. Nobels FR, Kwekkeboom DJ, Coopmans W, Hoekstra R, De Herder WW, Bouillon R, Lamberts SW. A comparison between the diagnostic value of gonadotropins, alpha- subunit, and chromogranin-A and their response to thyrotropin- releasing hormone in clinically nonfunctioning, alpha-subunit- secreting, and gonadotroph pituitary adenomas. J Clin Endocrinol Metab 1993; 77:784–789.
54. Snyder PJ, Bashey HM, Kim SU, Chappel SC. Secretion of uncombined subunits of luteinizing hormone by gonadotroph cell adenomas. J Clin Endocrinol Metab 1984; 59:1169–1175.
55. Daneshdoost L, Gennarelli TA, Bashey HM, Savino PJ, Sergott RC, Bosley TM, Snyder PJ. Recognition of gonadotroph adenomas in women. N Engl J Med 1991; 324:589–594.
56. Daneshdoost L, Gennarelli TA, Bashey HM, Savino PJ, Sergott RC, Bosley TM, Snyder PJ. Identification of gonadotroph adenomas in men with clinically nonfunctioning adenomas by the luteinizing hormone beta subunit response to thyrotropin-releasing hormone. J Clin Endocrinol Metab 1993; 77:1352–1355.
57. Arafah BM. Reversible hypopituitarism in patients with large nonfunctioning pituitary adenomas. J Clin Endocrinol Metab 1986; 62:1173–1179.
58. Arafah BM, Brodkey JS, Manni A, Velasco ME, Kaufman B, Pearson OH. Recovery of pituitary function following surgical removal of large nonfunctioning pituitary adenomas. Clin Endocrinol 1982; 17:213–222.
59. Ebersold MJ, Quast LM, Laws ER, Jr., Scheithauer B, Randall RV. Long-term results in transsphenoidal removal of nonfunctioning pituitary adenomas. J Neurosurg 1986; 64:713–719.
60. Nelson AT, Tucker HS, Becker DP. Residual anterior pituitary function following transsphenoidal resection of pituitary macroadenomas. J Neurosurg 1984; 61:577–580.
61. Wakai S, Fukushima T, Teramoto A, Sano K. Pituitary apoplexy: its incidence and clinical significance. J Neurosurg 1981; 55:187–193.

62. Heseltine D, White MC, Kendall-Taylor P, De Kretser DM, Kelly W. Testicular enlargement and elevated serum inhibin concentrations occur in patients with pituitary macroadenomas secreting follicle stimulating hormone. Clin Endocrinol 1989; 31:411–423.
63. Peterson RE, Kourides IA, Horwith M, Vaughan E, Jr., Saxena BB, Fraser RA. Luteinizing hormone- and alpha-subunit-secreting pituitary tumor: positive feedback of estrogen. J Clin Endocrinol Metab 1981; 52:692–698.
64. Faggiano M, Criscuolo T, Perrone L, Quarto C, Sinisi AA. Sexual precocity in a boy due to hypersecretion of LH and prolactin by a pituitary adenoma. Acta Endocrinol 1983; (Copenh) 102:167–172.
65. Ambrosi B, Bassetti M, Ferrario R, Medri G, Giannattasio G, Faglia G. Precocious puberty in a boy with a PRL-, LH- and FSH-secreting pituitary tumour: hormonal and immunocytochemical studies. Acta Endocrinol (Copenh) 1990; 122:569–576.
66. Harman SM, Tsitouras PD, Costa PT, Blackman MR. Reproductive hormones in aging men. II. Basal pituitary gonadotropins and gonadotropin responses to luteinizing hormone-releasing hormone. J Clin Endocrinol Metab 1982; 54:547–551.
67. Gray A, Feldman HA, McKinlay JB, Longcope C. Age, disease, and changing sex hormone levels in middle-aged men: results of the Massachusetts Male Aging Study. J Clin Endocrinol Metab 1991; 73:1016–1025.
68. Crowley WF, Whitcomb RW, Jameson JL, Weiss J, Finkelstein JS, O'Dea LS. Neuroendocrine control of human reproduction in the male. Recent Prog Horm Res 1991; 47:27–67.
69. Klibanski A, Jameson JL, Biller BM, Crowley WF, Jr., Zervas NT, Rivier J, Vale WW, Bikkal H. Gonadotropin and alpha-subunit responses to chronic gonadotropin- releasing hormone analog administration in patients with glycoprotein hormone-secreting pituitary tumors. J Clin Endocrinol Metab 1989; 68:81–86.
70. Samuels MH, Henry P, Kleinschmidt-Demasters BK, Lillehei K, Ridgway EC. Pulsatile glycoprotein hormone secretion in glycoprotein-producing pituitary tumors. J Clin Endocrinol Metab 1991; 73:1281–1288.
71. Ridgway EC, Klibanski A, Ladenson PW, Clemmons D, Beitins IZ, McArthur JW, Martorana MA, Zervas NT. Pure alpha-secreting pituitary adenomas. N Engl J Med 1981; 304:1254–1259.
72. Djerassi A, Coutifaris C, West VA, Asa SL, Kapoor SC, Pavlou SN, Snyder PJ. Gonadotroph adenoma in a premenopausal woman secreting follicle-stimulating hormone and causing ovarian hyperstimulation. J Clin Endocrinol Metab 1995; 80:591–594.
73. Cook DM, Watkins S, Snyder PJ. Gonadotrophin-secreting pituitary adenomas masquerading as primary ovarian failure. Clin Endocrinol (Oxf) 1986; 25:729–738.
74. Cunningham GR, Huckins C. An FSH and prolactin-secreting pituitary tumor: pituitary dynamics and testicular histology. J Clin Endocrinol Metab 1977; 44:248–253.
75. Friend JN, Judge DM, Sherman BM, Santen RJ. FSH-secreting pituitary adenomas: stimulation and suppression studies in two patients. J Clin Endocrinol Metab 1976; 43:650–657.
76. Chapman AJ, MacFarlane IA, Shalet SM, Beardwell CG, Dutton J, Sutton ML. Discordant serum alpha-subunit and FSH concentrations in a woman with a pituitary tumour. Clin Endocrinol (Oxf) 1984; 21:123–129.
77. MacFarlane IA, Beardwell CG, Shalet SM, Ainslie G, Rankin E. Glycoprotein hormone alpha-subunit secretion in patients with pituitary adenomas: influence of TRH, LRH and bromocriptine. Acta Endocrinol (Copenh) 1982; 99:487–492.
78. Gil-del-Alamo P, Pettersson KS, Saccomanno K, Spada A, Faglia G, Beck-Peccoz P. Abnormal response of luteinizing hormone beta subunit to thyrotrophin-releasing hormone in patients with non-functioning pituitary adenoma. Clin Endocrinol 1994; 41:661–666.
79. Steel JH, Van Noorden S, Ballesta J, Gibson SJ, Ghatei MA, Burrin J, Leonhardt U, Domin J, Bloom SR, Polak JM. Localization of 7B2, neuromedin B, and neuromedin U in specific cell types of rat, mouse, and human pituitary, in rat hypothalamus, and in 30 human pituitary and extrapituitary tumors. Endocrinology 1988; 122:270–282.
80. Natori S, Iguchi H, Ohashi M, Chretien M, Nawata H. LHRH increases plasma 7B2 concentration in normal human subjects. Endocrinol Jpn 1989; 36:367–371.
81. Iguchi H, Demura R, Yasuda D, Wakasugi H. Effect of LHRH on plasma 7B2 in patients with gonadotropin-producing pituitary adenomas. Horm Metab Res 1992; 24:31–33.
82. Venetikou MS, Ghatei MA, Burrin JM, Latif S, Bloom SR. 7B2, a new protein secreted by human functionless pituitary tumours, in vitro. Acta Endocrinol 1988; 118:521–527.

83. Lloyd RV, Wilson BS, Kovacs K, Ryan N. Immunohistochemical localization of chromogranin in human hypophyses and pituitary adenomas. Arch Pathol Lab Med 1985; 109:515–517.
84. Deftos LJ, O'Connor DT, Wilson CB, Fitzgerald PA. Human pituitary tumors secrete chromogranin-A. J Clin Endocrinol Metab 1989; 68:869–872.
85. Song JY, Jin L, Chandler WF, England BG, Smart JB, Landefeld TD, Lloyd RV. Gonadotropin-releasing hormone regulates gonadotropin beta-subunit and chromogranin-B messenger ribonucleic acids in cultured chromogranin-A-positive pituitary adenomas. J Clin Endocrinol Metab 1990; 71:622–630.
86. Snyder PJ. Gonadotrope adenoma. In: DeGroot LJ, ed. Endocrinology. W. B. Saunders, Philadelphia, PA, 1995, pp. 259–265.
87. Sassolas G, Trouillas J, Treluyer C, Perrin G. Management of nonfunctioning pituitary adenomas. Acta Endocrinol 1993; 1:21–26.
88. Arafah BM, Harrington JF, Madhoun ZT, Selman WR. Improvement of pituitary function after surgical decompression for pituitary tumor apoplexy. J Clin Endocrinol Metab 1990; 71:323–328.
89. Harris PE, Afshar F, Coates P, Doniach I, Wass JA, Besser GM, Grossman A. The effects of transsphenoidal surgery on endocrine function and visual fields in patients with functionless pituitary tumours. Q J Med 1989; 71:417–427.
90. Laws ER, Jr., Fode NC, Redmond MJ. Transsphenoidal surgery following unsuccessful prior therapy. An assessment of benefits and risks in 158 patients. J Neurosurg 1985; 63:823–829.
91. Beck-Peccoz P, Amr S, Menezes-Ferreira MM, Faglia G, Weintraub BD. Decreased receptor binding of biologically inactive thyrotropin in central hypothyroidism. Effect of treatment with thyrotropin-releasing hormone. N Engl J Med 1985; 312:1085–1090.
92. Ladenson PW, Levin AA, Ridgway EC, Daniels GH. Complications of surgery in hypothyroid patients. Am J Med 1984; 77:261–266.
93. Wilson CB. Role of surgery in the management of pituitary tumors. Neurosurg Clin North Am 1990; 1:139–159.
94. Melmed S. General aspects of the management of pituitary tumors by surgery or radiation therapy. In: DeGroot LJ, ed. Endocrinology. W. B. Saunders, Philadelphia, PA, 1995, pp. 497–503.
95. Black PM, Zervas NT, Candia GL. Incidence and complications of transspehenoidal operation for pituitary adenomas. Neurosurgery 1987; 20:920–924.
96. Klibanski A. Nonsecreting pituitary tumors. Endocrinol Metab Clin North Am 1987; 16:793–804.
97. Miller M, Moses AM. Potentiation of vasopressin action by chlorpropamide in vivo. Endocrinology 1970; 86:1024–1027.
98. Bayliss PH. Vasopressin and its neurophysin. In: DeGroot LJ, ed. Endocrinology. W. B. Saunders, Philadelphia, PA, 1995, pp. 406–420.
99. Stephanian E, Lunsford LD, Coffey RJ, Bissonette DJ, Flickinger JC. Gamma knife surgery for sellar and suprasellar tumors. Neurosurg Clin N Am 1992; 3:207–218.
100. Flickinger JC, Nelson PB, Martinez AJ, Deutsch M, Taylor F. Radiotherapy of nonfunctional adenomas of the pituitary gland. Results with long-term follow-up. Cancer 1989; 63:2409–2414.
101. Littley MD, Shalet SM, Beardwell CG, Robinson EL, Sutton ML. Radiation-induced hypopituitarism is dose-dependent. Clin Endocrinol 1989; 31:363–373.
102. al-Mefty O, Kersh JE, Routh A, Smith RR. The long-term side effects of radiation therapy for benign brain tumors in adults. J Neurosurg 1990; 73:502–512.
103. Tachibana O, Yamaguchi N, Yamashima T, Yamashita J. Radiation necrosis of the optic chiasm, optic tract, hypothalamus, and upper pons after radiotherapy for pituitary adenoma, detected by gadolinium-enhanced, T1-weighted magnetic resonance imaging: case report. Neurosurgery 1990; 27:640–643.
104. Littley MD, Shalet SM, Beardwell CG, Ahmed SR, Applegate G, Sutton ML. Hypopituitarism following external radiotherapy for pituitary tumours in adults. Q J Med 1989; 70:145–160.
105. Snyder PJ, Fowble BF, Schatz NJ, Savino PJ, Gennarelli TA. Hypopituitarism following radiation therapy of pituitary adenomas. Am J Med 1986; 81:457–462.
106. Tsagarakis S, Grossman A, Plowman PN, Jones AE, Touzel R, Rees LH, Wass JA, Besser GM. Megavoltage pituitary irradiation in the management of prolactinomas: long-term follow-up. Clin Endocrinol 1991; 34:399–406.
107. Wood DF, Johnston JM, Johnston DG. Dopamine, the dopamine D2 receptor and pituitary tumours. Clin Endocrinol 1991; 35:455–66.
108. Bevan JS, Webster J, Burke CW, Scanlon MF. Dopamine agonists and pituitary tumor shrinkage. Endocr Rev 1992; 13:220–240.

109. Molitch ME. Management of prolactinomas. Annu Rev Med 1989; 40:225–232.
110. Klibanski A, Shupnik MA, Bikkal HA, Black PM, Kliman B, Zervas NT. Dopaminergic regulation of alpha-subunit secretion and messenger ribonucleic acid levels in alpha-secreting pituitary tumors. J Clin Endocrinol Metab 1988; 66:96–102.
111. Kwekkeboom DJ, Hofland LJ, van Koetsveld PM, Singh R, van den Berge JH, Lamberts SW. Bromocriptine increasingly suppresses the in vitro gonadotropin and alpha-subunit release from pituitary adenomas during long term culture. J Clin Endocrinol Metab 1990; 71:718–724.
112. Lamberts SW, Verleun T, Oosterom R, Hofland L, van Ginkel LA, Loeber JG, van Vroonhoven CC, Stefanko SZ, de Jong FH. The effects of bromocriptine, thyrotropin-releasing hormone, and gonadotropin-releasing hormone on hormone secretion by gonadotropin- secreting pituitary adenomas in vivo and in vitro. J Clin Endocrinol Metab 1987; 64:524–530.
113. Berezin M, Olchovsky D, Pines A, Tadmor R, Lunenfeld B. Reduction of follicle-stimulating hormone (FSH) secretion in FSH- producing pituitary adenoma by bromocriptine. J Clin Endocrinol Metab 1984; 59:1220–1223.
114. Vance ML, Ridgway EC, Thorner MO. Follicle-stimulating hormone- and alpha-subunit-secreting pituitary tumor treated with bromocriptine. J Clin Endocrinol Metab 1985; 61:580–584.
115. Johnston DG, Hall K, McGregor A, Ross WM, Kendall-Taylor P, Hall R. Bromocriptine therapy for "nonfunctioning" pituitary tumors. Am J Med 1981; 71:1059–1061.
116. Hedner P, Valdemarsson S. Reduced size of a hormonally silent pituitary adenoma during treatment with CV 205-502, a new dopamine agonist mainly stimulating D2 receptors. Neurosurgery 1989; 25:948–950.
117. Lamberts SW, Krenning EP, Reubi JC. The role of somatostatin and its analogs in the diagnosis and treatment of tumors. Endocr Rev 1991; 12:450–482.
118. Wynick D, Bloom SR. Clinical review 23: the use of the long-acting somatostatin analog octreotide in the treatment of gut neuroendocrine tumors. J Clin Endocrinol Metab 1991; 73:1–3.
119. Quabbe HJ, Plockinger U. Dose-response study and long term effect of the somatostatin analog octreotide in patients with therapy-resistant acromegaly. J Clin Endocrinol Metab 1989; 68:873–881.
120. Vance ML, Harris AG. Long-term treatment of 189 acromegalic patients with the somatostatin analog octreotide. Results of the International Multicenter Acromegaly Study Group. Arch Intern Med 1991; 151:1573–1578.
121. Liebow C, Reilly C, Serrano M, Schally AV. Somatostatin analogues inhibit growth of pancreatic cancer by stimulating tyrosine phosphatase. Proc Natl Acad Sci U S A 1989; 86:2003–2007.
122. Yamada Y, Reisine T, Law SF, Ihara Y, Kubota A, Kagimoto S, Seino M, Seino Y, Bell GI, Seino S. Somatostatin receptors, an expanding gene family: cloning and functional characterization of human SSTR3, a protein coupled to adenylyl cyclase. Mol Endocrinol 1992; 6:2136–2142.
123. Buscail L, Delesque N, Esteve JP, Saint-Laurent N, Prats H, Clerc P, Robberecht P, Bell GI, Liebow C, Schally AV, et al. Stimulation of tyrosine phosphatase and inhibition of cell proliferation by somatostatin analogues: mediation by human somatostatin receptor subtypes SSTR1 and SSTR2. Proc Natl Acad Sci U S A 1994; 91:2315–2319.
124. Bell GI, Reisine T. Molecular biology of somatostatin receptors. Trends Neurosci 1993; 16:34–38.
125. Miller GM, Alexander JM, Bikkal HA, Katznelson L, Zervas NT, Klibanski A. Somatostatin receptor subtype gene expression in pituitary adenomas. J Clin Endocrinol Metab 1995; 80:1386–1392.
126. Faglia G, Bazzoni N, Spada A, Arosio M, Ambrosi B, Spinelli F, Sara R, Bonino C, Lunghi F. In vivo detection of somatostatin receptors in patients with functionless pituitary adenomas by means of a radioiodinated analog of somatostatin ([123I]SDZ 204-090). J Clin Endocrinol Metab 1991; 73:850–856.
127. Klibanski A, Alexander JM, Bikkal HA, Hsu DW, Swearingen B, Zervas NT. Somatostatin regulation of glycoprotein hormone and free subunit secretion in clinically nonfunctioning and somatotroph adenomas in vitro. J Clin Endocrinol Metab 1991; 73:1248–1255.
128. Katznelson L, Oppenheim DS, Coughlin JF, Kliman B, Schoenfeld DA, Klibanski A. Chronic somatostatin analog administration in patients with alpha- subunit-secreting pituitary tumors. J Clin Endocrinol Metab 1992; 75:1318–1325.
129. Warnet A. The role of octreotide (Sandostatin) in non-growth hormone-, non- thyroid-stimulating hormone-, and non-prolactin-secreting adenomas. Metabolism 1992; 41:59–61.
130. Vos P, Croughs RJ, Thijssen JH, van 't Verlaat JW, van Ginkel LA. Response of luteinizing hormone secreting pituitary adenoma to a long-acting somatostatin analogue. Acta Endocrinol 1988; 118:587–590.

131. Sassolas G, Serusclat P, Claustrat B, Trouillas J, Merabet S, Cohen R, Souquet JC. Plasma alpha-subunit levels during the treatment of pituitary adenomas with the somatostatin analog (SMS 201-995). Horm Res 1988; 29:124–128.
132. Daniels M, Newland P, Dunn J, Kendall-Taylor P, White MC. Long-term effects of a gonadotrophin-releasing hormone agonist ([D- Ser(But)6]GnRH(1-9)nonapeptide-ethylamide) on gonadotrophin secretion from human pituitary gonadotroph cell adenomas in vitro. J Endocrinol 1988; 118:491–496.
133. Damjanovic S, Micic D, Popovic V, Petakov M, Kendereski A, Sumarac M, Manojlovic D, Micic J. Follicle stimulating hormone-secreting pituitary adenoma: inappropriate secretion and effect of pulsatile luteinizing hormone releasing hormone analogue (buserelin) administration. J Endocrinol Invest 1991; 14:299–304.
134. Sassolas G, Lejeune H, Trouillas J, Forest MG, Claustrat B, Lahlou N, Loras B. Gonadotropin-releasing hormone agonists are unsuccessful in reducing tumoral gonadotropin secretion in two patients with gonadotropin- secreting pituitary adenomas. J Clin Endocrinol Metab 1988; 67:180–185.
135. Roman SH, Goldstein M, Kourides IA, Comite F, Bardin CW, Krieger DT. The luteinizing hormone-releasing hormone (LHRH) agonist [D-Trp6-Pro9- NEt]LHRH increased rather than lowered LH and alpha-subunit levels in a patient with an LH-secreting pituitary tumor. J Clin Endocrinol Metab 1984; 58:313–319.
136. Colombo P, Ambrosi B, Saccomanno K, Bassetti M, Cortelazzi D, Faglia G. Effects of long-term treatment with the gonadotropin-releasing hormone analog nafarelin in patients with non-functioning pituitary adenomas. Eur J Endocrinol 1994; 130:339–345.
137. Hall JE, Brodie TD, Badger TM, Rivier J, Vale W, Conn PM, Schoenfeld D, Crowley WF, Jr. Evidence of differential control of FSH and LH secretion by gonadotropin-releasing hormone (GnRH) from the use of a GnRH antagonist. J Clin Endocrinol Metab 1988; 67:524–531.
138. Pavlou SN, Wakefield GB, Island DP, Hoffman PG, LePage ME, Chan RL, Nerenberg CA, Kovacs WJ. Suppression of pituitary-gonadal function by a potent new luteinizing hormone-releasing hormone antagonist in normal men. J Clin Endocrinol Metab 1987; 64:931–936.
139. Leal JA, Williams RF, Danforth DR, Gordon K, Hodgen GD. Prolonged duration of gonadotropin inhibition by a third generation GnRH antagonist. J Clin Endocrinol Metab 1988; 67:1325–1327.
140. McGrath GA, Goncalves RJ, Udupa JK, Grossman RI, Pavlou SN, Molitch ME, Rivier J, Vale WW, Snyder PJ. New technique for quantitation of pituitary adenoma size: use in evaluating treatment of gonadotroph adenomas with a gonadotropin- releasing hormone antagonist. J Clin Endocrinol Metab 1993; 76:1363–1368.
141. Daneshdoost L, Pavlou SN, Molitch ME, Gennarelli TA, Savino PJ, Sergott RC, Bosley TM, River JE, Vale WW, Snyder PJ. Inhibition of follicle-stimulating hormone secretion from gonadotroph adenomas by repetitive administration of a gonadotropin-releasing hormone antagonist. J Clin Endocrinol Metab 1990; 71:92–97.
142. Chanson P, Lahlou N, Warnet A, Roger M, Sassolas G, Lubetzi J, Schaison G, Bouchard P. Responses to gonadotropin releasing hormone agonist and antagonist administration in patients with gonadotroph cell adenomas. J Endocrinol Invest 1994; 17:91–98.

13 Alpha-Subunit Secreting Pituitary Tumors

Tamis M. Bright, MD
and E. Chester Ridgway, MD

CONTENTS

INTRODUCTION

The pituitary glycoprotein hormones, TSH, FSH, and LH are comprised of two separate noncovalently bound subunits, alpha and beta. The alpha subunit is identi cal in all of the hormones. The β-subunit is unique for each and confers the specific immunologic and functional activity. The alpha and beta mRNAs are transcribed from two different genes and translated. The proteins are then glycosylated and non-covalently associate to form the intact dimeric molecules, which are secreted from gonadotrophs and thyrotrophs *(1)*. The free α-subunit proteins are secreted in excess of the β-subunits, but neither subunit has activity alone *(2)*. Free α-subunit is measurable in normal serum by radioimmunoassay and immunometric assays in the range of 0.1–1.6 ng/mL in premenopausal women, 1.0–4.0 ng/mL in post-menopausal women, and 0.1–1.0 ng/mL in men. Administration of TRH and GnRH will increase serum α-subunit levels in normal subjects *(3)*. States of increased thyrotropin or gonadotropin secretion such as primary hypothyoidism or menopause will cause the serum α-subunit levels to increase *(4,5)*.

From: *Contemporary Endocrinology, Vol. 3: Diseases of the Pituitary: Diagnosis and Treatment*
Edited by M. E. Wierman Humana Press Inc., Totowa, NJ

PREVALENCE

Approximately 30% of pituitary tumors were historically classified as nonsecreting or null cell tumors *(6)*. In contrast to the patients with PRL, GH, TSH, or ACTH secreting tumors, who present with symptoms of hormone excess, patients with these tumors present with symptoms of mass effects such as headaches, visual field defects, or pituitary insufficiency *(7,8)*. As techniques in immunocytochemistry and radioimmunoassay have advanced, these tumors have now been shown to synthesize a wide variety of hormones. The majority of these tumors synthesize intact glycoproteins or their free α- and β-subunits *(9,10)*. FSH, FSHβ, and α-subunit are the most commonly found products of these tumors *(9,11)*.

Pure alpha secreting tumors were first described by Ridgway et al. in two male subjects with large pituitary tumors *(12)*. Subsequently, pure alpha secreting tumors were found in approximately 7% of nonfunctioning tumors *(9,10)*. However, when the immunocytochemical staining for glycoproteins is studied, up to 25% of the tumors stain for the α-subunit alone *(13,14)*. Much more commonly, α-subunit is produced and secreted in conjunction with one or more of the intact glycoproteins. As many as 48% of glycoprotein tumors will cosecrete α-subunit with FSH or LH as measured in the serum by radioimmunoassay and 27–88% will stain for α-subunit in conjunction with the other glycoproteins on pathological specimens *(10,14–16)*.

Alpha-subunit has also been found to be secreted with the other pituitary hormones. Almost all TSH tumors cosecrete free α-subunit. Growth hormone secreting tumors also cosecrete α-subunit in 9–37%, and up to 59% stain positive for both growth hormone and α-subunit *(17,18)*. In one study, 11% of prolactinomas cosecreted α-subunit with prolactin in the serum *(17)*. The ACTH secreting tumors have also been reported to secrete free α-subunit *(17)*.

PATHOGENESIS

Tumor formation may be monoclonal or polyclonal in origin. Monoclonal expansion arises secondary to a mutation, rearrangement, or amplification of a single copy of a normal gene resulting in activation of a dominant oncogene, or inactivation of recessive tumor suppressor genes resulting from mutations of both copies of the gene. Polyclonal expansion of tumors is usually secondary to a stimulation factor *(19)*. X-linked restriction fragment length polymorphism studies have been done on nonfunctional pituitary tumors that all had at least one gonadotropin by immunocytochemistry, and 83% had alpha staining. All six tumors had a monoclonal pattern of X-inactivation, which gives convincing evidence that monoclonal somatic mutations are the cause of nonfunctioning pituitary tumor formation *(20)*.

MEN-1 (multiple endocrine neoplasia-1) syndrome pituitary tumors and sporadic somatotropinomas have been shown to have an allelic loss in the long arm of chromosome 11 *(21)*. In a study of 88 pituitary tumors of all types, chromosome 11 deletions were discovered in 18% of the tumors including 20% of nonfunctional tumors *(19)*. The authors concluded that at least 20% of sporadic tumors are secondary to allele loss on chromosome 11.

In GH secreting tumors a mutation in the α-subunit of the GTP binding protein that regulates adenylate cyclase has been described *(22)*. This suggests a constitutively

Table 1
Clinical Features of 35 Men and 28 Women with Clinically Nonfunctioning Pituitary Adenomas

Clinical feature	*No. men (%)*	*No. women (%)*
Macroadenoma[a]	35 (100)	27 (96)
Visual field defect[b]	29 (83)	24 (86)
Hypogonadism[c]	27 (77)	9/11 (89)
Hyperprolactinemia	26 (74)	20 (71)
Headache	16 (46)	7 (25)
Central hypoadrenalism at presentation	10 (29)	1 (4)
Central hypothyroidism at presentation	9 (26)	4 (14)
Pituitary apoplexy at presentation	3 (9)	2 (7)
Incidental finding	2 (6)	1 (4)

[a] > 10 mm on CT or MRI scanning.
[b] On formal neurophthalmological examination.
[c] Decreased sexual function and serum testosterone < 10.4 nmol/L (300 ng/dL) in men; oligo/amenorrhea in premenopausal women.

activated GHRH signaling pathway causing tumor growth and/or hormone secretion. Tordjman et al. investigated this mutation in nonfunctional tumors and showed two of 21 tumors also had a point mutation in the G_s alpha gene *(23)*. In Boggild's study, 36% of somatotropinomas had G_s alpha mutations, but none of the other subtypes of pituitary tumors had this mutation. Overall, these recent studies provide evidence for a monoclonal origin of sporadic pituitary tumors including the nonfunctional pituitary tumors. Unfortunately, the exact genetic defect for these tumors remains an unsolved problem in pituitary tumorogenesis.

DIAGNOSIS

If the tumor is cosecreting α-subunit with prolactin, growth hormone, ACTH, or TSH then the clinical syndromes of hyperprolactinemia, acromegaly/giantism, Cushing's disease, or hyperthyroidism will be apparent and can be worked up accordingly. Most studies have found the majority of nonfunctional tumors occur in men and in patients over 50 yr old *(6)*. However, most women with nonfunctioning pituitary adenomas are postmenopausal, and the elevated gonadotropin and α-subunit levels found normally in menopausal women make the diagnosis of this tumor difficult. In a recent study of 63 nonfunctioning tumors, 60% of patients were over 50 and only 56% were men *(24)*. Nonfunctioning tumors may be more frequent in women than previously suggested and go undiagnosed particularly in the menopausal period.

There is no clinical syndrome that accompanies the nonfunctioning pituitary tumors. Consequently, patients present with symptoms of mass effect from large tumor bulk, most commonly visual field defects and headaches *(7,24,25)* (Table 1). Magnetic resonance imaging (MRI) studies usually show large macroadenomas. Pituitary "incidentalomas" are also frequently found on CT and MRI scans done for other reasons *(26)*. These incidentalomas are most commonly pituitary adenomas that are usually asymptomatic *(26)*.

Once a pituitary mass has been documented, serum measurements of α-subunit or the gonadotropins may or may not elucidate the type of hormone or hormones produced, which will aid in the differential diagnosis. As these tumors have no clinical syndrome, they must be differentiated from other intracranial lesions such as craniopharyngiomas, meningiomas, granulomatous disease, and so on. Since elevated serum concentrations of α-subunit are not universally present, Kwekkeboom has advocated using an elevated α-subunit /gonadotropin ratio as a possible additional diagnostic tool in differentiating nonfunctional tumors from other lesions. This increased their percentage of patients with elevated hormone values from 23 to 55% *(15)*. Similarly an elevated α-subunit/TSH ratio is very common in TSH secreting tumors.

Because of the compression of the normal pituitary tissue by these large tumor masses, the patients often present with partial or complete hypopituitarism *(10)*. Secondary thyroid or adrenal insufficiency may by detected in 81% and 62% of patients, respectively *(27)*. Hyperprolactinemia may also be present secondary to stalk compression *(10)*. Hypogonadism is found in as many as 96% of patients *(24,27,28)*.

TRH Stimulation Tests

In normal subjects, TRH will increase serum α-subunit and TSH levels but not gonadotropins. In patients with nonfunctioning tumors, 40–72% will show an increase in gonadotropin and/or free subunit levels after TRH administration *(10,15)*. The TRH may also increase FSH levels in 50% of patients with FSH secreting pituitary tumors *(9)*. The TRH incubation in vitro can stimulate alpha and gonadotropin release. The TRH testing may help identify gonadotropin tumors, particularly in postmenopausal women. In pure alpha secreting tumors, there is a variable response to TRH stimulation. Thirty-three percent of pure alpha secreting tumors increased serum alpha levels with TRH administration *(29)*. Also of note, alpha secretion was nonsuppressible with T3 administration.

GnRH Stimulation Tests

In normal subjects, GnRH administration will increase serum gonadotropin levels. In patients with glycoprotein tumors, less than 50% will show this increase *(9,11,15)*. In normal subjects, repetitive GnRH administration will downregulate the receptors and lead to a decrease in gonadotropin levels. Patients with adenomas have persistent elevations in free α-subunit levels with repetitive GnRH administration *(30)*. In fact, some cases show a further increment above baseline with chronic GnRH administration. In vitro incubation of these tumors with GnRH stimulates release of gonadotropins in only 30% *(9,15)*.

TREATMENT

Surgery

The mainstay of treatment for pure α-subunit secreting tumors and those that cosecrete other intact hormones is surgical resection by either a transsphenoidal hypophysectomy or occasionally by a transfrontal approach. The success rate of pituitary surgery will vary depending on the expertise of the surgeon, the size of the tumor, and the extent upon which it encroaches other structures. Even if the entire tumor is not removed, debulking the majority of the mass can provide adequate control of these tumors since they usually grow slowly. In onc study of 100 patients with surgically resected nonfunctional pituitary tumors, of those who had no adjuvant X-ray therapy, 12% had a recurrence in a mean follow-up of 73.4 mo whereas 18% had a recurrence after 4000–5000 rad of conventional pituitary irradiation. Thus, pituitary irradiation may not offer a distinct advantage to these patients *(7)*. In patients who had elevated levels of gonadotropins and/or α-subunit preoperatively, surgery decreased the levels *(12,29)*. However, not all patients will have values which return to normal. Any future increase in levels should prompt a work-up for tumor recurrence.

Radiotherapy

Radiation therapy can be used as primary therapy or in conjunction with surgery. In 112 patients receiving radiation therapy for nonfunctional pituitary adenomas, 78% did so after surgery and 22% as a primary therapy. The progression-free survival at 5,10,15, and 20 yr was reported as 97, 89, 87, and 76%, respectively. The only complications occurred in patients receiving 5000 cGy. One patient developed a glioblastoma occurring 7.5 yr after radiation therapy and one developed optic neuropathy *(25)*. This higher dose has previously been reported to be associated with optic neuropathy *(31)*. Doses lower than 5000 cGy were not associated with any complications. Therefore, doses less than 4750c Gy in 25 fractions were found to be effective and safe *(25)*.

Medical Therapy

There is currently no universally effective medical therapy for gonadotropin or alpha secreting tumors. However, various agents are under investigation *(32)*. Somatostatin receptors have been found on nonfunctional pituitary tumors *(33–35)*. Miller et al. recently examined tissue from 4 normal pituitaries, 8 somatotroph, 8 lactotroph, 5 corticotroph, and 11 nonfunctional pituitary tumors for somatostatin receptor subtype mRNA. Messenger RNA was present for somatostatin receptor subtypes 1, 2, and 5 in normal pituitary and adenoma tissue. None had mRNA for subtype 4 and only one somatotroph adenoma had mRNA for subtype 3 *(36)*.

Cell cultures from nonfunctioning pituitary adenomas incubated with somatostatin showed an inhibition of intact glycoprotein or free subunit secretion in the majority of tumors studied. Alpha-subunit secretion was suppressed in 17% *(37)*. Multiplc small studies have been done on patients with gonadotropin, alpha, and nonsecreting tumors. The studies show heterogeneous results, with cases of improved visual fields, decreased levels of alpha and/ or gonadotropins and a few patients with decreased size of the tumor *(28,38–41)* (Table 2). When multiple series are examined, approximately 50% of patients will have a decrease in their serum hormone or subunit levels with octreotide therapy (Table 2).

Due to the promising results of some of the studies, somatostatin analogs might be considered as an adjuvant therapy in patients with residual tumor following surgery or radiotherapy. Patients who refuse surgery or radiotherapy, or patients in whom surgery is contraindicated could also be considered for a trial of somatostatin analog therapy. However, many patients had no response, so somatostatin should not be considered a first line therapy. Future studies with somatostatin analogs that are somatostatin receptor subtype-specific may improve the effect and specificity of this medical therapy.

Table 2
Octreotide Treatment of Nonfunctional and Alpha-Subunit Pituitary Tumors

Study	*Dose*	*Tumor*	*Decreased hormone*	*Tumor size decreased*	*Visual field improved*
DeBruin *(41)*	100 μg × 1	4 NF/2 Alpha	0/6	ND	ND
DeBruin *(41)*	1200 μg/d × 3–6 mo	4 NF	0/4	NC	3/4
Merolo *(38)*	150–300 μg/d × 1–12 mo	10 Alpha	6/10	NC	1/10
Katznelson *(28)*	500 μg/h	4 Alpha	2/4	ND	ND
	× 4 h	2 Alpha/TSH	2/2	ND	ND
	100 μg bid × 8 wk	5 GT/1 Alpha/TSH	2/6	2/6	1/6
Katznelson *(28)*	250 μg/d × 8 wk	2 GT/1 Alpha/TSH	1/3	1/3	NC
Sassolas *(40)*	250 μg/d × 14 mo	1 Alpha	1/1	1/1	ND
Total			18/36	4/10	6/20

NF, nonfunctioning; GT, gonadotropin; TSH, thyrotropin; ND, not done; NC, no change.

Table 3
Bromocryptine Treatment of Nonfunctioning and Glycoprotein Hormone Pituitary Tumors

Study	*Dose*	*Tumor*	*Decreased hormone*	*Tumor size decreased*	*Visual field improved*
Kwekkeboom *(15)*	2.5 mg × 1	3 NF	1/3	ND	ND
Kwekkeboom *(44)*	CV205-502[a]	2 Alpha	2/2	NC	1/2
	(300 μg/d × 1 yr)	2 NF	2/2	NC	1/2
		1 GT	0/1	1/1	NC
Vance *(46)*	2.5 mg × 1 yr	1 GT	1/1	NC	1/1
Lamberts *(47)*	2.5 mg × 1 yr	2 Alpha	2/2	ND	ND
		2 NF	2/2	ND	ND
Klibanski *(45)*	10 mg/d × 6 wk	4 Alpha	3/4	2/4	ND
Klibanski *(45)*	4 μg/kg/min × 4 h	2 Alpha	1/2	ND	ND
Total			14/19	3/5	3/5

NF, nonfunctioning; GT, gonadotropin; ND, not done; NC, no change.
[a]Equivalent to 30 mg bromocriptine.

Dopamine receptors have been reported on nonfunctional pituitary adenoma tissue *(42)*. In vitro incubation of gonadotroph and/or α-subunit secreting adenomas with bromocriptine decreased gonadotropin and α-subunit levels *(43)*. Based on these findings, a number of small studies on patients with gonadotropin and/or alpha secreting tumors have been done with dopamine and dopamine agonists in vivo. There are reports of improvement in visual fields, decrease in gonadotropin and alpha levels, and occasional cases of decreasing tumor mass *(15,44–47)*. Reduction in serum hormone levels

Table 4
GnRH Agonist Therapy of Nonfunctioning and Glycoprotein Pituitary Tumors

Study	*Dose*	*Tumor*	*Increased α-subunit*	*Tumor size decreased*	*Visual field improved*
Klibanski *(30)*	8–32 μg/kg/d[a] × 4–8 wk	4 GT 1 TSH/GH	5/5	NC	NC
Roman *(48)*	200 μg/d[a] × 3 wk	1 GT	1/1	ND	ND
Damjanovic *(49)*	Buserelin[b]	1 GT	1/1	ND	ND
Oppenheim *(32,50)*	32 μg/kg/d[a] × 24 d	6 PM	6/6	ND	ND

GT, gonadotropin; TSH, thyrotropin; GH, growth hormone; PM, postmenopausal; ND, not done; NC, no change.
[a] D-Trp6-Pro9-NEt-LHRH.
[b] D-Ser(TBu)6-GnRH.

Table 5
GnRH Antagonist Therapy of Postmenopausal Women and Glycoprotein Pituitary Tumors

Study	*Dose*	*Tumor*	*Decreased hormone*	*Tumor size decreased*	*Visual field improved*
Andreyko *(52)*	Detireli × 5–20 mg × 1	6 PM	6/6	ND	ND
Couzinet *(51)*	Nal-Glu 5 mg × 1	9 PM	9/9	ND	ND
McGrath *(53)*	Nal-Glu 5 mg bid	5 GT	5/5	NC	1/5↓

PM, postmenopausal; GT, gonadotropin; ND, not done; NC, no change.

was seen in 75% of cases and decreases in tumor mass ranged from 0 to 50%. Dopamine agonist doses were variable and the studies lasted from 1 to 12 mo. Although the studies are not uniform in improvement of biochemical markers or decreases in tumor size, dopamine agonist therapy can be used in patients with recurrence or who are not surgical candidates (Table 3).

In normal subjects, GnRH analogs initially stimulate gonadotropin secretion by binding to GnRH receptors, but then cause GnRH receptor downregulation and decreases in gonadotropin secretion. A few patents with gonadotropin tumors have been given GnRH agonists. Although some patients had a decrease in serum gonadotropins, others increased their levels, and all patients showed an alarming increase in α-subunit levels *(30,48)*. Consequently, GnRH analogs are not recommended for the treatment of gonadotropin or α-subunit secreting tumors (Table 4) *(49, 50)*.

GnRH antagonists have recently been developed that compete with GnRH at the GnRH receptor. Two studies using a GnRH antagonist in postmenopausal women showed a decrease in serum α-subunit levels *(51,52)*. The antagonist has also been given to five male patients with FSH secreting tumors in one study (Table 5). Although all normalized their serum FSH levels, α-subunit levels were not reported. No change in tumor size was demonstrated and one patient had worsening visual fields *(53)*. To date, no studies have been done using the antagonist to treat pure α-subunit secreting tumors. Although the data with FSH tumors appears promising, further studies will have to be done to assess the role of GnRH antagonists in gonadotropin and α-subunit secreting tumors.

FOLLOW-UP

Long-term follow-up is needed for patients who have a diagnosis of a pituitary adenoma. After primary treatment, yearly MRI scans should be done to assess any growth of the tumor. Visual fields should be examined and measurement of serum hormone levels should be done depending on which hormones the tumor secreted initially. In addition, the integrity of other pituitary function studies should be monitored annually to accurately assess possible hypopituitarism. If increasing levels of hormones or recurrence on MRI scanning occurs, radiation therapy should be considered. Repeat transsphenoidal surgery can also be undertaken for recurrences and trials of medical therapy can be considered.

SUMMARY

Previously, 30% of all pituitary adenomas were thought to be nonfunctional. With the improvement of immunocytochemical and specific hormone assays, many of these tumors have now been shown to be glycoprotein producing pituitary tumors. Approximately 7% of these are pure α-subunit secreting tumors. These tumors present with symptoms of mass effect and pituitary hypofunction. Treatment options include initial transsphenoidal surgery and/or radiation therapy. Dopamine agonist and somatostatin have been used with varying results on biochemical markers, symptoms, and tumor size. The GnRH agonist and antagonist therapy has been disappointing. There is no optimal medical therapy and treatment must be approached in an individual manner.

REFERENCES

1. Nagaya T, Jameson JL. Structural features of the glycoprotein hormone genes and their encoded proteins. In: Imura H, ed. The Pituitary Gland. 2nd ed., New York, 1994, pp. 63–83.
2. Samuels MH, Veldhuis JD, Henry P, Ridgway EC. Pathophysiology of pulsatile and co-pulsatile release of thyroid stimulation hormone, luteinizing hormone, follicle stimulating hormone and α-subunit. J Clin Endocrinol Metab 1990; 71:425–432.
3. Hagen C, McNeilly AS. Changes in circulating levels of LH, FSH, LHβ and α-subunit after gonadotropin-releasing hormone, and of TSH, LHβ- and α-subunit after thyrotropin-releasing hormone. J Clin Endocrinol Metab 1975; 41:466–471.
4. Kourides IA, Weintraub BD, Re RN, Ridgway EC, Maloof F. Thyroid hormone, oestrogen, and glucocorticoid effects on two different pituitary glycoprotein hormone α-subunit pools. Clin Endocrinol 1978; 9:535–542.
5. Kourides IA, Weintraub BD, Ridgway EC, Maloof F. Increase in the β-subunit of human TSH in hypothyroid serum after thyrotropin releasing hormone. J Clin Endocrinol Metab 1973; 37:836–840.
6. Samuels MH, Ridgway EC. Glycoprotein-secreting pituitary adenomas. In: Fagin J., ed., Bailliere's Clinical Endocrinology and Metabolism, vol 9, Baillière Tindall, London, 1995, pp. 337–358.
7. Ebersold MJ, Quast LM, Laws ER Jr, Scheithauer B, Randall RV. Long-term results in transsphenoidal removal of nonfunctioning pituitary adenomas. J Neurosurgery 1986; 64:713–719.
8. Oppenheim DS, Kana AR, Sangha JS, Klibanski A. Prevalence of α-subunit hypersecretion in patients with pituitary tumors: clinically nonfunctioning and somatotroph adenomas. J Clin Endocrinol Metab 1990; 70:859–864.
9. Synder PJ. Gonadotroph cell adenomas of the pituitary. Endocrine Rev 1985; 6:552–563.

10. Katznelson L, Alexander JM, Klibanski A. Clinically nonfunctioning pituitary adenomas. J Clin Endocrinol Metab 1993; 76:1089–1094.
11. Demura R, Jibiki K, Kubo O, Odagiri E, Demura H, Kitamura K, Shizume K. The significance of α-subunit as a tumor marker for gonadotropin-producing pituitary adenomas. J Clin Endocrinol Metab 1986; 63:564–569.
12. Ridgway EC, Klibanski A, Ladenson PW, Clemmons D, Beitins IZ, McArthur JW, Martorana MA, Zervas NT. Pure alpha-secreting pituitary adenomas. New Engl J Med 1981; 304:1254–1259.
13. Nobels FR, Kwekkeboom DJ, Coopmans W, Hoekstra R, De Herder WW, Bouillon R, Lamberts SW. A comparison between the diagnostic value of gonadotropins, α-subunit, and chromogranin-A and their response to thyrotropin-releasing hormone in clinically nonfunctioning, α-subunit-secreting, and gonadotroph pituitary adenomas. J Clin Endocrinol Metab 1993; 77:784–789.
14. Katznelson L, Alexander JM, Bikkal H, Jameson JL, Hsu DW, Klibanski A. Imbalanced follicle-stimulating hormone β-subunit hormone biosyntheses in human pituitary adenomas. J Clin Endocrinol Metab 1992; 74:1343–1451.
15. Kwekkeboom DJ, deJong FH, Lamberts SW. Gonadotropin release by clinically nonfunctioning and gonadotroph pituitary adenomas *in vivo* and *in vitro*: relation to sex and effects of thyrotropin-releasing hormone, gonadotropin-releasing hormone and bromocriptine. J Clin Endocrinol Metab 1989; 68:1128–1135.
16. Jameson JL, Klibanski A, Black PM, Zervas NT, Lindell CM, Hsu DW, Ridgway EC, Habener JF. Glycoprotein hormone genes are expressed in clinically nonfunctioning pituitary adenomas. J Clin Invest 1987; 80:1472–1478.
17. Ishibashi M, Yamaji, T, Takaku F, Teramoto A, Fukushima T. Secretion of glycoprotein hormone α-subunit by pituitary tumors. J Clin Endocrinol Metab 1987; 64: 1187–1193.
18. Kontogeorgos G, Asa SL, Kovacs K, Smyth HS, Singer W. Production of alpha-subunit of glycoprotein hormones by pituitary somatotroph adenomas in vitro. Acta Endocrinologica 1993; 129:565–572.
19. Boggild MD, Jenkinson S, Pistorello M, Boscaro M, Scanarini M, McTernan P, Perrett CW, Thakker RV, Clayton RN. Molecular genetic studies of sporadic pituitary tumors. J Clin Endocrinol Metab 1994; 78:387–392.
20. Alexander JM, Biller BM, Bikkal H, Zervas NT, Arnold A, Klibanski A. Clinically nonfunctioning pituitary tumors are monoclonal in origin. J Clin Invest 1990; 86:336–340.
21. Thakker RV, Pook MA, Wooding C, Boscaro M, Scanarini M, Clayton RN. Association of somatotrophinomas with loss of alleles on chromosome 11 and with gsp mutations. J Clin Invest 1993; 91:2815–2821.
22. Landis CA, Masters SB, Spada A, Pace AM, Bourne HR, Vallar L. GTPase inhibiting mutations activate the alpha chain of Gs and stimulate adenylyl cyclase in human pituitary tumors. Nature 1989; 340:692–696.
23. Tordjman K, Stern N, Ouaknine G, Yossiphov Y, Razon N, Nordenskjold M, Friedman E. Activating mutations of the Gs α-gene in nonfunctioning pituitary tumors. J Clin Endocrinol Metab 1993; 77:765–769.
24. Oppenheim DS. TSH-and other glycoprotein -producing pituitary adenomas: alpha-subunit as a tumor marker. Thyroid Today 1991; 14:1–11.
25. Flickinger JC, Nelson PB, Martinez AJ, Deutsch M, Taylor F. Radiotherapy of nonfunctional adenomas of the pituitary gland. Results with long-term follow-up. Cancer 1989; 63:2409–2414.
26. Molitch ME, Russell EJ. The pituitary "incidentaloma." Ann Int Med 1990; 112:925–931.
27. Arafah BM. Reversible hypopituitarism in patients with large nonfunctioning pituitary adenomas. J Clin Endocrinol and Metab 1986; 62:1173–1179.
28. Katznelson L, Oppenheim DS, Coughlin JF, Klibman B, Schoenfeld DA, Klibanski A. Chronic somatostatin analog administration in patients with α-subunit-secreting pituitary tumors. J Clin Endocrinol Metab 1992; 75:1318–1325.
29. Klibanski A, Ridgway EC, Zervas NT. Pure α-subunit-secreting pituitary tumors. J Neurosurgery 1983; 59:585–589.
30. Klibanski A, Jameson JL, Biller BM, Crowley WJ Jr, Zervas NT, Rivier J, Vale WW, Bikkal H. Gonadotropin and α-subunit responses to chronic gonadotropin-releasing hormone analog administration in patients with glycoprotein hormone-secreting pituitary tumors. J Clin Endocrinol Metab 1989; 68:81–86.
31. Aristizabal S, Caldwell WL, Avila J, Mayer EG. Relationship of time dose factors to tumor control and complications in treatment of Cushing's disease by irradiation. Int J Radiation Oncol, Biol, Phys 1977; 2:47–54.
32. Oppenheim DS, Klibanski A. Medical therapy of glycoprotein hormone-secreting pituitary tumors. Endocrinol Metab Clinics North America 1989; 18:339–358.
33. Ikuyama S, Nawata H, Kato K, Karashima T, Ibayashi H, Nakagaki H. Specific somatostatin receptors on human pituitary adenoma cell membranes. J Clin Endocrinol Metab 1985; 61:666–671.

34. Reubi J, Heitz P, Landolt A. Visualization of somatostatin receptors and correlation with immunoreactive growth hormone and prolactin in human pituitary adenomas: evidence for different tumor subclasses. J Endocrinol Metab 1981; 65:65–73.
35. Faglia G, Bazzoni N, Spada A, Arosio M, Ambrosi B, Spinelli F, Sara R, Bonino C, Lunghi F. *In vivo* detection of somatostatin receptors in patients with functionless pituitary adenomas by means of a radioiodinated analog of somatostatin ([^{123}I]SDZ 204-090), J Clin Endocrinol Metab 1991; 73:850–856.
36. Miller GM, Alexander JM, Bikkal HA, Katznelson L, Zervas NT, Klibanski A. Somatostatin receptor subtype gene expression in pituitary adenomas. J Clin Endocrinol Metab 1995; 80:1386–1392.
37. Klibanski A, Alexander JM, Bikkal HA, Hsu DW, Swearingen B, Zervas NT. Somatostatin regulation of glycoprotein hormone and free subunit secretion in clinically nonfunctioning and somatotroph adenomas *in vitro*. J Clin Endocrinol Metab 1991; 73:1248–1255.
38. Merola B, Colao A, Ferone D, Selleri A, DiSarno A, Marzullo P, Biondi B, Spazianti R, Rossi E, Lombardi G. Effects of a chronic treatment with octreotide in patients with functionless pituitary adenomas. Hormone Res 1993; 40:149–155.
39. Gasperi M, Petrini L, Pilosu R, Nardi M, Marcello A, Mastio F, Bartalena L, Martino E. Octreotide treatment does not affect the size of most non-functioning pituitary adenomas. J Endocrinol Invest 1993; 16:541–543.
40. Sassolas G, Serusclat P, Claustrat B, Trouillas J, Merabet S, Cohen R, Souquet JC. Plasma alpha-subunit levels during the treatment of pituitary adenomas with the somatostatin analog (SMS 201-995). Hormone Res 1988; 29:124–128.
41. de Bruin TW, Kwekkeboom DJ, Verlaat JW, Reubi JC, Krenning EP, Lamberts SW, Croughs RJ. Clinically nonfunctioning pituitary adenoma and octreotide response to long term high dose treatment, and studies in vitro. J Clin Endocrinol Metab 1992; 75:1310–1317.
42. Lloyd RV, Anagnostou D, Chandler WF. Dopamine receptors in immunohistochemically characterized null cell adenomas and normal human pituitaries. Mod Pathol 1988; 1:51–56.
43. Kwekkeboom DJ, Hofland LJ, van Koetsveld PM, Singh R, van den Berge JH, Lamberts SW. Bromocriptine increasingly suppresses the *in vitro* gonadotropin and α-subunit release from pituitary adenomas during long term culture. J Clin Endocrinol Metab 1990; 71:718–724.
44. Kwekkeboom DJ, Lamberts SW. Long-term treatment with the dopamine agonist CV205-502 of patients with a clinically non-functioning, gonadotroph, or α-subunit secreting pituitary adenoma. Clin Endocrinol 1992; 36:171–176.
45. Klibanski A, Shupnik MA, Bikkal HA, Black PM, Kliman B, Zervas NT. Dopaminergic regulation of α-subunit secretion and messenger ribonucleic acid levels in α-secreting pituitary tumors. J Clin Endocrinol Metab 1988; 66:96–102.
46. Vance ML, Ridgway EC, Thorner MO. Follicle-stimulating hormone-and α-subunit-secreting pituitary tumor treated with bromocriptine. J Clin Endocrinol Metab 1985; 61: 580–584.
47. Lamberts SW, Verleun T, Oosterom R, Hofland L, van Ginkel LA, Loeber JG, van Vroonhoven CC, Stefanko SZ, de Jong FH. The effects of bromocriptine, thyrotropin-releasing hormone, and gonadotropin-releasing hormone on hormone secretion by gonadotropin-secreting pituitary adenomas *in vivo* and *in vitro*. J Clin Endocrinol Metab 1987; 64:524–530.
48. Roman SH, Goldstein M, Kourides IA, Comite F, Bardin CW, Krieger DT. The luteinizing hormone-releasing hormone (LHRH) agonist [D-Trp^6-Pro^9-NEt]LHRH increased rather than lowered LH and α-subunit levels in a patient with an LH-secreting pituitary tumor. J Clin Endocrinol Metab 1984; 58:313–319.
49. Damjanovic S, Micic D, Popovic V, Petakov M, Kendereski A, Sumarac M, Manojlovic D, Micic J. Follicle stimulating hormone-secreting pituitary adenoma: inappropriate secretion and effect of pulsatile luteinizing hormone releasing hormone analogue (buserelin) administration. J Endocrinol Invest 1991; 14:299–304.
50. Oppenheim DS, Bikkal H, Crowley Jr WF, Klibanski A. Effects of chronic GnRH analog administration on gonadotropins and α-subunit secretion in postmenopausal women. Clin Endocrinol 1992; 36:559–564.
51. Couzinet B, Lahlou N, Thomas G, Thalabard JC, Bouchard P, Roger M, Schaison G. Effects of gonadotropin releasing hormone antagonist and agonist on the pulsatile release of gonadotropins and α-subunit in postmenopausal women. Clin Endocrinol 1991; 34:477–483.
52. Andreyko JL, Monroe SE, Marshall LA, Fluker MR, Nerenberg CA, Jaffe RB. Concordant suppression of serum immunoreactive luteinizing hormone (LH), follicle-stimulating hormone, α-subunit, bioactive LH, and testosterone in postmenopausal women by a potent gonadotropin releasing hormone antagonist (detirelix). J Clin Endocrinol Metab 1992; 74:399–405.
53. McGrath GA, Goncalves, RJ, Udupa JK, Grossman RI, Pavlou SN, Molitch ME, Rivier J, Vale WW, Snyder PJ. (1993) New technique for quantitation of pituitary adenoma size: use in evaluating treatment of gonadotroph adenomas with a gonadotropin-releasing hormone antagonist. J Clin Endocrinol Metab 1993; 76:1363–1368.

14 TSH

Normal Physiology

Joshua D. Safer, MD,
and Fredric E. Wondisford, MD

CONTENTS

INTRODUCTION

Central regulation of thyrotropin (TSH) synthesis and secretion is critical for the normal control of thyroid function and hormone synthesis. Thyrotropin is one of the five trophic hormones synthesized in the anterior pituitary. TSH-producing cells are referred to as thyrotrophs and are basophilic on hematoxylin and eosin (H&E) staining.

SYNTHESIS

Thyrotropin is a 28-kDa glycoprotein made up of two subunits. The α subunit is common to the luteinizing hormone (LH), follicle-stimulating hormone (FSH), and human chorionic gonadotropin (hCG). The β-subunit confers specificity, carrying the unique binding information which differentiates the four related hormones. The α- and β-subunits of thyrotropin are synthesized in parallel ways although the α-subunit is synthesized in excess of the β-subunit in the thyrotroph. Detection of α and β "pre" subunits in cell free systems yields proteins 2.5–3 kDa larger than the final proteins owing to the size of the respective leader peptides *(1–5)*. Intact cell systems reveal a pre α-subunit of either 18 or 21 kDa, depending on whether they contain one or two carbohydrate chains. The pre β-subunit is 18 kDa, reflecting the addition of one carbohydrate chain. Treatment of both proteins with endoglycosidase H, which removes glycosylation side-chains, results in 11-kDa products *(6)*. The crystallographic structure of intact hCG has recently been described. In this structure, the β-subunit surrounds part of the

From: *Contemporary Endocrinology, Vol. 3: Diseases of the Pituitary: Diagnosis and Treatment*
Edited by M. E. Wierman Humana Press Inc., Totowa, NJ

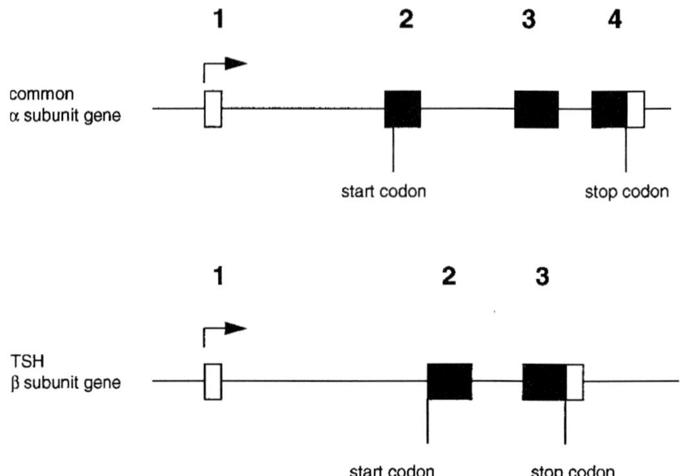

Fig. 1. Schematic representation of the human TSH subunit genes. Coding exons are denoted by black boxes and untranslated regions by white boxes. Stop and start sites are approximate. The bent arrow is at the transcription start site.

α-subunit through disulfide bonds and maintains the combination. A model of TSH structure based on these data has been proposed *(7)*.

Gene Structure

The α-subunit gene is found on chromosome 6 *(8)*. Although the amino acid sequence of the α subunit is the same in all pituitary and placental glycoproteins, the carbohydrate structures may vary due to different conformations induced by different β subunits and different carbohydrate processing enzymes in different cells *(9–11)*. The human α-subunit is 92 amino acids. The gene is 9.4 kb including four exons, coding for the protein and three introns, which are untranslated (Fig. 1). The introns are 6.4, 1.7, and 0.4 kb, respectively *(8)*. The α-subunit TATA box is located at -26 base pairs within the promoter. The gene also includes the sequence TGACGTCA, a palindromic sequence known to confer cyclic adenosin monophosphate (cAMP) responsiveness *(12,13)*. In addition, two thyroid hormone response elements (TREs) have been localized upstream of the α-subunit start site *(14,15)*.

The sequence for the unique TSHβ-subunit gene is found on chromosome 1 *(16)*. It includes three exons, coding for the protein (Fig. 1). In mice and rats, transcription from a downstream TATA box is increased in hypothyroid states *(17,18)*. An upstream TATA box is not affected. In humans, only the downstream TATA box site has been found *(19)*. Two TSHβ-subunit mutations have been described which result in loss of heterodimerization with the α-subunit in vitro and TSH deficiency in vivo *(20,21)*. A third mutation, a bioinactive form of TSH resulting from a C-terminus mutation in the β-subunit, has recently been described *(17)*.

Posttranslational Processing

As with other glycoproteins, carbohydrate chains are added to TSH subunits and modified in the rough endoplasmic reticulum and Golgi apparatus. The carbohydrate chains are covalently bound to asparagine residues on the α-subunit (residues 52 and

78) and the β-subunit (residue 23). The carbohydrates include mannose, fucose, *N*-acetylglucosamine, galactose, *N*-acetylgalactosamine, and sialic acid *(9,10)*. Glycosylation of the subunits plays a role in their navigation through the thyrotroph as well as TSH's final bioactivity and biological half-life. Deglycosylated TSH is less bioactive, more quickly degraded metabolically, and more quickly excreted by the kidney *(22)*. In TSH, the oligosaccharide side-chains may terminate in either sulfate or sialic acid residues *(10,23,24)*. A pathway for their synthesis has been proposed.

Aspects of glycosylation have been associated with varying thyroid status. Increased sialylation is associated with hypothyroidism and neonatal status. In rats for example, sialylation is increased relative to sulfation both in hypothyroidism *(25)* and in the neonatal period *(26,27)*. Adult rats show an increase in sialylated oligosaccharides only after prolonged hypothyroidism *(28)*. A possible functional consequence of these differences is suggested by the decreased renal clearance of more sialylated TSH *(25,28)*. Recombinant TSH is more sialylated than endogenous TSH. Although recombinant TSH has accordingly decreased renal clearance, it is also less potent owing to the incorporation of sialylic acid residues *(29,30)*.

Oligosaccharide side-chains may have one (biantennary), two (triantennary), or more (multiantennary) branching points. Attempts have been made to associate carbohydrate structure with function. TRH treatment is associated with a higher biantennary to triantennary ratio among TSH oligosaccharides *(31,32)* and increased TSH bioactivity. By contrast, nonthyroidal illness and aggressive pituitary adenomas are associated with relative increases in multiantennary oligosaccharides *(33)*.

ACTION

Thyrotropin binds to its unique receptor on the plasma membrane initiating two cascades (Fig. 2). The first is the activation of adenylyl cyclase resulting in an increase in cAMP *(34)*. Second, TSH activates phospholipase C with the consequent hydrolysis of phosphatidylinositol 4,5 bisphosphate (PIP_2) *(35)*.

TSH Receptor

The gene for the human TSH receptor (TSH-R) is greater than 60 kb in length. It is located on chromosome 14 *(36,37)* and contains 10 exons which code for a 764-amino acid protein *(38,39)*. The TSH receptor is of the seven transmembrane spanning domain superfamily *(40)* and is coupled to a stimulating guanine nucleotide binding protein (G_s protein). Ligand (TSH) binding causes an increase in G-protein activity, which in turn results in increased adenylyl cyclase activity and increased production of cAMP *(41,42)*.

Cyclic AMP Pathway

The rise in cAMP associated with TSH results in a dissociation of the inhibitory and catalytic subunits of cAMP-dependent protein kinase (protein kinase A). Disinhibited protein kinase A then phosphorylates various proteins and modulates cellular activities. Two subtypes of protein kinase A are described, type I and type II *(43,44)*. In dog thyroid cells, both enzymes play roles in iodide transport, thyroid hormone synthesis, thyroid hormone secretion, and DNA synthesis. The latter is more sensitive to changes in the activity of the type I enzyme. TSH dephosphorylates a number of proteins also, presumably via a cAMP-mediated phosphoprotein phosphatase *(45)*.

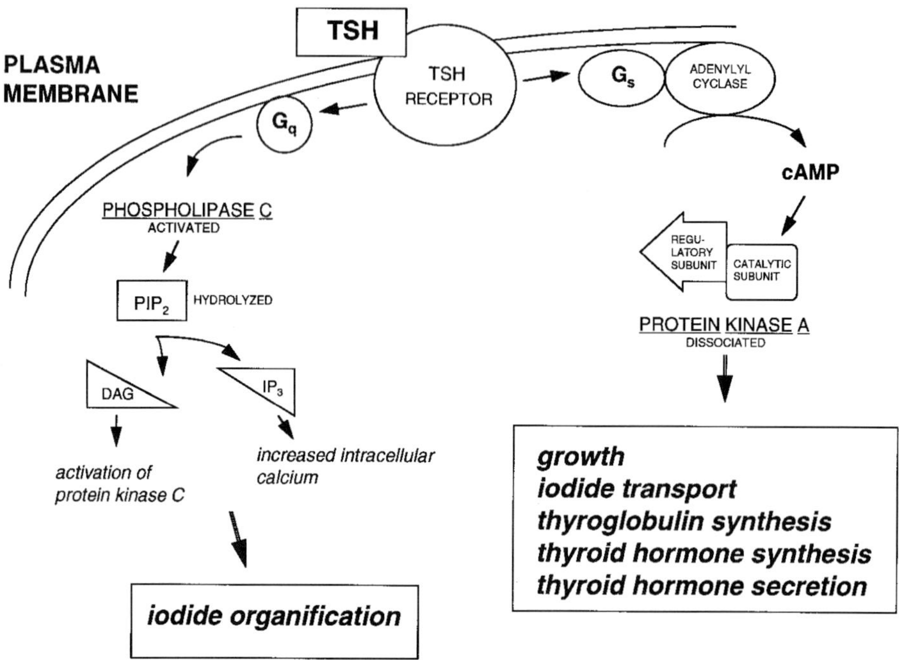

Fig. 2. Schematic outline of the two pathways by which TSH exerts its action.

Several factors have been noted to modulate the TSH cAMP pathway. IGF-1 augments a TSH-induced increase in DNA synthesis in thyroid follicular cells *(46,47)*. Because IGF-1 does not increase cAMP's sensitivity and response to TSH, a different mechanism must exist. Pertussis toxin abolishes the effect of an inhibitory guanine nucleotide binding protein (G_i), augmenting TSH stimulation of adenylyl cyclase. Catecholamines increase the activity of cAMP phosphodiesterase, diminishing the impact of TSH *(48)*.

Phospholipase C Pathway

Phosphorylation of some proteins by TSH is not cAMP-dependent *(35)*. The action of protein kinase C may be involved in these phosphorylations. The hydrolysis of PIP_2 by TSH-activated phospholipase C results in the formation of diacylgycerol (DAG) and inositol tris-phosphate (IP_3). DAG activates a Ca^{2+}-phospholipid-dependent protein kinase (protein kinase C). IP_3 is associated with an increase in intracellular Ca^{2+}. Because the quantity of TSH required for hydrolysis of PIP_2 is great, the physiological significance of this pathway in normal follicular cell function is debated. A role in iodination of thyroglobulin, however, has been claimed. In thyroid follicular cells, PIP_2 stimulates apical thyroid hormone peroxidase. Luminal iodine and thyroglobulin and their product are accordingly increased *(49)*. Further, the rise in H_2O_2 required for iodide organification is mediated by PIP_2 hydrolysis rather than cAMP *(50)*. A role for increased intracellular calcium in signal transduction within the thyroid is contradictory *(35)*. Thus, both the existence of the calcium shift and the physiological consequence remain topics for further study.

TSH Action

Thyroid morphology is rapidly altered by TSH *(51)*. Administration of TSH results in formation of microvilli and pseudopods at the apex of thyroid follicular cells. The effect of TSH on the cytoskeleton has been investigated in vitro. These cAMP-mediated changes have been noted to differ from those caused by phorbol esters (which induce protein kinase C via its rapid translation to the plasma membrane) *(52)*.

Although the mechanisms are not entirely elucidated, in vitro experimentation reveals TSH impact on a number of cell actions: TSH increases the activities of thyroid peroxidase *(53–55)*, lysosomal *N*-acetylglucosaminidase, β-galactosidase, leucyl-β-naphthylaminidase, glucose-6-phosphate dehydrogenase, NAD kinase, and RNA polymerase *(56)*. Thyroglobulin synthesis is increased in the presence of TSH *(57)*. Increased DNA synthesis in general is reported.

Metabolically, TSH increases glucose uptake, glucose oxidation, and anaerobic metabolism product formation in experiments using beef thyroid slices *(58)*. Although the glucose uptake is cAMP-mediated, the glucose oxidation seems related to increased NADP as a result of the increased NAD kinase activity *(54,55)*.

Iodine and TSH share a complex relationship. Thyrotropin initially decreases iodine transport but augments the transport, after several hours *(60,61)*. Cyclic AMP, under TSH stimulation, has been shown to inhibit iodine incorporation into T_4, T_3, diiodotyrosine, and mono-iodotyrosine *(62)*. By contrast, PIP_2 hydrolysis activates thyroglobulin iodination *(63)*. Conversely, the cAMP cascade enhances thyroid hormone secretion. The PIP_2 cascade has either no effect or even inhibits thyroid hormone secretion *(63)*.

MODULATION

General Considerations

Thyrotropin release follows a circadian rhythm. Its rise begins before sleep with a peak achieved between 11 PM and 4 AM. Both amplitude and frequency are maximal at this time *(64–66)*. Sleep itself decreases the pulse amplitude but not the frequency *(67)*. A trough in TSH secretion occurs between 10 AM and 2 PM *(68)*. Primary control over TSH is exerted by thyrotropin releasing hormone (TRH) and triiodothyronine (T_3) (Fig. 3).

Triiodothyronine Effect

Thyroid hormone rapidly and profoundly reduces the transcriptional rate of both the α- and TSHβ-subunits *(69–72)*. According to in vitro mRNA studies, TSHβ is altered more rapidly and to a greater degree by thyroid hormone than is α-subunit. With maximal thyroid hormone treatment, TSHβ gene transcription is virtually 100% suppressed, whereas α-subunit gene transcription is only 75% suppressed. Conversely, in hypothyroid mice, TSHβ rises to a greater degree than the common α-subunit.

In rats, T_3 causes TSH to fall to 10% of its basal level in 5 h *(73,74)*. Use of a fourth generation TSH assay reveals the onset of human TSH suppression by T_3 at approximately 50 min *(68)*. This action follows the binding of T_3 to its receptor and the combination, including yet ill-defined factors, causes a decrease in TSH gene expression through binding to *cis*-acting response elements near the transcription start sites of the

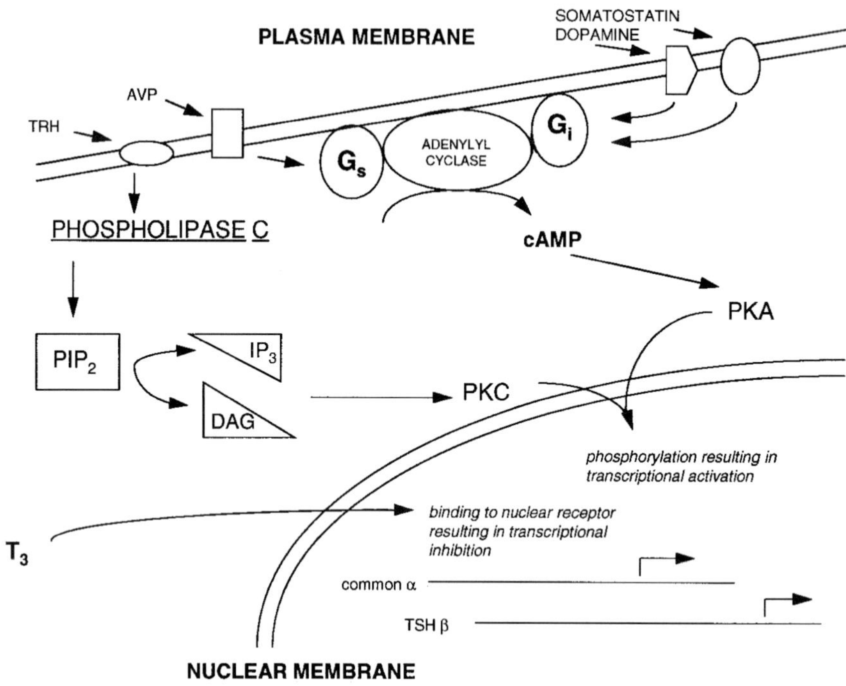

Fig. 3 Regulation of human TSH subunit biosynthesis. PKC, protein kinase C; PKA, protein kinase A; AVP, arginine vasopressin.

TSH subunit genes *(65)*. Exposure to T_3 also results in a decrease in the number of TRH receptors on the thyrotrophs *(75,76)*. Paradoxically, early or low dose replacement therapy for hypothyroidism may result in a temporary rise in the TSH *(77)*.

Thyrotropin Releasing Hormone Effect

TRH exerts its influence on TSH through several mechanisms. The TSH response to TRH is biphasic, a result of a TRH effect on both TSH stores and synthesis. Intravenous administration of TRH results in a detectable TSH response in 2–5 min *(78,79)*. Peak response occurs after 20–30 min and activity is no longer detectable after 2–5 h. Evidence for increased TSH synthesis in response to TRH is also evident.

TRH is documented to play a part in posttranslational processing of TSH. The need for appropriate glycosylation of TSH for full activity is well documented. Evidence exists for TRH influence on sialylation and sulfation *(80)* of TSH as noted above. Modification of other carbohydrate components of TSH has also been demonstrated *(32,81)*.

In tissue culture, TRH exerts its action on TSH through two cis-acting elements *(82,83)*. One is located between –128 and –60 bp and the other between –28 and +8 bp. Pit-1 is a necessary cofactor for TSH stimulation by TRH *(84)*. TRH activates phospholipase C, which hydrolyzes PIP_2 to DAG and IP_3. DAG activates protein kinase C, which presumably phosphorylates nuclear factors necessary for TSH gene expression. A cAMP pathway for TSH control is also documented. Increased cAMP raises TSH-β and α-subunit transcription via proximal 5′ flanking DNA sequences *(83)*.

Other Thyrotropin Inhibitors

Glucocorticoids are well known to cause a fall in serum TSH levels. Interestingly, however, TSH mRNA levels do not fall, suggesting that the impact is translational or posttranslational *(85,86)*.

Somatostatin causes a decrease in TSH as documented in tissue culture *(87)* and in humans *(88,89)*. The decrease is presumably caused by somatostatin binding to the TSH receptor and, by coupling to the G_i, reducing adenylyl cyclase activity. The importance of the effect is not clear because chronic somatostatin use does not result in hypothyroidism in humans *(90)*. Growth hormone administration also results in a fall in TSH *(91)*. The degree to which this is independent of the resulting somatostatin rise is unclear.

Dopamine decreases TSH through several pathways. In rat pituitary cells, dopamine administration has been associated with decreased TSH subunit gene transcription, decreased mRNA production, and decreased secretion of TSH *(79)*. Overall, dopamine may decrease TSH mRNA levels by as much as 50% *(92)*. Hypothyroidism results in greater TSH sensitivity to dopamine *(93)*.

Several additional factors are associated with a reduction in TSH: Stress and severe disease states are thought to decrease TSH via increases in glucocorticoids, tumor necrosis factor, or interleukin 1β. The latter two are known to decrease TSH independent of glucocorticoids *(94–98)*. Increasing age as well as starvation result in lower TSH *(99)*, although the mechanisms have yet to be elucidated. The finding has been reversed in rats with the use of somatostatin antibodies *(100)*. The human consequence of these data is not clear.

Other Thyrotropin Stimulators

Catecholamine stimulation of TSH can be almost as powerful as that of TRH. The most striking effect is in the setting of hypothyroidism *(93,101)*. Stimulation occurs via α_2 pathways. Inhibition can be effected by α_1 pathways. Arginine vasopressin has been used for in vitro study and is found to increase TSH release *(102)*. A rise in TSH in the winter has been noted in patients on levothyroxine replacement therapy. Cold *per se* has been implicated in an adrenergic response resulting in an increase in TRH and then TSH *(103)*.

REFERENCES

1. Chin WW, Habener JF, Kieffer JD, Maloof F. Cell-free translation of the messenger RNA coding for the α-subunit of thyroid-stimulating hormone. J Biol Chem 1978;253:7985
2. Giudice LC, Waxdal MJ, Weintraub BD. Comparison of bovine and mouse pituitary glycoprotein hormone pre-α subunits synthesized *in vitro*. Proc Natl Acad Sci USA 1979;76:4798.
3. Giudice LC, Weintraub BD. Evidence for conformational differences between precursor and processed forms of TSH-β subunit. J Biol Chem 1979;254:12679.
4. Kourides IA, Vamvakopoulos NC, Maniatis GM. mRNA directed biosynthesis of α- and β-subunits of thyrotropin. J Biol Chem 1979;254:11106.
5. Kourides IA, Weintraub BD. mRNA directed biosynthesis of α-subunit of thyrotropin: translation in cell-free and whole-cell systems. Proc Natl Acad Sci USA 1979;76:298.
6. Chin WW, Maloof F, Habener JF. Thyroid-stimulating hormone biosynthesis. J Biol Chem 1981;256:3059.
7. Medeiros-Neto G, Herodotou DT, Rajan S, Kommareddi S, de Lacerda L, Sandrini R, Boguszewski MCS, Hollenberg AN, Radovick S, Wondisford FE. A circulating biologically inactive thyrotropin caused by a mutation in the beta subunit gene. J Clin Invest 1996;97:1250.

8. Fiddes JC, Goodman HM. The gene encoding the common alpha subunit of the four human glycoprotein hormones. J Mol Appl Genet 1981;1:3.
9. Green ED, Baenziger JU. Asparagine-linked oligosaccarides on lutropin, follitropin, and thyrotropin. I. Structural elucidation of the sulfated and sialylated oligosaccharides on bovine, ovine, and human pituitary glycoprotein hormones.. J Biol Chem 1988;263:25.
10. Green ED, Baenziger JU. Asparagine-linked oligosaccarides on lutropin, follitropin, and thyrotropin. II. Distributions of sulfated and sialylated oligosaccharides on bovine, ovine, and human pituitary glycoprotein hormones. J Biol Chem 1988;263:36.
11. Green ED, Gruenebaum GK, Bielinska M, Baenziger JU, Boime I. Sulfation of lutropin oligosaccharides with a cell-free system. Proc Natl Acad Sci USA 1984;81:5320.
12. Deutch PC, Jameson JL, Habener JF. Cyclic AMP responsiveness of human gonadotropin a gene transcription is directed by a repeated 10-bp enhancer. J Biol Chem 1987;262:12169.
13. Silver BJ, Bokar JA, Virgin JB, Vallen EA, Milstead A, Nilson JH. Cyclic AMP regulation of the human glycoprotein hormone α subunit is mediated by an 18-bp element. Proc Natl Acad Sci USA 1987;84:2198.
14. Chatterjee VKK, Lee J-K, Rentoumis A, Jameson JL. Negative regulation of the thyroid-stimulating hormone α gene by thyroid hormone: receptor interaction adjacent to the TATA box. Proc Natl Acad Sci USA 1989;86:9114.
15. Pennathur S, Madison LD, Kay TW, Jameson JL. Localization of promoter sequences required for thyrotropin-releasing hormone and thyroid hormone responsiveness of the glycoprotein hormone alpha-gene in primary cultures of rat pituitary cells. Mol Endocrinol 1993;7:797.
16. Dracopoli NC, Retting WJ, Whitfield GK, et al. Assignment of the gene for the β subunit of thyroid-stimulating hormone to the short arm of human chromosome 1. Proc Natl Acad Sci 1986;83:1822.
17. Carr FE, Heed LR, Chin WW. Isolation and characterization of the rat thyrotropin β subunit gene: differential regulation of two transcriptional start sites by thyroid hormone. J Biol Chem 1987;262:981.
18. Gordon DF, Wood WM, Ridgway EC. Organization and nucleotide sequence of the gene encoding the β subunit of murine thyrotropin. DNA 1988;7:17.
19. Wondisford FE, Radovick S, Moates JM, Usala SJ, Weintraub BD. Isolation and characterization of the human thyrotropin β subunit gene. J Biol Chem 1988;262:12538.
20. Dacou-Voutekakis C, Feltquate DM, Drakopoulou M, Kourides IA, Dracopoli NC. Familial hypothyroidism caused by a nonsense mutation in the thyroid-stimulating hormone β subunit gene. Am J Hum Genet 1990;16:998.
21. Hayashizaki Y, Hiraoka Y, Tatsumi K, et al. Desoxyribonucleic acid analyses of five families with familial interited thyroid stimulating hormone deficiency. J Clin Endocrinol Metab 1990;71:792.
22. Magner JA. Thyroid-stimulating hormone: biosynthesis, cell biology and bioactivity. Endocrine Reviews 1990;11:354.
23. Gesundheit N, Magner JA, Chen T, Weintraub BD. Differential sulfation and sialylation of secreted mouse thyrotropin (TSH) subunits: regulation by TSH-releasing hormone. Endocrinology 1986;119:455.
24. Parsons TF, Pierce JG. Oligosaccharide moities of glycoprotein hormones: bovine lutropin resists enzymatic deglycosylation because of terminal O-sulfated N-acetylhexosamines. Proc Natl Acad Sci USA 1980;77:7089.
25. DeCherney GS, Gesundheit N, Gyves PW, Showalter CR, Weintraub BD. Alterations in the sialylation and sulfation of secreted mouse thyrotropin in primary hypothyroidism. Biochem Biophys Res Comun 1989;159:755.
26. Gyves PW, Gesundheit N, Stannard BS, DeCherney GS, Weintraub BD. Alterations in the glycosylation of secreted thyrotropin during ontogenesis: analysis of sialylated and sulfated oligosaccharides. J Biol Chem 1989;264:6104.
27. Gyves PW, Gesundheit N, Taylor T, Butler J, Weintraub BD. Changes in thyrotropin (TSH) carbohydrate structure and response to TSH-releasing hormone during postnatal ontogeny: analysis by concanavalin A chromatography. Endocrinology 1987;121:133.
28. Gyves PW, Gesundheit N, Thotakura NR,Stannard BS, DeCherney GS, Weintraub BD. Changes in the sialylation and sulfation of secreted thyrotropin in congenital hypothyroidism. Proc Natl Acad Sci USA 1990;87:3792.
29. Thotakura NR, Desai RK, Bates LG, Cole ES, Pratt BM, Weintraub BD. Biological activity and metabolic clearance of a recombinant human thyrotropin produced in Chinese hamster ovary cells. Endocrinology 1991;128:341.

30. Wondisford FE, Usala SJ, DeCherney SG, et al. Cloning of the human thyrotropin beta subunit gene and transient expression of biologically active human thyrotropin after gene transfection. Mol Endocrinol 1988;2:32.
31. Gesundheit N, Fink DL, Silverman LA, Weintraub BD. Effect of thyrotropin-releasing hormone on the carbohydrate structure of secreted mouse thyrotropin: analysis by lectin affinity chromatography. J Biol Chem 1987;262:5197.
32. Taylor T, Gesundheit N, Weintraub BD. Effects of *in vivo* bolus versus continuous TRH administration on TSH secretion, biosynthesis and glycosylation in normal and hypothyroid rats. Mol Cell Endocrinol 1986;46:253.
33. Ronin C, Stannard BS, Weintraub BD. Differential processing and regulation of thyroid-stimulating hormone subunit carbohydrate chains in thyrotropic tumors and in normal and hypothyroid pituitaries. Biochemistry 1985;24:562.
34. Meinkoth JL, Alberts AS, Went W, Fantozzi D, Taylor SS, Hagiwara M, Montminy M, Feramisco JR. Signal transduction through the cAMP-dependent protein kinase. Mol Cell Biochem 1993;127/128:179.
35. Jacquemin C. Glycosyl phosphatidylinositol in thyroid: cell signalling or protein anchor? Biochimie 1991;73:37.
36. Libert F, Passage E, Lefort A, Vassart G, Mattei M-G. Localization of human thyrotropin receptor gene to chromosome region 14q31 by *in situ* hybridization. Cytogenet Cell Genet 1990;54:82.
37. Rousseau-Merck MF, Misrahi M, Loosfelt H, Atger M, Milgrom E, Berger R. Assignement of the human thyroid stimulating hormone receptor (TSHR) gene to chromosome 14_q31. Genomics 1990;8:233.
38. Nagayama Y, Kaufman KD, Seto P, Rapoport B. Molecular cloning, sequence and functional expression of the cDNA for the human thyrotropin receptor. Biochem Biophys Res Commun 1989;165:1184.
39. Nagayama Y, Rapoport B. The thyrotropin receptor 25 after its discovery: new insight after its molecular cloning. Mol Endocrinol 1992;6:145.
40. Gross B, Misrahi M, Sar S, Milgrom E. Composite structure of the human thyrotropin receptor gene. Biochem Biophys Res Commun 1991;177:679.
41. Adams SR, Harootunian AT, Buechler YJ, Taylor SS, Tsien RY. Fluorescence ratio imaging of cyclic AMP in single cells. Nature 1991;349:694.
42. Meinkoth JL, Ji Y, Taylor SS, Feramisco JR. Dynamics of the distribution of cyclic AMP-dependent protein kinase in living cells. Nature 1991;349:694.
43. Breton MF, Roger PP, Omri B, Dumont JE, Palovic-Hournae M. Thyrotropin but not epidermal growth factor down regulates the isoenzymes I (PkaI) of cyclic AMP-dependent protein kinases in dog thyroid cells in primary culture. Mol Cell Endocrinol 1989;61:49.
44. Van Sande J, Lefort A, Beebe S, et al. Pairs of cyclic AMP analogues that are specifically synergistic for type I and type II cAMP dependent protein kinase mimic thyrotropin effects on the function, differentiation expression and mitogenesis of dog thyroid cells. Eur J Biochem 1989;183:699.
45. Kasai K, Field JB. Discrimination of multiple forms of phosphoprotein phosphatase in bovine thyroid. Metabolism 1983;32:296.
46. Brenner-Gati L, Berg KA, Gershengorn MC. Insulin-like growth factor I potentiates thyrotropin stimulation of adenylyl cyclase in FRTL-5 cells. Endocrinology 1989;125:1315.
47. Tramontano D, Moses AC, Veneziani BM, Ingbar SH. Adenosine 3′5′-monophosphate mediates the mitogenic effect of thyrotropin and its ability to amplify the response to insulin-like growth factor I in FRTL-5 cells. Endocrinology 1988;122:127.
48. Berman MI, Jerdack G, Thomas CG Jr., Nayfeh SN. Adrenergic regulation of TSH-stimulated cyclic AMP accumulation in rat thyroid cells. Arch Biochem Biophys 1987;253:249.
49. Taurog A, Dorris M, Doerge DR. Evidence for a mechanism in peroxidase-catalyzed coupling. I. Steady-state experiments with various peroxidases. Arch Biochem Biophys. 1994;315:82.
50. Bjorkman V, Ekholm R. Generation of H_2O in isolated porcine thyroid follicles. Endocrinology 1984;115:392.
51. Ericson LE, Johanson BR. Early effects of thyroid stimulatory hormone (TSH) on exocytosis and endocytosis in the thyroid. Acta Endocrinol (Copenh) 1977;86:112.
52. Yoshimura Y, Dekker A, Ferdows M, Rani CSS, Field JB. Effect of phorbol esters on metabolic variables in the thyroid. Endocrinology 1986;119:2018.
53. Damante G, Chazenbalk G, Russo D, Rapoport B, Foti D, Filetti S. Thyrotropin regulation of thyroid peroxidase messenger ribonucleic acid levels in cultured rat thyroid cells: evidence for involvement of a nontranscriptional mechanism. Endocrinology 1989;124:2889.

54. Gerard CM, Lefort A, Libert F, Christophe D, Dumont JE, Vassart G. Transcriptional regulation of the thyroperoxydase gene by thyrotropin and forskolin. Mol Cell Endocrinol 1988;60:239.
55. Perrild H, Loveridge N, Reader SCJ, Robertson WR. Acute stimulation of thyroidal NAD+ kinase, NADPH reoxidation and peroxidase activities by physiological concentrations of thyroid stimulating hormone acting in vitro: a quantitative cytochemical study. Endocrinology 1988;123:2499.
56. Perrild H, Hoyer PE, Loveridge N, Reader SCJ, Robertson WR. Acute in vitro thyrotropin regulation of lysosomal enzyme activity in the thyroid follicular cell. Mol Cell Endocrinol 1989;65:75.
57. Nagayama Y, Yamashita S, Hirayu H, et al. Regulation of thyroid peroxide and throglobulin gene expression by thyrotropin in cultured human thyroid cells. J Clin Endocrinol Metab 1989;68:1155.
58. Gillman AG, Rall TW. Factors influencing adenosine 3′5′-phosphate accumulation in bovine thyroid slices. J Biol Chem 1968;243:5817.
59. Pastan I, Johnson P, Kendig E, Field JB. Pyridine nucleotides in the thyroid. II. The effect of thyroid stimulating hormone, epinephrine, serotonin, acetylcholine, menadione and glucose concentration on the levels of TPN and TPNH. J Biol Chem 1963;238:3366.
60. Knopp J, Stolc V, Tong W. Evidence for the induction of iodide transport in bovine thyroid cells treated with thyroid stimulating hormone or dibutyryl cyclic adenosine 3′5′ monophosphate. J Biol Chem 1970;245:4403.
61. Manley SW, Bourke JR, Hawker RW. Kinetic aspects of the depression of 131 iodide concentration by thyrotropin in thyroid tissue in vitro. J Endocrinol 1972;54:387.
62. Ahn CS, Rosenberg IN. Prompt stimulation of the organic binding of iodine in the thyroid by adenosine 3′5′-phosphate in vivo. Proc Natl Acad Sci USA 1968;60:830.
63. Corvilain B, Laurent E, Lecomte M, Vansande, Dumont JE. Role of the cyclic adenosine 3′5′-monophosphate and the phosphatidylinositol-Ca^{2+} cascades in mediating the effects of thyrotropin and iodide on hormone synthesis and secretion in human thyroid slices. J Clin Endocrinol Metab 1994; 79:152.
64. Brabant G, Ranft U, Ocran K, Hesch RD, Muhlen A. Thyrotropin: an episodically secreted hormone. Acta Endocrinol 1986;112:315.
65. Brabant G, Brabant A, Ranft U, et al. Circadian and pulsatile thyrotropin secretion in euthyroid man under the influence of thyroid hormone and glucocorticoid administration. J Clin Endocrinol Metab 1987;65:83.
66. Greenspan SL, Klibanski A, Schoenfeld D, Ridgway EC. Pulsatile secretion of thyrotropin in man. J Clin Endocrinol Metab 1986;63:661.
67. Brabant G, Frank K, Ranft U, et al. Physiological regulation of circadian and pulsatile thyrotropin secretion in normal man and woman. J Clin Endocrinol Metab 1990;70:403.
68. Nicoloff JT, Spencer CA. Integration of thyroid hormones with hypothalamic factors on pituitary TSH secretion. Acta Medica Austriaca 1992;19(suppl):68.
69. Gurr JA, Kourides IA. Thyroid hormone regulation of thyrotropin α and β subunit gene transcription. DNA 1985;4:301.
70. Sheppard MC, Franklyn JA, Yarwood NJ, Gurr JA. Thyroid hormone regulation of human pituitary α subunit gene expression. Acta Medica Austriaca 1992;19 Suppl:66.
71. Shupnik MA, Chin WW, Habener JF, Ridgeway EC. Transcriptional regulation of of the thyrotropin subunit genes by thyroid hormone. J Biol Chem 1985;260:2900.
72. Shupnik MA, Ridgway EC, MacVeigh MS. Triiodothyronine rapidly decreases transcription of the thyrotropin subunit genes in thyrotropic tumor explants. Endocrinology 1985;117:1940.
73. Surks L, Oppenheimer IH. Incomplete suppression of thyrotropin secretion after single injection of large L-triodothyronine doses into hypothyroid rats. Endocrinology 1976;99:1432.
74. Surks MI, Lifschits BM. Biphasic thyrotropin suppression in euthyroid and hypothyroid rats. Endocrinology 1977;101:769.
75. De Lean A, Ferland L, Drouin J, et al. Modulation of pituitary thyrotropin releasing hormone receptor levels by oestrogens and thyroid hormones. Endocrinology 1977;100:1496.
76. Hinkle PM, Perrone MH, Schonbrunn A. Mechanism of thyroid hormone inhibition of thyrotropin-releasing hormone action. Endocrinology 1981;108:199.
77. Ridgway EC, Kourides IA, Chin WW, Cooper DS, Maloof F. Augmentation of pituitary thyrotropin response to TRH during subphysiological tri-iodothyronine therapy in hypothyroidism. Clin Endocrinol 1979;10:343.
78. Carr FE, Shupnik MA, Burnside J, Chin WW. Thyrotropin-releasing hormone stimulates the activity of the rat thyrotropin β-subunit gene promoter transfected into pituitary cells. Mol Endocrinol 1989;3:717.

79. Shupnik MA, Greenspan SL, Ridgway EC. Transcriptional regulation of thyrotropin subunit genes by thyrotropin-releasing hormone and dopamine in pituitary cell culture. J Biol Chem 1986;261:12675.
80. Gesundheit N, Weintraub BD. Mechanisms and regulation of TSH glycosylation. Adv Exp Med Biol 1986;205:87.
81. Taylor T, Weintraub BD. Thyrotropin (TSH)-releasing hormone regulation of TSH subunit biosynthesis and glycosylation in normal and hypothyroid rat pituitaries. Endocrinology 1985;116:1968.
82. Hollenberg AN, Monden T, Flynn TR, Boers M, Cohen O, Wondisford FE. The human thyrotropin-releasing hormone gene is regulated by thyroid hormone through two distinct classes of negative thyroid hormone response elements. Molecular Endocrinology 1995;9:540.
83. Weintraub BD, Wondisford FE, Farr EA, et al. Pre-translational and post-translational regulation of TSH synthesis in normal and neoplastic thyrotrophs. Horm Res 1989;32:22.
84. Cohen LE, Wondisford FE, Salvatoni A, Maghnie M, Brucker-Davis F, Weintraub BD, Radovick S. A "Hot Spot" in the Pit-1 gene responsible for combined pituitary hormone deficiency: clinical and molecular correlates. J Clin Endocrinol Metab 1995;80:679.
85. Re RN, Kourides IA, Ridgway EC. The effect of glucocorticoid administration on human pituitary secretion of thyrotropin and prolactin. J Clin Endocrinol Metab 1976;43:338.
86. Ross DS, Ellis MF, Milbury P, Ridgway EC. A comparison of changes in plasma thyrotropin and subunits, and mouse thyrotropic tumor thyrotropin and subunit mRNA concentrations after in vivo dexamethasone or T_3 administration. Metabolism 1987;36:799.
87. Vale W, Brazeau P, Rivier C, et al. Somatostatin. Recent Prog Horm Res 1975;31:365.
88. Lucke C, Hoffken B, Von Zur Muhlen A. The effect of somatostatin on TSH levels in patients with primary hypothyroidism. J Clin Endocrinol Metab 1975;41:1082.
89. Siler TM, Yen SSC, Vale W, Guillemin R. Inhibition by somatostatin of the release of TSH induced in man by thyrotropin-releasing factor. J Clin Endocrinol Metab 1974;38:742.
90. Page MD, Milward ME, Hourihan M, Hall R, Scanlon MF. Long-term treatment of acromegaly with a long-acting analogue of somatostatin, Octeotide. J Med 1990;74:189.
91. Lippe BM, Van Herle AJ, Lafranchi SH, et al. Reversible hypothyroidism in growth-hormone deficient children treated with growth hormone. J Clin Endoctinol Metab 1975;40:143.
92. Cooper DS, Klibanski A, Ridgway EC. Dopaminergic modulation of TSH and its subunits: in vivo and in vitro studies. Clin Endocrinol (Oxf) 1983;18:265.
93. Scanlon MF, Chan V, Heath M, et al. Dopaminergic control of thyrotropin, alpha-subunit and prolactin in euthyroidism and hypothyroidism: dissociated responses to dopamine receptor blockade with metoclopramide in euthyroid and hypothyroid subjects. J Clin Endocrinol Metab 1981;53:360.
94. Dubuis JM, Dayar JM, Siegrist-Kaiser CA, Burger AG. Human recombinant interleukin-1 β decreases plasma thyroid hormone and thyroid stimulating hormone levels in rats. Endocrinology 1988;123:2175
95. Kehlet H, Klauber PV, Weeke J. Thyrotropin, free and total triodothyronine, and thyroxine in serum during surgery. Clin Endocrinol 1979;10:131.
96. Pang XP, Hershman JM, Mirell CJ, Pekary AE. Impairment of hypothalamic-pituitary-thyroid function in rats treated with juman recombinant tumour necrosis factor-α (cachectin). Endocrinology 1989;125:76.
97. Pokroy N, Epstein S, Hendricks S, Pimstone B. Thyrotropin response to intravenous thyrotropin releasing hormone in patients with hepatic and renal disease. Horm Metab Res 1974;6:132.
98. Zalaga GP, Chernow B, Smallridge RC, et al. A longitudinal evaluation of thyroid function in critically ill surgical patients. Ann Surg 1985;201:456.
99. Van Coeverden A, Laurent E, DeCoster C, et al. Decreased basal and stimulated thyrotropin secretion in healthy elderly men. J Clin Endocrinol Metab 1989;69:177.
100. Hugues JN, Enjalbert A, Moyse E, et al. Differential effects of passive immunization with somatostatin antiserum on adenohypophysial hormone secretions in starved rats. J Endocrinol 1986;109:169.
101. Foord SM, Peters JR, Dieguez C, Jasani B, Hall R, Scanlon MF. Hypothyroid pituitary cells in culture: an analysis of TSH and PRL responses to dopamine and dopamine receptor binding. Endocrinology 1984;115:407.
102. Lumpkin MD, Samson WK, McCann SM. Arginine vasopressin as a thyrotropin releasing hormone. Science 1987;235:1070.
103. Morley JE. Neuroendocrine control of thyrotropin secretion. Endocr Rev 1981;2:396.

15 Thyrotropin-Secreting Pituitary Tumors

Differential Diagnosis and Treatment

Mary H. Samuels, MD

CONTENTS

INTRODUCTION

Thyroid stimulating hormone (TSH), or thyrotropin, is a glycoprotein normally secreted by the thyrotroph cells of the anterior pituitary gland. Like the other pituitary glycoproteins, TSH is composed of an alpha (α) and a beta (β) subunit. The α-subunit is identical among the glycoprotein hormones, whereas the unique TSH β-subunit confers biological specificity to the hormone. The TSH α and β subunits are glycosylated in specific patterns that determine subunit combination, clearance rates, and bioactivity.

Pituitary tumors that secrete TSH are rare, representing < 3% of all pituitary adenomas in large neurosurgical series *(1)*. However, with the recent advent of highly sensitive TSH assays, these tumors may be recognized with increasing frequency. This, in turn, may result in earlier diagnosis and improved cure rates for patients with TSH-secreting tumors.

CLINICAL PRESENTATION OF TSH-SECRETING TUMORS

To date, there have been over 140 published cases of patients with TSH tumors *(2–4)*. The age range of these patients is 11–76 yr, although the majority of patients present in early to mid adulthood. There is no male or female predominance in patients with TSH-secreting tumors, in contrast to Graves' disease, which is more common in women. Pa-

From: *Contemporary Endocrinology, Vol. 3: Diseases of the Pituitary: Diagnosis and Treatment*
Edited by M. E. Wierman Humana Press Inc., Totowa, NJ

tients with TSH-secreting tumors usually present with symptoms due to hyperthyroidism, including heat intolerance, sweating, nervousness, tremor, weight loss, increased appetite, and palpitations. These symptoms are indistinguishable from those caused by Graves' disease, excessive thyroid hormone therapy, or other causes of hyperthyroidism. Almost all patients have a goiter on physical examination, which is usually diffuse but rarely can be multinodular.

Since the signs and symptoms of hyperthyroidism are nonspecific in patients with TSH-secreting tumors, it is important to search for clinical clues that distinguish these patients from those with typical Graves' disease. TSH-secreting tumors are usually large when diagnosed, and patients may have headaches and/or visual field abnormalities, as well as symptoms due to deficiencies in other pituitary hormones (for example, ACTH). On the other hand, patients with Graves' disease often have associated autoimmune eye and skin changes that are not found in patients with TSH-secreting tumors. Therefore, the presence of exophthalmos favors the diagnosis of Graves' disease. However, it should be noted that unilateral proptosis has been described as a consequence of a large TSH secreting tumor *(2)*.

A significant subset of patients with TSH-secreting tumors also have acromegaly (22%) or amenorrhea/galactorrhea (10%), owing to cosecretion of growth hormone or prolactin from the tumor *(2)*. Additional patients have nonspecific prolactin elevations resulting from pituitary stalk compression by the large tumor. Occasional patients have been described with TSH-secreting tumors that also produce ACTH, FSH, and/or LH *(2,5–7)*. TSH-secreting tumors have been reported in families with multiple endocrine neoplasia type 1 (MEN1) *(8)*; such patients may also have hyperparathyroidism and pancreatic tumors. One patient with McCune-Albright syndrome (polyostotic fibrous dysplasia, cafe-au-lait pigmentation, and autonomous hyperfunction of multiple endocrine systems) has been described with a combined growth hormone, prolactin, and TSH secreting pituitary tumor *(9)*. Finally, one patient has been described with an aggressive TSH secreting carcinoma with bone and pulmonary metastases *(10)*.

DIFFERENTIAL DIAGNOSIS OF TSH-INDUCED HYPERTHYROIDISM

Many patients with TSH-secreting tumors are initially misdiagnosed as having Graves' disease, due to the presence of hyperthyroidism and a diffuse goiter. This may lead to inappropriate treatment directed toward the thyroid gland, which allows continued tumor growth and compromises ultimate cure rates *(2)*. To avoid this scenario, it is important to remember that patients with Graves' disease (or any other primary thyroid disorder that causes hyperthyroidism) should have undetectable serum TSH concentrations using a sensitive immunometric TSH assay. Any hyperthyroid patient with a measurable TSH level should be further evaluated for a possible TSH tumor.

All patients with TSH tumors have elevated serum levels of thyroid hormones and an inappropriately detectable serum TSH concentration. However, there are other diagnostic possibilities that can also explain this combination of laboratory findings (Table 1) *(7)*.

1. Excess thyroid hormone binding proteins;
2. Iodine-containing drugs;
3. Endogenously produced antibodies that interfere with hormone assays;

Table 1
Differential Diagnosis of Elevated Thyroid Hormone Levels and Nonsuppressed TSH Levels

Condition	*Clinical thyroid status*
Excess thyroid binding proteins	Euthyroid
Endogenous antibodies that interfere with TSH or T_4 assays	Euthyroid
Iodine containing drugs	Variable
Intermittent compliance with T_4 therapy	Variable
Initiation of antithyroid therapy in hypothyroid patient	Variable
Thyroid hormone resistance syndromes	
Generalized (GRTH)	Variable
Pituitary (PRTH)	Hyperthyroid
TSH secreting tumor	Hyperthyroid

4. Intermittent compliance in a patient receiving thyroid hormone therapy, or recent initiation of antithyroid treatment in a hyperthyroid patient;
5. Thyroid hormone resistance.

In a patient with excess thyroid hormone binding proteins, total thyroxine levels are elevated, whereas TSH levels are normal. Unlike patients with TSH-secreting tumors, these patients appear euthyroid, since there is no derangement of the hypothalamic-pituitary-thyroid axis, and serum free thyroxine levels are normal. Therefore, to exclude this entity, a serum free thyroxine level (ideally measured by equilibrium dialysis) can be obtained in patients with elevated total thyroxine levels and normal TSH levels.

In a patient with antibodies that interfere with hormone assays, falsely elevated serum TSH or thyroxine concentrations occur due to the presence of antibodies in the patient's serum that bind to the immunoglobulins used in the assay kits. The specific pattern of thyroid hormone levels depends on the type of antibody produced by the patient and the assay utilized for hormone measurement. The patient is euthyroid unless there is concomitant autoimmune thyroid disease. If this entity is suspected, further laboratory testing of the patient's serum is indicated.

Iodine containing drugs or contrast agents can produce a variety of alterations in thy roid hormone tests, including an elevated thyroxine level and a detectable TSH level. Patients are generally euthyroid, although the iodine load can lead to hypothyroidism or hyperthyroidism.

In patients receiving exogenous thyroid hormone therapy, intermittent compliance can cause elevated serum thyroxine and free thyroxine levels (due to recent ingestion of thyroxine), together with elevated or nonsuppressed TSH levels (due to past noncompliance). Similarly, patients with Graves' disease who initiate antithyroid hormone therapy may have a confusing combination of thyroid function tests until they achieve equilibrium. These patients may appear hypothyroid, euthyroid, or hyperthyroid, depending on the amount of thyroxine recently ingested or the time since initiation of antithyroid therapy.

The syndromes of thyroid hormone resistance are rare conditions associated with elevated thyroid hormone levels, nonsuppressed or overtly elevated TSH levels, and variable tissue resistance to thyroid hormone effects *(2,7,11–13)*. These syndromes are divided into two main types: generalized resistance to thyroid hormones (GRTH), and selective pituitary resistance to thyroid hormones (PRTH). Patients with GRTH may appear hypothyroid, euthyroid, or hyperthyroid, depending on the relative tissue resistance in different organs. It is now clear that GRTH is caused by mutations in the thyroid hormone nuclear receptor gene. Patients with PRTH appear hyperthyroid, since extrapituitary tissues respond to the excess circulating thyroid hormones. The etiology of PRTH is unclear; some authors suggest that there is clinical overlap between GRTH and PRTH, and mutations have been found in the thyroid hormone receptor gene in patients with PRTH that are similar to those found in GRTH. Thus, it is possible that GRTH and PRTH represent a spectrum of abnormalities of the thyroid hormone receptor.

In a clinically and biochemically hyperthyroid patient with nonsuppressed TSH levels, the main diagnostic problem is to distinguish PRTH from a TSH secreting tumor. These two conditions can be distinguished by the following tests *(2,7,11,12)*:

1. The molar ratio of free α-subunit to TSH is greater than unity in 90% of TSH tumors, and is usually less than unity in PRTH. This ratio can be calculated by multiplying the concentration of α-subunit in ng/mL by 10, and then dividing by the concentration of TSH in mU/L. Note that this test cannot be used in postmenopausal women or other patients with primary hypogonadism, since α-subunit is also derived from LH and FSH.
2. The serum TSH response to exogenous TRH is blunted (less than doubling of the basal TSH) in 80% of TSH tumors, and is exaggerated in PRTH.
3. Administration of suppressive doses of triiodothyronine (T_3) decreases TSH levels in 95% of patients with PRTH, but does not decrease serum TSH levels in 80% of patients with TSH-secreting tumors.
4. Radiologic imaging of the pituitary gland is positive in TSH tumors, and negative in PRTH. This is owing to the fact that, to date, most TSH-secreting tumors have been large and easily imaged by CT or MRI of the sella. However, there is a report of a patient with an initial negative study of the sella who subsequently developed a TSH-secreting tumor *(7)*. This scenario may become more common, as widespread use of sensitive TSH testing identifies more patients with small pituitary tumors.
5. Peck-Peccoz et al. have proposed that the measurement of serum sex hormone-binding globulin (SHBG) can distinguish between PRTH or GRTH and TSH-secreting tumors *(14)*. SHBG is elevated in most patients with the common types of hyperthyroidism and in patients with TSH-secreting tumors, but appears to be normal in patients with PRTH or GRTH.

ETIOLOGY OF TSH-SECRETING TUMORS

Primary Hypothyroidism

Patients with long-standing primary hypothyroidism, especially children, may develop compensatory pituitary enlargement due to thyrotroph hyperplasia *(15)*. Such patients may have headaches and visual field abnormalities, which mimic a pituitary tumor. However, there is usually an impressive response to thyroid hormone replacement, confirming that the pituitary enlargement is not due to neoplastic transformation. There are only a few cases of proven TSH adenomas in patients with long-standing, inadequately treated congenital hypothyroidism *(16)*. Such patients are hypothyroid, rather than hyperthyroid, and should be easily distinguished from previously euthyroid patients who develop TSH-secreting tumors.

Molecular Pathogenesis

If TSH tumors are similar to other pituitary adenomas, they represent a clonal expansion of abnormal cells, but sufficient cases have not been studied to determine clonality. Recent studies have attempted to define specific somatic mutations in pituitary adenomas; the following data summarize reports that pertain specifically to TSH tumors:

1. One report did not identify any allelic deletions on chromosome 11 (the site of the multiple endocrine neoplasia type 1 gene) in one TSH secreting tumor *(17)*.
2. No major alterations in the retinoblastoma gene (a tumor suppressor gene) have been found in 15 adenomas with positive immunostaining for TSH, although none of these patients was hyperthyroid *(18,19)*.
3. Molecular probes for other oncogenes, including *ras, myc, fos,* and *myb,* have not revealed alterations in expression levels or major gene deletions in three adenomas with positive immunostaining for TSH *(20,21)*.
4. The transcription factor Pit-1 has been found in five tumors with positive immunostaining for TSH, but Pit-1 sequence and expression levels appear to be normal *(22–24)*.

These limited studies are too preliminary to draw any conclusions regarding specific molecular abnormalities in TSH-secreting tumors.

Other molecular studies have focused on possible alterations in TSHα- and β-subunit gene transcription in TSH-secreting tumors. The unbalanced subunit secretion does not appear to be due to aberrantly initiated mRNAs, since the subunits are similar in length to those in normal thyrotrophs. Furthermore, the transcriptional initiation site of the TSHβ-subunit gene has been mapped in human TSH tumors and is consistent with the authentic start site of normal TSHβ-subunit gene transcription *(25,26)*. Therefore, the molecular alterations responsible for TSH tumor growth and hormone secretion remain obscure.

PATTERNS OF TSH PRODUCTION IN TSH-SECRETING TUMORS

TSH tumors secrete a combination of intact TSH and uncombined α- and TSHβ-subunits. Most secrete excess α-subunit, and 95% have elevated molar ratios of α-subunit to intact TSH in the serum *(2)*.

In patients with TSH tumors, the degree of hyperthyroidism and the serum TSH level may be poorly correlated, and some patients have normal TSH levels *(2)*. Recent studies show altered posttranslational processing of TSH in human TSH tumors, which causes abnormal TSH glycosylation and may alter bioactivity. This effect could explain why some patients with normal TSH levels are hyperthyroid *(7,27,28)*.

In patients with TSH tumors, TSH and α-subunit are secreted in a pulsatile fashion, as in healthy individuals *(29,30)* (Fig. 1). The TSH and α-subunit pulse frequency is relatively preserved, although pulse amplitude varies widely, and the normal circadian variation in TSH levels is altered. Thus, moderate changes in serum TSH or α-subunit levels may not signify changes in clinical status in patients with TSH-secreting tumors.

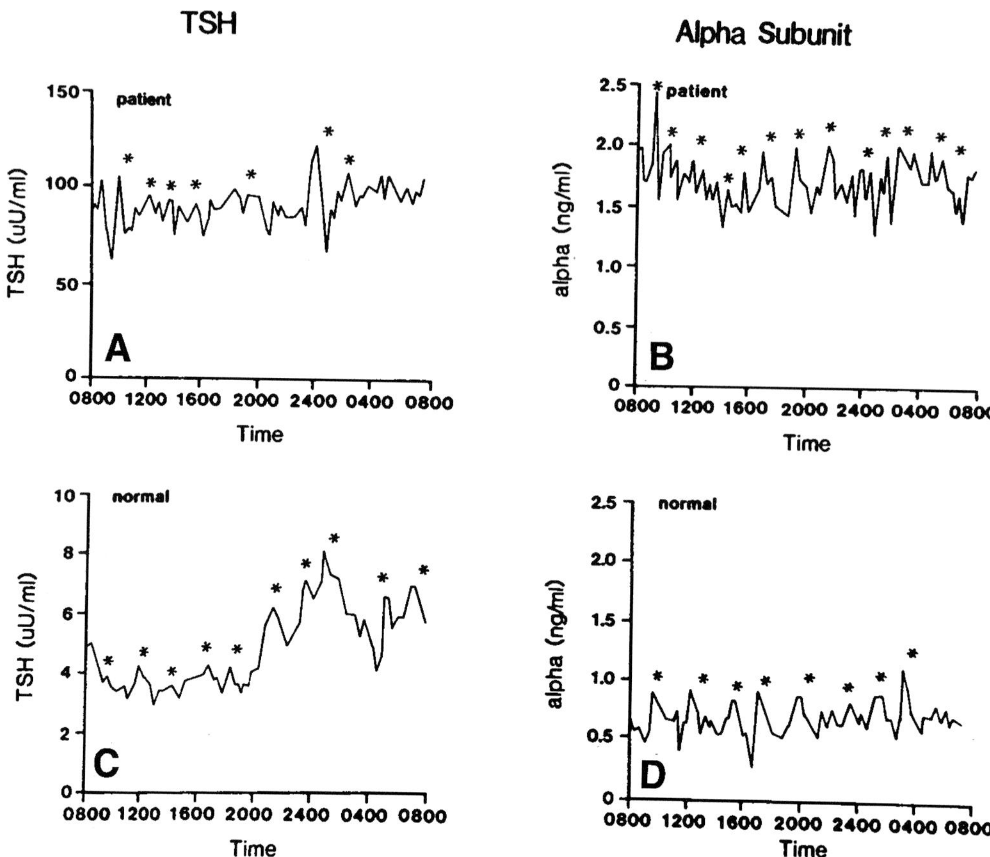

Fig. 1. Serum TSH (**A,C**) and α-subunit (**B,D**) levels in a patient with a TSH secreting tumor (**A,B**), compared to a healthy subject (**C,D**). The TSH and α-subunit levels were measured every 15 min for 24 h. Significant hormone pulses are indicated by asterisks. Note the different scales for serum TSH in the patient compared to the normal subject. Reproduced from ref. *25* with permission.

DYNAMIC TESTS OF SERUM TSH IN TSH-SECRETING TUMORS

Responses to Exogenous TRH

In vivo, 80% of patients with TSH tumors do not have the usual increases in serum TSH or α-subunit levels following TRH administration *(2,11)*. This contrasts with PRTH patients, who invariably have positive TRH tests. Thus, a lack of response to TRH is helpful in the diagnosis of these tumors, but a positive test does not exclude a tumor. In vitro, approximately half of TSH tumors do not respond to TRH, although only a small number of tumors have been studied. TRH-unresponsive tumors may lack TRH receptors, although this has only been studied in a few cases *(31,32)*.

Responses to Thyroid Hormones

The TSH levels in most patients with TSH tumors are resistant to the usual suppressive effects of exogenous thyroid hormone *(2,11)*. On the other hand, if endogenous thyroid hormones are lowered by antithyroid drugs, thyroid surgery, or radioactive iodine, further elevations in TSH levels are often seen. Due to this phenomenon, long-term treatment directed toward the thyroid gland is not recommended unless control of tumor size has been obtained, since there is a theoretical risk of accelerating tumor growth by removing this negative feedback.

Responses to Glucocorticoids

In the small number of patients studied, the normal suppressive effects of glucocorticoids are usually preserved in TSH tumors, and decreases in serum TSH levels occur following glucocorticoid administration in 80% of patients *(2)*. However, α-subunit levels are relatively unaffected, and possible effects on tumor size are unknown. In any case, chronic glucocorticoid therapy of TSH tumors is not recommended, due to the significant adverse effects of glucocorticoid excess.

Responses to Dopamine Agonists

Although dopamine suppresses TSH secretion from normal thyrotrophs, its effects on tumorous TSH secretion are variable *(2)*. In vivo and in vitro studies of dopamine agonist administration usually show a lack of suppressive effect on serum TSH concentrations, with occasional paradoxic stimulation of TSH secretion *(33,34)*.

Responses to Somatostatin

Somatostatin and its analogs decrease TSH secretion from normal thyrotrophs. Many TSH tumors contain somatostatin receptors, although their density is variable *(34,35)*. In most cases studied to date, in vitro incubation of TSH tumors with somatostatin or its analogs suppresses basal or TRH-induced TSH and α-subunit secretion *(36)*. In vivo, acute injections of somatostatin or its analogs lead to rapid decreases in TSH levels in most patients, by a mean of 60% *(15)*.

TREATMENT OF TSH-SECRETING TUMORS

Optimal treatment of TSH tumors is directed toward the clinical manifestations of hyperthyroidism, as well as the tumor itself. These tumors are often large and invasive, and a combined surgical, radiotherapy, and medical approach is often necessary for treatment. Short-term β-blockade and antithyroid drug therapy is recommended prior to pituitary surgery to optimize patient safety, but long-term antithyroid therapy or thyroid gland ablation are not recommended unless therapies directed at the pituitary gland are unsuccessful. The following options exist for treatment directed at the pituitary gland.

Surgery

Unless there is a contraindication to surgery, the initial management of TSH tumors should be surgical. Success rates of transsphenoidal surgery for TSH tumors are difficult to calculate, since these tumors are so rare. A recent review reports that approximately 38% of patients are cured by surgery; success rates probably depend on tumor size *(2,37)*. As smaller TSH tumors are discovered utilizing sensitive TSH assays, surgical cure rates may improve.

In most cases of successful surgery for TSH tumors, patients are euthyroid following surgery. However, patients should be monitored for the possible development of transient postsurgical hypothyroidism due to suppression of the normal thyrotrophs *(38)*.

Radiation Therapy

Because the effects of irradiation on hormonally active pituitary tumors occur slowly, the utility of this modality for initial management of TSH tumors is limited. Radiation therapy has been used in conjunction with surgery to improve long-term cure rates in patients with TSH tumors. It appears that the success rate of this combined modality is approximately 35%, although earlier diagnosis may improve cure rates *(2)*. The success rates of combined surgery and radiation therapy cannot be compared to those of surgery alone, since patients who received both therapies were more likely to have large, aggressive tumors.

Medical Therapy

Dopamine Agonist Therapy

As discussed, most TSH-secreting tumors do not respond to dopamine in vitro. However, occasional patients have a clinical response to dopamine agonists, and they can be tried if other treatment modalities are not effective. In one case, dopamine agonist therapy was used successfully over an 8-yr period in a woman with a large TSH secreting tumor. TSH and α-subunit levels decreased, but did not normalize, and there was no change in tumor size *(39)*.

Somatostatin Analog Therapy

As discussed above, most TSH-secreting tumors respond to somatostatin administration. Of interest, somatostatin analog therapy may also alter TSH glycosylation in TSH tumors, reducing its bioactivity *(40)*. Based on these findings, a number of patients with TSH tumors have been given the somatostatin analog octreotide, usually following pituitary surgery *(2,41,42)*. Octreotide therapy has been continued for up to 5 yr, with an efficacy rate of 76% in terms of decreasing serum TSH levels. Close to 100% of patients have shown a fall in serum T4 levels. Reduction in tumor volume has been noted in 40% of patients; extent of tumor shrinkage ranged from minimal to 70%. Reduction or disappearance of goiter and improvement of visual fields have been reported. Many patients have responded to a dose of 100 μg t.i.d., which is usually associated with tolerable side-effects. Rare patients have developed tachyphylaxis during therapy, which usually responded to increased octreotide doses. Based on these results, octreotide is the therapy of choice following surgery and/or radiation therapy for TSH tumors. Whether this treatment has a role as an alternative to surgery in selected patients has not been determined.

REFERENCES

1. Mindermann T, Wilson CB. Thyrotropin-producing pituitary adenomas. J Neurosurg 1993;79:521–527.
2. Smallridge RC. Thyrotropin-secreting tumors. In: Mazzaferri EL, Samaan NA, eds. Endocrine Tumors. Blackwell, Boston, 1993, pp. 136–151.
3. Gesundheit N, Petrick PA, Nissim M. Thyrotropin-secreting pituitary adenomas: clinical and biochemical heterogeneity. Ann Int Med 1989; 111:827–835.

4. Beckers A, Abs R, Mahler C, et al. Thyrotropin-secreting pituitary adenomas: report of seven cases. J Clin Endocrinol Metab 1991; 72:477–483.
5. Felix I, Asa SL, Kovacs K, et al. Recurrent plurihormonal bimorphous pituitary adenoma producing growth hormone, thyrotropin, and prolactin. Arch Pathol Lab Med 1994; 118:66–70.
6. Patrick AW, Atkin SL, MacKenzie, et al. Hyperthyroidism secondary to a pituitary adenoma secreting TSH, FSH, alpha-subunit and GH. Clin Endocrinol 1994; 40:275–278.
7. Magner J. TSH-mediated hyperthyroidism. The Endocrinologist 1993; 3:289–296.
8. Burgess JR, Shepherd JJ, Greenaway TM. Thyrotropinomas in multiple endocrine neoplasia type 1 (MEN-1). Aust NZ J Med 1994; 24:740–1.
9. Gessl A, Freissmuth M, Czech T, et al. Growth hormone-prolactin-thyrotropin-secreting pituitary adenoma in atypical McCune-Albright syndrome with functionally normal $G_{s\alpha}$ protein. J Clin Endocrinol Metab 1994; 79:1128–1134.
10. Mixsen AJ, Friedman TC, Katz DA. Thyrotropin-secreting pituitary carcinoma. J Clin Endocrinol Metab 1993; 76:529–533.
11. Refetoff S. Resistance to thyroid hormone revisited. Thyroid Today 1990; 13:1–11.
12. Beck-Peccoz P, Chatterjee KK. The variable clinical phenotype in thyroid hormone resistance syndrome. Thyroid 1994; 4:225–232.
13. Usula SJ. Molecular diagnosis and characterization of thyroid hormone resistance syndromes. Thyroid 1991; 1:361–367.
14. Beck-Peccoz P, Roncoroni R, Mariotti S et al. Sex hormone-binding globulin measurement in patients with inappropriate secretion of thyrotropin (IST): evidence against selective pituitary thyroid hormone resistance in nonneoplastic IST. J Clin Endocrinol Metab 1990; 71:19–25.
15. Smallridge RC. Thyrotropin-secreting pituitary tumors. Endocrinology and Metabolism Clinics 1987; 16:765–792.
16. Fatourechi V, Gharib H, Scheithauer BW. et al. Pituitary thyrotropic adenoma associated with congenital hypothyroidism. Am J Med 1984; 76:725–728.
17. Boggild MD, Jenkinson S, Pistorello M. et al. Molecular genetic studies of sporadic pituitary tumors. J Clin Endocrinol Metab 1994; 78:387–392.
18. Cryns VL, Alexander JM, Klibanski A, Arnold A. The retinoblastoma gene in human pituitary tumors. J Clin Endocrinol Metab 1993; 77:644–646.
19. Zhu J, Leon SP, Beggs AH. et al. Human pituitary adenomas show no loss of heterozygosity at the retinoblastoma gene locus. J Clin Endocrinol Metab 1994; 78:922–927.
20. Karga HJ, Alexander JM, Hedley-White ET. et al. Ras mutations in human pituitary tumors. J Clin Endocrinol Metab 1992; 74:914–919.
21. Woloschak M, Roberts JL, Post K. C-myc, c-fos, and c-myb gene expression in human pituitary adenomas. J Clin Endocrinol Metab 1994; 79:253–7.
22. Pellegrini I, Barlier A, Gunz G. et al. Pit-1 gene expression in the human pituitary and pituitary adenomas. J Clin Endocrinol Metab 1994; 79:189–96.
23. Asa SL, Puy LA, Lew AM. et al. Cell type-specific expression of the pituitary transcription activator Pit-1 in the human pituitary and pituitary adenomas. J Clin Endocrinol Metab 1993; 77:1275–80.
24. Friend KE, Chiou YK, Laws ER. et al. Pit-1 messenger ribonucleic acid is differentially expressed in human pituitary adenomas. J Clin Endocrinol Metab 1993; 77:1281–6.
25. Samuels MH, Wood WM, Gordon DF. et al. Clinical and molecular studies of a thyrotropin-secreting pituitary adenoma. J Clin Endocrinol Metab 1989; 68:1211–1215.
26. Wondisford FE, Radovick S, Moates JM. et al. Isolation and characterization of the human thyrotropin β-subunit gene. J Biol Chem 1988; 263:12,538–12,542
27. Magner J, Klibanski A, Fein H. et al. Ricin and lentil lectin-affinity chromatography reveals oligosaccharide heterogeneity of thyrotropin secreted by 12 human pituitary tumors. Metabolism 1992; 41:1009–1015.
28. Papandreou MJ, Persani L, Asteria C. et al. Variable carbohydrate structures of circulating thyrotropin as studied by lectin affinity chromatography in different clinical conditions. J Clin Endocrinol Metab 1993; 77:393–398.
29. Samuels MH, Henry P, Kleinschmidt-DeMasters BK. et al. Pulsatile glycoprotein hormone secretion in glycoprotein-producing pituitary tumors. J Clin Endocrinol Metab 1991; 73:1281–1288.
30. Adriaanse R, Brabant G, Endert E. et al. Pulsatile thyrotropin and prolactin secretion in a patient with a mixed thyrotropin- and prolactin-secreting pituitary adenoma. Eur J Endocrinol 1994; 130:113–20.

31. Chanson R, Li JY, LeDafniet M, et al. Absence of receptors for thyrotropin (TSH)-releasing hormone in human TSH-secreting pituitary adenomas associated with hyperthyroidism. J Clin Endocrinol Metab 1988; 66:447–450.
32. Le Dafniet M, Brandi AM, Kujas M, et al. Thyrotropin-releasing hormone (TRH) binding sites and thyrotropin response to TRH are regulated by thyroid hormones in human thyrotropic adenomas. Eur J Endocrinol 1994; 130:559–564.
33. Chanson P, Orgiazzi J, Derome PJ, et al. Paradoxical response of thyrotropin to l-dopa and presence of dopaminergic receptors in a thyrotropin-secreting pituitary adenoma. J Clin Endocrinol Metab 1984; 59:542–546.
34. Spada A, Bassetti M, Martino E. et al. In vitro studies on TSH secretion and adenylate cyclase activity in a human TSH-secreting pituitary adenoma. Effects of somatostatin and dopamine. J Endocrinol Invest 1985; 8:193–198.
35. Bertherat J, Brue T, Enjalbert A. et al. Somatostatin receptors on thyrotropin-secreting pituitary adenomas: comparison with the inhibitory effects of octreotide upon in vivo and in vitro hormonal secretions. J Clin Endocrinol Metab 1992; 75:540–546.
36. Takano K, Ajima M, Teramoto A. et al. Mechanisms of action of somatostatin on human TSH-secreting adenoma cells. Am J Physiol 1995; 268:E558–64.
37. McCutcheon IE, Weintraub BD, Oldfield EH. Surgical treatment of thyrotropin-secreting pituitary adenomas. J Neurosurg 1990; 73:674–683.
38. Jackson JA, Smigiel M. Hypothyroidism and thyrotropin-secreting pituitary microadenomectomy. Ann Int Med 1990; 112:388.
39. Karlsson FA, Burman P, Kampe O. et al. Large somatostatin-insensitive thyrotropin-secreting pituitary tumour responsive to d-thyroxine and dopamine agonists. Acta Endocrinol 1993; 129:291–295.
40. Francis TB, Smallridge RC, Kane J, Magner JA. Octreotide changes serum thyrotropin (TSH) glycoisomer distribution as assessed by lectin chromatography in a TSH macroadenoma patient. J Clin Endocrinol Metab 1993; 77:183–7.
41. Comi RJ, Gesundheit N, Murray L. et al. Response of thyrotropin-secreting pituitary adenomas to a long-acting somatostatin analogue. N Engl J Med 1981; 317:12–17.
42. Chanson P, Weintraub BD, Harris AG. Octreotide therapy for thyroid-stimulating hormone-secreting pituitary adenomas. A follow-up of 52 patients. Ann Int Med 1993; 119:236–240.

16 Infiltrative Diseases of the Pituitary Gland

Michael T. McDermott, MD

CONTENTS

INTRODUCTION

The human pituitary gland consists of the anterior pituitary (adenohypophysis), which is embryologically derived from the stomodeum (oropharynx); and the posterior pituitary (neurohypophysis), which arises as an evagination of the diencephalon (hypothalamus). During development, these two structures migrate toward one another and become collocated within the bony sella turcica. The anterior pituitary is a composite of five distinct cell types: somatotrophs, lactotrophs, thyrotrophs, gonadotrophs, and corticotrophs. These cells synthesize and secrete, respectively, growth hormone (GH), prolactin, thyrotropin (TSH), follicle-stimulating hormone (FSH) and luteinizing hormone (LH), and corticotropin (ACTH). The posterior pituitary consists of axons whose nerve cell bodies and nuclei lie within the supraoptic and paraventricular nuclei of the hypothalamus. It secretes oxytocin and vasopressin (antidiuretic hormone or ADH), both of which are synthesized in the hypothalamus and migrate to the neurohypophysis in association with carrier proteins called neurophysins. The blood supply to the anterior pituitary is predominantly from the hypophyseal portal vessels, a relatively slow flowing venous system derived from the superior hypophyseal artery. The posterior pituitary is supplied almost entirely by arterial blood from the inferior

From: *Contemporary Endocrinology, Vol. 3: Diseases of the Pituitary: Diagnosis and Treatment*
Edited by M. E. Wierman Humana Press Inc., Totowa, NJ

Table 1
Infiltrative Diseases of the Pituitary

Inflammatory
Sarcoidosis
Langerhans cell histiocytosis
Lymphocytic hypophysitis
Granulomatous hypophysitis
Wegener's granulomatosis
Necrotizing infundibulo-hypophysitis
Infectious
Tuberculosis
Syphilis
Suppurative hypophysitis
Fungi
Parasites
Virusus
Neoplastic
Metastatic carcinoma
Lymphoma
Leukemia
Miscellaneous
Iron overload
Amyloidosis
Snakebite coagulopathy

hypophyseal artery. These differences in tissue derivation or in blood flow may partly explain the predilection of some disorders to preferentially involve either the adenohypophysis or neurohypophysis.

Infiltrative diseases of the pituitary may be defined as the presence of cells or the deposition of substances that are not normally found in the pituitary parenchyma. The reported etiologies are shown in Table 1. These disorders may be asymptomatic, but frequently present with features of pituitary enlargement or of deficient secretion of one or more pituitary hormones. Diagnosis is often inferred by the association of these findings with one of the systemic illnesses listed in Table 1. However, some of the disorders have characteristic features on computed tomography (CT) or magnetic resonance imaging (MRI) and others may occasionally require tissue histology for an accurate diagnosis. Therapy generally consists of treatment of the primary systemic illness and replacement of any deficient hormones.

SARCOIDOSIS

Sarcoidosis is characterized by the development of noncaseating epithelioid granulomas in various organs throughout the body. The etiology is uncertain, but it is known that macrophages and activated T-lymphocytes participate in the development of granulomatous parenchymal inflammation, which eventually resolves or progresses to fibrosis. The disease most commonly affects the lungs, lymph nodes, skin, and eyes, but may be found in any tissue *(1,2)*. The hypothalamus is infiltrated by moderate to extensive

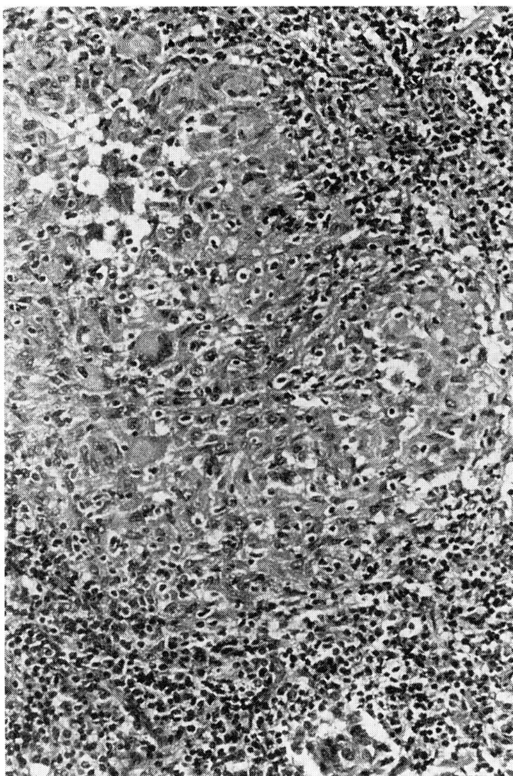

Fig. 1. Pituitary sarcoidosis. Epithelioid granuloma with a central multinucleated giant cell. H&E, ×145. Reproduced from ref. *2a* with permission.

granulomatous inflammation in up to 5% of cases of sarcoidosis, but the pituitary gland is involved less frequently (Fig. 1) *(3–6)*. These patients have extensive multisystem disease, but occasionally isolated hypothalamic or pituitary involvement occurs *(7,8)*. The posterior pituitary gland is affected more frequently than the anterior pituitary.

Disorders of water metabolism are the most common clinical manifestations of hypothalamic-pituitary sarcoidosis. Diabetes insipidus (ADH deficiency) may occur owing to loss of the ADH secreting neurons of the posterior pituitary, destruction of the ADH producing hypothalamic nuclei, or dysfunction of the regulatory osmoreceptor *(9–11)*. Primary polydipsia may sometimes result from lowering of the osmostat thirst threshold *(11)*. The syndrome of inappropriate ADH secretion (SIADH) has also been reported *(12)*.

Anterior pituitary hormone deficiency, causing growth failure, hypogonadism, hypothyroidism, and adrenal insufficiency, alone or in combination, is a less frequent but well recognized complication of sarcoidosis. Although there has occasionally been evidence of primary pituitary damage *(13)*, in most cases pituitary dysfunction appears to be owing to hypothalamic involvement with diminished production of the regulatory hypothalamic-releasing hormones *(6,14,15)*. Further evidence of this is the finding of hyperprolactinemia, suggesting decreased production of hypothalamic prolactin inhibiting factor, in some but not all studies *(16–18)*.

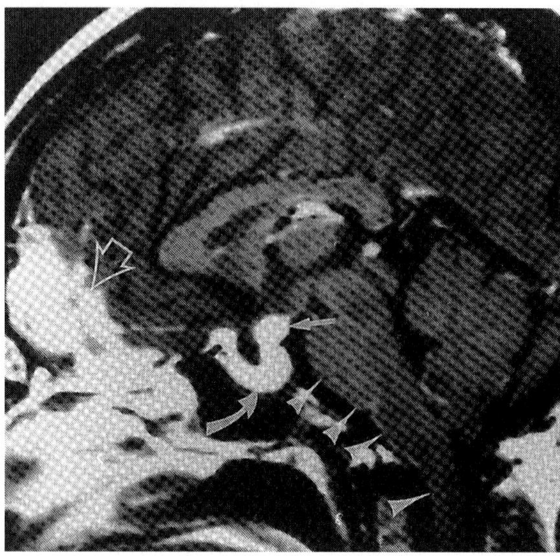

Fig. 2. Pituitary sarcoidosis. Midsagittal T-1 weighted MRI with contrast shows marked enhancement of the pituitary (curved white arrow), chiasm, infundibulum and tuber cinereum (straight white arrow). Reproduced from ref. *20a* with permission.

Imaging of the pituitary gland has recently proved helpful in confirming a diagnosis of hypothalamic-pituitary sarcoidosis. Computed tomography scanning generally reveals slightly hyperdense regions that enhance with contrast administration *(19,20)*. Magnetic resonance imaging often shows hyperintense lesions (Fig. 2) *(20)*.

Treatment consists mainly of hormone replacement therapy although improvement in pituitary function has occasionally been reported with corticosteroid administration *(6,21)*.

LANGERHANS CELL HISTIOCYTOSIS

Histiocytes originate in the bone marrow, first appear in the blood as circulating monocytes, and later migrate into the tissues to become phagocytic tissue macrophages. As they take up residence in peripheral tissues, histiocytes mature into several subclasses: dermal Langerhans cells, hepatic Kupffer cells, pulmonary alveolar macrophages, osteoclasts, and probably neuronal microglial cells. Histiocytes occasionally proliferate abnormally, fuse into multinucleated giant cells, and form tissue granulomas. Langerhans cell histiocytosis, which was formerly termed histiocytosis X, consists of a group of disorders in which Langerhans cells proliferate aggressively, infiltrate tissues, and coalesce to form granulomas, producing tissue damage. Although the classification remains a subject of disagreement and change, Langerhans cell histiocytosis (histiocytosis X) has usually been considered as comprising three somewhat overlapping entities: Langerhans cell granulomatosis, Hand-Schüller-Christian disease, and Letterer-Siwè disease.

Langerhans cell granulomatosis is also known as eosinophilic granulomatosis because of the coexisting tissue infiltration with eosinophils, probably due to the elaboration of eosinophil chemotactic factors by the proliferating histiocytes. It affects

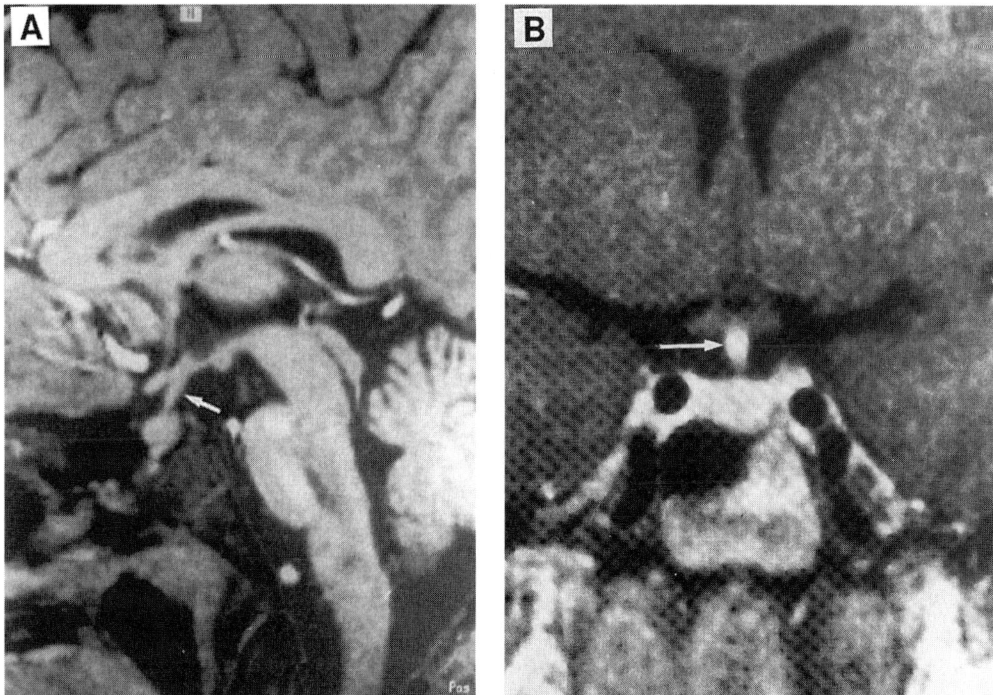

Fig. 3. Langerhans cell histiocytosis with diabetes insipidus. T-1 weighted sagittal (**A**) and coronal (**B**) MRI shows a thickened pituitary stalk (white arrow) and an absent posterior pituitary bright signal. Reproduced from ref. *34* with permission.

predominantly young males, causing lytic lesions of bone, interstitial pulmonary disease and, less commonly, involvement of the hypothalamus, pituitary, skin, liver, spleen, and lymph nodes. Hand-Schüller-Christian disease, which produces the classic triad of diabetes insipidus, exophthalmos, and lytic bone lesions is probably just a variant of Langerhans cell granulomatosis, occurring mainly in adults. Letterer Siwè disease is a more fulminant and often fatal form affecting the liver, spleen, lymph nodes, lung, bones, skin, and sometimes the hypothalamus or pituitary gland in very young children.

Langerhans cell histiocytosis involving the hypothalamic-pituitary region, like sarcoidosis, most often presents with diabetes insipidus or other disorders of water metabolism *(22–27)*. Although destruction of the hypothalamus or posterior pituitary gland is usually responsible for this syndrome, autoantibodies to ADH secreting neurons have been reported in some patients with Hand-Schüller-Christian disease, suggesting that autoimmunity may also play a role *(28)*. Growth failure is the most frequent manifestation of anterior pituitary involvement, but hypogonadism, hypothyroidism, adrenal insufficiency, and hyperprolactinemia sometimes occur *(22,27,29–32)*. As in sarcoidosis, anterior pituitary dysfunction appears to be owing mainly to hypothalamic destruction with loss of regulation by hypothalamic releasing and inhibiting hormones *(22,24,31)*.

Computed tomography scanning usually reveals contrast enhancing mass lesions, whereas MRI often shows pituitary stalk thickening *(25,26,32,35)* associated with a diminished or absent posterior pituitary bright signal (Figs. 3 and 4) in patients with

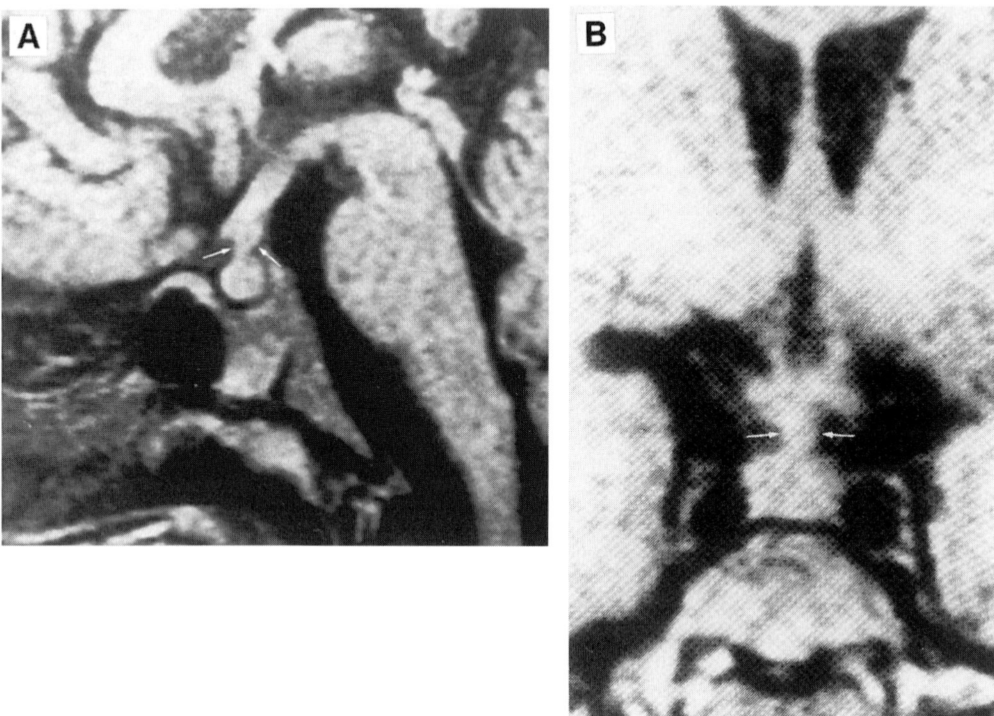

Fig. 4. Langerhans cell histiocytosis with diabetes insipidus. T-1 weighted MRI demonstrates thick pituitary stalk and no posterior pituitary bright signal. Reproduced from ref. *34* with permission.

evolving or overt diabetes insipidus *(33–35)* and prolonged enhancement of affected anterior lobes *(26,27,35)*. Hormone replacement is the primary therapy for hypothalamic-pituitary Langerhans cell histiocytosis, but corticosteroids, cytotoxic agents, and radiotherapy have sometimes been helpful *(22,23,36–38)*.

LYMPHOCYTIC HYPOPHYSITIS

Lymphocytic hypophysitis is characterized by lymphocyte infiltration, atrophy, and eventual destruction of the anterior pituitary gland *(39–44)*. It occurs mainly during pregnancy or the postpartum period, but has been reported in nonpregnant women *(42)* and in a man *(43)*. An autoimmune pathogenesis has been suggested, since approximately 30% of reported patients have had other coexisting autoimmune disorders such as Hashimoto's disease, Addison's disease, hypoparathyroidism, atrophic gastritis, and pernicious anemia *(39)*. Interestingly, a case has also been reported in a patient with pulmonary sarcoidosis *(44)*.

This disorder presents as a pituitary mass lesion causing headaches and visual defects or as clinical deficiency of one or more anterior pituitary hormones. The first clue may be failure to lactate postpartum due to prolactin deficiency. CT and MRI usually show mass lesions with contrast enhancement (Fig. 5). Histologic specimens show extensive lymphocyte infiltration, loss of normal pituitary cells, and fibrosis (Fig. 6) *(39,40)*.

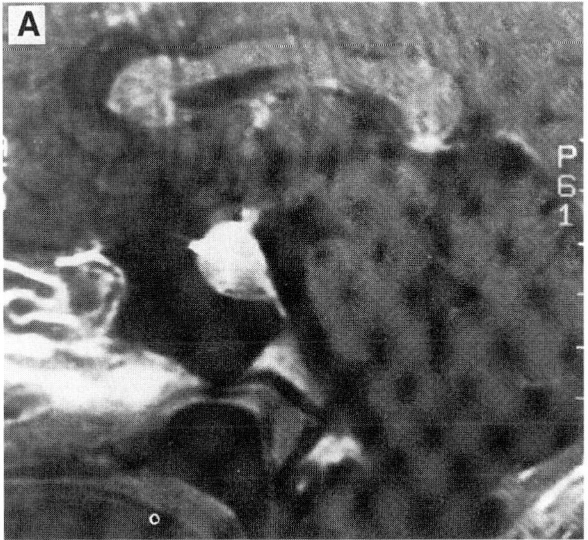

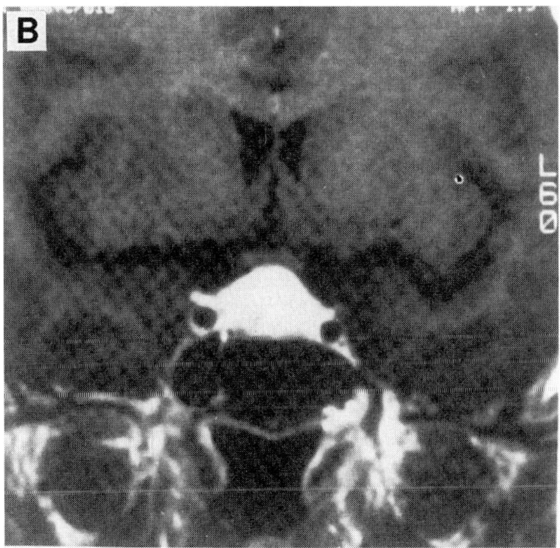

Fig. 5. Lymphocytic hypophysitis. T-1 weighted MRI shows a sellar mass with suprasellar extension. **(A)** Sagittal view, **(B)** coronal cut. Reproduced from ref. *44a* with permission.

Hormone deficiencies should be treated with appropriate replacement regimens. Observation with serial imaging studies and visual field examinations is indicated if the mass effects are mild. When mass effects are severe or progressive, transsphenoidal surgical visualization and biopsy are indicated. If the mass is clearly hypophysitis, decompression without hypophysectomy is the treatment of choice, whereas uncertainty as to the presence of an adenoma may warrant gland removal *(39)*.

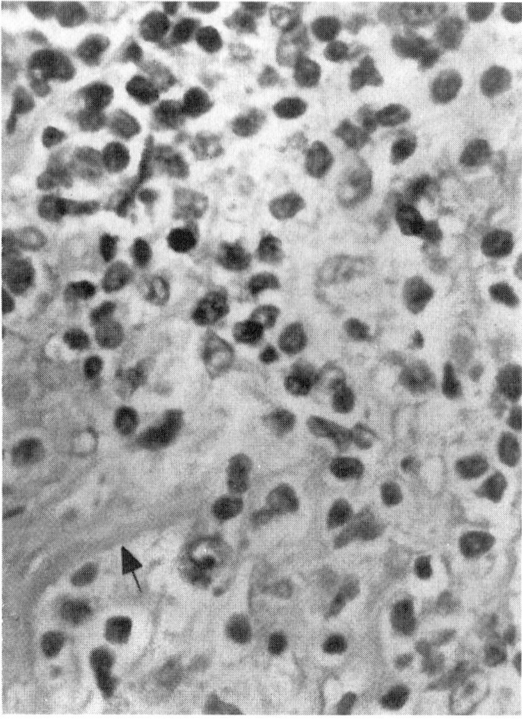

Fig. 6. Lymphocytic hypophysitis. Section shows diffuse lymphocyte infiltration, occasional anterior pituitary cells and some fibrosis (arrow). H&E, ×400. Reproduced with permission from ref. *39*.

OTHER INFLAMMATORY DISORDERS

Granulomatous hypophysitis is a rare pituitary disorder characterized by infiltration of the pituitary with plasma cells, lymphocytes, and multinucleated giant cells and by granuloma formation with areas of necrosis *(45–50)*. Giant cell granuloma, a subset of granulomatous hypophysitis, has been reported to be associated with panhypopituitarism in 66% and with diabetes insipidus in 9% of 23 cases *(51,52)*. Wegener's granulomatosis may rarely involve the posterior pituitary *(53,54)* and has been found in one case to cause anterior pituitary dysfunction *(55)*. Finally, there have been two reported cases of necrotizing infundibulo-hypophysitis, characterized by chronic inflammation, fibrosis, and necrosis throughout the pituitary gland and stalk *(56)*. Clinical features include headaches, diabetes insipidus, hypopituitarism, and pituitary mass lesions on imaging studies.

INFECTIOUS DISEASES

Infections of the pituitary gland *(57)* may be caused by a variety of organisms including bacteria, fungi, viruses, and parasites. Infection may occur by the hematogenous route or by invasion from the contiguous paranasal sinuses, cavernous sinus, meninges, and brain parenchyma. The most frequent clinical manifestations are fever, headaches, visual loss, and extraocular nerve palsies, due to invasion and compression of surrounding structures; less commonly, patients may present with deficiencies of one or more pi-

Table 2
Bacteria Causing Suppurative Hypophysitis

Pneumococcus	*Escherichia coli*
Group A *Streptococcus*	*Citrobacter diversus*
Staphylococcus aureus	*Diphtheroids*
Staphylococcus epidermidis	Anaerobes
Enterococcus	*Actinomyces*
Neisseria	

tuitary hormones. A remarkable number of cases are asymptomatic and discovered only at autopsy. Imaging studies usually reveal a nonspecific mass in the sella turcica. The diagnosis rests on histological recognition or microbiological isolation of an organism from pituitary tissue, although this may not be necessary if the appropriate clinical features are associated with a known systemic infection. The prognosis is generally good provided effective therapy is instituted.

Mycobacterium tuberculosis may infect the pituitary gland in up to 4% of patients with disseminated disease *(58)*, although it is clinically recognized much less frequently. Pituitary tuberculomas usually present as sellar mass lesions with associated fever, headaches, visual loss, and/or ophthalmoplegia, and sometimes with anterior or posterior pituitary insufficiency *(59–62)*. Tuberculous meningitis, which has a predilection for the basilar meninges, may cause pituitary deficiencies in approximately 3% of patients in the proximal postinfectious period *(63,64)*; but one study, employing dynamic endocrine testing, found abnormal endocrine function in 10 of 49 patients (20%) after a mean follow-up of 17.5 yr *(65)*. In half of these cases, a primary hypothalamic defect was suggested as the cause. *Mycobacterium avium intracellulare* and *Mycobacterium fortuitum* have both been reported to infect the pituitary in patients with the acquired immune deficiency syndrome (AIDS) *(66)*.

Both congenital and acquired syphilis may involve the pituitary gland *(57,67–73)*. Congenital disease is often characterized by interstitial inflammation or multiple small gummas in the anterior pituitary, whereas the acquired form more often produces large solitary pituitary gummas. Most cases are asymptomatic but cranial nerve III palsies, visual loss, sellar erosion, anterior pituitary hormone deficiency, and diabetes insipidus may also occur.

Acute bacterial hypophysitis with abscess formation *(57,74–76)* may result from infection by a number of different pyogenic organisms (Table 2). Most cases are associated with preexisting pituitary tumors, craniopharyngiomas, or Rathke's cleft cysts, which have presumably eroded into the sphenoid sinus. Occasionally, the infection may occur as a postoperative complication. The clinical features include fevers, headaches, visual loss, ophthalmoplegia, and hypopituitarism, often in association with sphenoid sinusitis. Imaging studies reveal sellar enlargement and bony erosion. The treatment of choice is surgical drainage with appropriate antibiotic coverage *(77,78)*.

Fungal infection of the pituitary may occur in patients with histoplasmosis, blastomycosis, coccidioidomycosis, candidiasis, aspergillosis, and sporotrichosis *(57)*. Treatment generally consists of surgery and systemic antifungal therapy. Reported par-

Table 3
Viruses That Infect the Pituitary

Encephalitis viruses	Rubella virus
Influenza type A virus	Varicella virus
Herpes simplex virus	Variola virus
Coxsackie B virus	Measles virus
Poliomyelitis virus	Mumps virus
Cytomegalovirus	Rabies virus
Korean hemorrhagic fever virus	HIV virus

asitic pituitary infections include toxoplasmosis, amebiasis, malaria, cysticercosis, and echinococcosis *(57)*. Appropriate drugs and/or surgery may be required for cure.

The pituitary and/or hypothalamus may be affected by a wide variety of viruses (Table 3). Such viral involvement may produce inflammation and necrosis with transient or permanent hypopituitarism *(57)*. Korean (epidemic) hemorrhagic fever is associated with pituitary atrophy, necrosis, and dysfunction in as many as half of infected patients *(79–81)*. The human immunodeficiency virus (HIV) may directly infect the pituitary or predispose it to infection by several opportunistic pathogens such as cytomegalovirus, *Pneumocystis carinii, Toxoplasma gondii*, and *Cryptococcus neoformans (82–84)*. A variety of anterior and posterior pituitary dysfunction syndromes have been described in HIV-infected patients *(84–94)*.

METASTATIC CANCER

Autopsy studies of patients dying of metastatic cancer have revealed that 1–4% of such patients have pituitary metastases *(95–97)*. The most common primary tumor sites are breast, lung, and prostate *(95–98)*. The posterior pituitary is involved with metastases 3–5 times more often than is the anterior pituitary *(95–98)*. Clinical manifestations include headaches, extraocular nerve palsies, visual loss, and pituitary dysfunction. Diabetes insipidus occurs in approximately 7% of cases, whereas anterior pituitary hormone deficiencies appear in only 1% *(99,100)*. Imaging studies cannot reliably distinguish metastatic tumor masses from primary pituitary adenomas, and thus the diagnosis relies primarily on clinical features *(97)*. Treatment often includes radiation therapy and hormone replacement, when indicated.

IRON OVERLOAD

Prolonged, excessive iron intake or absorption leads to iron deposition in tissues, causing widespread organ damage. The most common etiologies are idiopathic hemochromatosis (IH), multiple blood transfusions, and chronic ingestion of iron supplements. Idiopathic hemochromatosis is an autosomal recessive genetic disorder in which intestinal iron absorption chronically exceeds normal metabolic needs, resulting in tissue iron overload. This disorder is highly prevalent in the population; 1 out of 10 whites is heterozygous and 1 out of 300–400 is homozygous for the disease. The most common manifestations of iron overload are bronze skin, diabetes mellitus, cirrhosis, cardiomyopathy, and sexual dysfunction. The latter may sometimes be the sole presenting feature.

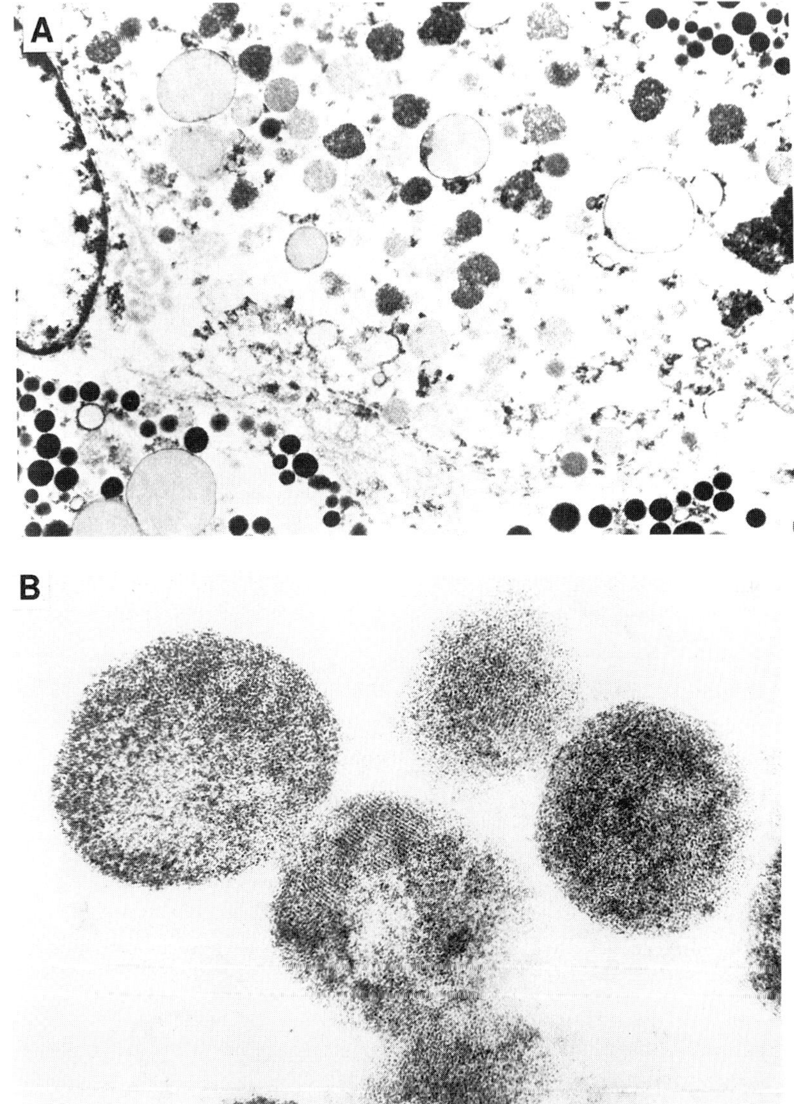

Fig. 7. Hemochromatosis. Anterior pituitary cell (**A**), probably a gonadotrope, with aggregates of hemosiderin and ferritin (magnified in **B**) and a reduced number of secretory granules. Portions of surrounding cells show normal granulation. Uranyl acetate, lead citrate, ×10,200. Reproduced from ref. *118* with permission.

Sexual dysfunction has, in most cases, resulted from secondary hypogonadism owing to deficient pituitary secretion of gonadotropins *(101–115)*; occasionally primary gonadal or hypothalamic involvement has also been reported *(102,104,106,108,115)*. The secretion of other anterior and posterior pituitary hormones is usually normal in adults *(101–104,101,112)*, although deficient prolactin responses to secretogogs have sometimes been found *(103,104,110,117)*. Consistent with this clinical picture are the histologic findings of iron deposition (Fig. 7) occurring predominantly in gonadotrophs and, to a lesser extent, lactotrophs of the ante-

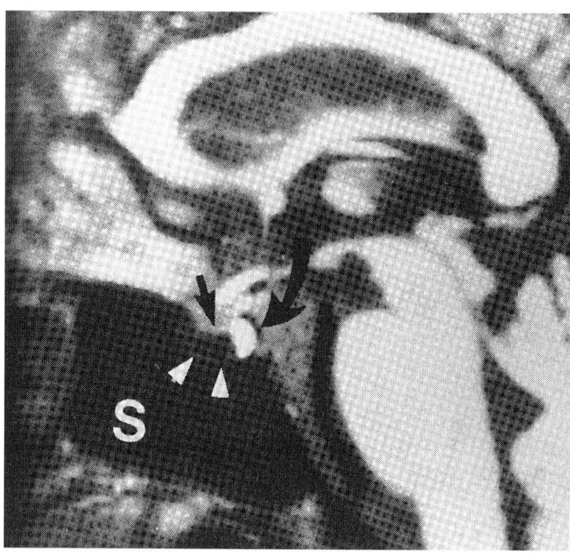

Fig. 8. Hemochromatosis. T-1 weighted sagittal MRI shows an absent anterior lobe signal (straight arrow) with a normal posterior pituitary bright signal (curved arrow). Reproduced from ref. *119* with permission.

rior pituitary gland *(118)*. Growth hormone deficiency has also been reported in children with transfusion-induced iron overload syndromes *(115)*.

Computed tomography scanning is often uninformative, but MRI may show markedly reduced or no signal intensity on T-1 weighted images of the anterior pituitary contrasted with the normally high signal from the posterior pituitary gland (Fig. 8) *(119)*. Treatment consists primarily of hormone replacement therapy. Reduction of body iron stores by serial phlebotomies, although usually unsuccessful *(105,110,112)*, has improved gonadal function in some patients *(106,107,116)*. Prophylactic iron chelation therapy in children who require multiple transfusions for anemia has also been advocated *(113)*.

AMYLOIDOSIS

Amyloid deposits have been observed in the pituitary glands of patients with various types of systemic amyloidosis (Fig. 9), both primary and secondary *(120)*. Pituitary function tends to remain normal, but hypopituitarism has been reported, affecting primarily anterior pituitary hormone secretion *(121)*. One study of familial amyloidotic polyneuropathy described subtle to severe abnormalities of either growth hormone or prolactin regulation in 71% and relatively low ADH levels in 17% of affected patients, respectively *(122)*. Hormone treatment is not usually necessary.

SNAKEBITE COAGULOPATHY

The venom of Russell's viper, an inhabitant of Burma, contains a powerful procoagulant, which leads to disseminated intravascular coagulopathy, acute renal failure, and death in snakebite victims. Autopsy studies of fatal cases have revealed fibrin deposits, hemorrhage, and necrosis of the anterior pituitary gland *(123)*, whereas studies of sur-

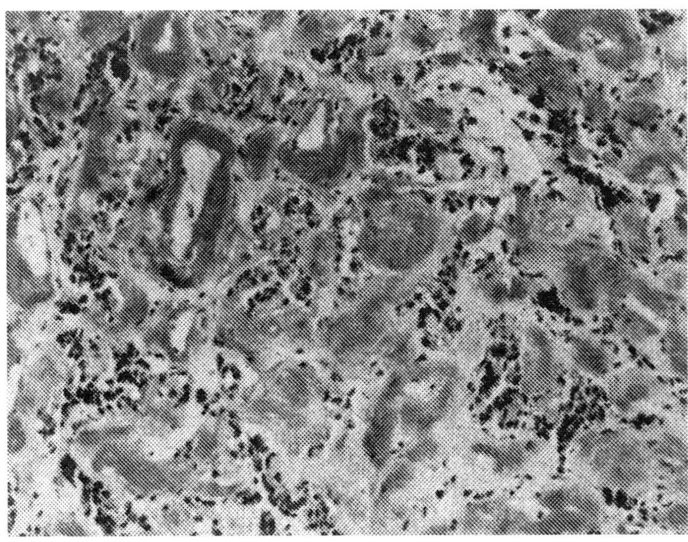

Fig. 9. Amyloidosis. Diffuse perivascular and parenchymal amyloid infiltration in the anterior pituitary gland. Reproduced from ref. *121* with permission.

vivors have revealed hypopituitarism to be a common sequela *(124,125)*. Chronic hormone replacement therapy is indicated in these patients.

REFERENCES

1. Carlson HE. Pituitary Function in Systemic Disorders. In: Melmed S, ed. The Pituitary. Blackwell, Cambridge, MA, 1995; pp. 595–605.
2. Bell NH. Endocrine complications of sarcoidosis. Endocrinol Metab Clin NA 1991; 20(3): 645–654.

2a. Lara Capellan JI, et al. Intrasellar mass with hypopituitarism as a manifestation of sarcoidosis. J Neurosurg 1990; 73:283–286.

3. Bleisch VR, Robbins SL. Sarcoid-like granulomata of pituitary gland: A cause of pituitary insufficiency. Arch Intern Med 1952; 89:877–892.
4. Dickinson ES. Sarcoidosis meningoencephalitis. Diagnostic difficulties encountered in two cases. Dis Nerv Syst 1971; 32:118–124.
5. Herrin AB, Urich H. Sarcoidosis of the central nervous system. J Neurol Sci 1969; 9:405–422.
6. Stuart CA, Neelon FA, Lebovitz HE. Hypothalamic insufficiency: The cause of hypopituitarism in sarcoidosis. Ann Intern Med 1978; 88:589–594.
7. Cariski AT. Isolated CNS sarcoidosis. JAMA 1981; 245:62–63.
8. Lawton FG, Beardwell CG, Shalet SM, Daws RA. Hypothalamicpituitary disease as the sole manifestation of sarcoidosis. Postgrad Med J 1982; 58:771–772.
9. Longcope WT, Freiman DG. A study of sarcoidosis: Based on a combined investigation of 160 cases including 30 autopsies from the Johns Hopkins Hospital and Massachusetts General Hospital. Medicine 1952; 31:1–132.
10. Winnacker JL, Becker KL, Katz S. Endocrine aspects of sarcoidosis (concluded). N Engl J Med 1968; 278:483–492.
11. Stuart CA, Neelon FA, Lebovitz HE. Disordered control of thirst in hypothalamic-pituitary sarcoidosis. N Engl J Med 1980; 303:1078–1082.
12. Kirkland JL, Pearson DJ, Goddard C, Davies I. Polyuria and inappropriate secretion of arginine vasopressin in hypothalamic sarcoidosis. J Clin Endocrinol Metab 1983; 56:269–272.
13. Scott IA, Stocks AE, Saines N. Hypothalamic/pituitary sarcoidosis. Aust N Z J Med 1987; 17:243–245.
14. Vesely DL, Maldonodo A, Levey GS. Partial hypopituitarism and possible hypothalamic involvement in sarcoidosis: report of a case and review of the literature. Am J Med 1977; 62:425–431.

15. Jawadi MH, Hanson TJ, Schemmel JL, Beck P. Katz FH. Hypothalamic sarcoidosis and hypopituitarism. Horm Res 1980; 12:1–9.
16. Turkington RW, MacIndoe JH. Hyperprolactinemia in sarcoidosis. Ann Intern Med 1972; 76:545–549.
17. Munt PW, Marshall RN, Underwood LE. Hyperprolactinemia in sarcoidosis. Incidence and utility in predicting hypothalamic involvement. Am Rev Resp Dis 1975; 112:269–272.
18. Nakao K, Noma K, Sato B et al. Serum prolactin levels in 80 patients with sarcoidosis. Eur J Clin Invest 1978; 8:37–40.
19. Brooks BS, El Gammal T. Hungerford GD, Acker J. Trevor RP, Russel W. Radiologic evaluation of neurosarcoidosis: role of computed tomography. AJNR 1982; 3:513–521.
20. Hayes WS, Sherman JL, Stern BJ, Citrin CM, Pulaski PD. MR and CT evaluation of intracranial sarcoidosis. AJNR 1987; 8:841–847.
20a. Sherman JL, Stern BJ. Sarcoidosis of the CNS: comparison of unenhanced and enhanced MR images. AJR 1990; 155:1293–1301.
21. Shealy CN, Kahana L, Engel FL, McPherson HT. Hypothalamicpituitary sarcoidosis. A report on four patients, one with prolonged remission of diabetes insipidus following steroid therapy. Am J Med 1961; 30:46–55.
22. Braunstein GD, Kohler PO. Endocrine manifestations of histiocytosis. Am J Ped Hematol Oncol 1981; 3:67–75.
23. Dunger DB, Broadbent V, Yeoman E et al. The frequency and natural history of diabetes insipidus in children with Langerhans-cell histiocytosis. N Engl J Med 1989; 321:1157–1162.
24. Rothman JG, Snyder PJ, Utiger RD. Hypothalamic endocrinopathy in Hand-Schüller-Christian disease. Ann Intern Med 1978; 88:512–513.
25. Tien RD, Newton TH, McDermott MW, Dillon WP, Kucharczyk J. Thickened pituitary stalk on MR images in patients with diabetes insipidus and Langerhans cell histiocytosis. AJNR 1990; 11:703–708.
26. Schmitt S. Wichmann W. Martin E, Zachmann M, Schoenle EJ. Pituitary stalk thickening with diabetes insipidus preceding typical manifestations of Langerhans cell histiocytosis in children. Eur J Pediatr 1993; 152:399–401.
27. Langer A, Fettes I. Multifocal eosinophilic granuloma with a pituitary stalk lesion. West J Med 1985; 142:829–831.
28. Scherbaum WA, Wass JAH, Besser GM, Bottazzo GF, Doniach D. Autoimmune cranial diabetes insipidus: its association with other endocrine diseases and with histiocytosis X. Clin Endocrinol 1986; 25:411–420.
29. Nishio S. Mizuno J. Barrow DL, Takei Y. Tindall GT. Isolated histiocytosis X of the pituitary gland: case report. Neurosurgery 1987; 21:718–721.
30. Dean HJ, Bishop A, Winter JS. Growth hormone deficiency in patients with histiocytosis X. J Pediatr 1986; 109:615–618.
31. Gelato MC, Loriaux DL, Merriam GR. Growth hormone responses to growth hormone-releasinig hormone in Hand-Schüller-Christian disease. Neuroendocrinology 1989; 50:259–264.
32. Graif M, Pennock JM. MR imaging of histiocytosis X in the central nervous system. AJNR 1986; 7:21–23.
33. Broadbent V, Dunger DB, Yeomans E, Kendall B. Anterior pituitary function and computed tomography/magnetic resonance imaging in patients with Langerhans cell histiocytosis and diabetes inisipidus. Med and Ped Oncol 1993; 21:649–654.
34. Maghnie M, Arico M, Villa A, Genovese E, Beluffi G. Severi F. MR of the hypothalamic-pituitary axis in Langerhans cell histiocytosis. Am J Neuroradiol 1992; 13:1365–1371.
35. Maghnie M, Genovese E, Arico M, Villa A, Beluffi G. Campani R. Severi F. Evolving pituitary hormone deficiency is associated with pituitary vasculopathy: Dynamic MR study in children with hypopituitarism, diabetes insipidus, and Langerhans cell histiocytosis. Radiology 1994; 193:493–499.
36. Forrest E, Gallacher SJ, Hadley D, Soukop M, Boyle IT. Central nervous system histiocytosis X - imaging and responses to chemotherapy. Scott Med J 1993; 38(5):148–149.
37. El-Sayed S. Brewin TB: Histiocytosis X. Does radiotherapy still have a role? Clin Oncol 1992; 4:27–31.
38. Minehan KJ, Chen MG, Zimmerman D, Su JQ, Colby TV, Shaw EG. Radiation therapy for diabetes insipidus caused by Langerhans cell histiocytosis. Int J Radiation Oncology Biol Phys 1992; 23:519–524.
39. Cosman F. Post KD, Holub DA, Wardlaw SL. Lymphocytic hypophysitis. Report of 3 new cases and review of the literature. Medicine 1989; 68:240–256.
40. Asa SL, Bilbao JM, Kovacs K, Josse RG, Kreines K. Lymphocytic hypophysitis of pregnancy resulting in hypopituitarism: a distinct clinicopathologic entity. Ann Intern Med 1981; 95:166–171.

41. Jensen MD, Handwerger BS, Scheithauer BW, Carpenter PC, Mirakian R. Banks PM. Lymphocytic hypophysitis with isolated corticotropin deficiency. Ann Intern Med 1986; 105:200–203.
42. Miura M, Ushio Y. Kuratsu J-i, Ikeda J-i, Kai Y. Yamashiro S. Lymphocytic adenohypophysitis: report of two cases. Surg Neurol 1989; 32:463–470.
43. Guay AT, Agnello V, Tronic BC, Gresham DG, Freidberg SR. Lymphocytic hypophysitis in a man. J Clin Endocrinol Metab 1987; 64:631–634.
44. Hayashi H. Yamada K, Kuroki T. Katayama M, Shigemori M, Kuramoto S. Nonaka K. Lymphocytic hypophysitis and pulmonary sarcoidosis. Report of a case. Am J Clin Pathol 1991; 95:506–511.
44a. Case records of the Massachusetts General Hospital. N Engl J Med 1995; 333:44–41.
45. Scully RE, Mark EJ, McNeely BU. Case records of the Massachusetts General Hospital. Weekly Clinicopathological Exercises. N Engl J Med 1985; 312:297–305.
46. del Pozo JM, Roda JE, Montoya JG, Iglesias JR, Hurtado A. Intrasellar granuloma: case report. J Neurosurg 1980; 53:717–719.
47. Holck S. Laursen H. Prolactinoma coexistent with granulomatous hypophysitis. Acta Neuropathol (Berl) 1983; 61:253–257.
48. Chanson P. Timsit J. Kuzas M, Violante A, Guillausseau PJ, Derome PJ, Warnet A, Lubetzki J. Pituitary granuloma and pyoderma gangrenosum. J Endocrinol Invest 1990; 13:677–681.
49. Hassoun P. Anayssi E, Salti I: A case of granulomatous hypophysitis with hypopituitarism and minimal pituitary enlargement. J Neurol Neurosurg Psychiatry 1985; 48:949–951.
50. Albini CH, MacGillivray MH, Fisher JE, Voorhess ML, Klein DM. Triad of hypopituitarism, granulomatous hypophysitis and ruptured Rathke's cleft cyst. Neurosurgery 1988; 22:133–136.
51. Rickards AG, Harvey PW. "Giant cell granuloma" and the other pituitary granulomata. Q J Med 1954; 23:425–439.
52. Doniach I, Wright EA. Two cases of giant-cell granuloma of the pituitary gland. J Pathol Bacteriol 1951; 63:69–79.
53. Hurst NP, Dunn NA, Chalmers TM. Wegener's granulomatosis complicated by diabetes insipidus. Ann Rheum Dis 1983; 42:600–601.
54. Haynes BF, Fauci AS. Diabetes insipidus associated with Wegener's granulomatosis successfully treated with cyclophosphamide. N Engl J Med 1978; 299:764.
55. Lohr K, Ryan LM, Toohill RJ, Anderson T. Anterior pituitary involvement in Wegener's granulomatosis. J Rheumatol 1988; 15:855–861.
56. Ahmed SR, Aiello DP, Page R. Hopper K, Towfighi J. Santen RJ. Necrotizing infundibulo-hypophysitis: a unique syndrome of diabetes insipidus and hypopituitarism. J Clin Endocrinol Metab 1993; 76:1499–1504.
57. Berger SA, Edberg SC, David G. Infectious disease in the sella turcica. Rev Infect Dis 1986; 8(5):747–755.
58. Slavin RE, Walsh TJ, Pollack AD. Late generalized tuberculosis: a clinical pathologic analysis and comparison of 100 cases in the preantibiotic and antibiotic eras. Medicine 1980; 59:352–366.
59. Flannery MT, Pattani S. Wallach PM, Warner E. Case report: hypothalamic tuberculoma associated with secondary panhypopituitarism. Am J Med Sci 1993; 306:101–103.
60. Esposito V, Fraioli B. Ferrante L, Palma L. Intrasellar tuberculoma: case report. Neurosurgery 1987; 21:721–723.
61. Delsedime M, Aguggia M, Cantello R et al. Isolated hypophyseal tuberculoma: case report. Clin Neuropathol 1988; 7:311–313.
62. Ranjan A, Chandy MJ: Intrasellar tuberculoma. Brit J Neurosurg 1994; 8:179–185.
63. Lanigan CJ, Buckley MP. Adult panhypopituitarism with normal stature following tuberculous meningitis: a case report. Irish Med J 1983; 76:353–354.
64. Garg SK, Bandyopadhyay PK, Dash RJ. Hypogonadotropic hypogonadism. An unusual complication of tuberculous meningitis. Trop Geogr Med 1987; 39:296–298.
65. Lam KSL, Sham MMK, Tam SCF, Ng MMT, Ma HTG. Hypopituitarism after tuberculous meningitis in childhood. Ann Intern Med 1993; 118:701–706.
66. Jacob CN, Henein SS, Heurich AE, Kamholz S. Nontuberculous mycobacterial infection of the central nervous system in patients with AIDS. South Med J 1993; 86(6):638.
67. Fink EB. Gumma of the hypophysis and hypothalamus. Arch Pathol 1933; 15:631–635.
68. Kennedy FS, Fisher JH. Syphilis of the pituitary body: a case report with review of literature. Am J Syphilis and Neurol 1934; 18:1223.

69. DeSchweinitz GE. Concerning the ocular symptoms in the subjects of hypophyseal disease with acquired syphilis; with illustrative cases. Arch Ophthamol 1921; 50:203–216.
70. Oelbaum MH. Hypopituitarism in male subjects due to syphilis. Q J Med 1952; 21:249–264.
71. Wood CE. Gumma of the pituitary body. JAMA 1909; 52:700–701.
72. Oelbaum MH, Wainwright J. Hypopituitarism in a male due to giant cell granuloma of the anterior pituitary. J Clin Pathol 1950; 3:122–129.
73. Daaboul JJ, Kartchner W. Jones KL: Neonatal hypoglycemia caused by hypopituitarism in infants with congenital syphilis. J Pediatr 1993; 123:983–985.
74. Askenasy HM, Israeli J. Karny H. Dujovny M. Intrasellar abscess simulating pituitary adenoma. Neurochirugica 1971; 14:34–37.
75. Domingue JN, Wilson CB. Pituitary abscesses. Report of seven cases and review of the literature. J Neurosurg 1977; 46:601–608.
76. Bjerre P. Riisheda J. Lindholm J. Pituitary abscess. Acta Neurochir (Wien) 1983; 68:187–193.
77. Whalley N. Abscess formation in a pituitary adenoma. J Neurol Neurosurg Psychiatr 1952; 15:66–67.
78. Zorub DS, Martinez AJ, Nelson PB, Lam M-T. Invasive pituitary adenoma with abscess formation: case report. Neurosurgery 1979; 5:718–722.
79. Wahle GH, Jr, McKay DG. Panhypopituitarism following epidemic hemorrhagic fever. II. Pathologic anatomy. Ann Intern Med 1955; 43:1320–1330.
80. Hullinhorst RL, Steer A. Pathology of epidemic hemorrhagic fever. Ann Intern Med 1953; 38:77–101.
81. Lim TH, Chang KH, Han MC, et al. Pituitary atrophy in Korean (epidemic) hemorrhagic fever: CT correlation with pituitary function and visual field. AJNR 1986; 7:633–637.
82. Ferreiro J. Vinters HV. Pathology of the pituitary gland in patients with the acquired immune deficiency syndrome (AIDS). Pathology 1988; 20:211–215.
83. Sano T. Kovacs K, Scheithauer BW, Rosenblum MK, Petito CK, Greco CM. Pituitary pathology in acquired immunodeficiency syndrome. Arch Pathol Lab Med 1989; 113:1066–1070.
84. Milligan SA, Katz MS, Craven PC, Strandberg DA, Russell IJ, Becker RA. Toxoplasmosis presenting as panhypopituitarism in a patient with the acquired immune deficiency syndrome. Am J Med 1984; 77:760–764.
85. Dobs AS, Dempsey MA, Ladenson PW, Polk BF. Endocrine disorders in men infected with human immunodeficiency virus. Am J Med 1987; 84:611–616.
86. Membreno L, Irony I, Dere W. Klein R. Biglieri EG, Cobb E. Adrenocortical function in acquired immunodeficiency syndrome (AIDS). J Clin Endocrinol Metab 1987; 65:482–487.
87. Root RK, Biglieri EG. Adrenocortical function in the acquired immunodeficiency syndrome (AIDS). West J Med 1988; 148:70–73.
88. Agarwal A, Soni A, Ciechanowsky M, Changer P. Treser G. Hyponatremia in patients with the acquired immunodeficiency syndrome. Nephron 1989; 53:317–321.
89. Croxson TS, Chapman WE, Miller LK, Levit CD, Senie R. Zumoff B. Changes in the hypothalamic-pituitary-gonadal axis in human immunodeficiency virus-infected homosexual men. J Clin Endocrinol Metal 1989; 68:317–321.
90. Lo Presti JS, Fried JC, Spencer CA, Nicoloff JT. Unique alterations of thyroid hormone indices in the acquired immunodeficiency syndrome (AIDS). Ann Intern Med 1989; 110:970–975.
91. Tang WW, Kaptein EM. Thyroid hormone levels in the acquired immunodeficiency syndrome (AIDS) or AIDS-related complex. West J Med 1989; 151:627–631.
92. Aron DC. Endocrine complications of the acquired immunodeficiency syndrome. Arch Intern Med 1989; 149:330–333.
93. Merenich JA, McDermott MT, Asp AA, Harrison SM, Kidd GS. Evidence of endocrine involvement early in the course of human immunodeficiency virus infection. J Clin Endocrinol Metab 1990; 70:566–571.
94. Dluhy RG. The growing spectrum of HIV-related endocrine abnormalities. J Clin Endocrinol Metab 1990; 70:563–565.
95. Abrams HL, Spiro R. Goldstein N. Metastases in carcinoma analysis of 1000 autopsied cases. Cancer 1950; 3:74–85.
96. Kovacs K. Metastatic cancer of the pituitary gland. Oncology 1973; 27:533–542.
97. Max MB, Deck MDF, Rottenberg DA. Pituitary metastasis: incidence in cancer patients and clinical differentiation from pituitary adenoma. Neurology 1981; 8:998–1002.
98. Hagerstrand I, Schonebeck J: Metastases to the pituitary gland. Acta Pathol Microbiol Scand 1969; 75:64–70.

99. Teears RJ, Silverman EM. Clinicopathologic review of 88 cases of carcinoma metastatic to the pituitary gland. Cancer 1975; 36:216–220.
100. Nugent JL, Bunn PA Jr, Matthews MJ et al. CNS metastases in small cell bronchogenic carcinoma. Cancer 1979; 44:1885–1893.
101. Schafer AI, Cheron RG, Dluhy R et al. Clinical consequences of acquired transfusional iron overload in adults. N Engl J Med 1981; 304:319–324.
102. Charbonnel B. Chupin M, LeGrand A, Guillon J. Pituitary function in idiopathic haemochromatosis: hormonal study in 36 male patients. Acta Endocrinol 1981; 98:178–183.
103. Walton C, Kelly WF, Laing I, Bu'lock DE. Endocrine abnormalities in idiopathic haemochromatosis. Q J Med 1983; 52:99–110.
104. McNeil LW, McKee LC Jr, Lorber D, Rabin D. The endocrine manifestations of hemochromatosis. Am J Med Sci 1983; 285:7–13.
105. Resnitzky P. Zuckerman H. Harpaz S. Hypophyseal gonadotropin insufficiency in a young woman with idiopathic hemochromatosis. Isr J Med Sci 1981; 17:359–366.
106. Kelly TM, Edwards CQ, Meikle AW, Kushner JP. Hypogonadism in hemochromatosis: reversal with iron depletion. Ann Intern Med 1984; 101:629–632.
107. Siemons LJ, Mahler CH. Hypogonadotropic hypogonadism in hemochromatosis: recovery of reproductive function after iron depletion. J Clin Endocrinol Metab 1987; 65:585–587.
108. Williams TC, Frohman LA. Hypothalamic dysfunction associated with hemochromatosis. Ann Intern Med 1985; 103:550–551.
109. Kley HK, Stremmel W. Niederau C et al. Androgen and estrogen response to adrenal and gonadal stimulation in idiopathic hemochromatosis: evidence for decreased estrogen formation. Hepatology 1985; 5:251–256.
110. Lufkin EG, Baldus WP, Bergstralh EJ, Kao PC. Influence of phlebotomy treatment on abnormal hypothalamic-pituitary function in genetic hemochromatosis. Mayo Clin Proc 1987; 62:473–479.
111. Stremmel W. Niederau C, Berger M, Kley H-K, Kruskemper H-L, Strohmeyer G. Abnormalities in estrogen, androgen, and insulin metabolism in idiopathic hemochromatosis. Ann N Y Acad Sci 1988; 526:209–223.
112. Wang C, Tso SC, Todd D. Hypogonadotropic hypogonadism in severe B-thalassemia: effect of chelation and pulsatile gonadotropin-releasing hormone therapy. J Clin Endocrinol Metab 1989; 68:511–516.
113. Bronspiegel-Weintrob N. Olivieri NF, Tyler B. Andrews DF, Freedman MH, Holland FJ. Effect of age at the start of iron chelation therapy on gonadal function in β-thalassemia major. N Engl J Med 1990; 323:713–719.
114. Duranteau L, Chanson P, Blumberg-Tick J. Thomas G. Brailly S. Lubetzki J. Schaison G. Bouchard P. Non-responsiveness of serum gonadotropins and testosterone to pulsatile GnRH in hemochromatosis suggesting a pituitary defect. Acta Endocrinologica 1993; 128:351–354.
115. Oerter KE, Kamp GA, Munson PJ, Nienhuis AQ, Cassorla FG, Manasco PK. Multiple hormone deficiencies in children with hemochromatosis. J Clin Endocrinol Metab 1993; 76:357–361.
116. Piperno A, Rivolta MR, D'Alba R. Fargion S. Rovelli F. Ghezzi A, Micheli M, Fiorelli G. Preclinical hypogonadism in genetic hemochromatosis in the early stage of the disease: evidence of hypothalamic dysfunction. J Endocrinol Invest 1992; 15:4238.
117. Levy CL, Carlson HE. Decreased prolactin reserve in hemochromatosis. J Clin Endocrinol Metab 1978; 47:444–446.
118. Bergeron C, Kovacs K. Pituitary siderosis: a histologic immunocytologic and ultrastructural study. Am J Pathol 1978; 93:295–306.
119. Fujisawa I, Morikawa M, Nakano Y. Konishi J. Hemochromatosis of the pituitary gland: MR imaging. Radiology 1988; 168:213–214.
120. Ishihara T. Nagasawa T. Yokota T. Gondo T. Takahashi M, Uchino F. Amyloid protein of vessels in leptomeninges, cortices, choroid plexuses and pituitary glands from patients with systemic amyloidosis. Hum Pathol 1989; 20:891–895.
121. Las MS, Sturks MI. Hypopituitarism associated with systemic amyloidosis. N Y State J Med 1983; 83:1183–1185.
122. Olofsson B-O, Grankvist K, Olsson T. Boman K, Forsberg K, Lafvas I, Lithner F. Assessment of hypothalamic-pituitary function in patients with familial amyloidotic polyneuropathy. J Intern Med 1991; 229:55–59.

123. Than-Than, Francis N. Tin-Nu-Swe et al. Contribution of focal haemorrhage and microvascular fibrin deposition to fatal envenoming by Russell's viper (Vipera russelli siamensis) in Burma. Acta Trop 1989; 46:23–38.
124. Tun-Pe, Warrell DA, Tin-Nu-Swe et al. Acute and chronic pituitary failure resembling Sheehan's syndrome following bites by Russell's viper in Burma. Lancet 1987; ii:763–767.
125. Proby C, Tha-Aung, Thet-Win, Hla-Mon, Burrin JM, Joplin GF. Immediate and long-term effects on hormone levels following bites by the Burmese Russell's viper. Q J Med 1989; 75:399–411.

17 Imaging of the Sella and Perisellar Region

John C. Stears, MD

Contents

NORMAL ANATOMY

The center of our attention is the sella turcica, the bony skeleton of which is a transverse hemicylinder open on either side and superiorly *(1)*. The anterior wall is perpendicular. The tuberculum sellae is a transverse interface between the anterior wall and the sphenoid plate or plane. Frequently this interface is a transverse groove between the anteriorly placed limbus sphenoidalis of the sphenoid plate and the tuberculum with the misnamed chiasmatic groove between, extending toward each intracranial optic canal orifice. The posterior convex wall (both superoinferiorly and side to side) is the dorsum sellae terminating superolaterally in the posterior clinoids which tend to be directed anteriorly. The anterior clinoids are more lateral and are projected posteriorly and somewhat medially. A thin plate of bone forms the roof of the optic canal (the operculum), extending from the top of the anterior clinoid to the sphenoid plate on each side. The floor of the optic canal is the optic strut, a triangular section of bone upon which touches the distal cavernous loop of the internal carotid artery inferiorly and the optic nerve su-

From: *Contemporary Endocrinology, Vol. 3: Diseases of the Pituitary: Diagnosis and Treatment*
Edited by M. E. Wierman Humana Press Inc., Totowa, NJ

periorly. In most skeletons, the cavernous internal carotid artery lies in a groove upon the superolateral aspect of the body of the sphenoid bone.

The dura forms a carpet over and into these structures. It covers the sphenoid plate and orbital roof and anterior clinoids, and covers the clivus and the anterior and posterior face of each temporal bone. The cavernous sinus forms the lateral wall of the sella turcica from the medial cavernous dura to the lateral cavernous dura. A relatively flat section of dura forms the superior surface of the cavernous sinus, the superior cavernous dura. This extends medially, usually into a small depression that is the diaphragma sellae. The latter is typically perforated by a small opening to accept the pituitary stalk (though frequently is larger and a sac of arachnoid enters into the exposed aspect of the intrasellar space). The superior cavernous dura is elevated laterally into an edge that passes in an elongated oval from one anterior clinoid process around the tentorial aperture to the other anterior clinoid process, forming the free edge of the tentorium. Other folds of dura extending from the temporal apex to this fold, and beneath this fold to the posterior clinoid and dorsum and clivus form an interlaced but continuous dural region.

The cavernous sinus as a general term contains two compartments, separated by a vertically oriented septum between the more medially placed venous compartment and the more laterally placed nerve compartment *(2)*. The lateral compartment contains the third, fourth, and the first division of fifth cranial nerves (the paracavernous space). The medial or venous compartment (better termed a plexus than a sinus) contains the cavernous internal carotid artery, its sympathetic plexus, and the cranial nerve VI. The venous compartment reaches to the medial cavernous dura and to the medial aspect of the superior cavernous dura. The lateral compartment reaches to the lateral cavernous dura. There are intrasellar channels connecting the two cavernous venous compartments, which are difficult to see on MR, are variable, but most typically are anterosuperior and posterosuperior relative to the pituitary gland. The superior and inferior ophthalmic veins enter the cavernous compartment through the superior orbital fissure. Also mid and inferior cerebral veins and the sphenoparietal sinus enter. The egress from the venous compartment is through superior and inferior petrosal sinuses and the clival plexus and the pterygoid plexus. There are normally small locules of fat within the cavernous sinus. The internal carotid artery traverses the cavernous sinus venous compartment from an average of 8 mm proximal to the proximal cavernous loop, to the beginning of the distal cavernous loop beneath the base of the anterior clinoid process. The proximal cavernous loop, varies widely from near 90° to more commonly in the order of 135°, and lies medially. The cavernous internal carotid artery then passes forward and laterally, and at the base of the anterior clinoid makes an average of a 145° turn, both medially and then superiorly around the medial aspect of the base of the anterior clinoid, to perforate the dura and become the subarachnoid internal carotid artery. It then passes superolaterally for an average of 30 mm to bifurcate into anterior and middle cerebral arteries (Fig. 1A,B).

The branches of the internal carotid artery are predominantly the meningohypophyseal trunk, which originates just proximal to the proximal cavernous loop, and the ophthalmic artery, which originates in 92% from the immediate proximal subarachnoid internal carotid artery on its inferomedial side. In the region of the base of the anterior clinoid, within the proximal aspect of the distal cavernous loop, the internal carotid

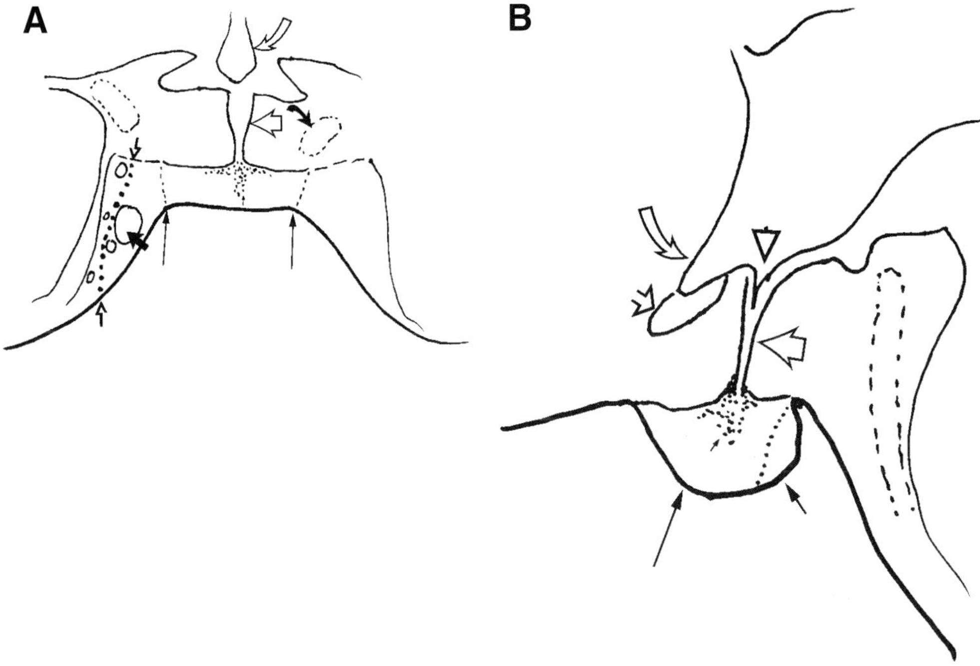

Fig. 1. These are line drawings—a mid pituitary coronal (**A**) section, and a midline sagittal (**B**) section of the perisellar region. The semi-open arrow on the right indicates the septation between the nerve and venous portions of the cavernous sinus. The small black arrows demonstrate anterior lobe (long stalk) and posterior lobe (short stalk). A triangular open arrow indicates the infundibular recess of the third ventricle. A curved open arrow indicates the supraoptic recess of the third ventricle. Note the "tuft" in the anterior pituitary lobe (smallest arrow).

Throughout the figures in this chapter there are some standard arrows:

1. A small triangular arrow with a long stalk denotes the lateral margin of the pituitary gland, or the pituitary gland itself.
2. A similar arrow with a shorter stalk denotes margins of a lesion.
3. A large closed arrow indicates cavernous internal carotid artery.
4. A medium-sized, closed arrow with a curved stem indicates subarachnoid internal carotid artery.
5. An open arrow with a short stalk, small, demonstrates the chiasm.
6. A large open arrow indicates the pituitary stalk.
7. A large open arrow with a curved stalk indicates the third ventricle.

artery becomes an extracavernous epidural structure for a short distance. In 8%, the ophthalmic artery arises from this segment. More distally along the horizontal segment of the cavernous internal carotid artery, the inferior lateral trunk (the artery of the inferior cavernous sinus) arises inferiorly *(3)*. A branch of the latter provides a potential collateral from the internal maxillary artery to the internal carotid artery via the foramen ovale. These branches supply local dura and cavernous cranial nerves. In 30% of the specimens there arises from the distal horizontal internal carotid artery segment inferior and anterior capsular arteries supplying the dura in the region of the sella. The superior hypophyseal artery, arises from the subarachnoid internal carotid artery as single or multiple origins, in 85% arising within 5 mm of the ophthalmic artery, and measuring in average of 0.22 mm in diameter (not usually visible on an-

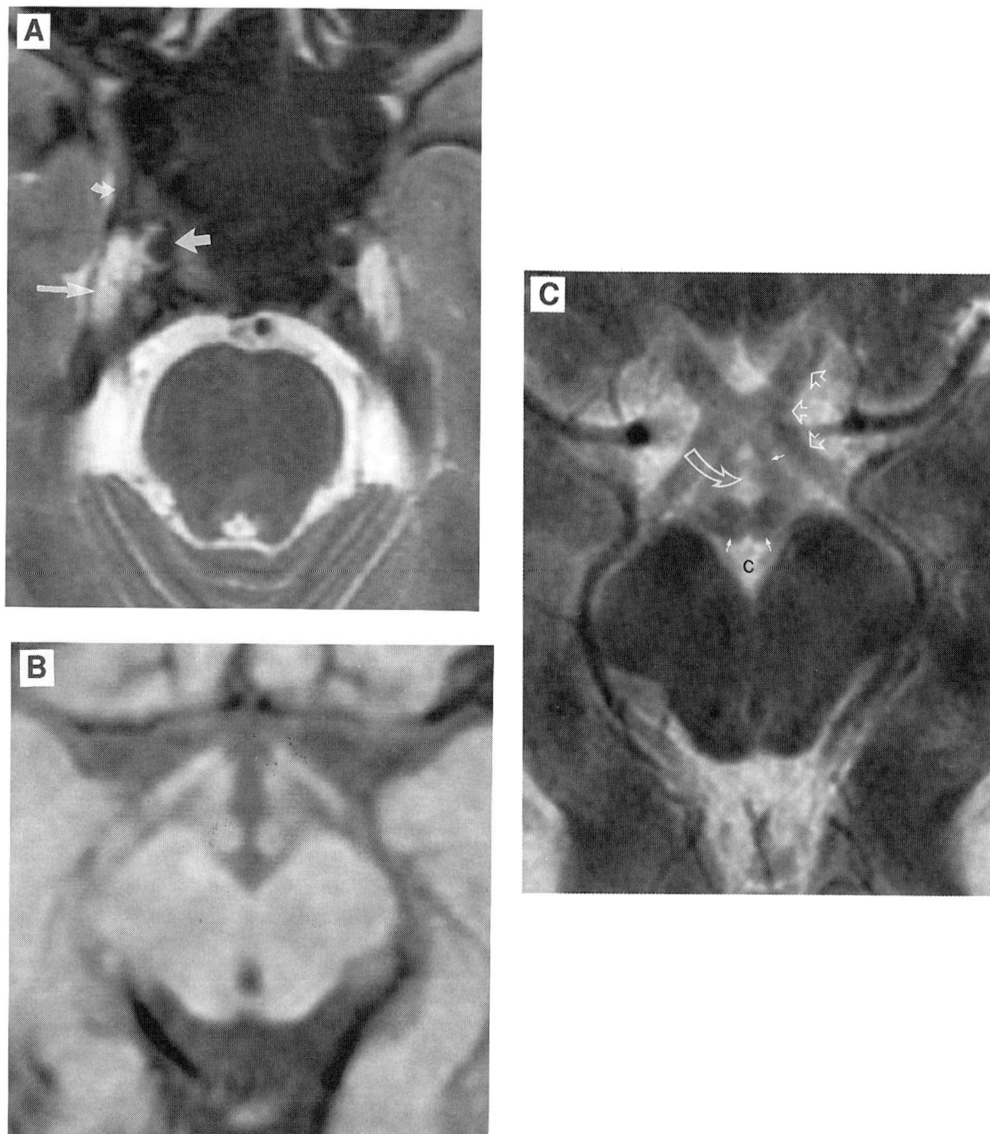

Fig. 2. (A) A T2-weighted MR axial section through the pons and the sphenoid sinus. The small arrow denotes the lateral margin of the cavernous sinus, the intermediate-sized arrow the trigeminal cistern, and the large arrow the proximal aspect of the cavernous internal carotid artery. **(B)** A T1-weighted axial section through the midbrain and suprasellar cistern. **(C)** A T2-weighted section at the same level. The open arrows with short stems demonstrate optic nerve, chiasm, and optic tract. The curved open arrow indicates the third ventricle. Short arrows demonstrate anteriorly the lateral margin of the ventral hypothalamus, and posteriorly the mammillary bodies.

giography) *(4)*. This supplies the pituitary stalk, partially the ventral hypothalamus, with branches descending into the anterior pituitary lobe, and supplies the optic nerves and chiasm in part. However, the anterior lobe receives its dominant circulation from the hypophyseal portal venous system, which passes inferiorly to the lobe.

A more direct blood supply to the posterior lobe comes from the inferior lateral trunk. The horizontal segment of the cavernous internal carotid artery lies 1–2 mm lateral to the medial cavernous dura or interface. Indentation as a normal variant or as a result of atherosclerotic disease may cause this horizontal segment to loop or to enlarge and bulge into the sella and to indent the pituitary gland, sometimes severely. This might be a major problem for transsphenoidal surgery.

The trigeminal nerve (cranial nerve V) arising from the lateral surface of the pons passes anteriorly and mildly laterally through the pontine cistern, passes through a bony trough within the temporal apex dura, and enters an arachnoid-lined space termed the trigeminal cistern (Meckel's cave). This cistern lies lateral to the vertical limb and the proximal cavernous loop of the internal carotid artery (Fig. 2A). The trigeminal cistern is posteroinferior to the nerve component of the cavernous sinus, and is lateral to the venous compartment. The first division exits from the arc-like coalescence of the fifth nerve fascicles (the gasserian ganglion), and runs within the nerve compartment inferiorly and slightly laterally with respect to the fourth nerve *(4a)*. The second division is inferolateral and traverses only the posterior portion of the cavernous compartment, leaving to exit through the foramen rotundum. The third division does not enter the cavernous sinus, passing inferolaterally and anteriorly from the ganglion to exit via the foramen ovale into the infratemporal fossa. Cranial nerve III (oculomotor nerve) exits from the midbrain-pons junction near the midline, and runs anterolaterally and slightly inferiorly through the ventral cistern, passing between the posterior cerebral and superior cerebellar artery branches of the basilar artery, to pierce the lateral aspect of the superior cavernous dura. A short sheath of cerebrospinal fluid may accompany this entry. The third nerve is the most superolateral nerve in the cavernous sinus. Cranial nerve IV exits from the dorsal surface of the midbrain just caudal to the inferior colliculus within the superior medullary velum, passes forward and subsequently laterally and inferiorly in the circumesencephalic and interpeduncular cistern to enter the most posterolateral aspect of the superior cavernous dura or the adjacent clival dura, beneath the more superior elevated free edge of the tentorium. In the cavernous sinus, nerve compartment, the fourth nerve is inferior and slightly lateral but close to the third nerve. Cranial nerve VI (abducens) passes superiorly and slightly laterally from the ventral pontomedullary junction. In the cisternal segment, the nerve passes superiorly and slightly laterally to enter the clival dura at approximately the junction of its upper one-third and lower two-thirds (Dorello's canal). It enters the venous compartment and runs forward to the superior orbital fissure, medial to the first division of five and inferomedial to the fourth cranial nerve. The optic nerve emerges from the optic canal at the intracranial end of the optic canal, and pass obliquely posteriorly and slightly superiorly to form the optic chiasm, then divides into optic tracts that follow the choroidal fissure superior to the parahippocampal gyrus to the lateral geniculate bodies, and then to Meyer's loop and the optic radiation. The very close relationship of the subarachnoid optic nerve to the subarachnoid internal carotid artery is to be noted, there being virtually no space between them for the width of the optic nerve, and often the internal carotid artery indents the optic nerve from inferiorly. This relationship is clearly seen on thin T2-weighted fast spin echo coronal images.

The subarachnoid cisterns surround this central anatomy. A cistern between the lateral cavernous dura and the temporal lobe, is usually relatively planar. The suprasellar cistern extends in a five- to six-sided shape from the gyrus rectus anteriorly to the rostral

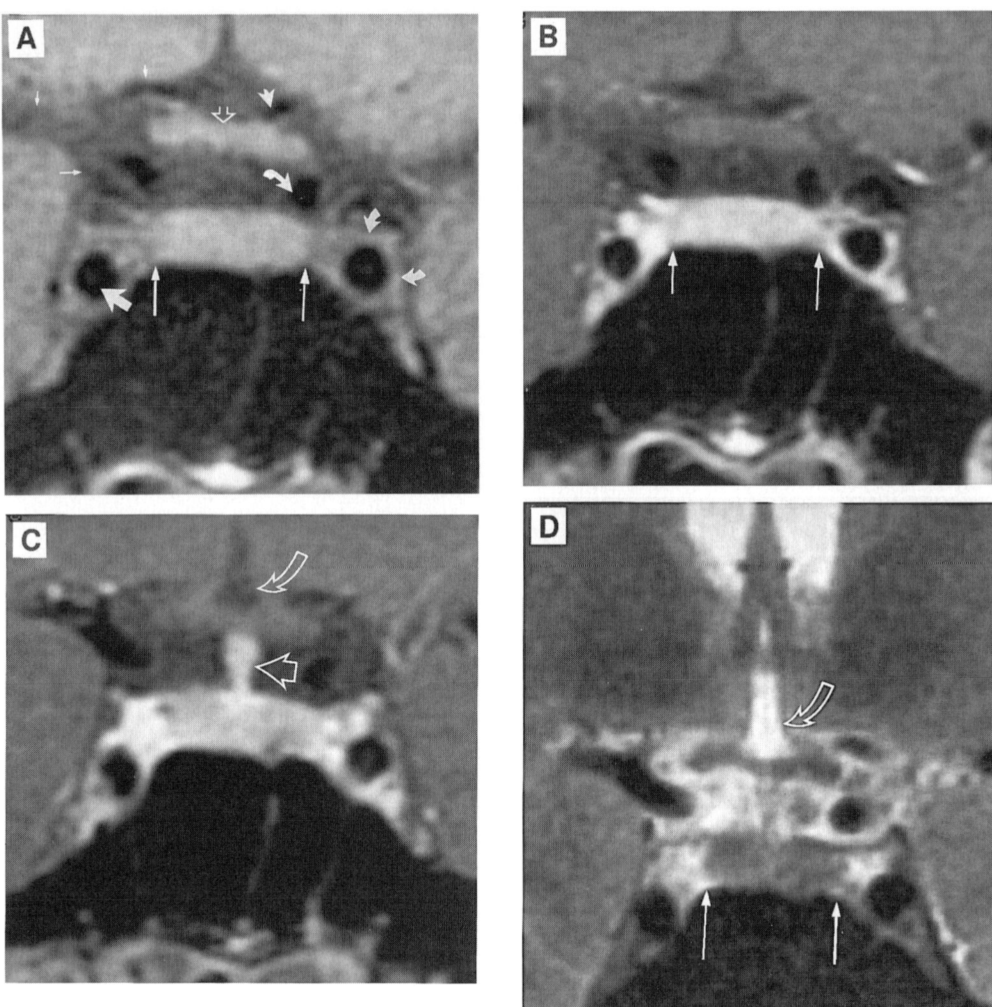

Fig. 3. **(A)** Normal unenhanced T1-weighted MR coronal section through the mid-pituitary gland. **(B)** Same level, postcontrast enhancement MR. **(C)** Åimately 4 mm posterior to **(B)**, enhanced. **(D)** A T2-weighted midpituitary coronal section, same patient.

pons and cerebral peduncles posteriorly and laterally to the medial surface of each temporal lobe. It contains the subarachnoid carotid arteries through their bifurcations into anterior and middle cerebral arteries. The middle cerebral artery stem enters the tubular first portion of the sylvian fissure. The anterior cerebral arteries (A1 segments) usually lie directed superiorly and medially over the optic nerves but occasionally are as far posterior as the chiasm. The distal basilar artery and its branches are in this cistern, the branching occurring inferior to the posterior aspect of the ventral hypothalamus. Centrally, the ventral surface of the hypothalamus, extending from the pituitary stalk posteriorly to the ventral midbrain, through the mammillary bodies, forms the roof of the cistern (Fig. 2B,C). The third ventricle terminates anteriorly in a supraoptic recess above the chiasm and an infundibular recess beneath the chiasm, the latter entering for a distance into the stalk commonly.

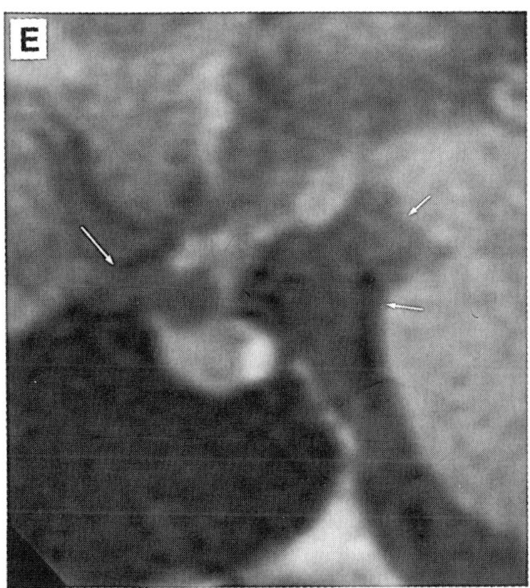

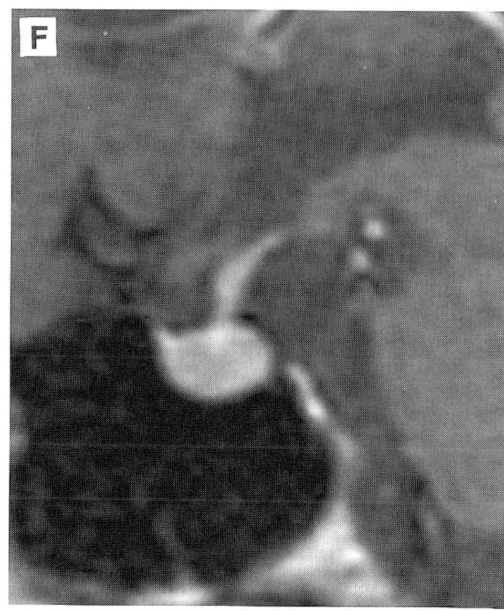

Fig. 3 (continued) **(E)** A midsagittal T1-weighted section of the pituitary gland, suprasellar cistern, and anterior third ventricle, unenhanced. **(F)** Same, postcontrast enhancement.

The pituitary gland lies within the sella *(1,5)*. It extends from the medial cavernous interface (dura) from one side to the other, so that the cavernous sinus and its contents form its total lateral margin. The superior cavernous dura usually is elevated above the flat or somewhat concave superior surface of the pituitary gland. The pituitary stalk typically enters the gland in the posterior 50% of the tuberculum-dorsum plane, in the midline. The stalk tends to be wider superiorly than centrally and again slightly wider as it approaches the pituitary gland (Fig. 3A–E). A venous plexus is seen with contrast enhancement extending from the enhancing stalk onto the surface of the diaphragm and radiating downward centrally in the anterior lobe. The anterior lobe typically occupies approximately 75% of the intrasellar pituitary volume. The anterior lobe has a pars tuberalis extending superiorly along the anterior surface of the infundibulum, the two components forming the stalk, and being inseparable by imaging. Anatomists tend to use the term "pars distalis" to describe the dominant portion of the adenohypophysis. The pars intermedia is vestigial in humans and can be viewed in imaging only when it becomes hypointense and that is probably cystic. There has been reported a cell distribution within the anterior lobe with the lactotrophs and somatotrophs tending to be lateralized, and the gonadotrophs corticotrophs and thyrotrophs being more central. The clinical correlation is that smaller prolactinomas do tend to be lateralized and to displace the residual pituitary gland contralaterally and superolaterally. Otherwise the relation to tumor location is not appreciated. With imaging, the anterior lobe is typically isodense on all sequences with brain tissue, but the posterior lobe in the majority of adults (90%) is hyperintense on T1 weighting, and is less well seen after contrast enhancement because of the greater though slightly slower enhancement of the anterior lobe. The infundibulum extends to the posterior lobe. The neurohypophysis consists of the posterior lobe, the infundibulum, and the median eminence, the latter lies in the ventral hypothalamus at and anterior to the infundibulum. The posterior lobe typically is spherical when seen in a coronal view, with posterior extension of the anterior lobe around it, particularly laterally.

In the first 2 mo of life, the pituitary gland has a convex superior surface and is hyperintense on T1 weighting to brain *(5)*. In a child older than 2 mo, there is a slow growth of the pituitary gland but its superior surface becomes flat or slightly concave downward, with a height of 2–6 mm. At puberty, the gland enlarges, often becomes convex upward, and reaches a height of 10 mm in the female and 8 mm in the male. On axial imaging, the convex superior surface of the pituitary may be seen in the ventral aspect of the suprasellar cistern, frequently causes concern, but is almost always normal in the asymptomatic adult patient. Occasionally, however, coronal imaging by MR is suggested as a follow-up. In pregnancy the gland becomes much larger again, enlarging progressively through pregnancy to reach a height of 10 mm (from 5 to 9 mm) in the third trimester with a convex superior surface and sometimes an increase in T1-weighted signal above brain signal. The maximum enlargement is during the first 1–2 wk postpartum when the gland measures up to 12 mm in height but thereafter rapidly regresses in height. Except for pregnancy, the pituitary gland until at least age 50 is stable. Changes in size during the menstrual cycle are too small to evaluate, and are not a problem. Beyond the 50s, the gland becomes smaller, frequently having a height of 2–4 mm, but rarely is this indicative of overt dysfunction.

An autopsy study (without imaging) of 1000 pituitary glands (without history or features of pituitary disease) found 61 focal abnormalities that were greater than 2 mm in size, i.e., 6% *(6)*. Of these, 30% were adenomas (all chemically nonsecretory), and 61% were Rathke cleft cysts, and there were a very small number of miscellaneous other causes.

A study using MR, T1-weighted unenhanced, coronal sections, on 52 healthy volunteers, demonstrated a hypointensity in the pituitary gland 2–5 mm in diameter in 20 of the 52, i.e., 38% *(7)*. These volunteers had serum assessments of pertinent pituitary hormones and these were all normal. Had contrast medium been given, the percentage would probably have been greater. The conclusion from these two studies would appear to be that careful correlation of the imaging observation of a focal pituitary gland lesion need be made with endocrinologic data.

IMAGING TECHNIQUES

The MR is the procedure of choice when a macroadenoma or other perisellar lesion is suspected. This is also true when the suspicion is toward a microadenoma. The CT technique requires thin sections, 2 mm or less in thickness, performed coronally, pre and post intravenous (iodinated) enhancement.

The MR technique includes a small field of view (16 cm), thin sections (3 mm with 0–1 interspace) imaging. These are performed in T1 weighting (TR 600, TE 15 m), coronal sections from mid sphenoid sinus to upper clivus and in sagittal sections medial temporal to medial temporal T1 weighted (12 images), each before and after intravenous Gadolinium enhancement. Proton density and T2-weighted fast spin echo coronal series yields 18 images each and requires 4.5 min. This totals 16.5 min.

Typically, the adenoma is slightly hypointense to normal gland on T1 weighting, but on T2 weighting, less than half are hyperintense to normal gland and the remainder isointense. Coronal fast spin echo T2-weighted similar coronal sections are routine in our protocol. Axial sections of the perisellar area are valuable for perisellar lesions, but infrequently valuable for intrasellar lesions, and therefore are used selectively.

Dynamic imaging of the pituitary gland is not used routinely. Rather, it is used for definition of a small intrasellar lesion, either previously suspected, or picked up on monitoring of the pre-enhancement series (and always for Cushing's disease). The dynamic series is coronal fast spin echo (TR 700, TE18, echo time 8, 3 mm thick with 0 gap, 256 × 192 matrix). Four images are performed in 18 s, the four images placed through the pituitary gland. This sequence is performed six times; that is, once before contrast injection and five times after contrast injection, using the 18-s sequence with a 3-s period between the sequences. These are printed out as six images in a block, the average timing after contrast injection for each series would be pre, 9, 30, 51, 72, and 93 s. Thus, the time for the dynamic series is approximately 2.5 min.

Simultaneous bilateral transjugular catheterization of the inferior petrosal sinuses, is used to diagnose and to attempt to lateralize a corticotroph adenoma, with venous sampling being performed before and after corticotropin releasing hormone stimulation *(8,9)*. The diagnosis is usually confirmed but the lateralization is only correct in 65% cases.

PITUITARY ADENOMA

At autopsy, small adenomas are detected, as are small pars intermedia cysts, infarcts, metastases, or other tiny lesions *(10,11)*. These would usually be impossible to differentiate from a microadenoma, in life. Thus, the interpretation of a focal small lesion (in the millimeter range) must be associated with a pertinent endocrinologic abnormality, if a microadenoma is to be diagnosed.

This is the most common tumor in this perisellar area in the adult, arising from the anterior lobe of the pituitary. They also constitute in the order of 10% of all intracranial adult neoplasms, and are frequently found incidentally at autopsy. Approximately 70% of adenomas are overtly secretory of one or more hormonal products. These are most commonly prolactin, though growth hormone, FSH and LH, ACTH, and uncommonly TSH may be produced. The imaging features of these different adenomas are identical, that is, one cannot predict from imaging the secretory function. This is however determined clinically or by the immune chemistry reaction of the resected tissue. Note that there is often a discrepancy between the production of these hormones and their release to become clinically active.

The secreting adenomas tend to be smaller than the nonsecreting lesions, because of the ability to reach clinical detection earlier. The most common adenoma is the prolactin secreting adenoma (with amenorrhea, galactorrhea, decreased libido, impotence, infertility), which tends to be of any size, and tends to be larger and less common in males. The growth hormone secreting tumors, however, tend to be clinically delayed in their diagnosis and therefore are often large tumors. The ACTH secreting tumors (causing hypercortisolism) are usually in the order of millimeters in diameter, and are the most difficult for imaging diagnosis *(12)*. Thus, the diagnosis of the adenoma depends on clinical features of the hypersecretion, or on the intrasellar or extrasellar hypervolumia of the lesion itself (and this is usually in terms of growth from the sella into the suprasellar cistern with visual system compression, and occasionally of obstructive ventriculomegaly at the cisternal or foramen of Monro level; that is, presentation with elevated intracranial pressure). Hypothalamic symptoms also occur.

The imaging of the pituitary adenoma is relatively specific, and classically divides the lesion into the microadenoma and macroadenoma, with a diameter of 10 mm being the dividing point. The size is precisely defined by imaging, and varies from probably 2 mm (as the smallest detectable size) to several centimeters. Computed tomography, which historically was the initial study, tends to show surface features and bone change. The MR, which is now the study of choice, better shows the content of the lesion and better defines relationships to skull base and brain. We tend to use both T1 weighting and T2 weighting, and with the former pre- and post-Gadolinium imaging. Note that the generic intracranial tumor reaction to Gadolinium is to become brighter than its environment; although the adenoma may enhance, its diagnosis is (to the contrary) made by relatively less enhancement of the adenoma than of the pituitary gland itself. This is particularly important with respect to the small tumors that tend to be predominantly intrasellar only (Fig. 4A–E). Volume changes are also important. As the tumor grows it enlarges the sella, the floor, anterior wall, and posterior wall often being asymmetrically enlarged and advanced along the margin of the tumor. These bone changes are visible on MR as well. The common route of extrasellar growth relates to elevation and stretching of the diaphragma sellae and ultimately to rupture through the diaphragma sellae into the suprasellar cistern. The chiasm is most commonly elevated over the dome of the tumor, resembling a beret or cap. Occasionally, the growth occurs superiorly between the optic nerves or, less commonly, between the optic tracts, resulting in either the nerves or tracts being displaced around the waist of the tumor. In large tumors, the chiasm may not be identified, but the general course can be predicted from parasagittal images demonstrating the optic nerves. Growth from the sella into the sphenoid sinus, diffuse or focal, usually preserves thinned dura and bone. Posterior extension through the dorsum and occasionally inferiorly through the clivus will yield epidural tumor referable to the clival dura and this occasionally will lead to deformity of the pons or midbrain. Thus, one can differentiate between direct suprasellar, anterior suprasellar-subfrontal, and posterior suprasellar-interpeduncular and pontine cistern growth. Gross filling of the third ventricle and gross deformity of the frontal lobes may occur in the very large tumors. Rarely, inferior growth will breach the pharyngeal aspect of the skull base and produce a mass in the nasopharynx, introducing the risk of meningitis. The involvement of the cavernous sinus is frequent, either as a diffuse bulge (Fig. 5A,B) against the medial cavernous dura, or of invasion of the cavernous sinus through breaches in this dura. The differentiation may be difficult, but if tissue characteristic of the intrasellar tumor reaches to the mid cavernous internal carotid artery or more laterally, or with artery encompassment, invasion is present (Fig. 6A,B). Surprisingly, however, symptomatic involvement of the cavernous cranial nerves is quite uncommon. The internal carotid artery in its cavernous segment may be displaced, encased, reduced in cross-sectional size, but rarely occluded. Displacement of, but rarely encasement of, the distal basilar artery is seen also with the posterior suprasellar growth. The ability to see the medial cavernous dura (the interface between cavernous sinus and gland) is often possible. Thus, on T1-weighted images, the cavernous sinus is slightly less intense (darker) than the pituitary gland. On T2 weighting, the medial cavernous sinus (to the interface) is more intense than the pituitary gland and than the more lateral cavernous sinus. With contrast enhancement, the cavernous sinus tends to enhance slightly more than the pituitary gland, again creating the visibility of the interface. The importance of these growth routes and character relates to the choice of the surgical approach to the adenoma, whether transsphenoidal, or transcranial.

Dynamic scanning of the pituitary has recently become possible, using a multiplanar gradient echo sequence *(13)*. This is based on the observation that enhancement of the pituitary gland occurs maximally between 1 and 3 min, but the microadenoma enhances somewhat more slowly, the crossover probably occurs between 2 and 3 min. Thus, the scans before this crossover point may demonstrate the microadenoma better (as more hypointense focus). Thus, based on these differential rates of enhancement, early scans may show the adenoma better. This procedure is indicated particularly for Cushing's disease in which the detection of a tiny adenoma may otherwise be impos-sible. Thus, we use this technique for Cushing's disease, and otherwise when the pre-enhancement T1-weighted sections are nondiagnostic. An attempt to evaluate the ability to detect an ACTH secreting adenoma, was 47% by CT and 55% by MR (most of which were not enhanced) *(12)*. However with both modalities, the correlation with the surgical localization was only approximately 50%. There is an insensitivity to differentiate nonadenomatous focal lesions from microadenoma. The detection rate for the ACTH secreting microadenoma is < 50%. The other features used are displacement of the pituitary stalk to one side, usually indicating that the gland is displaced laterally or occasionally anterolaterally. This contralateral displacement of the stalk associated with ipsilateral increased volume, associated with a local hypoenhancing area is often the basis of diagnosis of the micro tumors. Current MR techniques demonstrate pituitary microadenomas (other than ACTH producing) probably 60–80% of the time, and contrast enhancement increases sensitivity by 5–10%. Dynamic contrast enhanced images increase detection an additional 5–20%, therefore suggesting an overall sensitivity of 80–90%. The apparent benefit of dynamic imaging in microadenomas is reported to be 9–16% *(14)*.

Cystic features are seen in adenomas, often in the larger ones. The cystic content is somewhat hypointense on T1 weighting and hyperintense on T2 weighting, both of these being equal to CSF, or higher protein in nature than CSF. However a noncystic adenoma is uncommonly identical to CSF on MR. The adenoma may appear hyperintense on T1 weighting, and in some this is related to acute hemorrhage, although in some it is unexplained.

The information desired from the imaging, in the prolactinoma suspect, is exclusion of other disease affecting the stalk or otherwise, and a baseline size of the adenoma for future comparison on Bromocriptine therapy. The patient with symptoms of suprasellar extension, or of clinically important hypersecretion, are evaluated for the neurosurgeon. The surgeon's decision is between transsphenoidal and transcranial surgery. In the former, the nature of sphenoid sinus septation and of cavernous internal carotid arteries is important, as well as detail regarding the sellar and perisellar anatomy. In the latter, the location of the chiasm and subarachnoid internal carotid arteries is important.

The evaluation of the perisellar region after thorough surgery is usually difficult in terms of finding small islands of residual (functioning) tissue. Comparison to preoperative and to serial postoperative studies is important, using the 3-mo postoperative baseline as the first appropriate study. We have found small areas of residual tissue to occur related to the cavernous extension, along the visual system, or ventral hypothalamus. After surgery (and irradiation) of tumors that had markedly enlarged

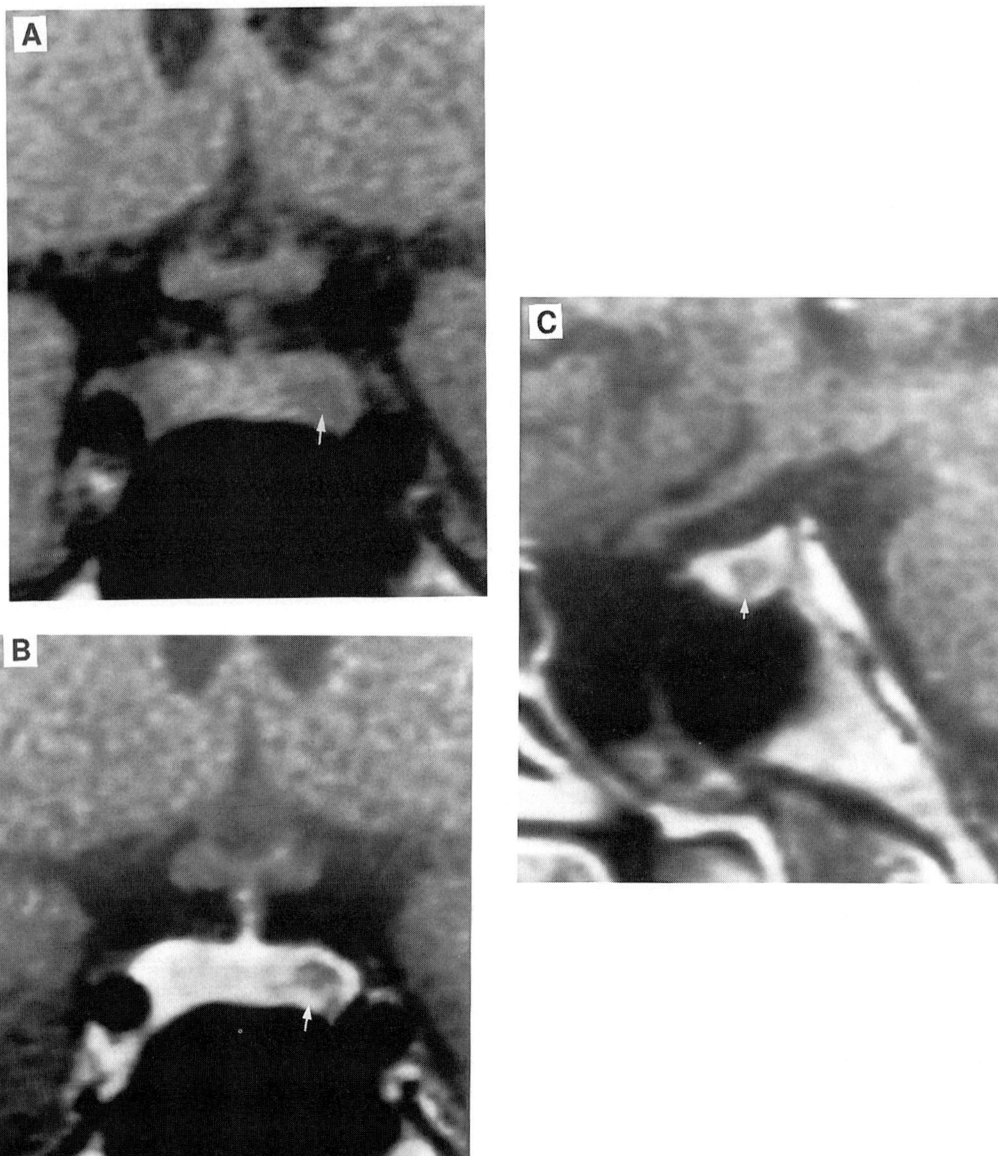

Fig. 4. **(A)** This is a patient with a 7-mm prolactinoma of the inferior lateral left side of the pituitary gland. Pre-enhancement, T1-weighted coronal. **(B)** Postenhancement T1-weighted, coronal. **(C)** Parasagittal postenhancement T1-weighted image through the lesion. Diagnosis on the sagittal image alone is dangerous because this type of lucency could be produced by imaging the medial edge of the cavernous internal carotid artery.

the sella, it is common to see descent of the hypothalamus and visual system into the enlarged sella, and to see minimal residual pituitary tissue. Overt hypopituitarism and/or recurrent visual symptoms are unusual. In general, differentiation of residual tumor within the sella from residual normal pituitary gland may be impossible.

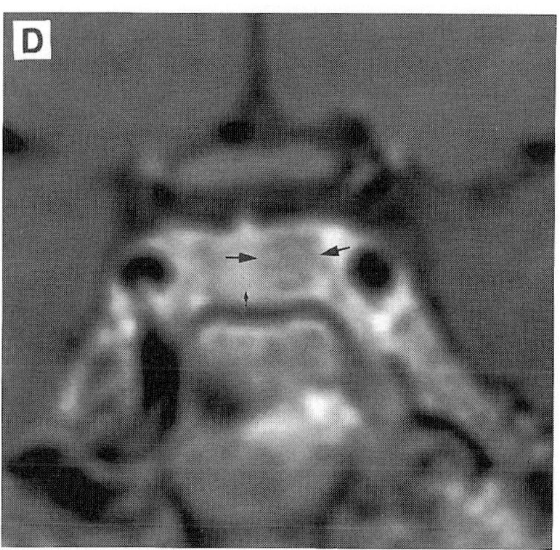

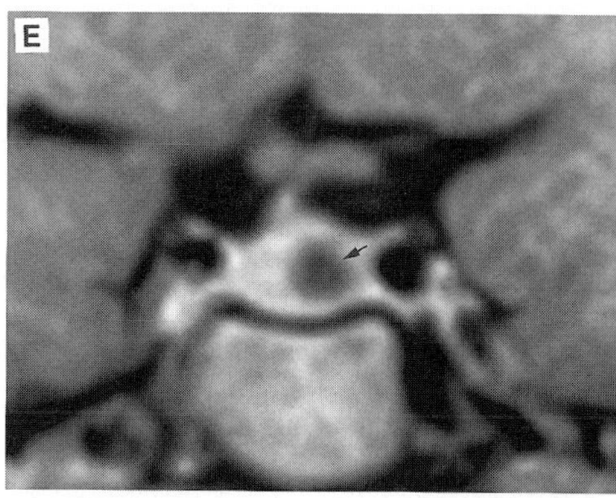

Fig. 4. (continued) (D) An enhanced, T1-weighted midpituitary coronal section, different patient. Note a 10-mm, slightly hypointense lesion in the left half of the gland displacing the tuft (tiny arrow) toward the right with the stalk. At operation this lesion had a nondiscrete margin and pathology is an ACTH producing tumor. **(E)** An unenhanced, T1-weighted coronal section through the pituitary gland demonstrates a 9-mm, unusually hypointense lesion of the gland on the left, which at operation was a noncystic null-cell adenoma. Note the displacement of the stalk toward the right-sided normal gland.

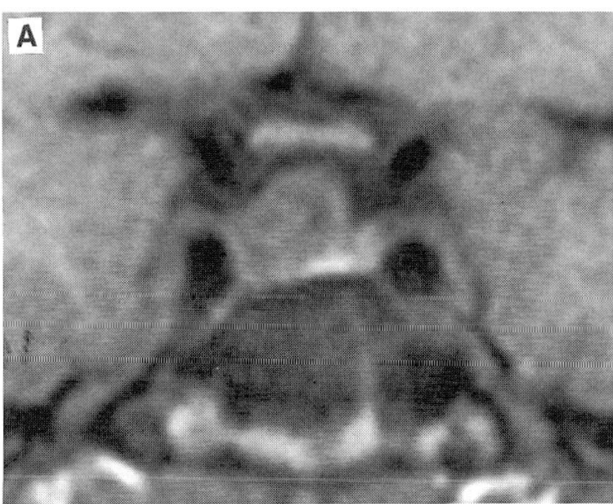

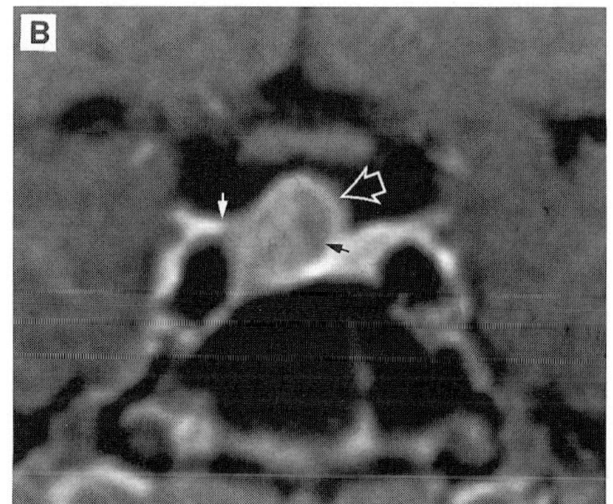

Fig. 5. Coronal images, T1-weighted through midsella preenhancement **(A)** and postenhancement **(B)**. This is a 16-mm diameter prolactinoma almost reaching the chiasm, reaching to and tending to obliterate the medial cavernous dura on the right (possible invasion) with the stalk displaced over the left surface of the tumor to the normal far-left pituitary gland.

It is now common for prolactinomas to be diagnosed by endocrine information and by MR imaging. In the less compressive adenoma, therapy (without biopsy) commonly begins with a dopamine receptor agonist such as Bromocriptine *(15)*. Size reduction occurs rapidly, and almost always persists during therapy. Failure to diminish size, or to maintain the reduction, suggests noncompliance. Also the T2-weighted signal often becomes more hyperintense suggesting increased water content. Rapid (a few weeks) recurrence of tumor size to original occurs with withdrawal of the drug.

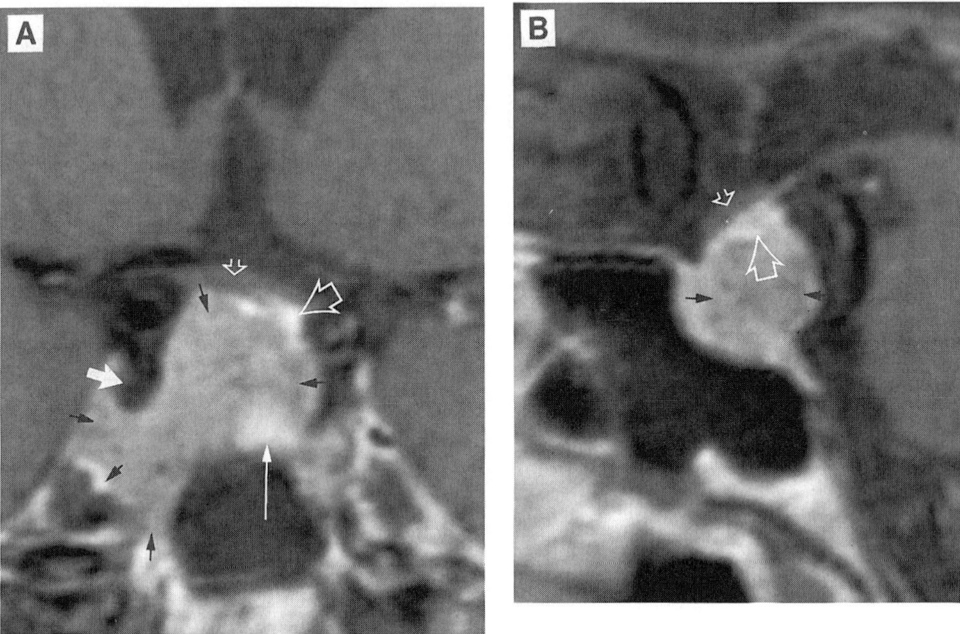

Fig. 6. Enhanced T1-weighted coronal **(A)** and enhanced, T1-weighted midsagittal **(B)** sections. This adenoma reaches and is showing moderate elevation and narrowing of the chiasm. Definite invasion throughout the right cavernous sinus, with indentation of the trigeminal cistern is seen on the right. The small arrows indicate tumor margins. The small white arrow with long stem shows the displaced posterior lobe. The stalk is displaced superiorly and to the left. The anterior lobe is anterior and left.

Hemorrhage into pituitary adenomas may be more common into prolactinomas, and may be more common in larger tumors (Fig. 7A–C). It would appear however that Bromocriptine correlates with this hemorrhage (45%, compared to 13% who did not receive Bromocriptine) *(16)*. In terms of hemorrhage into pituitary adenomas, it is probable that somewhat < 50% of the patients have resultant increased symptomatology in terms of new headache, new visual change, and so on *(17)*.

Pituitary adenoma in the age under 20 is uncommon, constituting approximately 6% of all proven pituitary adenomas *(18)*. Of this group, 23% occurred in the 0–11-yr old age group and 77% from the 12–19-yr old age group. Approximately two-thirds occurred during puberty. The prepubertal children were most likely to have ACTH releasing adenomas, whereas pubertal and postpubertal patients were most likely to have prolactinomas. Endocrine-inactive adenomas are quite unusual in this entire group (3% as compared to one-third in the adult).

CRANIOPHARYNGIOMAS

A cord of cells within the body of the sphenoid bone represents the obliterated craniopharyngeal canal, and tracks to the anterior lobe of the pituitary. The origin of these cells is disputed. However, along this track the Rathke cleft cyst or the craniopharyngioma forms. The tumor often centers on the pituitary stalk, but rarely tumors have been

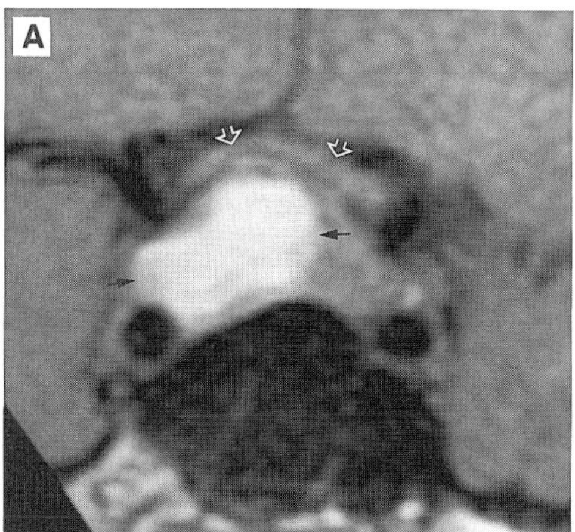

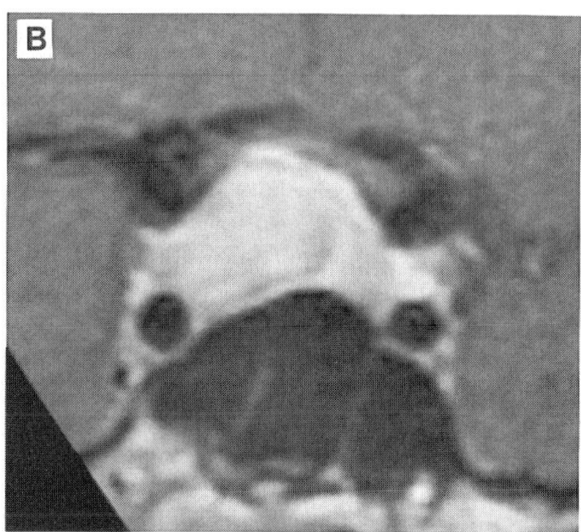

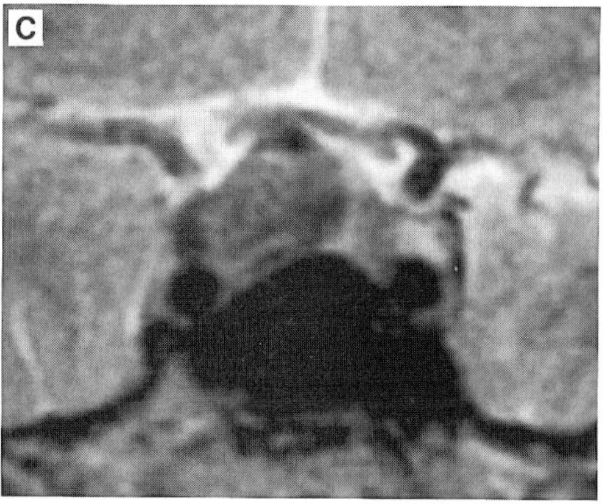

Fig. 7. These are coronal sections. **(A)** A T1-weighted, unenhanced. **(B)** T1-weighted, enhanced. **(C)** T2-weighted. A large hyperintense adenoma occupies all but the left side of the enlarged sella, with moderate elevation of the chiasm (more on the right) and with extension almost to the lateral margin of the cavernous sinus suggesting invasion. The lesion is T1-weighted hyperintense on 7a, and hypointense on its T2-weighting. Note chronic deformity of the sella floor towards the right. At operation, there were old blood products in the adenoma.

reported from the caudal end in the submucosal nasopharynx, to the third ventricle lumen. In two reports of the nasopharyngeal craniopharyngioma, there is curious tracking through the nose, to ethmoid and into the anterior cranial fossa with probably some involvement of the sellar contents *(19,20)*.

Over 50% of craniopharyngiomas arise in the first and early half of the second decade of life, and a smaller number occur in the 40–50 age range. They typically present as a large lesion in children and, therefore, their exact origin is uncertain. They probably however arise most commonly within the pituitary stalk (perhaps between the pars tuberalis of the anterior lobe of the pituitary and the infundibulum to the posterior lobe). They are also usually large in the adult where they present with pituitary insufficiency and visual symptoms. The lesions commonly are suprasellar cistern lesions, with probably < 20% involving the pituitary gland, and even less commonly associated with an enlargement of the sella because of the intrasellar involvement.

The CT characteristics of this mass is heterogeneity, partly because of calcification (with 70–90% calcifying in the pediatric age, but < 50% in the adult age). The calcification tends to be within the solid portions of lesion, and also within the mural portion of cysts.

As with other perisellar lesions, the examination method of choice is the MR. Here, heterogeneity of texture is again the important characteristic (Figs. 8A–8C). That is, there are solid and cystic portions often intermixed in a complex way, with variability in terms of which is the prominent component. On T1 weighting, the cystic portions vary from hypointense to isointense to hyperintense, with the solid portions being relatively isointense to brain *(21)*. On T2 weighting, the solid portions become hyperintense, and the cystic portions vary and often reverse their character from T1 weighting. Enhancement occurs often in a heterogeneous or speckled pattern within the solid portion and usually in the mural aspects of the cysts. The heterogeneous pattern probably corresponds to the calcification, within the solid portions (and not to vascularity). This overall heterogeneity is quite characteristic, tending not to be seen in other lesions in this region in this way. The distribution of the lesion most commonly brings it down to the diaphragma sellae, but ascends to usually obliterate the stalk, to elevate or engulf the visual system, and to usually deeply indent and to be surgically very adherent to the ventral hypothalamus and third ventricle. As with the pituitary adenoma, extension into the interpeduncular cistern, or extension into the subfrontal and frontal areas sometimes occurs, creating very large tumors. They may occasionally be present only within the third ventricle, adherent to the hypothalamic margins. With brain invasion there is an intense reaction making surgical resection difficult or impossible. At surgery, the content of the cyst is typically yellow to brown, contains cholesterol crystals, carotene, high protein material, and often necrosis, and occasionally hemorrhage *(21)*.

The craniopharyngioma permits long survival, and analysis of functional outcome and predictive factors regarding recurrence are of interest *(22,23)*. To be considered in the differential diagnosis are two entities, the hypothalamic/optic system glioma, and the pilocystic astrocytoma *(24)*. These may be the one and the same tumour. The former tend to be more homogeneous, they usually enhance less. The pilocystic astrocytoma very commonly involves the hypothalamus and extends into the frontal lobes, enhances well with contrast medium and may be somewhat heterogeneous (with cysts). Mural enhancing cysts are very characteristic of the craniopharyngioma, on periphery of the solid tumors, whereas in the other lesions (if they contain cysts), the cysts are contained centrally within the solid tumor.

RATHKE CLEFT CYST

Approximately 20% of these lesions are confined to a relatively disc-shaped lesion between the anterior and posterior lobes (Fig. 9A–C). The majority extend from here into the suprasellar cistern, after having compressed the posterior lobe into a thin, usually midline, posterior superior arc (which remains hyperintense on T1

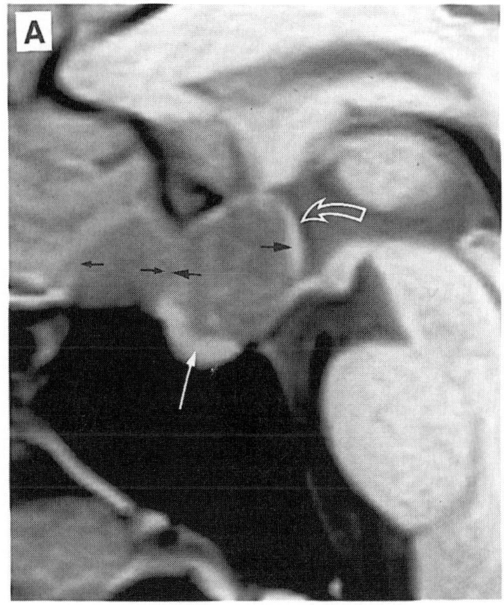

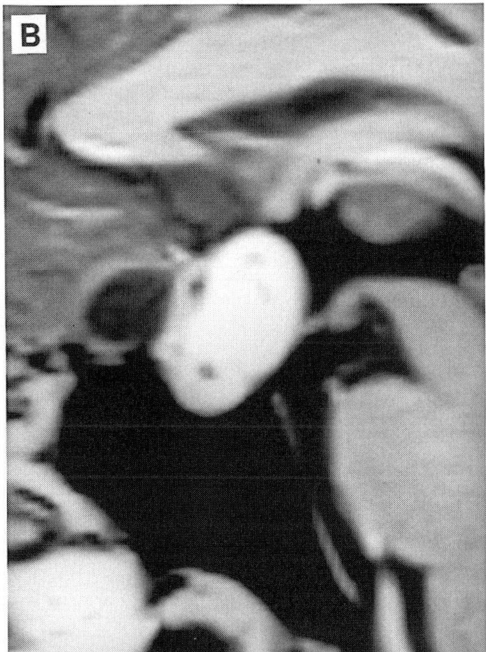

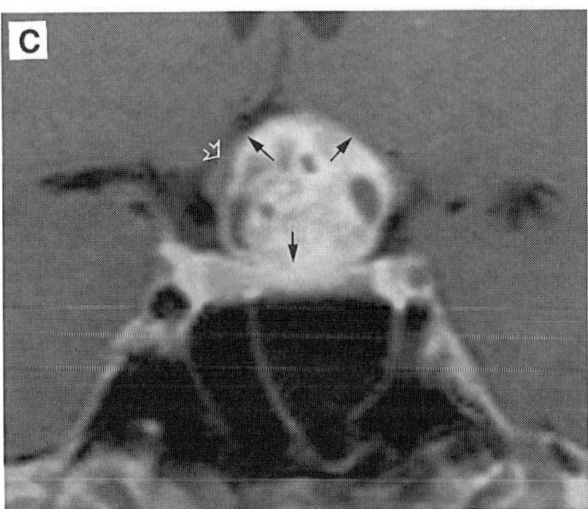

Fig. 8. **(A)** Midsagittal, unenhanced, T1-weighted section. **(B)** Postenhancement T1-weighted sagittal. **(C)** Midsellar coronal postenhancement. This is a craniopharyngioma with the anterior lobule (tiny arrows) being a cyst with mural enhancement and the larger posterior lobule (medium sized arrows) is a solid enhancing component. The chiasm is severely stretched over its dome and the pituitary gland beneath is compressed but probably not invaded.

weighting). Similarly, the anterior lobe is compressed into a thin arc anterosuperiorly but remains visible. The ascent into the suprasellar cistern occurs with pointing to the stalk, and evidence suggests it lies between the pars tuberalis and the infundibulum. The characteristic imaging features are a stalk which is anterior to the midpoint of the tuberculum/dorsum plane. In approximately 50%, there is flat shelf over the posterior aspect of the plane, with the superior extension and stalk being an-

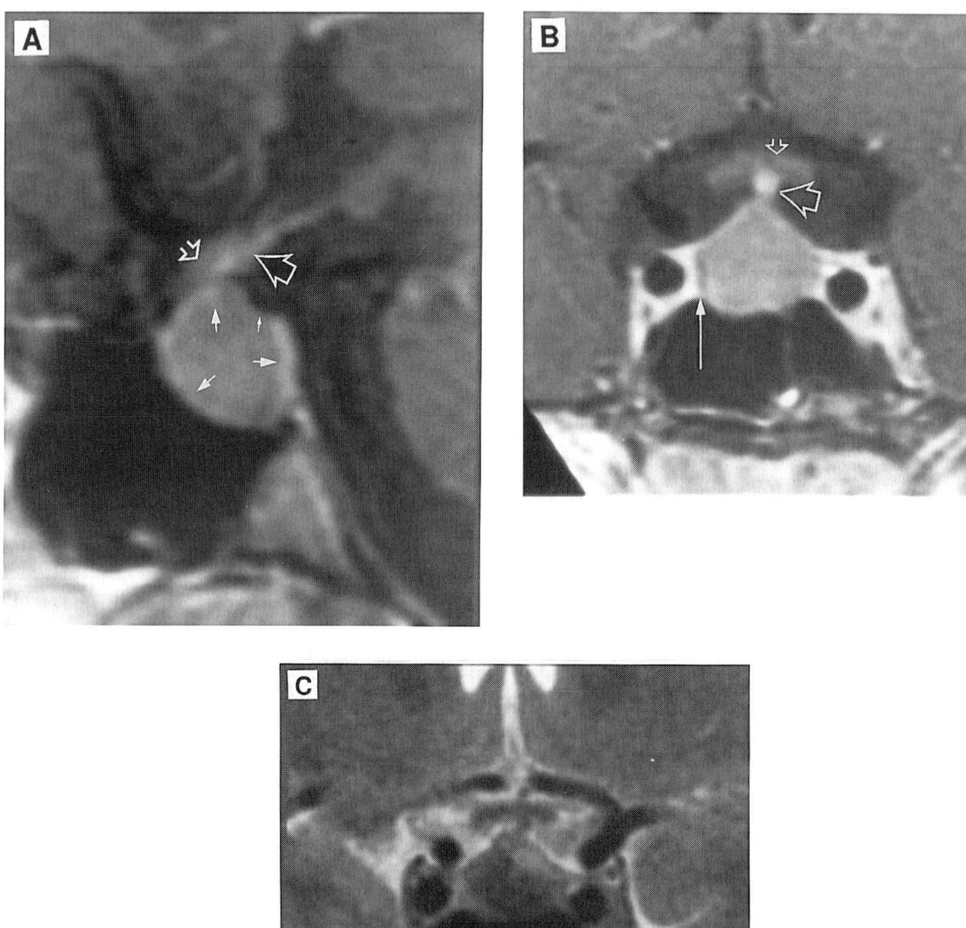

Fig. 9. (A) Midsagittal pre-enhancement, T1-weighted MR. **(B)** Postenhancement coronal midsella T1-weighted section. **(C)** T2-weighted coronal section at the same level. This is a Rathke cleft cyst, proven (surgically). The arrows demonstrate the margin of the cyst, the lack of indentation of the medial cavernous dura, the superior projection pointing toward the stalk which is anterior in its position. The tiny arrow shows the posterior shelf. Note the thin arced anterior and posterior lobes respectively anteriorly and posteriorly. The content is mostly hypointense to brain on T2 weighting, the small portion that is not is unexplained.

terior to this. The stalk is almost always in the midline. The dome as it ascends tends to be slightly anterior to perpendicular to the tuberculum-dorsum plane, whereas the adenoma tends to be slightly posterior to perpendicular to this plane. The Rathke cleft cyst is hypointense to the pituitary gland on T1 weighting, does not enhance, and approximately 75% are hypointense to the pituitary tissue on T2 weighting. A statistical analysis of these features with comparison to the pituitary adenoma should be coming from us in 1997 *(25–30)*.

MENINGIOMA

This ubiquitous tumor, over one-third of which occur along the skull base, can have origins from the sphenoid plate, sphenoid wing, orbital roof, any aspect of the margins of the middle fossa, along the free edge of the tentorium, from the diaphragma sellae, or from aspects of the cavernous surface. A common type originates from the sphenoid plate or tuberculum dura and grows posteriorly over or onto the diaphragma sellae, does not invade the pituitary gland until late, and can be distinguished by relatively uniform definite enhancement. The lesion may arise in the diaphragma sellae itself. These may produce bulky lesions on the intracranial surface of the diaphragma sellae either anterior (or posterior) to the pituitary stalk, and invasion of the pituitary gland would be unusual. A subgroup of diaphragma sellae meningioma (14 of 33 patients in one report) had a lesion that invaded the pituitary gland, probably arising from the inferior surface of the diaphragma sellae *(31)*. The differentiation of this latter type from a pituitary adenoma is based on the much brighter enhancement of the meningioma. Uncommonly does this lesion enter the cavernous sinus or clival region.

An apparently separate and common type of meningioma arises from the free edge of the tentorium, takes on a saddle-bag configuration with a portion descending into the middle fossa, and another portion descending medially onto the superior clival dura, with spread onto both superior and inferior leaves of the tentorium and often eventual extension to the dorsolateral and/or ventrolateral surfaces of the ipsilateral posterior cranial fossa (Fig. 10A–C). This type tends to invade the cavernous sinus and trigeminal cistern, to encompass and often narrow, and occasionally occlude the internal carotid artery (usually in its cavernous segment). Many cranial nerves are at risk in the cisterns or cavernous sinus. A rarer meningioma arises essentially extracranially within the paranasal sinuses, with little or no extension beyond the dura intracranially (Fig. 11A,B).

A common occurrence with meningioma is hyperostotic bone around its base, particularly around its vascular hilum and this is seen as a thickened black zone on all sequences of MR. With moderate frequency, vessels from the vascular hilum can be seen radiating into the tumor (T1-weighted hypointense arteries, and T1-weighted enhanced or T2-weighted hyperintense arteries). The meningioma can arise anywhere, but these are the common origins relating to the perisellar area.

OTHER INTRASELLAR ABNORMALITIES

There are numerous uncommon to rare abnormalities occurring in the sella. Metastasis to the pituitary gland is an uncommon clinical phenomenon, though it is seen in up to 5% of patients at autopsy *(32,33)*. These do not have characteristic imaging features, though they may progress to bone destruction. These enlarge more rapidly than a pituitary adenoma. One cause of a hyperintense T1-weighted signal of the pituitary fossa is a melanoma metastasis. The metastasis may be to clival marrow, beneath or into the pituitary gland.

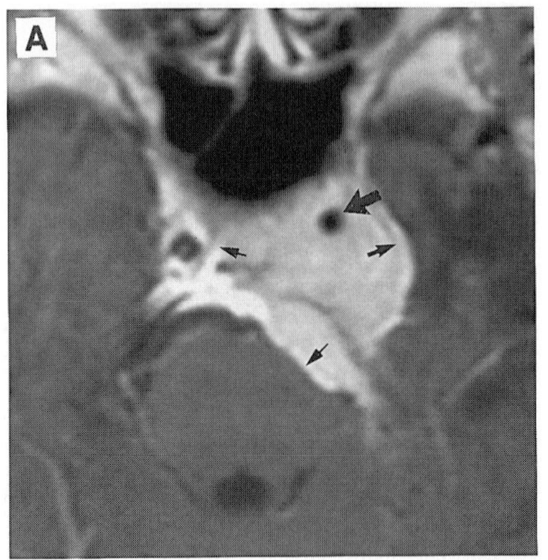

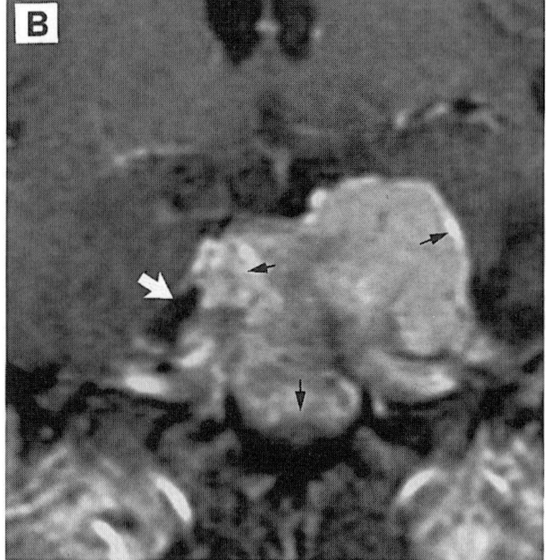

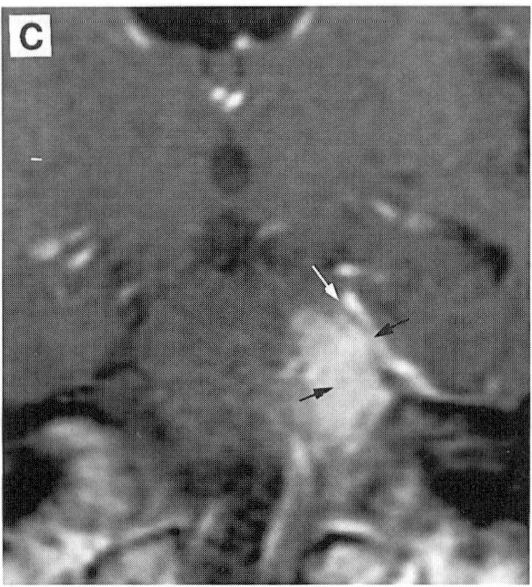

Fig. 10. (**A**) Enhanced, T1-weighted axial midsella image. (**B**) Posterior sella, T1-weighted, enhanced coronal. (**C**) Enhanced, retrosellar, T1-weighted coronal image. This is a meningioma invading the pituitary gland and the left cavernous sinus, arising from the left free edge of the tentorium, with tentorial invasion, and extension into the posterior cranial fossa. Large arrows indicate the slightly small cavernous internal carotid artery (black) and the normal right trigeminal cistern (white). The tentorium is indicated by a white arrow with a long stem.

A rare neoplasm termed granular cell tumor or myoblastoma occurs in the posterior pituitary lobe. This may extend to the hypothalamus. These are slow growing lesions. A pituicytoma is a neurohypophyseal astrocytoma *(34)*.

Pituitary abscess is a rare phenomenon related to spread from local sphenoid sinus or cavernous sinus infection, or hematogenous spread. On MR imaging, a peripheral rim

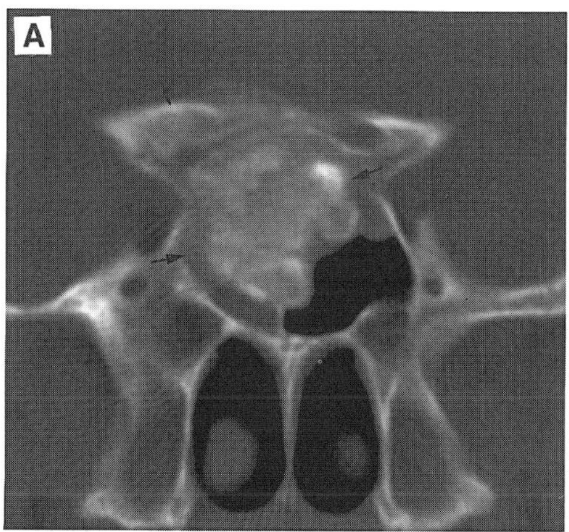

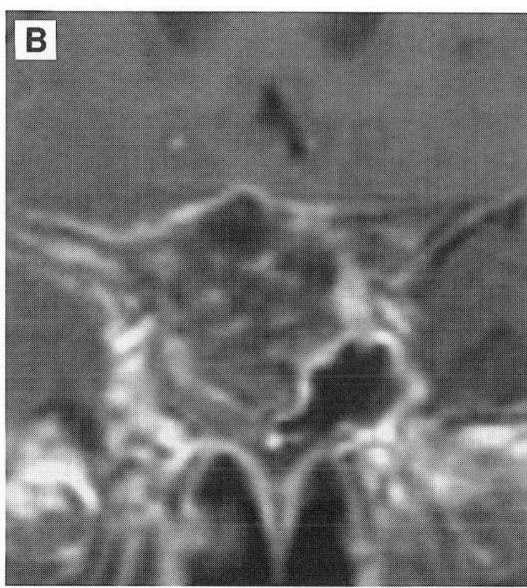

Fig. 11. **(A)** A CT coronal bone section, presellar, through the sphenoid sinus. **(B)** A section at the same level with T1-weighted, enhanced MR. This demonstrates a calcifying meningioma of the sphenoid sinus without entry into the sella or cavernous sinus.

enhancement around a low density center is suggestive, but not specific, when compared to the pituitary adenoma. A history of an immunocompromised state would suggest that an abscess may be fungal in origin *(35)*. Infections also may complicate a pre-existent intrasellar lesion of any sort.

Lymphocytic hypophysitis produces diffuse homogeneous enlargement of the anterior lobe which enhances, which is reported to enlarge the stalk, but is not separable by imaging from an adenoma *(36–38)*. It consists of lymphocyte and plasma cell infiltration, occurs in late pregnancy and in the weeks or months postpartum, and is probably an autoimmune disease. It is rare in males. The patients present with anterior pituitary deficiency and in some, diabetes insipidus. Response to steroid therapy has been noted. Spontaneous regression is not reported.

There are several congenital abnormalities of the perisellar region. The first is typically termed empty sella, better termed "diaphragma sellae anomaly with intrasellar arachnocele" *(39)*. The sella may be enlarged superoinferiorly with symmetrical inferior concave cupping of the floor (wasp nest configuration). In the days before CT and MR imaging, this sellar enlargement could be predicted to represent the diaphragma anomaly, but many pneumoencephalograms were performed to exclude tumor. The pituitary gland is spread along the floor particularly inferiorly. The pituitary stalk reaches down to this tissue, especially to the posterior aspect, and the optic chiasm is often found (anterior to the pituitary stalk) forming a "V" shape as it and the hypothalamus descend into the sella (Fig. 12A–C). The optic nerves then pass inferiorly and medially to reach the chiasm, and on route may be compressed over the proximal subarachnoid internal carotid arteries or against the bone of the intracranial optic canal orifice. In spite of the visual system deformity and of the small pituitary gland, overt endocrine abnormality is uncommon, and visual symptoms are

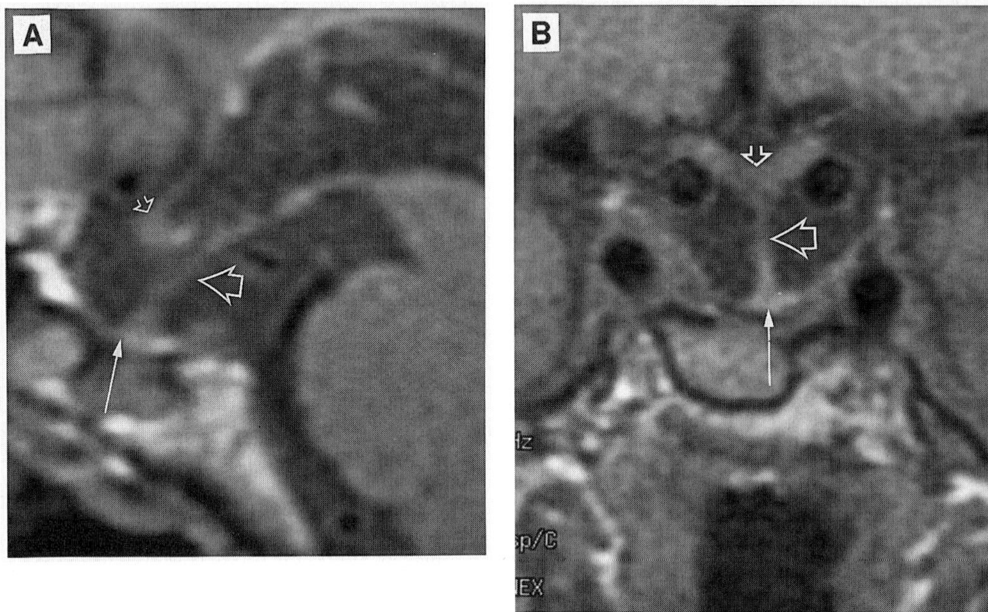

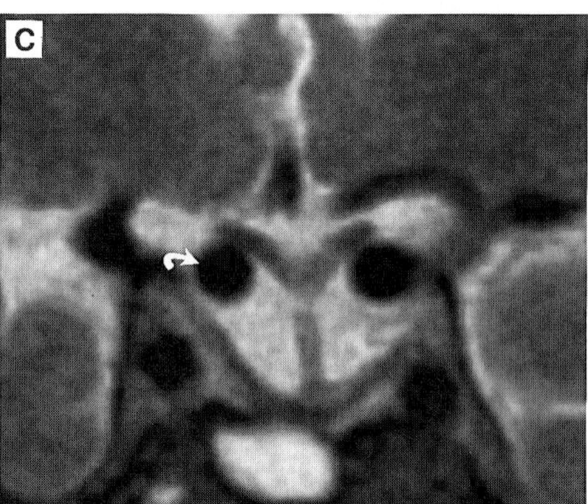

Fig. 12. **(A)** Unenhanced midsagittal section demonstrating a large sella. **(B)** Unenhanced, T1-weighted, midsellar coronal section. **(C)** T2-weighted coronal section at the same level. There is descent in a "V" shape of optic nerves and chiasm and hypothalamus, with the stalk descending in midsella to a very tiny pituitary gland. Note the course of the optic nerves over the subarachnoid internal carotid artery (curved arrow). This is a diaphragma sellae large congenital deficiency with intrasellar (communicating) arachnocele ("empty sella").

uncommon. The postoperative form of this configuration usually may be anatomically identical, but required initially a tumor with large sella and thorough treatment of the adenoma. Whether the diaphragma sellae was abnormal initially or whether it become abnormal as a result of stretching by the tumor is unclear and probably unimportant. Rarely this process may produce cerebrospinal fluid rhinorrhea. The transsphenoidal encephalocele is probably an extreme and rare example of the congenital intrasellar arachnocele, and is usually associated with other midline anomalies involving the corpus callosum, palate, facial configuration, and so on. In these, the cyst reaches into the nasopharynx, carrying with it the hypothalamus and visual system. A true noncommunicating arachnoid cyst can occur sellar/suprasellar, and displace normal structures, as does any other hypervolumic lesion. Confusion with a communicating arachnocele would be unusual, but occasionally a water-soluble cisternogram would clarify.

Septo-optic dysplasia involves hypoplasia of the visual system, and usually of the infundibulum and posterior gland, and is associated with absence of the septum pellucidum.

Hypoplasia or maldevelopment of the pituitary gland is rare. In one form it may represent a small gland in a small sella. This may be associated with other midline anomalies of the brain, skull, orbit, and palate. In another form, the anterior lobe is small and hypofunctioning within a small sella turcica, and the posterior lobe appears to be ectopic, seen on the unenhanced T1-weighted studies as a hyperintensity along the stalk toward the ventral hypothalamus *(40)*. The pituitary stalk inferior to this signal is either small or absent (Fig. 13A–D). This phenomenon is referred to as pituitary dwarfism, this being the most obvious manifestation. Note that this constellation may represent stalk transection in the neonate. Acute stalk transection from closed head injury at an older age results in coma, diabetes insipidus, and later to anterior lobe hypofunction. There may be no visualization of a hyperintense hypothalamic area on T1 weighting. Acute pituitary stalk transection from trauma is associated with severe pituitary dysfunction and hypothalamic dysfunction (diabetes insipidus).

Central diabetes insipidus is caused by hypothalamic dysfunction, and in over half can be related to sellar or suprasellar trauma, neoplasm, and so on, and is seen after surgery to the area. The posterior pituitary hyperintense signal on T1 weighting is absent.

Approximately 90% of healthy subjects have a hyperintense T1-weighted signal in the posterior pituitary. Absence of this hyperintensity is seen with nephrogenic diabetes insipidus, with anorexia nervosa, in central diabetes insipidus (in whom ADH levels are low), and also in patients with elevated ADH in patients undergoing hemodialysis *(41)*.

Pituitary gland hyperplasia produces enlargement secondary to end-organ failure, usually of the thyroid gland. The enlargement is moderate, and the entire anterior lobe is involved, without residual normal gland as would be seen in adenomas of comparable size typically.

Pituitary adenoma may occur as a component of certain rare syndromes such as Forbes-Albright syndrome, Chiari-Frommel syndrome, and Werner syndrome (multiple endocrine neoplasia Type I).

Other unusual inflammatory lesions can involve the pituitary gland, such as cysticercosis, sarcoidosis, Erdheim-Chester disease, blastomycosis, Wegener granulomatosis, Tolosa-Hunt syndrome, and tuberculosis. Deposits can also occur within the pituitary gland in amyloidosis, hemochromatosis (with a very dark hypointensity on all MR sequences, and associated with thyroid, liver, and spleen hypointensity on MR) and in Hurler syndrome. Also vascular lesions may invaginate the sella such as an aneurysm projecting from the cavernous internal carotid

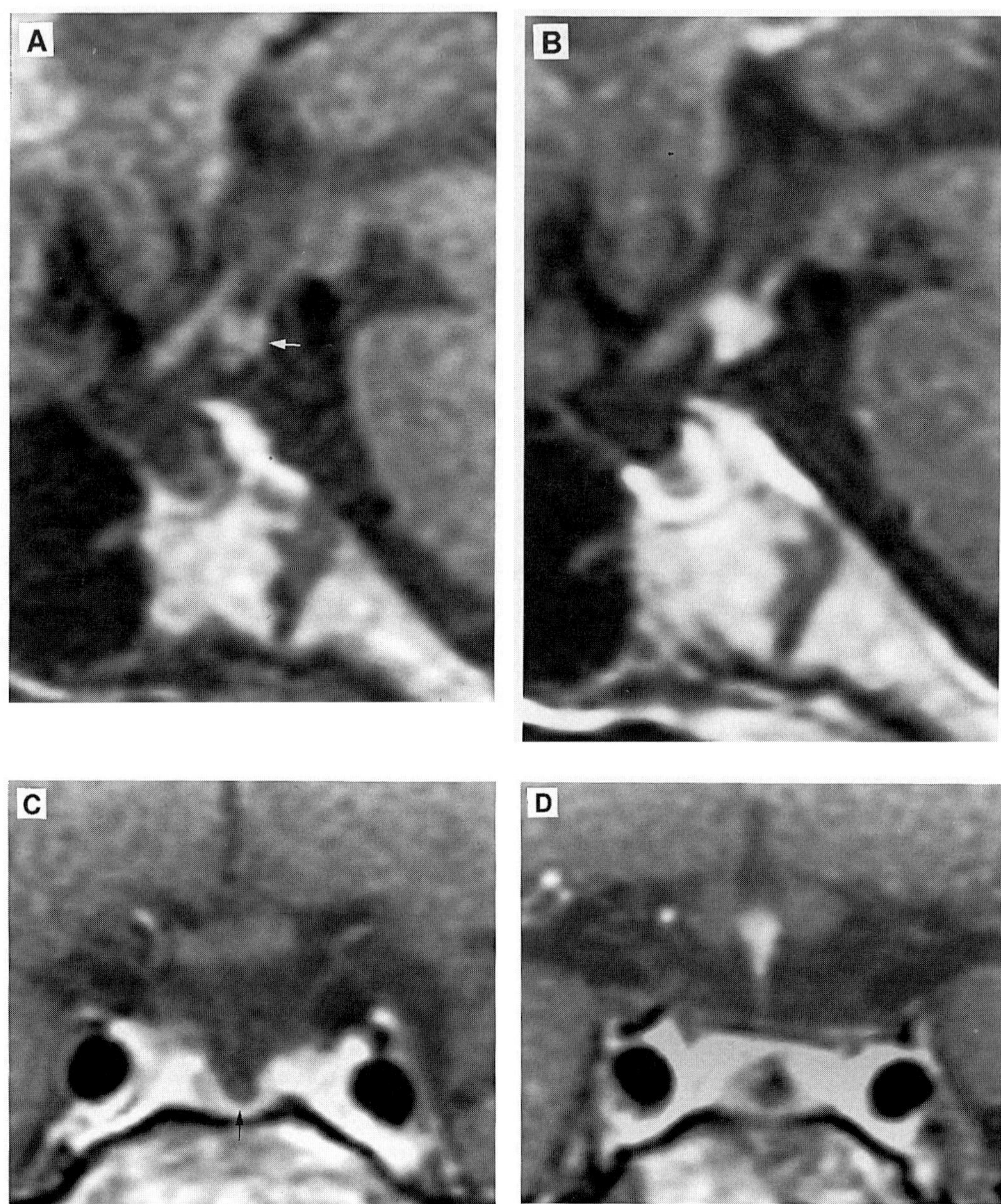

Fig. 13. **(A)** Midsagittal unenhanced, T1-weighted section. **(B)** Same postenhancement. **(C)** T1-weighted, postenhancement midsellar coronal section. **(D)** Same, slightly posterior to (C). Note the small sella, the small pituitary gland, the enhancing 7-mm lobule of tissue beneath the chiasm along the rostral stalk. The stalk is tiny, but may continue to the pituitary. This is a 33-yr-old pituitary dwarf with hypotestosteronism. The posterior pituitary lobe is ectopic in rostral stalk.

artery, an intrasellar trigeminal artery, and possibly channels related to a dural carotid cavernous fistula. Rarely, transsellar arterial channels are present in which one cavernous internal carotid artery supplies the more proximal hypoplastic or absent opposite internal carotid artery *(42)*. Note that prominent medial curvature of the cavernous internal carotid arteries (usually both) may seriously compress the pituitary gland; in lesser cases, they will on a sagittal view produce a hypointensity not to be confused with an intrinsic pituitary lesion. In liver failure, a slightly large and T1-weighted hyperintense pituitary gland is seen (along with similar centrosylvian brain change).

GIANT INTRACRANIAL ANEURYSM

These aneurysms, usually over 15 mm in diameter, must always be considered in the differential diagnosis of lesions in the cavernous sinus or in the suprasellar cistern, and also in the ventral posterior fossa cisterns. On T1-weighted MR, these appear to be isointense or hyperintense to brain. On CT, there is frequently calcification within the wall. On either modality the lumen component of the aneurysm enhances (Fig. 14A–F). The large majority contain thrombus, which makes up the nonenhancing or nonluminal portion. This latter is very characteristically hypointense on T2 weighting, a relatively unique feature. These arise from the distal basilar artery, or from the cavernous or subarachnoid internal carotid artery including its bifurcation, and more peripherally and less commonly from the first portions of the anterior and middle cerebral arteries, and from the anterior communicating artery area. In the pre-CT era when perisellar lesions were detected by skull films or tomopneumoencephalography, angiography was invariably used to exclude the diagnosis of aneurysm. Now, angiography is rarely needed.

LESIONS PREDOMINANTLY OF THE SUPRASELLAR CISTERN

Numerous lesions involve the hypothalamus, visual system, pituitary stalk, in varied combinations, and some in association with more remote dissemination or multifocality. The imaging is not usually specific to differentiate these lesions, but clinical features and evidence of systemic manifestations may be helpful.

The most common adult lesion is the metastasis from systemic neoplasia. This may be isolated to the hypothalamus, stalk, or pituitary gland (Fig. 15A,B). There may be other deposits in the parenchyma of the brain, and/or subarachnoid space diffuse dissemination.

Chronic meningitides affect these areas. Sarcoidosis tends to be diffuse in the pia-arachnoid, and may extend to the ependymal surfaces. The patients present with hypothalamic symptoms and/or multiple cranial nerve abnormalities. It is common to have associated systemic sarcoidosis. Other lesions of similar nature are cryptococcosis, tuberculosis, syphilis, and perhaps viral infections of the meninges (varicella zoster).

Histiocytosis (Langerhans cell) clinically consists of diabetes insipidus, exophthalmus, and lytic bone lesions *(43,44)*. It may involve bone only or may extend to involve the temporal bone and hypothalamus and pituitary gland. A thickened and enhancing pituitary stalk is noted. These patients are children, and soft tissues masses and interstitial lung disease, are part of the picture.

Wegener granulomatosis appears by imaging to be a similar disease in the adult, male more commonly *(45,46)*. Patients have lesions in the lung, upper respiratory tract, kid-

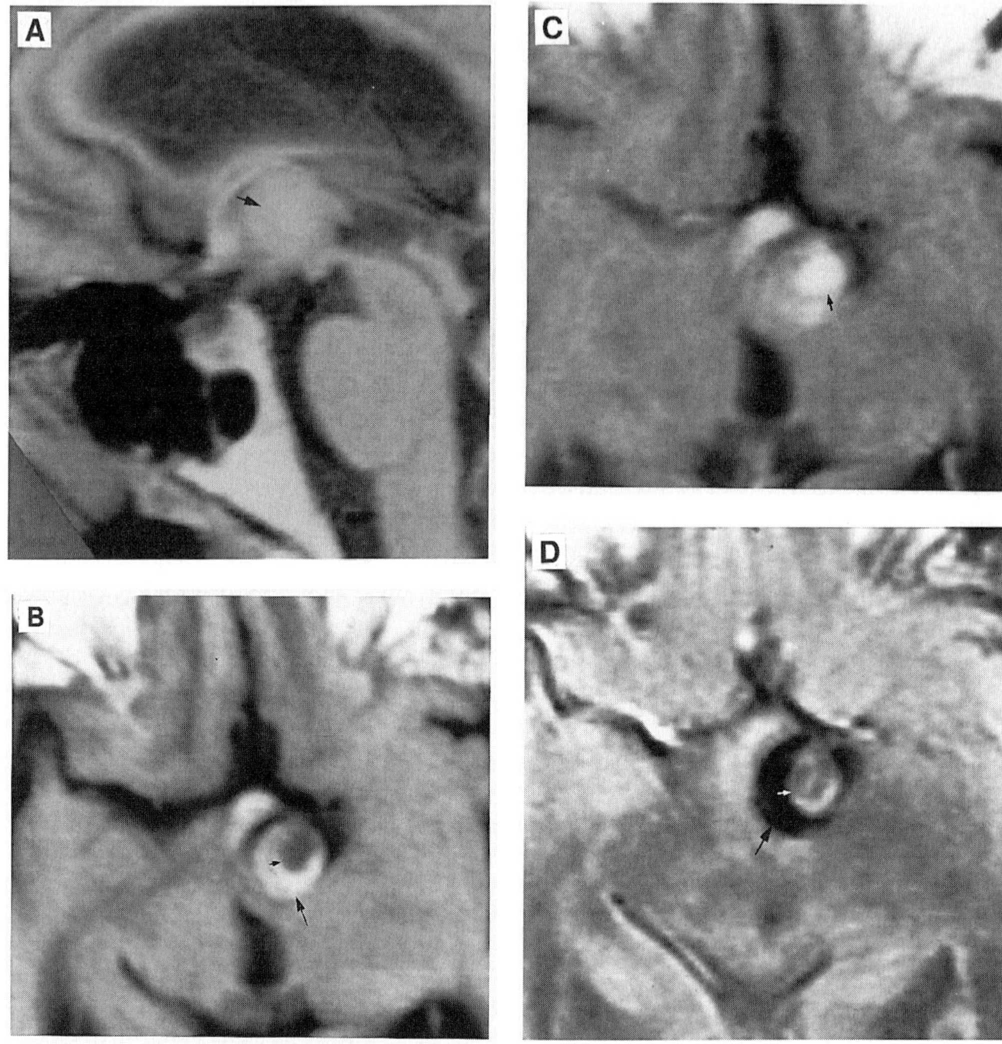

Fig. 14. **(A)** Midsagittal, unenhanced, T1-weighted image showing deformity of the third ventricle by a lesion lying to its left side and indenting it. **(B)** T1-weighted, unenhanced axial image of the suprasellar cistern. **(C)** Same, postenhancement. **(D)** Same, T2-weighted.

ney, mastoid, and within hypothalamus, stalk, and pituitary gland. This may be a hypersensitivity disorder. The etiology is granulomatous, and a necrotizing vasculitis. Central diabetes insipidus may result as well as anterior lobe functional abnormality. Diffuse meningeal involvement has been reported.

A recent publication from Italy suggested an entity termed, "hypophyseal microcirculatory vasculopathy" *(40)*. It is suggested that this occurs with or without inflammatory disease in the stalk region, results in delayed circulation through the stalk and to the posterior lobe (resulting in diabetes insipidus) and perhaps ultimately to delayed portal circulation to the anterior lobe with single or multiple hormonal deficiencies resulting. This can be evaluated by dynamic MR imaging, observing the relative and absolute rates of enhancement of these tissues.

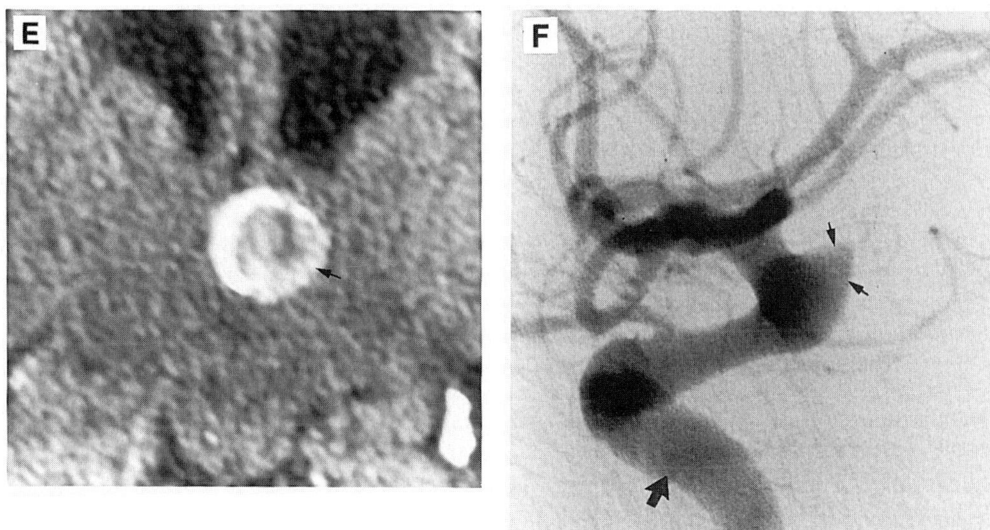

Fig. 14. (continued) (E) Unenhanced axial CT through the superior aspect of the suprasellar cistern. **(F)** Lateral view of a left internal carotid angiogram. The small arrows demonstrate the small lumen of this predominantly thrombosed giant aneurysm and larger arrows the outer margin. Note the lumen enhancement between (B) and (C). Note the lesion is hyperintense to T1 weighting and hypointense to T2 weighting and has a calcified rim. The giant aneurysm arises from the subarachnoid internal carotid artery.

The germinoma usually occurs in the testis or ovary in young people. It probably arises from primitive germ cells. The lesion primarily occurs also in the quadrigeminal cistern, and in the suprasellar cistern *(47)*. It may be multifocal, or subtly continuous between these areas (and elsewhere particularly along the frontal aspect of the ventricles; thus the term, central brain germinoma). As is common in this group, these lesions enhance well and appear to have infiltrating margins. An unusual feature of the germinoma is that it resembles brain tissue on all MR sequences, unlike many tumors that become hyperintense on T2 weighting (Fig. 16A–C).

The lymphoma, which also is parenchymal and/or pia-arachnoid in its distribution, frequently involves the suprasellar cistern, as an enhancing lesion. This is becoming a common lesion, especially in patients with HIV infection.

Gliomas occur either in the visual system or in the hypothalamus or in both (Fig. 17A,B). These are usually homogeneous and poorly enhance. They do not calcify. Occasionally, however, these can become very heterogeneous and may tend to resemble the craniopharyngioma, though the discrete enhancing cyst walls tend to be encompassed in the tumor with the glioma, rather than peripheral as in the craniopharyngioma. Some of these gliomas will enhance. Their pathologic grade is quite variable. Neurofibromatosis is associated with some of these lesions. The pilocystic astrocytoma tends to occur in young children, enhances very well, and tends to involve the frontal lobe, centrosylvian brain, and suprasellar areas.

The hypothalamic hamartoma occurs in the midline of the ventral hypothalamus projecting inferiorly into the cistern, usually small, is bright on T2 weighting, and nonen-

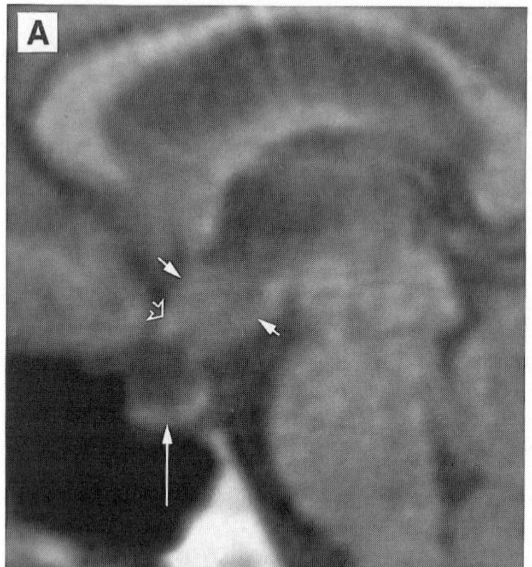

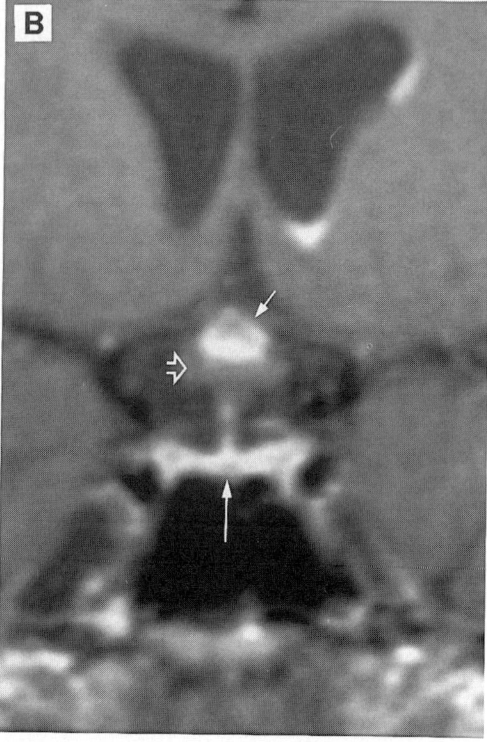

Fig. 15. **(A)** Unenhanced, midsagittal, T1-weighted section showing a large mass, partially involving the chiasm, involving the rostral stalk and ventral hypothalamus. **(B)** Enhanced, T1-weighted coronal section showing enhancement in the ventral hypothalamus as well as subependymally. This is metastatic disease from a systemic cancer.

hancing *(48)*. Histologically, the hamartoma resembles gray matter, is thought to be nonneoplastic, but rather to be heterotopic or hyperplastic tissue. These seem to be associated with a specific syndrome of precocious puberty (74%), gelastic (48%) and generalized epilepsy, and with behavioral disturbances. Other congenital abnormalities may coexist. Rarely the lesions may be prechiasmatic or may appear to be free in the interpeduncular cistern.

In a recent paper concerning 26 children with precocious puberty, the hypothalamic hamartoma was the cause in three, a pineal tumor in one, an "empty sella" in one, and idiopathic in 21 *(49)*. In any of the categories, an increased height and volume of the pituitary gland is seen. This suggests hypothalamic-pituitary-gonadal activation.

The epidermoid or dermoid inclusion cyst has predilection to the ventral basal cisterns as well as to intraventricular locations (especially in the third and fourth ventricles). The epidermoid resembles cerebrospinal fluid fairly closely on MR imaging, has sharp, lobulated margins and usually a granular or particulate content and does not enhance to contrast medium (Fig. 18). These insinuate into brain parenchyma and may resemble primary parenchymal lesions. They tend to occur in the cisterns, which may include the suprasellar cistern, and often they are eccentric. The dermoid tends to be hyperintense on all sequences because of its oil content,

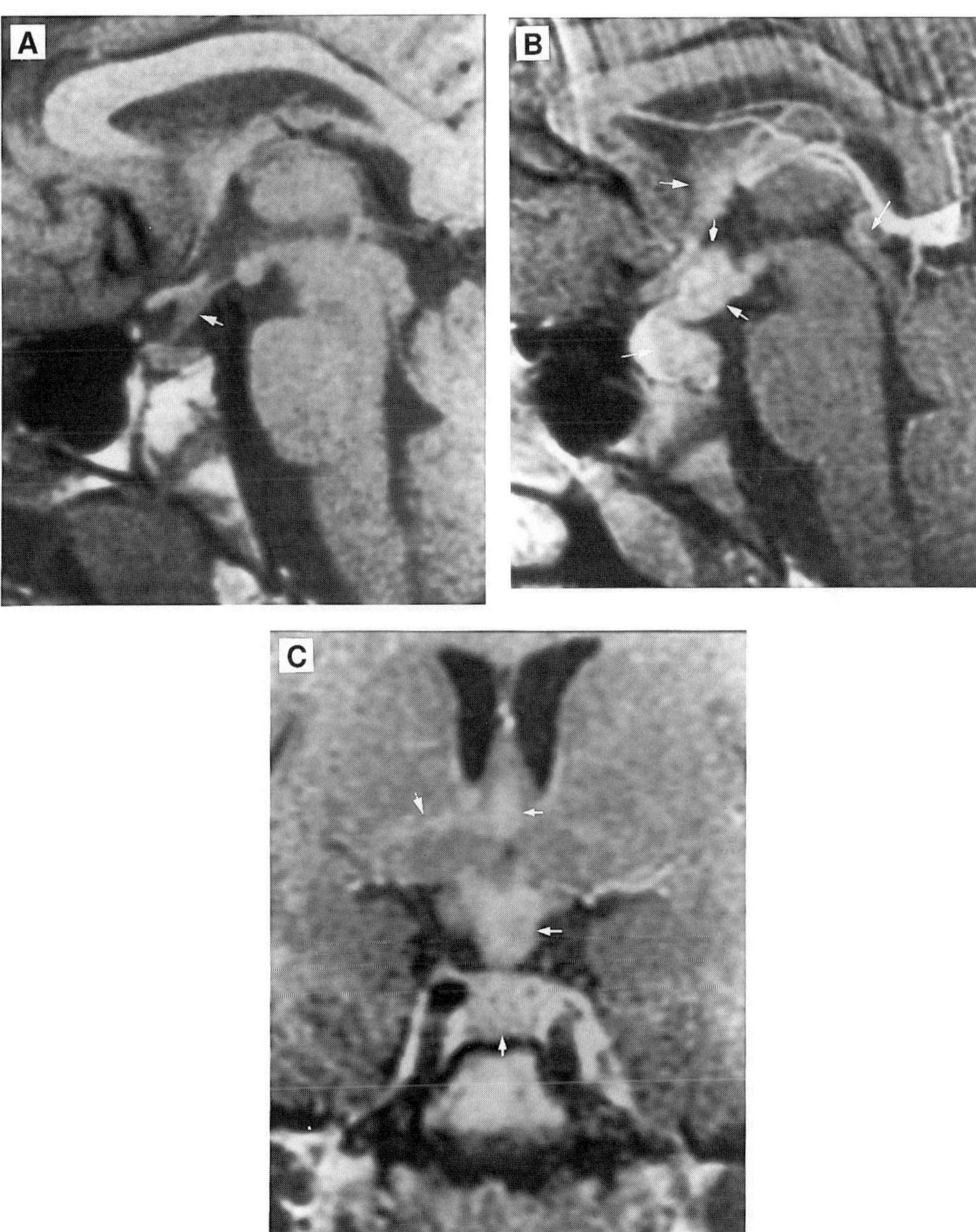

Fig. 16. **(A)** Midsagittal, T1-weighted, unenhanced section. **(B)** Similar section but postenhancement 4 yr later. **(C)** Postenhancement, T1-weighted coronal section through the midsella, same date as **(B)**. Note the slightly enlarged pituitary stalk on (A) (contrast medium was not used); the marked enlargement of stalk, ventral hypothalamus, and the majority of the pituitary gland on (B), with invasion of the region of the anterior commissure; and on (C) invasion of the ventral hypothalamus and into the centrosylvian brain. This is the natural history of an untreated germinoma. There is probably also neoplasm along the anterior aspect of the corpus callosum, and in the quadrigeminal cistern.

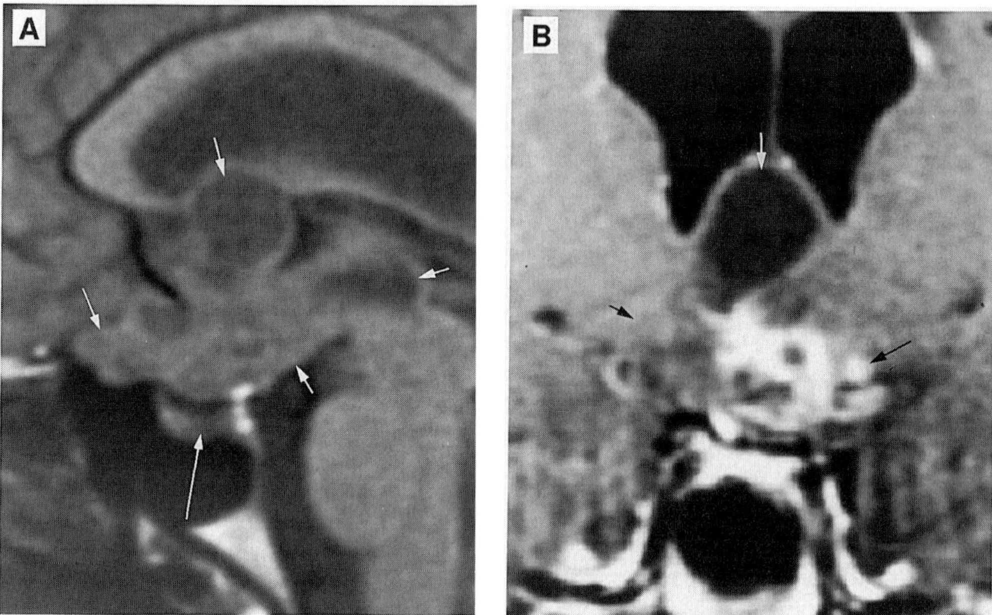

Fig. 17. **(A)** Unenhanced, midsagittal, T1-weighted MR section demonstrating a large suprasellar lesion with cystic portions invaginating the anterior third ventricle to the foramen of Monro (with obstructive ventriculomegaly) and a posterior cyst deeply and eccentrically invaginating the posterior third ventricle and rostral midbrain. **(B)** T1-weighted coronal section demonstrates enhancement irregularly within part of the lesion. The pituitary gland is normal. This is an optic system-hypothalamic glioma.

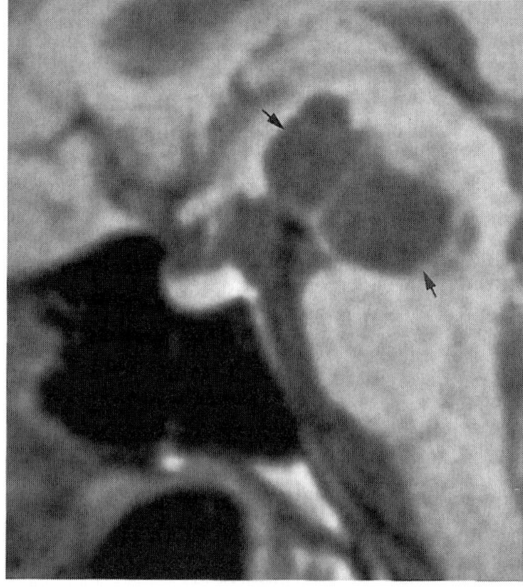

Fig. 18. Unenhanced, midsagittal, T1-weighted section demonstrates a lesion severely affecting, from the left side, the midbrain and hypothalamus; this is a posterior fossa to supratentorial epidermoid inclusion cyst.

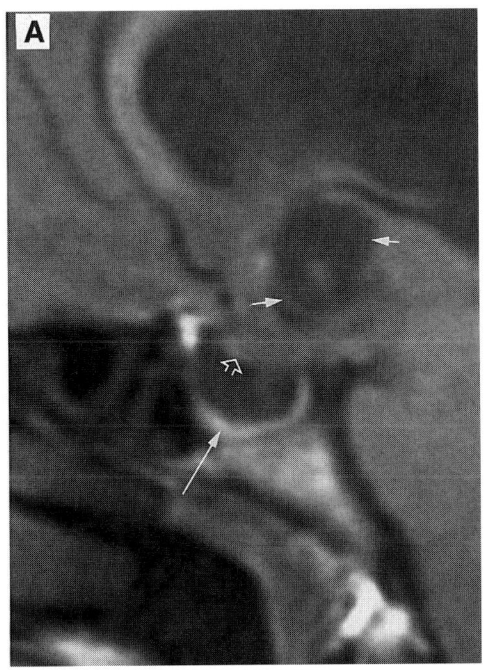

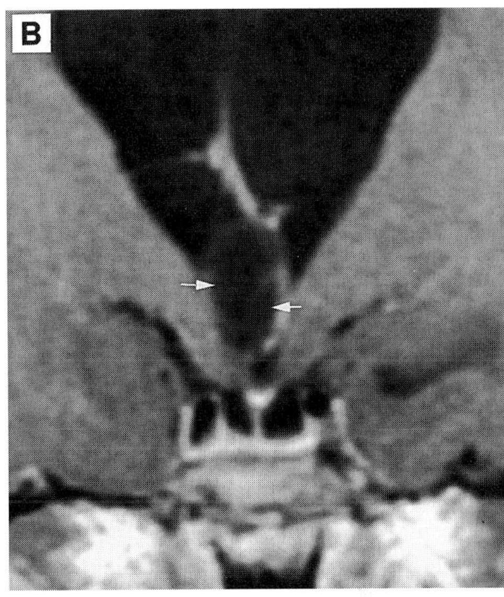

Fig. 19. The images are T1-weighted midline, unenhanced, sagittal (**A**) and a midsellar postenhancement coronal view (**B**). This represents a small pituitary gland with a diaphragma sellae congenital anomaly, partly enlarged (compressed) ventral hypothalamus and chiasm, caused by a cysticercosis cyst within the third ventricle producing obstructive ventriculomegaly at the foramen of Monro.

and appears to be more apt to rupture and distribute this fat-like material into the cisterns.

Many types of lesions of the paranasal sinuses and nose may extend into the intracranial space, especially into the anterior cranial fossa *(50–54)*. These include benign fibro-osseous lesions (ossifying fibroma, fibrous dysplasia, and intraosseous hemangioma), inverted papilloma, and malignancies.

Lesions primarily within the third ventricle may affect the hypothalamus by compression or invasion (Fig. 19A,B). These include the ependymoma, craniopharyngioma, and even less common entities such as a cysticercosis cyst *(55)*. These commonly produce obstructive ventriculomegaly, which may then lead to hypothalamic symptoms. The colloid cyst may have the latter feature as well.

LESIONS OF THE CAVERNOUS SINUS

Cavernous sinus may be home for primary lesions which include Schwannoma, epidermoid, or dermoid inclusion cyst (Fig. 20A,B), hemangioma (cavernous vascular malformation), and atherosclerotic aneurysm or congenital aneurysm of the internal carotid artery *(56)*. The cavernous sinus may be the recipient of lesions arising elsewhere (for example from the sphenoid sinus, from the cavernous dura, from an intrasellar lesion, from the nasopharynx, and so on). The common presen-

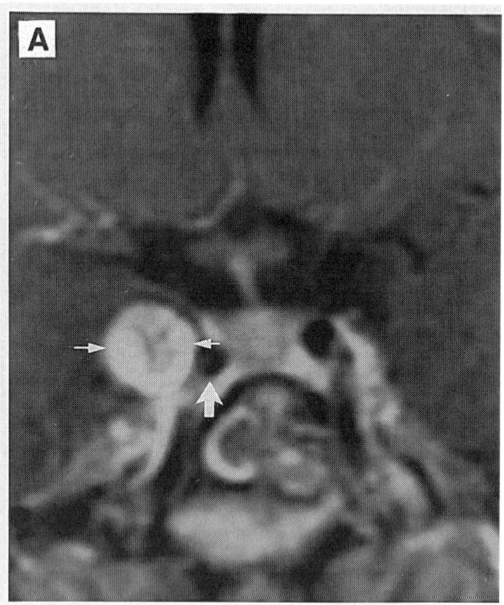

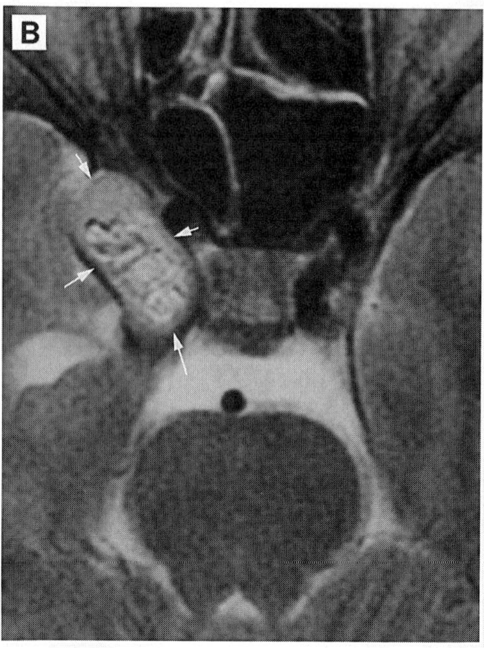

Fig. 20. **(A)** Midsellar, T1-weighted, postenhancement coronal section. **(B)** Midsellar, T2-weighted, axial section. The lesion is an intracavernous (nerve compartment) dermoid. Note the characteristic MR signal features. The pituitary gland is normal. This patient presented with sixth nerve palsy.

tation is a deficit in the extraocular muscle innervation, especially cranial nerve III or VI *(57–59)*.

The Schwannoma occurs most commonly in this area from cranial nerve V and less commonly from cranial nerve III. These may be in the cavernous sinus, in the trigeminal cistern, or peripherally along the fifth nerve branches or within the orbit. The atherosclerotic internal carotid aneurysm of the cavernous segment will have calcified walls. Hematogenous metastases locate here, and also lymphoma.

The Tolosa-Hunt syndrome is an inflammatory granuloma occurring in the orbital apex, superior orbital fissure, or cavernous sinus. This is often not seen on standardimaging, and its mimic would be lymphoma. Painful ophthalmoplegia is its clinical characteristic.

An uncommon phenomenon is cavernous sinus thrombosis, producing severe inflammatory proptosis and extraocular muscle palsy, usually unilateral. The septic process may originate from infections in the face or paranasal sinuses. Orbital and soft tissue eyelid swelling, chemosis, and dilatation of the superior ophthalmic vein may be seen.

Similar findings but with less inflammatory signs are associated with carotid-cavernous (arteriovenous) fistula. The added feature of a bruit would lead this patient to angiography, to precise localization of the lesion, and often to endovascular therapy.

Lesions affecting cranial nerve I may coexist with or be independent from cavernous sinus lesions *(49,60)*.

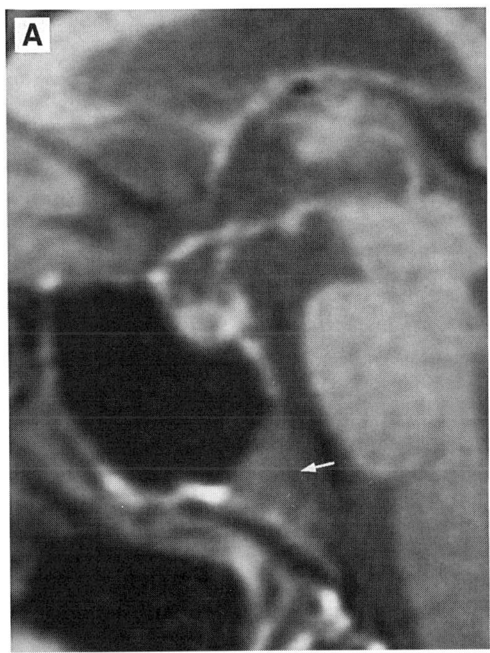

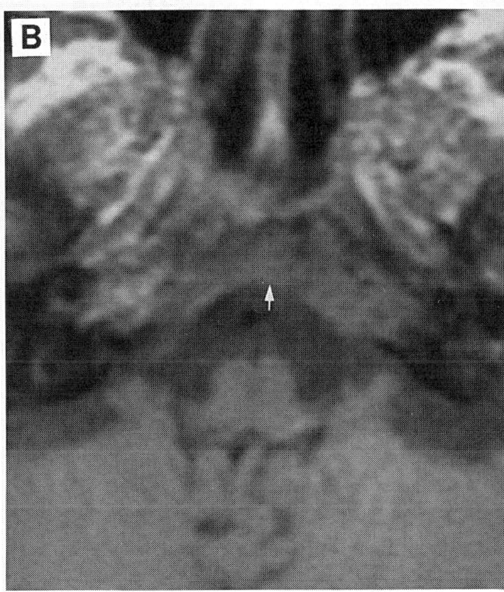

Fig. 21. **(A)** This is a patient with sixth nerve palsy. The clival marrow on T1-weighted, unenhanced midsagittal section is hypointense, very apt to be abnormal. **(B,C)** T1-weighted, axial sections through the caudal clivus showing clival hypointensity on the unenhanced (B) and irregular clival enhancement on (C).

SKULL BASE LESIONS

There are many skull base lesions that affect the clivus, sphenoid sinus, cavernous sinus, middle cranial fossa, and the intrasellar space. There are few differentiating features on imaging. The imaging serves to demonstrate the exact distribution of the neoplasm, so that a biopsy may be best planned. In many, a transsphenoidal biopsy provides the safest route to biopsy. The lesions involved include chordoma, chondroma, chrondosarcoma, metastasis (Fig. 21A–D), rhabdomyosarcoma, juvenile angiofibroma, and primary tumors of the sphenoid sinus, nose, and nasopharynx *(61)*. Involvement of a synchondrosis (especially the clivo-temporal synchondrosis) favors the cartilage tumor (Fig. 22A–C). The chordoma often has calcification or bone spicules within it. The metastasis tends to be the most osteolytic. In most of these skull base/clival lesions, the pituitary is elevated, and invasion often partial.

SUMMARY

Lesions within the perisellar area have many anatomic variations and many pathologic variations. The role of imaging is to precisely define the extent of the lesion, and if possible, the origin of the lesion. Relationships of the lesion are important especially with respect to the intrasellar pituitary gland, the cavernous sinus, the pituitary

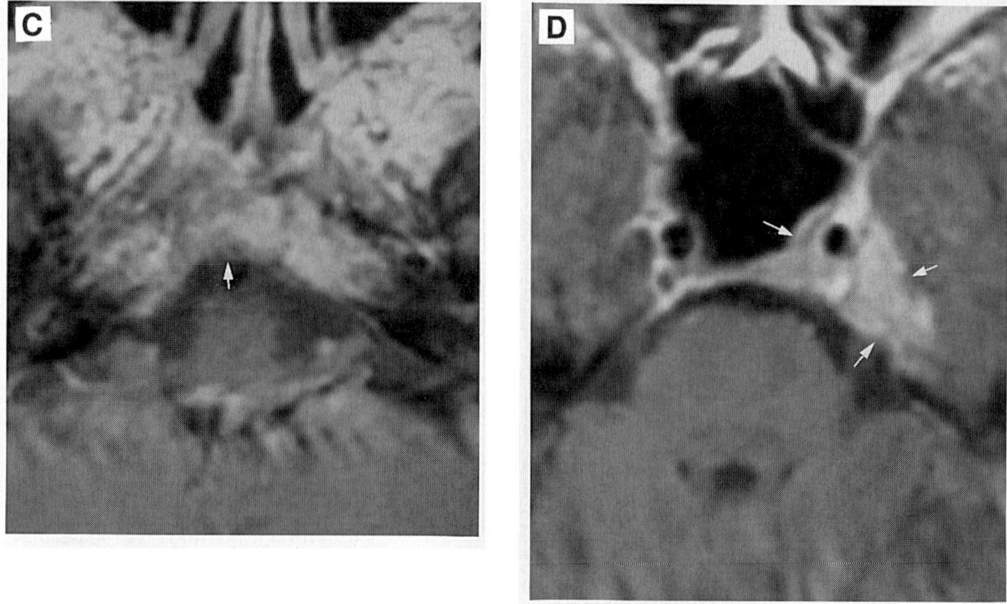

Fig. 21. (continued) (C) Such marrow is abnormal. **(D)** Enhanced, T1-weighted, axial section through the sphenoid sinus and trigeminal cistern. The left trigeminal cistern and the dura around it are replaced by enhancing tissue, which probably involves the proximal cavernous sinus into the sphenoid sinus. This is metastatic prostate carcinoma.

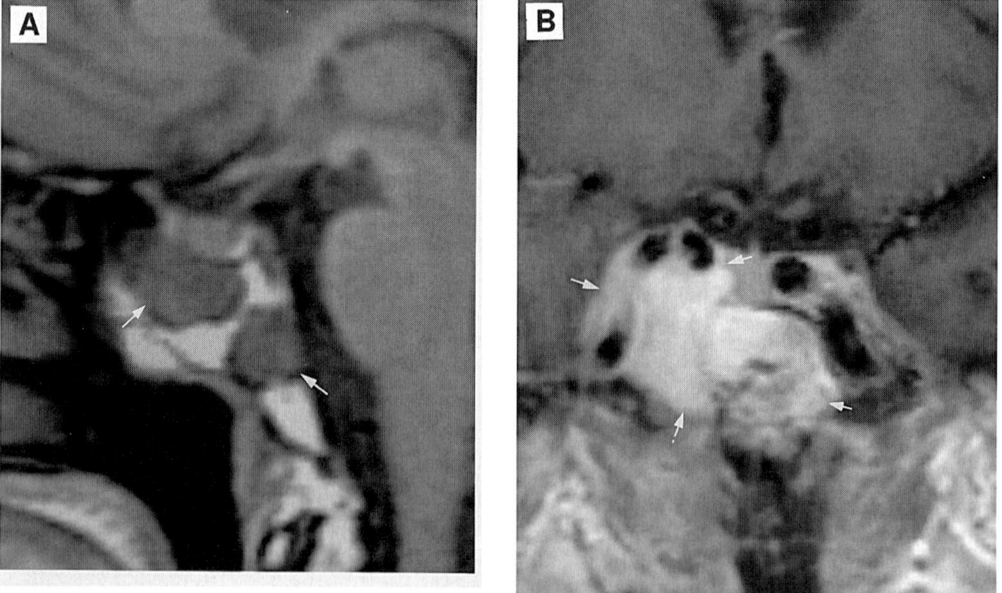

Fig. 22. (A) Unenhanced, T1-weighted, midsagittal section. **(B)** Midsellar, postenhancement, T1-weighted coronal section.

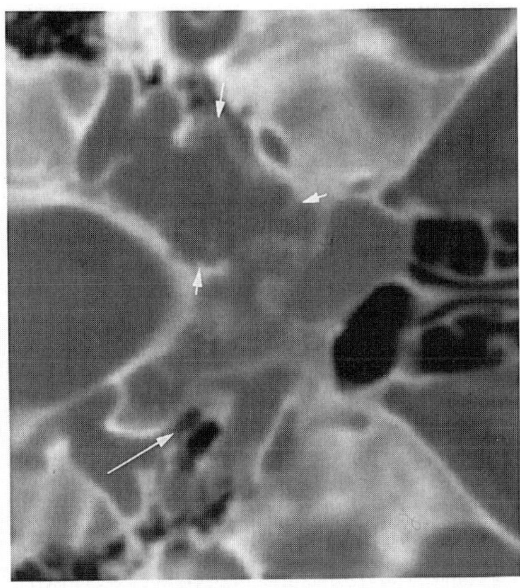

Fig. 22. (continued) **(C)** Skull base CT (bone algorithm). Note heterogeneous replacement of clivus and sphenoid sinus and cavernous sinus by T1-weighted hypointense and densely enhancing tissue. This is causing bone destruction especially along the clivo-temporal fissure. This is a chondrosarcoma in a woman with sixth nerve palsy as the presentation.

stalk, the hypothalamus, the cisterns, the brain, and the bony skull base. The imaging directs the surgeon's approach to the definitive surgery or biopsy. For all of these lesions, the MR is almost invariably the best study, and almost always requires Gadolinium enhancement. The multiple projections of the MR and the multiple pulse sequences are very helpful in defining anatomic disturbances, and the characteristics of the tissue.

REFERENCES

1. Rhoton AL Jr., Hardy DG. Microsurgical anatomy of the sphenoid bone, cavernous sinus, and sellar region. Clinical Management of Pituitary Disorders. Raven, New York, 1979; pp. 1–73.
2. Dolenc VV. Anatomy and Surgery of the Cavernous Sinus. Springer-Verlag, Wien, 1989.
3. Krisht A, Barnett DW, Barrow DL, Bonner G. The blood supply of the intracavernous cranial nerves: an anatomic study. Neurosurgery 1994;34:275–279.
4. Krisht AF, Barrow DL, Barnett DW, Bonner GD, Shengalaia G. The microsurgical anatomy of the superior hypophyseal artery. Neurosurgery 1994;35:899–903.

4a. Rubinstein D, Stears RLG, Stears JC. Trigeminal nerve and ganglion in the Meckel cave: appearance at CT and MR imaging. Radiology 1994;193:155–159.

5. Elster AD. Modern imaging of the pituitary. Radiology 1993;187:1–14.
6. Teramoto A, Hirakawa K, Sanno N, Osamura Y. Incidental pituitary lesions in 1,000 unselected autopsy specimens. Radiology 1994;193:161–164.
7. Chong BW, Kucharczyk W, Singer W, George S. Pituitary gland MR: a comparative study of healthy volunteers and patients with microadenomas. AJNR Am J Neuroradiol 1994;15:675–679.
8. Gebarski SS, Gebarski KS. Inferior petrosal sinus: imaging-anatomic correlation. Radiology 1995;194:239–247.
9. Miller DL, Doppman JL, Chang R. Anatomy of the junction of the inferior petrosal sinus and the internal jugular vein. AJNR Am J Neuroradiol 1993;14:1075–1083.

10. Johnsen DE, Woodruff WW, Allen IS, Cera PJ, Funkhouser GR, Coleman LL. MR imaging of the sellar and juxtasellar regions. RadioGraphics 1991;11:727–758.
11. Chong BW, Newton TH. Hypothalamic and pituitary pathology. Radiologic Clin North Am 1993;31:1147–1183.
12. Buchfelder M, Nistor R, Fahlbusch R, Huk WJ. The accuracy of CT and MR evaluation of the sella turcica for detection of adrenocorticotropic hormone-secreting adenomas in Cushing disease. AJNR Am J Neuroradiol 1993;14:1183–1190.
13. Kucharczyk W, Bishop JE, Plewes DB, Keller MA, George S. Detection of pituitary microadenomas: comparison of dynamic keyhole fast spin-echo, unenhanced, and conventional contrast-enhanced MR imaging. AJR Am J Roentgenol 1994;163:671–679.
14. Elster AD. High-resolution, dynamic pituitary MR imaging: standard of care or academic planning. AJR Am J Roentgenol 1994;163:680–682.
15. Lundin P, Bergstrom K, Nyman R, Lundberg PO, Muhr C. Macroprolactinomas: serial MR imaging in long-term bromocriptine therapy. AJNR Am J Neuroradiol 1992;13:1279–1291.
16. Yousem DM, Arrington JA, Zinreich SJ, Kumar AJ, Bryan RN. Pituitary adenomas: possible role of bromocriptine in intratumoral hemorrhage. Radiology 1989;170:239–243.
17. Ostrov SG, Quencer RM, Hoffman JC, Davis PC, Hasso AN, David NJ. Hemorrhage within pituitary adenomas: how often associated with pituitary apoplexy syndrome? AJR Am J Roentgenol 1989; 153:153–160.
18. Mindermann T, Wilson CB. Pediatric pituitary adenomas. Neurosurgery 1995;36:259–269.
19. Kanungo N, Just N, Black M, Mohr G, Glikstein R, Rochon L. Nasopharyngeal craniopharyngioma in an unusual location. AJNR Am J Neuroradiol 1995;16:1372–1374.
20. Graziani N, Donnet A, Bugha TN, Dufour H, Figarella–Branger D, Grisoli F. Ectopic basisphenoidal craniopharyngioma: case report and review of the literature. Neurosurgery 1994;34:346–349.
21. Ahmadi J, Destian S, Apuzzo MLJ, Segall HD, Zee CS. Cystic fluid in craniopharyngiomas: MR imaging and quantitative analysis. Radiology 1992;182:783–785.
22. Weiner HL, Wisoff JH, Rosenberg ME, et al. Craniopharyngiomas: a clinicopathological analysis of factors predictive of recurrence and functional outcome. Neurosurgery 1994;35:1001–1011.
23. Thapar K, Stefaneanu L, Kovacs K et al. Estrogen receptor gene expression in craniopharyngiomas: an in situ hybridization study. Neurosurgery 1994;35:1012–1017.
24. Millar WS, Tartaglino LM, Sergott RC, Friedman DP, Flanders AE. MR of malignant optic glioma of adulthood. AJNR Am J Neuroradiol 1995;16:1673–1676.
25. Maggio WW, Cail WS, Brookeman JR, Persing JA, Jane JA. Rathke's cleft cyst: computed tomographic and magnetic resonance imaging appearances. Neurosurgery 1987;21:60–62.
26. Kucharczyk W, Peck WW, Kelly WM, Norman D, Newton TH. Rathke cleft cysts: CT, MR imaging, and pathologic features. Radiology 1987;165:491–495.
27. Asari S, Ito T, Tsuchida S, Tsutsui T. MR appearance and cyst content of Rathke cleft cysts. J Comput Assist Tomogr 1990;14:532–535.
28. Voelker JL, Campbell RL, Muller J. Clinical, radiographic, and pathological features of symptomatic Rathke's cleft cysts. J Neurosurg 1991;74:535–544.
29. Ross DA, Norman D, Wilson CB. Radiologic characteristics and results of surgical management of Rathke's cysts in 43 patients. Neurosurgery 1992;30:173–179.
30. Sumida M, Uozumi T, Mukada K, Arita K, Kurisu K, Eguchi K. Rathke cleft cysts: correlation of enhanced MR and surgical findings. AJNR Am J Neuroradiol 1994;15:525–532.
31. Kinjo T, Al-Mefty O, Ciric I. Diaphragma sellae meningiomas. Neurosurgery 1995;36:1082–1092.
32. Koshimoto Y, Maeda M, Naiki H, Nakakuki K, Ishii Y. MR of pituitary metastasis in a patient with diabetes insipidus. AJNR Am J Neuroradiol 1995;16:971–974.
33. Mitchell CS, Wood BP, Shimada H. Neonatal disseminated primitive neuroectodermal tumor. AJR Am J Roentgenol 1994;162:1160.
34. Hurley TR, D'Angelo CM, Clasen RA, Wilkinson SB, Passavoy RD. Magnetic resonance imaging and pathological analysis of a pituicytoma: case report. Neurosurgery 1994:35;314–317.
35. Heary RF, Maniker AH, Wolansky LJ. Candidal pituitary abscess: case report. Neurosurgery 1995;36:1009–1013.
36. Lee JH, Laws Jr. ER, Guthrie BL, Dina TS, Nochomovitz LE. Lymphocytic hypophysitis: occurrence in two men. Neurosurgery 1994;34:159–163.

37. Beressi N, Cohen R, Beressi JP et al. Pseudotumoral lymphocytic hypophysitis successfully treated by corticosteroid alone: first case report. Neurosurgery 1994;35:505–508.
38. Abe T, Matsumoto K, Sanno N, Osamura Y. Lymphocytic hypophysitis: case report. Neurosurgery 1995;36:1016–1019.
39. Kaufman B, Tomsak RL, Kaufman BA et al. Herniation of the suprasellar visual system and third ventricle into empty sella: morphologic and clinical considerations. AJR Am J Roentgenol 1989;152:597–608.
40. Kelly WM, Kucharczyk W, Kucharczyk J et al. Posterior pituitary ectopia: an MR feature of pituitary dwarfism. AJNR Am J Neuroradiol 1988;9:453–460.
41. Maghnie M, Genovese E, Arico M et al. Evolving pituitary hormone deficiency is associated with pituitary vasculopathy: dynamic MR study in children with hypopituitarism, diabetes insipidus, and Langerhans cell histiocytosis. Radiology 1994;193:493–499.
42. Midkiff RB, Boykin MW, McFarland DR, Bauman JA. Agenesis of the internal carotid artery with intercavernous anastomosis. AJNR Am J Neuroradiol 1995;16:1356–1359.
43. Meyer JS, Harty MP, Mahboubi S et al. Langerhans cell histiocytosis: presentation and evolution of radiologic findings with clinical correlation. RadioGraphics 1995;15:1135–1146.
44. Stromberg JS, Wang AM, Huang TE, Vicini FA, Nowak PA. Langerhans cell histiocytosis involving the sphenoid sinus and superior orbital fissure. AJNR Am J Neuroradiol 1995;16:964–967.
45. Tishler S, Williamson T, Mirra SS, Lichtman JB, Gismondi P, Kibble MB. Wegener granulomatosis with meningeal involvement. AJNR Am J Neuroradiol 1993;14:1248–1252.
46. Czarnecki EJ, Spickler EM. MR demonstration of Wegener granulomatosis of the infundibulum, a cause of diabetes insipidus. AJNR Am J Neuroradiol 1995;16:968–970.
47. Moon WK, Chang KH, Kim IO et al. Germinomas of the basal ganglia and thalamus: MR findings and a comparison between MR and CT. AJR Am J Roentgenol 1994;162:1413–1417.
48. Valdueza JM, Cristante L, Dammann O et al. Hypothalamic hamartomas: with special reference to gelastic epilepsy and surgery. Neurosurgery 1994;34:949–958.
49. Sharafuddin MJA, Luisiri A, Garibaldi LR et al. MR imaging diagnosis of central precocious puberty: importance of changes in the shape and size of the pituitary gland. AJR Am J Roentgenol 1994; 162:1167–1173.
50. Woodruff WW, Vrabec DP. Inverted papilloma of the nasal vault and paranasal sinuses: spectrum of CT findings. AJR Am J Roentgenol 1994;162:419–423.
51. Kim HJ, Kim JH, Kim JH, Hwang EG. Bone erosion caused by sinonasal cavernous hemangioma: CT findings in two patients. AJNR Am J Neuroradiol 1995;16:1176–1178.
52. Allbery SM, Chaljub G, Cho NL, Rassekh CH, John SD, Guinto FC. MR imaging of nasal masses. RadioGraphics 1995;15:1311–1327.
53. Nakagawa K, Takasato Y, Ito Y, Yamada K. Ossifying fibroma involving the paranasal sinuses, orbit, and anterior cranial fossa: case report. Neurosurgery 1995;36:1192–1195.
54. Banerji D, Inao S, Sugita K, Kaur A, Chhabra DK. Primary intraosseous orbital hemangioma: a case report and review of the literature. Neurosurgery 1994;35:1131–1134.
55. Oppenheim JS, Strauss RC, Mormino J, Sachdev VP, Rothman AS. Ependymomas of the third ventricle. Neurosurgery 1994;34:350–353.
56. Cusimano MD, Sekhar LN, Sen CN et al. The results of surgery for benign tumors of the cavernous sinus. Neurosurgery 1995;37:1–10.
57. Blake PY, Mark AS, Kattah J, Kolsky M. MR of oculomotor nerve palsy. AJNR Am J Neuroradiol 1995;16:1665–1672.
58. Morard M, Tcherekayev V, de Tribolet N. The superior orbital fissure: a microanatomical study. Neurosurgery 1994;35:1087–1093.
59. Natori Y, Rhoton Jr. AL. Microsurgical anatomy of the superior orbital fissure. Neurosurgery 1995;36:762–775.
60. Majoie CBLM, Verbeeten Jr. B, Dol JA, Peeters FLM. Trigeminal neuropathy: evaluation with MR imaging. RadioGraphics 1995;15:795–811.
61. Gay E, Sekhar LN, Rubinstein E et al. Chordomas and chondrosarcomas of the cranial base: results and follow-up of 60 patients. Neurosurgery 1995;36:887–897.

18 Neurosurgical Approach to Pituitary Adenomas

Kevin O. Lillehei, MD

CONTENTS

INTRODUCTION

The diagnosis and treatment of pituitary adenomas is a field in continuous evolution, spurred on by new advancements in radiographic imaging, microneurosurgery, and clinical pharmacology. As our armamentarium for the treatment of these lesions is increasing, the role of surgery needs to be carefully reevaluated.

This chapter addresses the role of surgery in the treatment of endocrine active and inactive tumors, including a discussion of the expected outcomes from surgical intervention for specific tumor types. Also included is a discussion of the presenting signs and symptoms of pituitary region tumors, the differential diagnosis of a parasellar mass, and the indications for a transsphenoidal vs a transcranial surgical approach. A short history of the evolution of pituitary surgery is included as a historical perspective.

HISTORICAL PERSPECTIVE

The first recorded attempt to surgically remove a pituitary tumor was performed by Paul in 1893 in Liverpool, England *(1,2)*. This was performed in an acromegalic patient using a lateral subtemporal approach recommended by Sir Victor Horsley. At surgery, a bony temporal decompression was performed with the dura mater found to be extremely tense. For fear of brain herniation, the dura was never opened, and the pituitary tumor was never visualized. In 1904, Sir Victor Horsley performed the first successful removal of a pituitary tumor *(3,4)*, using a lateral middle fossa approach. From 1904 to

From: *Contemporary Endocrinology, Vol. 3: Diseases of the Pituitary: Diagnosis and Treatment*
Edited by M. E. Wierman Humana Press Inc., Totowa, NJ

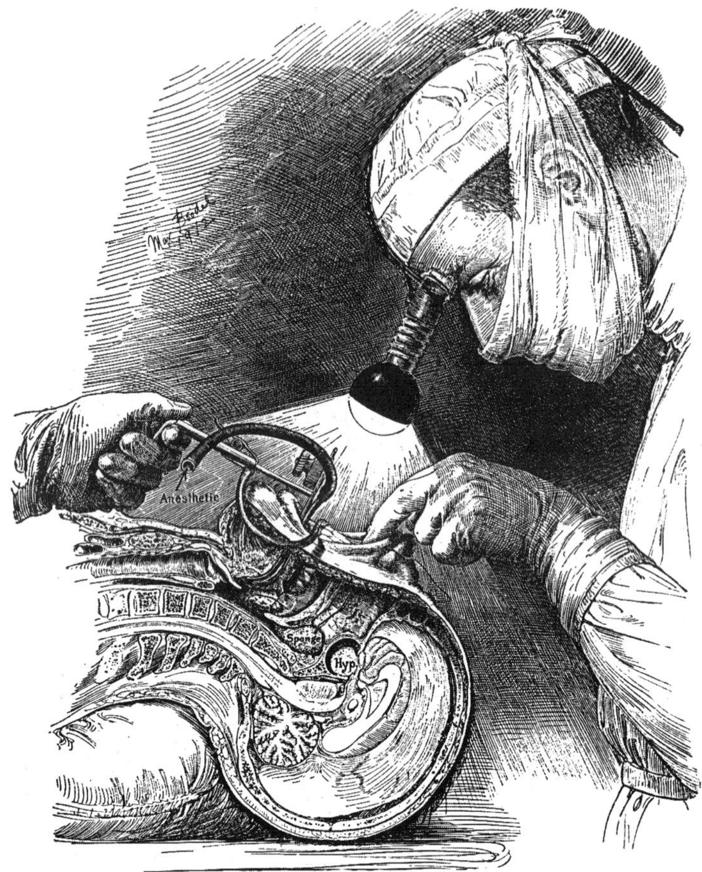

Fig. 1. Cushing's operative approach to the pituitary sella using the sublabial transsphenoidal route. This photograph is reproduced from his original article in *The Journal of the American Medical Association*, 1914 (Reproduced with permission from ref. *3*).

1906 he operated on an additional 9 patients, achieving a successful result in 8 of the 10 patients with pituitary tumors using this technique *(5)*. Schloffer, an Innsbruck rhinologist, is credited with having performed the first successful transsphenoidal operation on the pituitary gland in 1907 *(3,6)*. This initial crude approach involved surgically rotating the nose off of the midline of the face with removal of the septum and the turbinates bilaterally. From 1907 to 1910, this approach was gradually refined, ultimately leading to the technique described by Cushing *(3)* (Fig. 1). Cushing, employing Hirsch's endonasal approach, Halstead's sublabial incision, Eiselberg and Kocher's submucous resection of the septum, and Kanavel's headlight to improve visualization, operated transsphenoidally on a total of 231 pituitary tumors between 1910 and 1925 with an operative mortality of only 5.6% *(3,7)*. This is surprising considering the lack of endotracheal anesthesia, operative magnification, intraoperative X-ray, and the absence of steroid replacement. Although clearly having advantages over the craniotomy, the transsphenoidal approach due to its limited visibility, had an unacceptably high rate of symptomatic recurrence. Because of this, it was abandoned in favor of the transcranial route from 1920 until the latter part of the 1960s. Interest in the use of the transsphenoidal route, however, was rekindled by Guiot and Hardy, who adapted the use of the operating microscope and intraoperative fluoroscopy to the procedure. With these two major innovations, the transsphenoidal route was demonstrated to be as effective as transcranial surgery in removing most large pituitary tumors, and more effective for the treatment of small adenomas. In addition, transsphenoidal surgery carried an inherently lower risk than craniotomy. Since then, transsphenoidal surgery has become the procedure of choice in the treatment of the majority of pituitary tumors.

CLINICAL SIGNS AND SYMPTOMS ASSOCIATED WITH PITUITARY ADENOMAS

The clinical presentation of patients with tumors of the pituitary region is generally related either to the signs and symptoms of mass effect or those associated with hormone hypersecretion. In patients who develop signs and symptoms of mass effect, the tumor is generally > 1 cm in size. Lesions this size or larger can extend into the suprasellar cistern resulting in the classically described vertex headache from distention of the diaphragma sella or a bitemporal hemianopsia from upward distention of the optic chiasm. Rarely, in very large lesions, hydrocephalus may occur from tumor extension into the third ventricle and obstruction of the foramen of Monroe. Extension of tumor laterally into the cavernous sinus may cause compression of the cranial nerves contained within this structure, resulting in blurred or double vision from involvement of cranial nerves III, IV, and/or VI, or ipsilateral facial numbness from involvement of the first and second divisions of the trigeminal nerve. Extension of tumor far laterally into the temporal lobe can occasionally result in the patient presenting with seizures, usually of the uncinate or partial complex variety. Extension of tumor inferiorly into the sphenoid sinus is often asymptomatic until the tumor reaches a very large size at which time the patient may present with recurrent sinusitis or a spontaneous cerebrospinal fluid leak.

As tumors enlarge, there is also progressive compression of the normal pituitary gland which ultimately will lead to a loss of normal pituitary function. As the anterior gland becomes compressed, loss of hormone function generally follows a reproducible pattern with growth hormone secretion disrupted first, followed by LH, FSH, TSH, ACTH, and, lastly, prolactin *(8)*. Progressive compression of the pituitary stalk, in addition, can lead to loss of prolactin inhibitory factor (PIF) from the hypothalamus and, instead of prolactin secretion dropping, it may rise, a phenomenon known as the "stalk effect." Prolactin elevation from stalk effect rarely exceeds 125–150 pg/mL. If prolactin is found exceeding this level, a prolactin secreting tumor must be considered. Loss of normal posterior pituitary function from a pituitary adenoma is rare and if present, is usually the last stage of panhypopituitarism. A patient who presents with diabetes insipidus as an early symptom will rarely harbor a pituitary adenoma, but rather a lesion which preferentially involves the pituitary stalk or hypothalamus as seen with craniopharyngiomas or inflammatory lesions (i.e., sarcoidosis, histiocytosis X).

Patients may also present with excess hormone secretion from "functional" pituitary adenomas. These hypersecretory syndromes include Cushing's disease (ACTH hypersecretion), acromegaly (GH hypersecretion), amenorrhea/galactorrhea (prolactin hy-

Table 1
Differential Diagnosis of Sellar and Parasellar Lesions

Tumors	
	Pituitary adenomas
	Pituitary carcinoma (rare)
	Craniopharyngioma
	Meningioma
	Germinoma
	Chordoma
	Sarcoma
	Granular cell tumor (choristoma)
	Neuroma (usually arising from cranial nerve V)
	Metastatic tumor
	Optic nerve glioma
	Dermoid tumor
	Epidermoid tumor
	Infundibuloma
	Hypothalamic glioma
	Esthesioneuroblastoma
	Lymphoma (usually of the hypothalamus)
Cysts	
	Rathke's cleft cyst
	Benign pituitary cyst
	Arachnoid cyst
	Mucocele of sphenoid sinus
Inflammatory Lesions	
	Bacterial abscess
	Sarcoidosis
	Eosinophilic granuloma (Histiocytosis X)
	Tuberculosis
	Lymphocytic hypophysitis
	Granulomatous hypophysitis
	Mycoses
Aneurysm	
Empty Sella Syndrome	
Pituitary Apoplexy	

persecretion), and Nelson's syndrome (ACTH hypersecretion after adrenalectomy). Adenomas in patients with Cushing's disease and in females with hyperprolactinemia tend to be small, < 1 cm. Those patients with acromegaly, Nelson's syndrome, and males with hyperprolactinemia, however, tend to have large adenomas, > 1 cm. The pituitary hypersecretion syndromes and their endocrine evaluation are discussed in detail in Chapters 4, 7, and 9 and will not be addressed further here. The reader is referred to this earlier discussion.

DIFFERENTIAL DIAGNOSIS

Although the most common parasellar lesion encountered by the neurosurgeon is the adenoma, not infrequently other lesions will be encountered. It is imperative that the surgeon have some familiarity with these more unusual lesions in order to provide appropriate treatment at the time of the initial surgical exploration. The spectrum of lesions that may occur in the sella and parasellar region are listed in Table 1.

In my 10-yr experience at the University of Colorado, I have performed 237 transsphenoidal operations. Of these precedures: 196 were for adenomas; 16 for Rathke's Cleft cysts *(9)*; 4 for craniopharygiomas; 2 for intrasellar and suprasellar meningiomas; and one each for intrasellar germinoma, granulomatous hypophysitis (a suspected tuberculus abscess), lymphocytic hypophysitis *(10)*, an intermediate grade chondrosarcoma, nasopharyngeal carcinoma, esthesioneuroblastoma, metastatic tumor, and an arachnoid cyst. With current day radiographic imaging and sophisticated endocrinologic testing, it is unusual for the surgeon to be suprised by the intraoperative findings. Nevertheless, he or she must be prepared to deal with some of these more unusual histologies.

SURGICAL TREATMENT AND RESULTS

Preoperative assessment

Patients felt to be candidates for pituitary exploration are:

1. Those with suspected nonsecretory pituitary adenomas, usually > 1 cm in size causing symptoms secondary to mass effect;
2. Hypersecretory adenomas, including prolactinomas in patients who are unresponsive to or cannot tolerate dopamine agonists; and
3. The occasional unusual parasellar lesion which is symptomatic and in which the diagnosis is unclear.

The endocrinologic work-up in patients with suspected pituitary lesions is covered extensively in the previous chapters. From a neurosurgical standpoint, however, once the decision to operate has been made, it is imperative to know the hormone status of the adrenal and thyroid axis. If deficient, and proper hormone replacement can be instituted prior to surgery, this is strongly advised. All patients with macroadenomas, whether they require hormone replacement or not, should be assumed to have a compromised pituitary-adrenal axis in response to stress. Therefore, the routine use of stress dose steroids in the perioperative period is recommended. We routinely administer dexamethasone 4 mg iv or po the morning of surgery and then every 6 h thereafter on a tapering schedule for a total of 72 h. Prolonged use of steroids postoperatively is generally unnecessary unless there is a known preoperative deficiency or the surgeon is concerned with the amount of normal gland removed at the time of surgery.

One should always be aware of the occasional hypothyroid patient who presents with pituitary hyperplasia, mimicking a tumor. This pituitary enlargement will resolve dramatically with thyroid replacement and surgery is ill advised.

The preoperative radiographic study of choice is the MRI scan. We recommend sagittal and coronal images through the sella with and without gadolinium enhancement. These images not only assist in visualizing the size, shape, and suprasellar symmetry of the lesion, but also give information on the displacement within the sella of the normal gland, unusual parasellar or intrasellar vascularity, and any cystic or necrotic areas within the lesion. The MRI will delineate the extent of invasion of the lesion into the cavernous and/or sphenoid sinuses. The symmetry of the lesion and the degree of its intrasellar extension is crucial in deciding whether it should be approached transsphenoidally or via a subfrontal craniotomy. It is our philosophy to approach all tumors that arise within the sella and extend symmetrically into the suprasellar region, transsphenoidally, irregardless of size. Unusually large tumors extending into the third ventricle, with occasional obstructive hydrocephalus can be very adequately treated through the transsphenoidal route, occasionally requiring multiple "staged" transsphenoidal intracapsular debulkings (Fig. 2).

Surgical Approach

The three primary goals of pituitary surgery are to establish a diagnosis, decompress surrounding structures, and achieve a gross total resection of the tumor where possible. In endocrine inactive macroadenomas all three goals are sought, whereas in the hypersecretory microadenoma, surgery is aimed primarily at achieving a gross total resection. How these goals can best be achieved determines our operative approach.

The two most common surgical approaches to tumors of the pituitary region are the transsphenoidal route and the subfrontal craniotomy. Approximately 95% of pituitary tumors are approached using the transsphenoidal route. In the macroadenoma, the transsphenoidal approach allows tumor to be removed from beneath the optic chiasm, putting the optic system at least risk. In the microadenoma, the transsphenoidal approach allows the best view of the entire sella, allowing the surgeon to carefully dissect around and often within the normal gland to identify the adenoma. The transsphenoidal approach is usually accomplished using a sublabial incision with a submucosal midline approach through the nose to the anterior wall of the sphenoid sinus (Fig. 3). This requires temporary deviation of the cartilagenous nasal septum to one side and resection of the bony nasal septum. Once the sphenoid sinus is reached, it is opened widely using the operating microscope and the floor of the sella is visualized. Intraoperative X-ray flouroscopy is used to obtain a lateral view of the sella and help guide the surgeon directly to the sellar floor. In large tumors, this bony floor is generally very thin and at times may be totally dehiscent. In microadenomas, it may still be thick, requiring the use of a high speed drill for removal. Once the floor of the sella is removed, the dura is widely opened and in the macroadenoma, tumor tissue is usually readily evident. The tumor is removed using blunt microcurets and suction, with the suprasellar extent of the tumor delivered into the sella by the use of increased intracranial pressure, pushing the tumor down from above. This may be accomplished by the anesthesiologist raising the pCO_2 to around 40 mmHg and/or performing intermittent valsalva maneuvers. Occasionally air or saline can be infused intrathecally to raise intracranial pressure, through a previosly placed lumbar spinal catheter. In the microadenoma, the tumor may be evident on the surface of the gland or require careful disection around and often within the normal gland. Once found, the microadenoma is removed along with a small rim of normal gland to ensure a total resection.

Contraindications for use of the transsphenoidal approach are tumors which have significant intracranial extension into the subfrontal or middle fossa regions (Fig. 4), or the rare tumor which displays a normal-sized sella with the bulk of the tumor extending suprasellar. In the latter instance, this is often seen as an hourglass constriction at the level of the diaphragma sella, which prevents adequate exposure of the suprasellar tumor from a transsphenoidal route. In these instances, the subfrontal craniotomy ap-

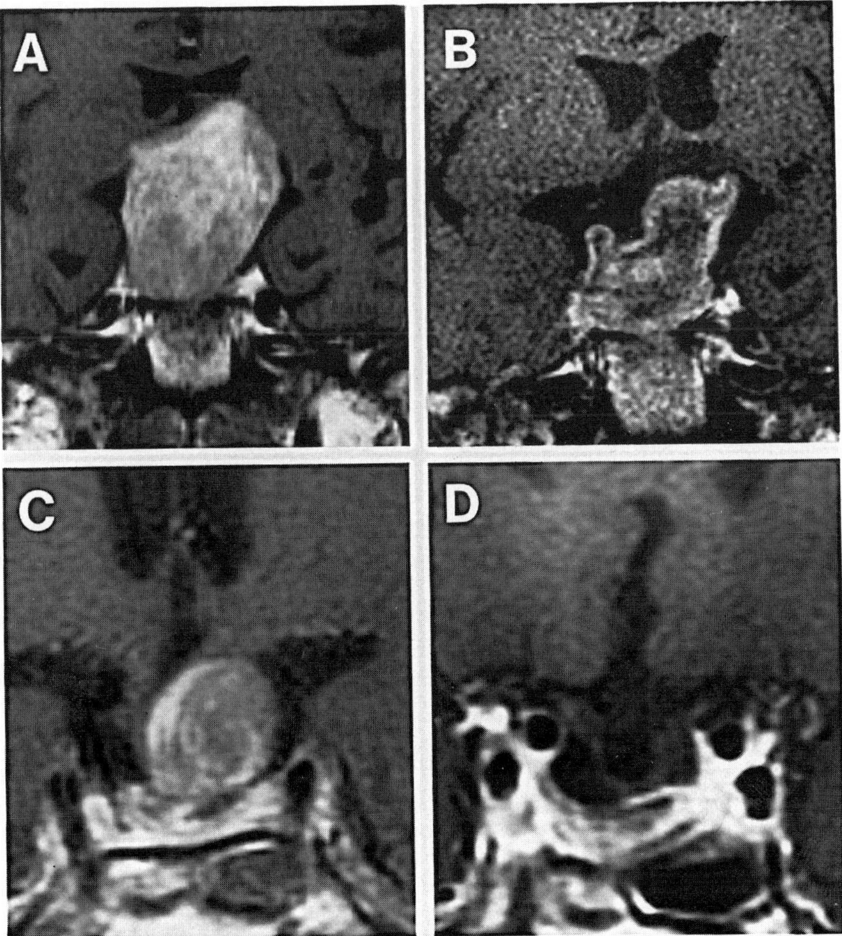

Fig. 2. Use of the staged transsphenoidal approach for removal of large pituitary adenomas. Shown is the preoperative, enhanced MRI scan **(A)**; the immediate postoperative, enhanced MRI scan **(B)**; a follow-up, enhanced MRI scan 6 mo later **(C)** (prior to the second transsphenoidal operation); and a final 3-mo postoperative, enhanced MRI scan following the second operation **(D)**. We recommend waiting at least 3 mo between surgeries to allow time for the tumor capsule to contract and gradually free itself from the surrounding brain.

proach is preferred. It is also the approach of preference in known meningiomas involving the sella and suprasellar region and most craniopharyngiomas (excepting those that are truly intrasellar with little suprasellar extension).

The three most common transcranial routes used for treatment of pituitary adenomas are the subfrontal approach, the pterional (or frontotemporal) approach and the subtemporal approach. The subfrontal craniotomy (Fig. 5) gives the most direct approach to the sella with good visualization of both optic nerves, bilateral internal carotid and anterior cerebral arteries, and the optic chiasm. Access to the third ventricle, if needed, may also be obtained through the lamina terminalis above the optic chiasm. If the chiasm however, is prefixed, visualization of the tumor through this route can be seriously limited and a more lateral approach may be preferable. The pterional approach is preferred in

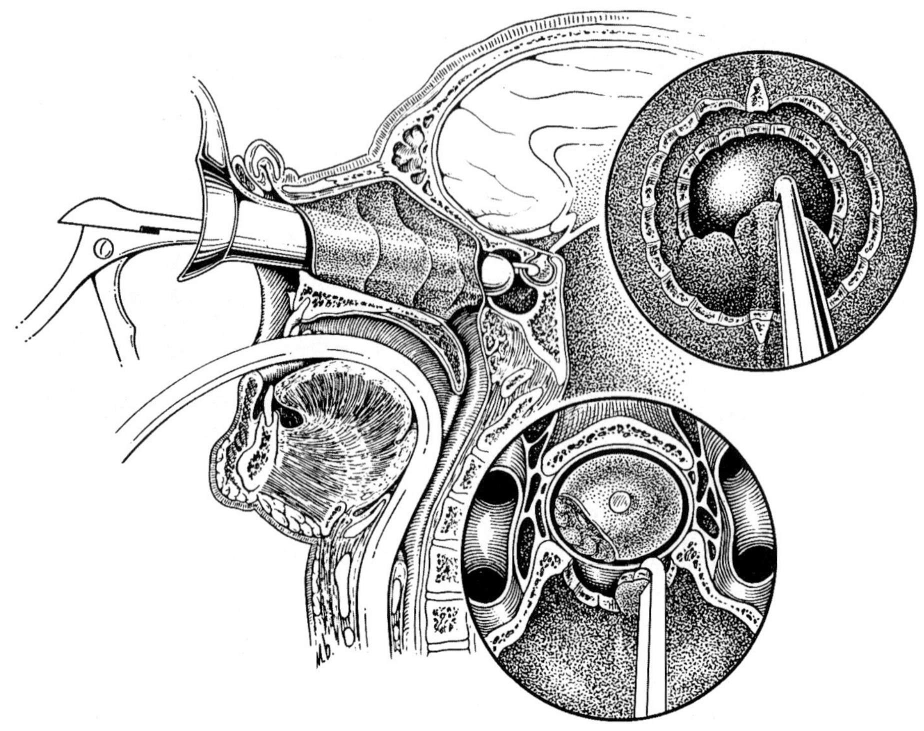

Fig. 3. The sublabial transsphenoidal approach. Shown is the speculum in place with exposure of the anterior dural surface of the pituitary gland. Visualization and illumination is provided by use of the operating microscope (not shown). Reproduced with permission from ref. *7a*.

this instance, allowing visualization of the suprasellar region through a space created between the optic nerve and tract superiorly and the internal carotid artery inferolaterally. Although allowing good decompression of the optic nerve and tract unilaterally, this approach does not give as good visualization of the sella nor the optic nerve and tract contralaterally. For the rare lesion that extends out of the sella and into the temporal lobe unilaterally, the subtemporal approach may be useful. It may also be useful in decompressing a tumor that has significant retrochiasmatic extension. This approach gives very poor visualization of the sella as well as limited exposure to the contralateral optic nerve and internal carotid artery.

Surgical Results

Endocrine-Inactive Adenomas

The term "endocrine-inactive" adenoma was coined by Charles Wilson *(11)* to describe those tumors that produce clinical effects as a direct consequence of their growth, without raising a clinical suspicion of endocrine activity. This term is preferable to "chromaphobe" adenoma in the current era of tumor immunohistochemistry, since almost all adenomas have some secretory ability but the hormones secreted are often inactive or cause no clinical symptoms. Endocrine-inactive adenomas include the true null-cell adenoma, the oncocytoma, the glycoprotein secreting adenomas (FSH, LH,

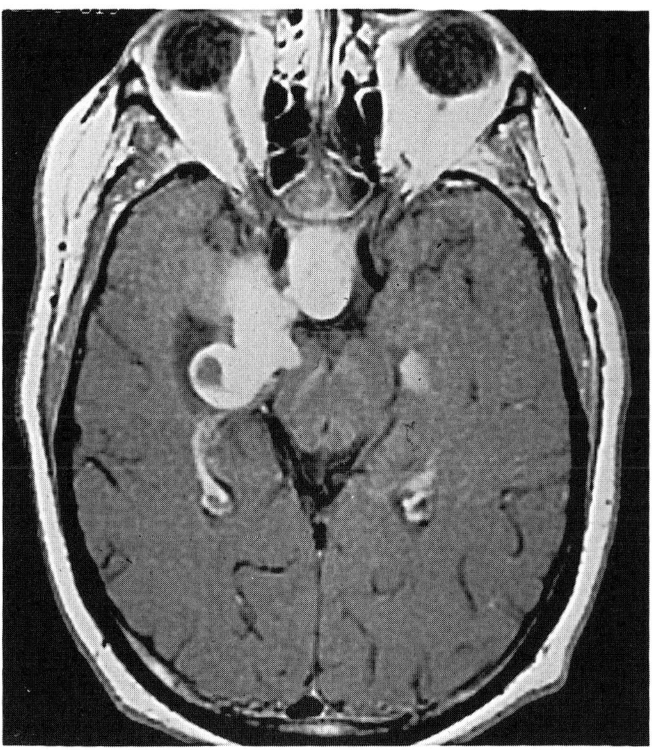

Fig. 4. An axial gadolinium-enhanced MRI scan through the suprasellar cistern, showing extension of adenoma into the medial temporal lobe. This patient presented with classic uncinate seizures consisting of olfactory hallucinations.

and α-subunit) and the occasional silent prolactin, GH, or ACTH secreting adenoma. These lesions are invariably > 1 cm at presentation and treatment is centered on establishing a diagnosis, decompressing surrounding structures (i.e., the optic chiasm and cranial nerves within the cavernous sinus), and an attempt at gross total resection. The first goal is usually easily accomplished, with immunohistochemical analysis revealing the majority of these lesions to be gonadotroph secreting adenomas (FSH, LH, and α-subunit). The second goal is also relatively easily accomplished with the vast majority of adenomas being soft in consistency and easily decompressed. Only rarely, (often following previous radiation therapy) will an adenoma be particularly fibrous, making decompression difficult. Success with decompression is evidenced by a 74–86% improvement in vision following transsphenoidal surgery *(11–13)*. Rarely do we see an improvement in endocrine function following surgery; however, the most frequent improvement seen is usually in the circulating serum testosterone levels in males. The third goal of total tumor resection is much more difficult to accomplish. In macroadenomas, it has been shown that 24% of tumors show evidence of gross invasiveness at surgery, with 88–94% of lesions showing evidence of microscopic dural invasion *(14)*. How this relates to actual tumor recurrence, however, is unclear. In an attempt to define the rate of tumor recurrence in patients with endocrine-inactive macroadenomas who underwent gross total tumor resection and did not recieve radiation therapy, we

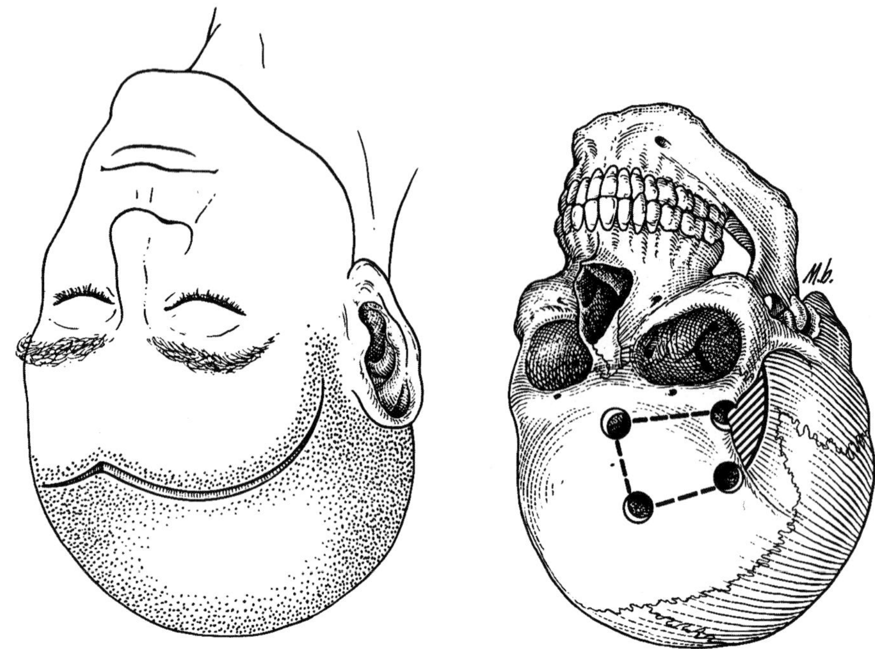

Fig. 5. Subfrontal craniotomy: The surgeon's view of the scalp incision and bone flap used for intracranial resection of parasellar lesions. Reproduced with permission from ref. *7a*.

followed a group of 32 patients treated at our institution for an average of 48.6 mo (4 yr). During this period of time, only two patients recurred (6.2%), both showing evidence of radiographic recurrence only and no recurrent clinical symptoms. Owing to the relatively low recurrence rate with generously resected macroadenomas, it has become the general trend among neurosurgeons, supported by the above data, to not give irradiation on initial presentation and to save this modality for evidence of recurrence. Obviously, this approach must be individualized to the patient. Radiation therapy should be strongly considered at first presentation in patients who are unreliable and unlikely to return for follow-up.

Cushing's Disease

The treatment of choice for pituitary-dependent hypercortisolism is transsphenoidal pituitary exploration. In 50–60% of the cases, the radiographic imaging will be normal requiring the surgeon to perform a careful and thorough exploration of the gland. If positive, the radiographic imaging will help in localizing the lesion within the gland, with inferior petrosal sinus sampling (IPSS) also being useful. In our hands, IPSS with CRF stimulation, has lateralized the adenoma correctly within the gland in only 60% of the cases, as opposed to the 71% accuracy previously reported *(15)*. At the time of surgery, if a tumor is not evident upon opening the dura and examining all surfaces of the gland, then incisions into the gland must be performed with an internal exploration carried out. ACTH microadenomas may occur anywhere in the pituitary, but 80–85% tend to be found in the lateral portions of the gland *(16,17)*. This becomes an important issue when, after exploring the gland, no tumor is readily visualized. It is our practice to then perform an approximately two-thirds resection of the gland, removing both lateral aspects of the gland (being more generous on the side of the IPSS lateralization), and the inferior portion of the gland. This leaves an area of residual gland surrounding the pituitary stalk and rarely results in hormonal dysfunction. Total hypophysectomy is also a possibility, but we generally reserve this option for the time of re-exploration if an initial cure has not been obtained.

In approximately 75% of patients explored, a microadenoma will be discovered *(16–20)*. When found, a cure can be expected in 88–96% of patients. Recurrence rates in this group tend to be approximately 5%. Macroadenomas are found in approximately 14% of patients with an initial remission rate of 61% *(21)*. At 5-yr follow-up, however, a 36% recurrence rate has been noted with these larger lesions *(21)*. In patients with macroadenomas, the use of postoperative radiation therapy can clearly improve the rate of recurrence, possibly avoiding the need for later adrenalectomy. When no adenoma is identified, as is the case in approximately 10–15% of patients explored *(20)*, and a partial or total hypophysectomy is performed, only approximately 60% of the patients will have a postoperative remission. In many of these patients, the origin of the ACTH hypersecretion remains in question and they should be followed closely for the appearance of a possible ectopic source later on.

Acromegaly

Like Cushing's disease, acromegaly is a life threatening condition. The number of deaths in patients with acromegaly are almost twice that expected from a general age-matched population *(22)*. In males, deaths tend to result from cardiovascular and respiratory disease; in women, it is from cerebrovascular and respiratory disease *(22)*. It is believed that treatment, with normalization of the GH and insulin-like growth factor I (IGF-I) levels favorably influences survival. Unfortunately, only 20–34% of GH secreting tumors are microadenomas, making surgical cure difficult. Surgery, however, remains the treatment of choice with the goal being to reduce symptoms associated with the tumor mass and to attain a biochemical cure. Cure is defined as a basal GH level < 5 ng/mL, normalization of IGF-I, and an oral glucose tolerance test (75–100 gm glucose) showing GH level supression to < 2 ng/mL. Using this strict criteria, the "cure" rate for transsphenoidal surgery is approximately 65–88% for microadenomas and 55–60% for macroadenomas *(23,24)*. Normalization of GH is more likely to result when a tumor is small, noninvasive, and the initial GH level is < 40 ng/mL *(24)*. Late recurrence rates vary from 4 to 14% *(23–25)*. It has been suggested that in large, invasive GH secreting adenomas, preoperative treatment with octreotide (a somatostatin analogue), 1–4 wk before surgery, helps soften the tumor, allowing better delineation of the adenoma from the surrounding normal gland *(26)* and results in an increased short-term cure rate *(27)*.

Radiation therapy has been shown to be a very useful adjunct in the treatment of acromegalic patients who have failed surgery. Unfortunately, it takes years for the GH level to respond. Eastman reported on 47 patients treated with conventional radiation therapy receiving between 4000–5000 cGy *(28)*. At 2 yr posttreatment, 17% had GH levels < 5 ng/mL. At 5 and 10 yr, the percentages were 42 and 69%, respectively. Associated with this, however, was a progressive risk of hypopituitarism with a 19% incidence of hypothyroidism, 38% risk of hypoadrenalism, and 58% incidence of hypogonadism in males and 50% in females at 10 yr. Therefore, radiation is a useful adjunct for the control of GH excess over time, but carries a significant risk of panhypopituitarism. In the interim, there is good rationale for use of bromocriptine or the somatostatin analogs to temporarily lower GH levels while awaiting the effects of radiation therapy. Bromocriptine has been shown to lower GH levels in 71% of patients, however, levels < 10 ng/mL were achieved in only 14% *(29)*. Octreotide in a recent randomized, multicenter trial was shown to lower growth hormone level to < 5 ng/mL in 53% of patients and bring IGF-1 levels to normal in 68% of patients receiving 100 μg sc three times a day *(30)*. Use of 250 μg sc three times a day proved to be of no greater biochemical benefit but did show an increased frequency of tumor shrinkage (19–37%).

PROLACTINOMAS

The treatment of the prolactin secreting pituitary adenoma has undergone a dramatic change in the past 20 yr. With the advent of bromocriptine and other dopamine agonists, a reasonably effective medical treatment for prolactinomas is now available. The availability of this medical alternative, along with surgery and radiation therapy, has resulted in a considerable controversy as to the most effective therapy for a particular lesion. Size of the adenoma is often a critical variable in deciding the effectiveness of each treatment modality and, therefore, macroadenomas and microadenomas will be discussed seperately.

Macroadenomas. Prolactin secreting pituitary macroadenomas often present with symptoms of mass effect (visual deterioration and headaches), only later to have the symptoms associated with hyperprolactinemia elucidated (amenorrhea, oligomenorrhea, galactorrhea, and impotence). Treatment is therefore aimed at decompression of the tumor and cure of the hyperprolactinemia. Surgery has been shown to be very effective in decompressing the visual system, improving vision in 80% of cases *(31)*. However, in tumors > 1 cm, or with serum prolactin levels > 200 ng/mL, surgery has been disappointing in its ability to normalize serum prolactin levels. Hardy *(32)* reporting on the surgical treatment of 355 patients with prolactinomas, was able to normalize only 29% of patients with PRL levels > 250 ng/mL, and only 34% of patients with tumors > 1 cm. Randall et al. *(31)* reporting on 100 patients, normalized prolactin level in only 28% of patients with macroadenomas. In the microadenomas, if the preoperative prolactin level was < 100 ng/mL, 88% were cured; however, if the prolactin level was > 100 ng/mL only 50% were cured.

Use of bromocriptine in the treatment of macroprolactinomas has been very successful. Prolactin levels have been shown to decrease in almost all patients, returning to normal in over 46% *(33)*. Tumor size decreases in over 90% of the tumors, often dramatically *(33)*. Patients presenting with visual deficits who are started on bromocriptine invariably start showing evidence of visual improvement within days of treatment, and it has been difficult to argue that surgery is superior to medical treatment in this instance. Unfortunately, bromocriptine is not tumoricidal and withdrawal of treatment will inevitably result in recurrent hyperprolactinemia and tumor enlargement, often quite rapidly. Long-term experience with the use of bromocriptine is now available and it does not appear to have significant adverse effects. It has not been shown to be teratogenic, and is being used more frequently throughout pregnancy in patients with macroadenomas. Pregnancy has clearly been shown to stimulate prolactinoma growth and in macroadenomas left untreated during pregnancy, 25% will enlarge.

Although radiation therapy has been shown to be effective in the treatment of macroprolactinomas *(34)*, its use is currently limited to invasive adenomas, which are unresponsive to dopamine agonist therapy. If a tumor is responsive to the dopamine agonists, we generally prefer to treat these lesions medically, avoiding the risk of radiation-induced hypopituitarism.

Based on the above information, our practice has been to initially treat all patients with macroadenomas with a trial of a dopamine agonist. In those patients unable or unwilling to tolerate the medicine or in the rare case where no radiographic or biochemical response is seen (the rare bromocriptine-resistent prolactinoma), we recommend surgical intervention. In this instance, surgery may offer a small possibility of cure and often will lower the prolactin level significantly. If prolactin levels remain above the normal range, the patient will once again require a dopamine agonist, usually at a lower dose, or need to consider radiation therapy. As stated, we rarely recommend the use of radiation therapy for prolactinomas, reserving its use for the invasive macroadenoma unresponsive to medical therapy.

Microadenomas. The surgical treatment of prolactin secreting microadenomas is more encouraging. Hardy reported a normalization of serum prolactin level in 77% of patients treated surgically *(32)*, Richards et al. *(35)* in 77%, Randall et al. *(31)* in 72%, and Landolt et al. *(36)* in 81%. Of interest, Landolt noted that in patients who had been on prolonged bromocriptine therapy prior to surgery, the success with surgical extirpation dropped to 33% *(36)*. He subsequently demonstrated that prolonged bromocriptine use resulted in significant intratumoral fibrosis, with the hypothesis being that the resultant firmer texture of the tumor made it more difficult to distinguish and therefore remove from the surrounding normal gland *(37)*. Use of medical therapy, therefore, although effective, may lessen the chance of a long-term surgical cure.

More recently, a substantial long-term hyperprolactinemia recurrence rate for surgically "cured" microadenomas has also been recognized. Charpentier et al. *(38)* reported a recurrence rate of 17%, Rodman et al. *(39)* a rate of 17%, and Serri et al. *(40)*, reporting on the long-term follow-up of Hardy's patients, a 50% recurrence rate after 4 yr. Of interest, in neither of the two latter studies was there evidence of radiographic tumor recurrence. With this recognition of high postoperative recurrence rates, pituitary surgeons are now tending to remove prolactin secreting lesions more aggressively, as has been done in the past with ACTH or GH secreting microadenomas, taking a small rim of surrounding normal appearing gland. This has led to improved initial cure rates in patients previously treated with bromocriptine (Landolt, personal communication) and inevitably will lead to a lower recurrence rate in patients treated solely with surgery. Another problem with proloactinomas has been deciding on what level of postoperative prolactin constitutes a cure. Merely to have prolactin in the normal range is probably not adequate. Postoperative serum prolactin levels in the high range of normal (> 10 ng/mL), along with a blunted response to thyrotropin releasing hormone (TRH), appear predictive of later recurrence. Stringent criteria for the assessment of cure in microprolactinomas, however, is lacking.

Do patients with hyperprolactinemia and an associated microadenoma necessarily need treatment? A limited study of the natural history of untreated microprolactinomas showed that over a period of 6 yr 80% showed no significant change in prolactin level or tumor size, with 10% showing an increase in size, requiring surgical intervention and an additional 10% showing spontaneous normalization of the prolactin level *(41)*. This would argue in favor of a very conservative approach to the treatment of prolactinomas. However, untreated hyperprolactinemia has since been shown to lead to progressive osteoporosis which in most cases is only partially reversible with treatment *(42,43)*. Our practice, at present, is to recommend treatment in all patients with hyperprolactinemia, beginning with a thorough discussion of the risks and benefits of surgery vs use of a dopamine agonist. In most instances, we begin with a trial of medical management. Surgery has generally been reserved for those patients who initially are unwilling to consider the possibility of prolonged medical management or those patients who after a trial of dopamine agonists, are unwilling or unable to continue medical management. These patients, being well informed, are then willing to accept the risk of surgery in exchange for the potential of a long-term cure.

REFERENCES

1. Caton R, Paul FT. Notes of a case of acromegaly treated by operation. Br Med J 1893; 2:1421–1423.
2. Weiss MHA. Surgery of the pituitary gland. Bull Los Angeles Neurol Soc. 1977; 42:190–200.
3. Cushing H. Surgical experiences with pituitary disorders. JAMA 1914; 63:1515–1525.
4. Nager FR. The paranasal approach to intrasellar tumors. J Laryngol Otol 1940; 55:361–381.
5. Cope UZ. The pituitary fossa and the methods of surgical approach thereto. Br J Surg 1916; 4:107–144.
6. Schloffer H. Erfolgreiche operation eines hypophysentumors auf nasalem wege. Wein Klin Wochenschr 1907; 20:621.
7. Henderson WR. The pituitary adenomata. A followup study of the surgical results in 338 cases (Dr. Harvey Cushing's series). Br J Surg 1939; 26: 1930; 811–921.

7a. Tindall GT, Barrow DL. Pituitary surgery, in Disorders of the pituitary. CV Mosby, St. Louis, 1986; 366, 379.

8. Abboud CF, Laws EF. Clinical endocrinologic approach to hypothalamic-pituitary disease. In: Laws ER, Randall RV, Kern EB, Abboud CF, eds. Management of Pituitary Adenomas and Related Lesions with Emphasis on Transsphenoidal Microsurgery. Appleton-Century-Crofts, New York, 1982, pp. 33–63.
9. Kleinschmidt-DeMasters BK, Lillehei KO, Stears JC. The pathologic, surgical and MR spectrum of Rathke's cleft cysts. Surg Neurol 1995; 44:19–27.
10. Reusch JEB, Kleinschmidt-DeMasters BK, Lillehei KO, Ruppe D, Gutierrez-Hartmann A. Pre-operative diagnosis of lymphocytic hypophysitis (Adenohypophysis) unresponsive to short course dexamethasone - Case report. Neurosurgery 1992; 30: 268–272.
11. Wilson CB. Endorine-inactive pituitary adenomas. In: Selman W, ed. Clinical Neurosurgery, vol 38. Williams and Wilkins, Baltimore, MD 1992, pp. 10–31.
12. Cohen AR, Cooper PR, Kupersmith MJ, Flamm ES, Ransohoff J. Visual recovery after transsphenoidal removal of pituitary adenomas. Neurosurg 1985; 17:446–452.
13. Ebersold MJ, Quast LM, Laws ER, Scheithauer B, Randall RV. Long-term results in transsphenoidal removal of nonfunctioning pituitary adenomas. J Neurosurg 1986; 64:713–719.
14. Selman WR, Laws ER, Scheithauer B, Carpenter SM. The occurrence of dural invasion in pituitary adenomas. J Neurosurg 1986; 64:402–407.
15. Oldfield EH, Doppman JL, Nieman LK, Chrousos GP, Miller DL, Katz DA, Cutler GB, Loriaux DL. Petrosal sinus sampling with and without corticotropin-releasing hormone for the differential diagnosis of Cushing's syndrome. N Engl J Med 1991; 325:897–905.
16. Boggan JE, Tyrrell JB, Wilson CB. Transsphenoidal microsurgical management of Cushing's disease. J Neurosurg 1983; 59:195–200.
17. Kuwayama A, Kageyama N. Current management of Cushing's disease - Part II. Contemp Neurosurg 1985; 7(3):1–6.
18. Hardy J: Cushing's disease. 50 years later. Can J Neurol Sci 1982; 9:375–380.

19. Salassa RM, Laws ER, Carpenter PC, Northcutt RC. Cushing's disease - 50 years later. Am Clin Climatol Assoc (Trans) 1982; 94:122–129.
20. Chandler WF, Schteingart DE, Lloyd RV, McKeever PE. Surgical treatment of Cushing's disease. J Neurosurg 1987; 66:204–212.
21. Zervas NT. Surgical results for pituitary adenomas: Results of an international survey. In: Black PM, Zervas NT, Ridgway EC, Martin JB, eds. Secretory Tumors of the Pituitary Gland. Raven, New York, 1984, pp. 377–385.
22. Wright AD, Hill DM, Lowy C, Fraser TR. Mortality in acromegaly. Q J Med 1970; 39:1.
23. Serri O, Somma M, Comtois R, Rasio E, Beauregard H, Jilwan N, Hardy J. Acromegaly: Biochemical assessment of cure after long term follow-up of transsphenoidal selective adenomectomy. J Clin Endocrinol Metab 1985; 61:1185–1189.
24. Laws ER. Neurosurgical management of acromegaly. In: Cooper PR, ed. Contemporary diagnosis and management of pituitary adenomas. Park Ridge, American Association of Neurological Surgeons, 1991, pp. 53–59.
25. Ross DA, Wilson CB. Results of transsphenoidal microsurgery for growth hormone-secreting pituitary adenoma in a series of 214 patients. J Neurosurg 1988; 68:854–867.
26. Spinas GA, Zapf J, Landolt AM. Pre-operative treatment of 5 acromegalics with a somatostatin analogue: endocrine and clinical observations. Acta Endocrinol (Copenh) 1987; 114:249–256.
27. Barkan AL, Lloyd RV, Chandler WF, Hatfield MK, Gebarski SS, Kelch RP, Beitins IZ. Pre-operative treatment of acromegaly with long-acting somatostatin analogue SMS 201-995: shrinkage of invasive pituitary macroadenomas and improved surgical remission rate. J Clin Endocrin Metab 1988; 67: 1040–1048.
28. Eastman RC, Gorden P, Roth J. Conventional supervoltage irradiation is an effective treatment for acromegaly. J Clin Endocrinol Metab 1979; 48:931–940.
29. Besser GM, Wass JAH. The medical management of acromegaly. In: Black PM, Zervas NT, Ridgway EC, Martin JB, eds. Secretory tumors of the pituitary gland. Raven, New York, 1984, pp. 155–168.
30. Ezzat S, Snyder PJ, Young WF, Boyajy LD, Newman C, Klibanski A, Molitch ME, Boyd AE, Sheeler L, Cook DM, Malarkey WB, Jackson I, Vance ML, Thorner MO, Barkan A, Frohman LA, Melmed S. Octreotide treatment of acromegaly: a randomized, multicenter study. Ann Intern Med 1992; 117:711–718.
31. Randall RV, Laws ER, Abboud CF, Ebersold MJ, Kao PC, Scheithauer BW. Transsphenoidal microsurgical treatment of prolactin-producing pituitary adenomas. Mayo Clin Proc 1983; 58:108–121.
32. Hardy J. Transsphenoidal microsurgery of prolactinomas. In: Black PM, Zervas NT, Ridgway EC, Martin JB, eds. Secretory tumors of the pituitary gland. Raven, New York, 1984, pp. 73–81.
33. Thorner MO, Evans WS, Vance ML. Medical management of prolactinomas: I. In: Black PM, Zervas NT, Ridgway EC, Martin JB, eds. Secretory tumors of the pituitary gland. Raven, New York, 1984, pp. 53–64.
34. Sheline GE, Grossman A, Jones AE, Besser GM. Radiation therapy for prolactinomas. In: Black PM, Zervas NT, Ridgway EC, Martin JB, eds. Secretory tumors of the pituitary gland. Raven, New York, 1984, pp. 93–108.
35. Richards AM, Bullock MRR, Teasdale GM, Thomson JA, Khan MI. Fertility and pregnancy after operation for a prolactinoma. Br J Obstet Gynecol 1986; 93:495–502.
36. Landolt AM, Keller PJ, Froesch ER, Mueller J. Bromocriptine: does it jeopardize the result of later surgery for prolactinomas? Lancet 1982; 1:657,658.
37. Landolt AM, Osterwalder V. Perivascular fibrosis in prolactinomas: is it increased by bromocryptine? J Clin Endocrinol Metab 1984; 58:1179–1183.
38. Charpentier G, dePlunkett T, Jedynak P, Peillon F, LeGentil P, Racadot J, Visot A, Derome P. Surgical treatment of prolactinomas. Short- and long-term results, prognostic factors. Horm Res 1985; 22:222–227.
39. Rodman EF, Molitch ME, Post KD, Biller BJ, Reichlin S. Long-term follow-up of transsphenoidal selective adenectomy for prolactinoma. JAMA 1984; 252:921–924.
40. Serri O, Rasio E, Beauregard H, Hardy J, Somma M. Recurrence of hyperprolactinemia after selective transsphenoidal adenomectomy in women with prolactinoma. N Engl J Med 1983; 309:280–283.
41. Weiss MH, Teal J, Gott P, Wycoff R, Yadley R, Apuzzo MLJ, Giannotta SL, Kletzky O, March C. Natural history of microprolactinomas: six-year follow-up. Neurosurgery 1983; 12:180–183.
42. Klibanski A, Greenspan SL. Increase in bone mass after treatment of hyperprolactinemic amenorrhea. N Engl J Med 1986; 315:542–546.
43. Klibanski A, Biller BMK, Rosenthal DI. Effects of prolactin and estrogen deficiency in amenorrheic bone loss. J Clin Endocrin Metab 1988; 67:124–130.

19 Immunohistochemistry of Pituitary Adenomas

B.K. Kleinschmidt-DeMasters, MD

CONTENTS

INTRODUCTION

The use of immunohistochemical staining has had a considerable impact on general surgical pathology, where it serves to clarify the diagnosis on confusing cases. In contrast, immunohistochemistry for pituitary adenomas is seldom necessary to make the diagnosis but has, along with transmission electron microscopy, served as the backbone for a modern classification system of adenoma subtypes. The surety with which most pituitary adenomas are diagnosed preoperatively via their clinical presentations, serum hormone values, and/or radio-graphic studies of the sellar region (usually magnetic resonance imaging) often make the role of the pathologist or neuropathologist who sees pituitary adenomas under the microscope one of confirmation *(1)*. Only occasionally do other sellar masses mimic pituitary adenomas preoperatively, and then the light microscopic appearance, either at the time of frozen or permanent histological section, is usually all that is necessary to identify the type of tumor. Rarely is it necessary to employ immunohistochemistry for the differential diagnosis of sellar region masses.

Most large pathology laboratories keep in stock the antibodies to all the common anterior pituitary hormones (growth hormone [GH], prolactin [PRL], adrenocorticotropic

From: *Contemporary Endocrinology, Vol. 3: Diseases of the Pituitary: Diagnosis and Treatment*
Edited by M. E. Wierman Humana Press Inc., Totowa, NJ

hormone [ACTH] and the β-subunits to follicle-stimulating hormone [FSH], luteinizing hormone [LH], thyroid-stimulating hormone [TSH], and the α-subunit [ASU] common to FSH, LH, and TSH). These are routinely applied to all pituitary adenoma specimens and along with transmission electron microscopy, serve to subclassify adenomas into approximately 13 categories. Despite this classification system, subtyping of adenomas has as yet been incompletely correlated with biological behavior of the tumors *(2)*. The presence or absence of specific hormone production by the adenoma corresponds minimally with microscopic dural invasion, macroscopic invasion of the sphenoid sinus or cavernous sinus, or metastasis in the rare pituitary carcinoma. With the possible exception of the sparsely granulated growth hormone cell adenoma, the uncommon acidophil stem cell adenoma, and the corticotroph cell adenomas in Nelson's syndrome, which have more aggressive biological behavior *(3)*, classification of pituitary adenomas into subtypes does not predict growth rate. Since adenoma subtype cannot be determined at the time of frozen section, subtyping has no influence on intraoperative management, which for any adenoma is as complete a surgical resection as possible, usually via the transphenoidal approach. The choice of postoperative external beam radiotherapy is largely dictated by quantity of residual adenoma or recurrence, and less by adenoma subtype. Although radiotherapy has a clearly established success in controlling acromegaly, its role in other hormone producing subtypes of pituitary adenomas still is debated *(4)*. The major impact of adenoma subtyping on patient management has been in the use of chemical agonists or antagonists such as bromocriptine (2-bromo-α-ergocryptine) for prolactin secreting pituitary adenomas, somatostatin analogs (octreotide) for growth hormone secreting adenomas, or octreotide for ACTH producing adenomas.

This chapter will begin with an overview of the principles of immunohistochemistry; the technical details have been reviewed elsewhere and will only be dealt with briefly *(5,6)*. The next two sections will deal with the use of immunohistochemistry in the differential diagnosis of sellar lesions or in small confusing specimens, and the section after that will deal with how immunohistochemistry characterizes subtypes of adenomas and why immunohistochemical staining does not correlate perfectly with serum hormone levels or clinical symptomology. The last brief section will talk about immunohistochemical detection of various oncoproteins or growth factors in pituitary adenomas.

OVERVIEW OF PRINCIPLES AND VARIABLES OF IMMUNOHISTOCHEMISTRY

Immunohistochemistry (IHC) is a staining technique by which various tissue antigens can be identified through the use of antibodies tagged to enzymes that can produce a colored precipitate at the site of antibody localization. Antibodies to the desired human antigen are raised in heterologous species, usually mouse or rabbit, and are linked to an enzyme through any of a number of linker molecules. The enzyme reacts with a colorless substrate (chromogen) to produce a colored precipitate, localizing the desired antigen to cells or other tissue structures. Most commonly utilized are either the peroxidase method or the alkaline phosphatase methods. The use of the chromogen 3 diaminobenzidine tetrahydrochloride (DAB) produces a brown colored precipitate, whereas 3 amino-9-

ethylcarbyzol (AEC) forms a rose-red end product. Hence, the color seen in tissue is dependent on which chromogen is chosen, not on the specificity of the antibody.

Several different staining methods can be employed. The original direct method linked the enzyme directly to the primary antibody. Whereas the direct method limited nonspecific reactions, signal amplification was relatively low and the direct method is now seldom utilized *(5)*. In contrast, two- and three-step indirect methods are now employed in which multiple layers of antibodies (either secondary or tertiary antibodies) are linked with the enzyme/chromogen and react directly to the primary antibody. The secondary and tertiary antigens have to be raised in a third species, usually goat (or swine), and multiple-labeled antibodies react with the mouse or rabbit primary immunoglobulin raised against the human antigen. The advantages of the indirect method are that it increases staining intensity and that it does not require the enzyme to be covalently linked to one specific primary antibody. How the antibody enzyme complex is formed can also be varied and the two most commonly used linkers are the peroxidase-antiperoxidase technique or the avidin–biotin method.

A variety of other parameters can be manipulated in IHC in addition to which enzyme linker or chromogen are used. These can lead to some differences in staining from laboratory to laboratory, but the differences are generally quantitative rather than qualitative. These variables include which dilutions of antibody are used, the temperature at which the reaction is conducted, and whether or not enzyme digestion of tissue (such as with pronase) to enhance antigen exposure is employed. The advancements in unmasking antigens, especially antigen retrieval in paraffin-embedded tissues via microwaving, have in fact made formalin-fixed tissues almost as useful as frozen tissues *(6)*. The original IHC techniques were developed for frozen tissues and used an immunofluorescent rather than immunoenzymatic reaction. However, immunofluorescent techniques necessitated that tissue be frozen at the time of tissue procurement. Most of the antibodies now utilized have been selected because of their adequate staining on paraffin-embedded, formalin-fixed tissues. The ability to use standardly processed tissues not only facilitates retrospective studies on archival material but also increases the ability of large laboratories to study outside referral specimens. Many smaller hospitals choose not to keep all the antibodies to pituitary hormones in stock in their laboratory and use reference laboratories for immunohistochemical typing of their pituitary adenomas.

A most important variable in IHC, however, is the source and specificity of the antibody. Whereas antibodies to the common anterior pituitary hormones are available commercially, some laboratories prefer noncommercial sources and feel such antibodies have superior specificity. Either monoclonal or polyclonal antibodies are available for most of the standard anterior pituitary hormones (GH, PRL, FSH, LH, TSH, ACTH, and ASU). Monoclonal antibodies are raised in mouse by injecting antigen, harvesting B-cell lymphocytes from the mouse spleen, fusing the lymphocytes with myeloma cells, and creating hybrid cells (hybridomas). These hybridoma cells can then be propagated in mice or in tissue culture and either ascitic or supernatant fluid, respectively, can be harvested to achieve high titers of MAb. These MAbs produced by clones of plasma cells have the advantage of homogeneity, absence of nonspecific contaminating antibodies, and no batch-to-batch variability. However, the pitfalls include the fact that the targeted antigenic epitope may not survive normal formalin fixation and that the targeted epitope, if small, may be shared by other unrelated antigens *(5)*. Hence, crossreactivity is a problem with MAbs. In contrast, polyclonal antibodies are produced by multiple different cells and react with a large variety of epitopes on the single antigen to which they are raised. The chance for nonspecific staining is higher with polyclonal rather than MAbs, but can be dealt with by absorption techniques.

Immunohistochemistry then is a technique that allows detection of small amounts of antigen through the use of antigen–antibody reactions, often in routinely processed formalin-fixed, paraffin-embedded tissues. Modifying the method, chromogen, fixation of tissues, or source and type of antibody can lead to some interlaboratory variation that is usually quantitative rather than qualitative.

USE OF GENERAL IMMUNOHISTOCHEMICAL MARKERS IN THE DIFFERENTIAL DIAGNOSIS OF SELLAR REGION MASSES

The diagnosis of pituitary adenoma is generally strongly suspected preoperatively by the endocrinologist or surgeon and straightforward for the pathologist at the time of intraoperative consultation whether he or she uses touch preparations or frozen section *(1)*. Difficulties in interpretation arise more in distinguishing normal, nonadenomatous anterior pituitary gland from adenoma than with the distinction between adenoma and other sellar neoplasms *(2)*. Only occasionally is another sellar region mass such as a meningioma, germinoma, or craniopharyngioma mistaken preoperatively for a pituitary adenoma. Histologically these tumors are sufficiently distinctive at the light microscopic level to the pathologist that immunohistochemistry is seldom needed. A table outlining the use of several different immunohistochemical stains in pituitary adenomas vs other sellar masses has recently been published and will only be summarized here *(2)*. Pituitary adenomas are positive for antibodies directed against cytokeratins, chromogranin, neuron-specific enolase, and synaptophysin. Low and intermediate molecular weight cytokeratins are present in GH, PRL, and ACTH cells *(8)* and their adenomas. Antibodies to chromogranin may be directed against several of the A, B, and C glycoproteins or specifically to one of the components *(7)*. Chromogranin A is found in null-cell adenomas and those that produce TSH or FSH/LH. Chromogranin B can be found in PRL, gonadotroph, and null-cell adenomas. Synaptophysin is a membrane protein present in neuronal synaptic vesicles and is found in many endocrine cells and, hence, can be demonstrated in all types of normal anterior pituitary cells and most pituitary adenomas *(7)*. NSE has limited value owing to its lack of specificity since it can be present in many nonneuroendocrine tumors *(8)*. The S100 protein is a marker for folliculostellate cells in the normal anterior pituitary gland; scattered S100-positive cells can be seen in many types of pituitary adenomas, especially gonadotrophic adenomas, but the adenoma cells themselves are usually not strongly S100-positive *(2)*. Other epithelial differentiation markers such as epithelial membrane antigen (EMA) or carcinoembryonic antigen (CEA) are negative in adenomas; negative immunostaining for vimentin, GFAP, and neurofilaments is also found.

The differential diagnosis between pituitary adenoma and other sellar region masses is usually raised only when pituitary adenomas display an unusual histological pattern. Histologic variations are particularly difficult to recognize for pathologists who see relatively few pituitary adenoma specimens. The common microscopic pattern for a pituitary adenoma is a sheet-like monotonous epithelial neoplasm punctuated by small

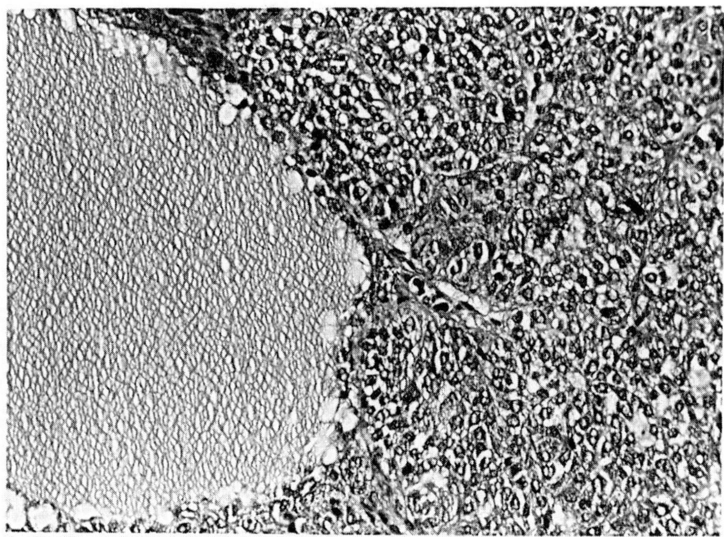

Fig. 1. Low photomicrograph of a chromophobic pituitary adenoma illustrates the sheet-like monotony of many adenomas, interrupted only by the delicate vasculature and occasional colloid containing microcysts (at left). (H&E, original magnification × 400.)

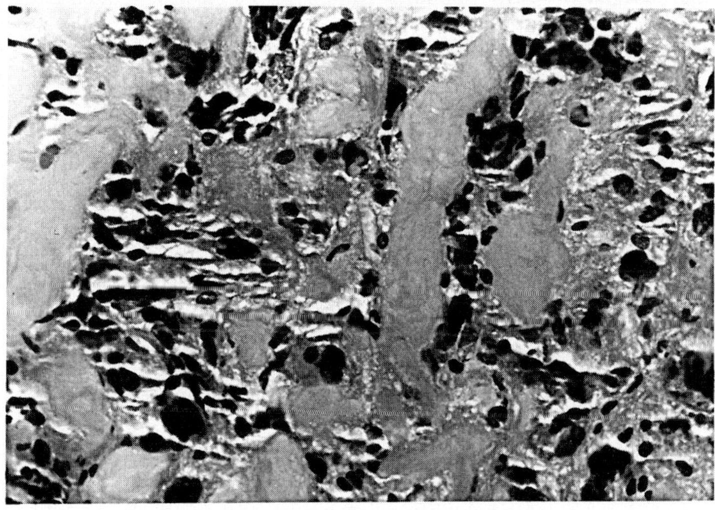

Fig. 2. Dense fibrosis obscures the cells population in this adenoma, which immunostaining confirmed as a prolactinoma. Although this patient was not treated with bromocriptine, such therapy can also result in fibrosis. (H&E, original magnification × 350).

blood vessels and occasional microcysts (Fig. 1). The adenoma usually lacks necrosis (except in cases of apoplexy) or high mitotic activity. The calcification, squamous or adamantinomatous epithelium, or cholesterol formation common to craniopharyngioma are seldom seen. If unusual features such as dense fibrosis (Fig. 2) or pleomorphism (Fig. 3A) are present in adenomas, immunohistochemistry can clarify the diagnosis (Fig. 3B). When adenoma cells are arranged in perivascular rosettes, a pitu-

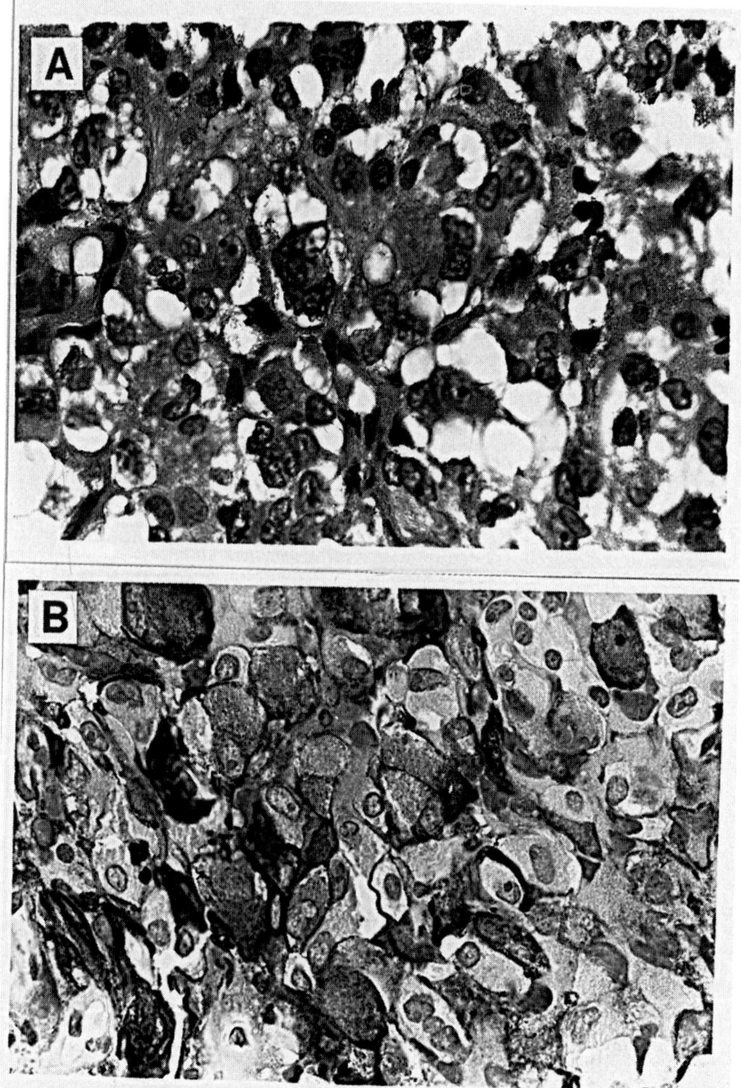

Fig. 3. **(A)** Pleomorphism in an adenoma can raise concerns by the pathologist about a metastatic carcinoma, as it did in this intrasellar mass from a 73-yr-old woman with known breast carcinoma. (H&E, original magnification × 525.) **(B)** The tumor was immunoreactive for alpha-subunit, as illustrated in this photomicrograph, as well as for LH, FSH, and very focally prolactin and TSH, identifying this tumor as a plurihormonal pituitary adenoma. Peroxidase-antiperoxidase technique for alpha subunit. (original magnification × 60.)

itary adenoma may vaguely simulate an ependymoma (Fig. 4). Diffuse S100 immunoreactivity and GFAP positivity in the ependymoma vs only scattered S100-positive cells and GFAP negativity in the pituitary adenoma would serve as distinguishing features. Usually, however, the radiographic demonstration of a tumor confined to the sella virtually excludes ependymoma or other glial neoplasms from practical consideration *(2)*.

Pituitary adenomas would only rarely be mistaken for a bland, poorly whorled meningothelial meningioma, but diffuse immunoreactivity for cytokeratins and

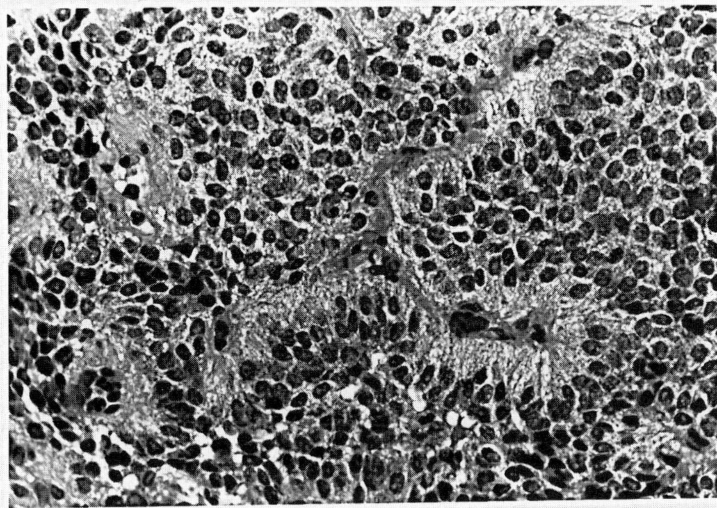

Fig. 4. Like other endocrine tumors, pituitary adenomas may show orientation of cells around the abundant blood vessels, vaguely simulating perivascular pseudorosettes; immunohistochemical staining would clarify this as a pituitary adenoma rather than an ependymoma. (H&E, original magnification × 350.)

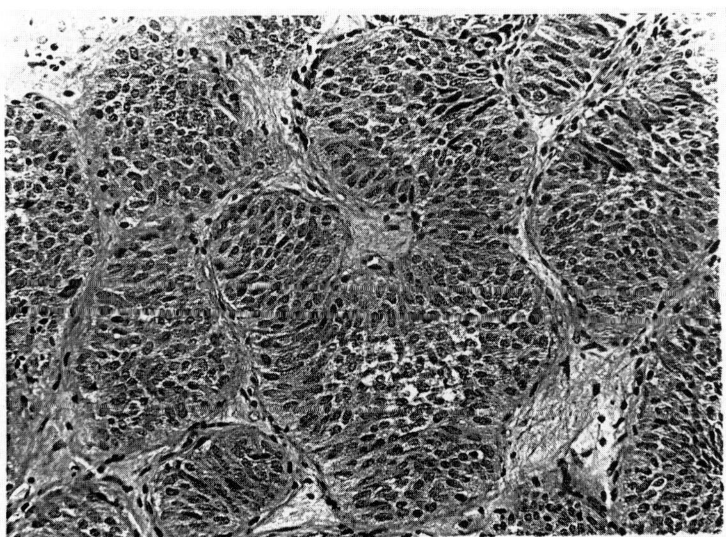

Fig. 5. The nested pattern in pituitary adenomas such as this one can simulate the appearance of neuroendocrine tumors, but immunohistochemical staining can clarify diagnosis. (H&E, original magnification × 175.)

negativity for EMA in an adenoma would contrast it with a meningioma. In adenomas that display a festooned or nested pattern, an olfactory neuroblastoma may come to mind, but negative immunoreactivity for neurofilaments in adenomas and positive immunoreactivity in olfactory neuroblastomas would be helpful (Fig. 5). In some cases, the pathologist may also mistake a festooned or pleomorphic pituitary adenoma for metastatic carcinoma. Although metastases involve the sellar region infrequently, either extension from skull base bony metastases into the sella or hematogenous metastases to the pituitary gland itself are occasionally seen *(9)*. Whereas immunostaining for cytokeratins would not distinguish between pituitary adenoma and most metastatic carcinomas, positivity for EMA or CEA would suggest metastatic carcinoma and immunoreactivity for chromogranin or synatophysin would indicate pituitary adenoma. Only in the rare condition of lymphocytic hypophysitis where an anterior pituitary gland is overrun by nonneoplastic lymphocytes and plasma cells might a consideration of germinoma, a lymphocytic-rich germ-cell tumor, be entertained. Germ-cell tumors would be negative for all of the markers seen in pituitary adenomas (except possibly focal cytokeratin positivity), and would be positive for placental alkaline phosphatase and/or β human chorionic gonadotrophin and α-fetoprotein *(2)*.

The distinction then between pituitary adenoma and other sellar region masses can be definitively made by immunohistochemistry, but it seldom needs to be employed.

IMMUNOHISTOCHEMISTRY FOR ANTERIOR PITUITARY HORMONES IN DOCUMENTING THE DIAGNOSIS OF PITUITARY ADENOMA IN SMALL OR CONFUSING SPECIMENS

The most common problem confronting a pathologist, as noted, is not the differential between pituitary adenoma and other sellar region masses, but rather between normal anterior pituitary gland and adenoma *(2)*. The mainstay of differential diagnosis for adenoma vs normal as well as for normal vs hyperplasia is the routine, nonimmunohistochemical reticulin stain. The normal anterior pituitary gland shows a nested or acinar appearance via this stain (Fig. 6A–C), whereas acini are disrupted or expanded in hyperplasia and usually lost entirely in the pituitary adenoma. IHC is only supplemental in the issues of normal anterior gland vs adenoma or normal anterior gland vs hyperplasia, but if utilized shows an assortment of anterior pituitary cell types in normal gland vs a relative monotony of IHC staining in many adenomas. A disclaimer to this, however, is the fact that the various hormone-producing cells are not equal in number nor are they regularly distributed throughout the normal anterior pituitary gland and concentrate by cell type either in the lateral wings or midline "mucoid wedge." GH-producing cells (50% of anterior pituitary cells) and PRL-producing cells (10–30%) are localized to the lateral wings. ACTH-producing cells (10–30% of normal anterior pituitary cells) and TSH-producing cells (5%) predominate in the mucoid wedge. FSH/LH-producing cells (a single cell type with dual hormonal production) (10%) are diffusely distributed throughout the anterior

Fig. 6. Although not an immunohistochemical stain, a reticulin stain is essential in the pathological work-up of pituitary adenomas. The normal acinar pattern of nonadenomatous anterior pituitary gland is seen in the upper left, whereas the acini are disrupted in the pituitary microadenoma at lower right. In the center of a macroadenoma as shown in **(B)**, there is virtually complete loss of reticulin except around vessels. Some adenomas such as in **(C)** may show reticulin staining with a somewhat nested pattern but it clearly differs from the reticulin pattern seen in the normal anterior pituitary gland. Gomori's reticulin stain. (original magnifications—A: × 175; B: × 90; C: × 175.)

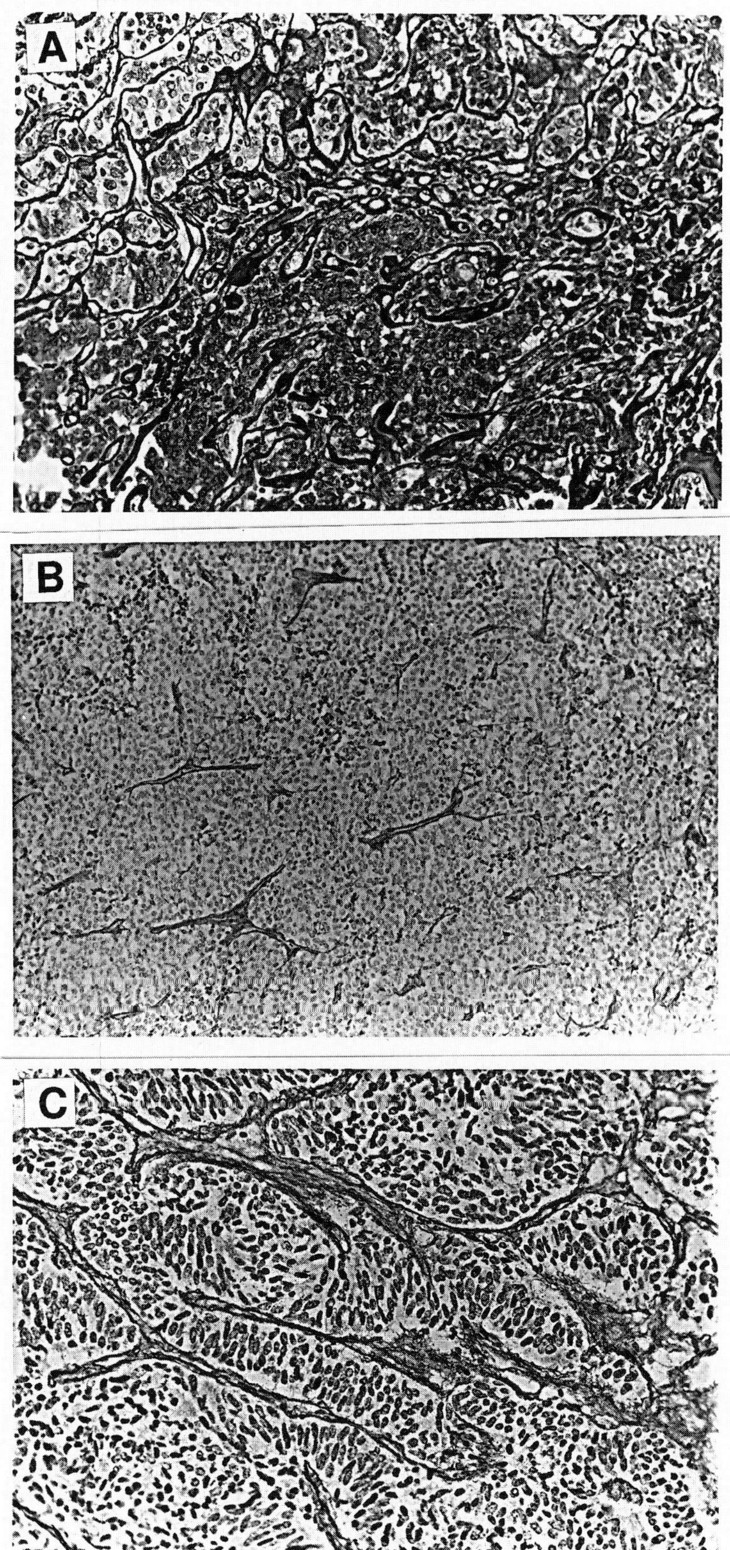
A
B
C

gland *(2)*. Hence, for example, if the pathologist attempts to use immunohistochemistry without reticulin staining on a small biopsy taken from the lateral wing, even in the normal gland a large number of GH and PRL staining cells will be seen and could be mistaken for a mixed GH-PRL adenoma. IHC can also be confusing if used at the midline junction between anterior and posterior pituitary glands. With advancing age, increasing numbers of basophils normally encroach in this area on the posterior pituitary gland ("basophil invasion"). If a small pituitary biopsy is taken from this site and immunohistochemistry is utilized without recognition of the posterior lobe location, the biopsy will be monotonously immunoreactive for ACTH and could erroneously suggest an ACTH adenoma.

Immunohistochemical staining can also be confusing at the edge of pituitary adenomas. Whereas most macroadenomas form sharply delineated pushing edges as they compress normal pituitary gland and surrounding structures, some microadenomas will encompass normal anterior pituitary cells at their growing edge. Such entrapped normal anterior pituitary cells within a microadenoma will stain for their respective hormones. At times it can be difficult to tell if these individual cells are normal cells engulfed by adenoma or represent a small alternately staining subpopulation with a plurihormonal tumor. Confinement of a few alternately staining cells to the edge of a couple of tissue fragments often suggests that they are entrapped cells rather than part of the adenoma.

IHC results then need to be interpreted in conjunction with the routine H&E and reticulin stains and with caution in regard to anatomic site and at the edges of microadenomas.

IHC for anterior pituitary hormones can be of help in identifying small or confusing collections of possible pituitary adenoma cells. The cells appear small and dark and cytoplasmic detail is often obscured when neoplastic or nonneoplastic anterior pituitary cells undergo crush artifact from compression *(2)*, or when small numbers of adenoma cells invade dura. Small, dark cells with cytoplasmic shrinkage can also be seen in pituitary adenomas following treatment of prolactinomas with the dopamine agonist bromocriptine. In each case, these small dark cells with virtually "naked nuclei" and a high nuclear-to-cytoplasmic ratio can simulate small-cell carcinoma or lymphocytes for the unwary pathologist. Whereas immunohistochemical staining is also generally reduced in these cells, some cytoplasmic staining may remain and can be a corroboration of the identity of these cells.

Another situation in which IHC for anterior pituitary hormones is helpful is one in which adenomas extend to, and/or present in, the sphenoid sinus or other parasellar sites (Fig. 7) or primarily arise in ectopic locations. Ectopic pituitary adenomas may develop anywhere along the migration pathway of Rathke's pouch including sphenoid sinus or third ventricle *(10)*. The IHC for anterior pituitary hormones can identify these tumors as pituitary adenomas.

IMMUNOHISTOCHEMISTRY FOR SUBCLASSIFYING PITUITARY ADENOMAS

Immunohistochemistry coupled with transmission electron microscopy forms the basis for subclassifying pituitary adenomas into approximately 13 subtypes. As

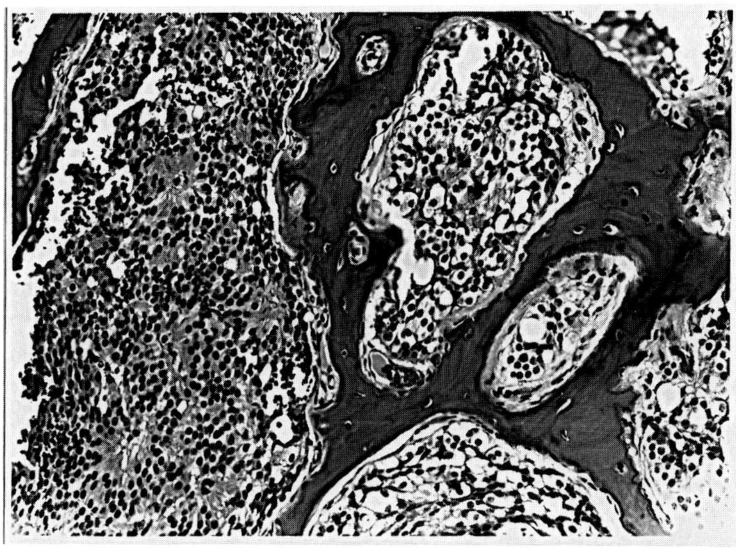

Fig. 7. When pituitary adenomas invade and/or present in the sphenoid sinus, or are ectopic in this location, diagnosis on morphologic grounds can be corroborated by immunohistochemical staining for anterior pituitary hormones. Note the boney trabeculae of the sphenoid sinus completely surrounded by this adenoma with focal clear-cell morphology. (H&E, original magnification × 350.)

noted in the introduction, such subclassification is of great interest in delineating origin of these tumors and correlating with patient presentation and serum hormone values *(1,2,8)*. Immunohistochemistry is a "static" marker for hormonal production, however, and says little about secretory rate for the hormone. Although in general, the intensity of the immunohistochemical staining for intracellular hormone product in pituitary adenomas correlates fairly well with the serum hormone values, tumor size and secretion parameters of hormone are also important variables. In the case of TSH-secreting adenomas for example, the immunohistochemical staining for TSH may be very weak and patchy, whereas staining for the α-subunit is much stronger; nevertheless, the patient demonstrates serum elevation of TSH. Presumably in such cases the TSH is rapidly secreted by the adenoma and little remains intracytoplasmically at any given time. Even more commonly, patchy or weak immunostaining is demonstrated for gonadotrophic hormones and minimal serum abnormalities of these hormones are found, suggesting secretion is slow and/or insufficient to raise plasma levels. Immunohistochemical staining furthermore is inhomogeneous throughout many pituitary adenomas, especially gonadotrophic adenomas *(8)*. Hence, if one is correlating immunohistochemical results done on paraffin-embedded histologic sections with hormone production in tissue culture samples taken from small areas of the tumor, there may be differences.

Several standard reference works *(2,7,11)* have detailed descriptions of the adenoma subtypes based on both immunohistochemistry and transmission electron microscopy (EM) and the classification is reproduced in Table 1. Whereas IHC alone classifies most adenomas into subtypes, for identifying some variants, EM is essential. This is particularly true in tumors of the GH/PRL line, such as the mixed GH-PRL adenoma vs the acidophil stem-cell or mammosomatotroph adenoma. Use of EM in plurihormonal adenomas helps to determine whether the plurihormonal secretion is arising from one or more cell types. Rare, silent corticotroph adenoma subtypes also necessitate EM to classify them into one of the three subtypes. In contrast, for most of the other subtypes of pituitary adenoma, EM largely supplements what is already strongly suspected based on IHC.

Whereas most series list prolactin-cell adenomas as the most frequent adenoma subtype, the advent of bromocriptine and nonsurgical treatment has greatly reduced the incidence of pure prolactinomas that come to the neurosurgeon or pathologist. The majority of prolactinomas are sparsely granulated and immunoreactive diffusely throughout the tumor for prolactin (Fig. 8). Null-cell adenomas have supplanted prolactinomas as the most frequent subtype of surgically removed adenomas. Perhaps better called nonsecretory or weakly secretory adenomas, some authors further subdivide null-cell adenomas into the oncocytic and nononcocytic types based on the number of mitochondria demonstrated by EM *(8)*. Mitochondria content, however, represents a spectrum and no specific number of mitochondria has been established to distinguish between these two subtypes of nonsecretory adenomas. When IHC is done on null-cell adenomas, many have scanty or very irregularly distributed immunoreactivity for FSH, LH, α-subunit, or TSH. By tissue culture studies, some null-cell adenomas secrete gonadotrophins *(13)*. Such findings suggest the presence of a spectrum between gonadotrophic adenomas and many null-cell adenomas, with distinction between the two based on clinical data and intensity of IHC staining, not on the histogenesis of the tumor.

The third most frequent type of pituitary adenoma is the GH-cell adenoma. There are roughly equal numbers of dense and sparsely granulated types. Interestingly, many GH-cell adenomas stain for α-subunit and a few for TSH, although hyperthyroidism is infrequent with such tumors *(8,14)*. The sparsely granulated GH adenomas can show very scanty immunopositivity for GH, again illustrating the fact that despite clinical acromegaly and elevated serum hormone levels, the immunostaining on tissue can be deceptively minimal. Coexpression of prolactin is seen in many growth hormone adenomas; bimodal tumors with two cell populations are quite common, whereas secretion of both hormones by the same cell type is seen only with the uncommon acidophil stem-cell or mammosomatotroph adenomas.

Corticotrophic adenomas generally secrete only ACTH (or other portions of the precursor ACTH molecule such as lipotropin/melanotropin, or beta-endorphin [*14*]), although occasional ACTH-producing adenomas may also make α-subunit, prolactin, or LH *(8,14)* (Fig. 9). Usually, the immunoreactivity for the additional hormone is very patchy and restricted. Infrequently, ACTH-immunoreactive pituitary adenomas may be unassociated with elevated serum ACTH levels or Cushing's disease and are designated "silent corticotroph adenomas." Three subtypes of these silent ACTH adenomas are distinguished on clinical or ultrastructural features *(8,12)*.

Functioning gonadotroph cell adenomas blend imperceptibly by light microscopy and immunohistochemical staining with the null-cell (nonsecretory group), although by definition serum hormone levels for FSH, LH, or α-subunit are elevated. Since elevations in serum FSH or LH can occur normally in older men and, especially, older postmenopausal women who do not have pituitary adenomas, these can be dif-

Table 1
Classification and Incidence of Surgically Removed Pituitary Adenomas

Type	*Frequency, %*
PRL-cell adenoma	20–30
GH-cell adenoma[a]	5
Densely granulated	3
Sparsely granulated	2
Mixed GH-cell/PRL-cell adenoma[a]	5
Mammosomatotroph-cell adenoma[a]	1
Acidophilic stem-cell adenoma[a]	2
Plurihormonal adenoma[a] (largely GH-PRL-TSH)	15
ACTH-cell adenoma	10–15
Endocrinologically active	13
Cushing's syndrome	12
Nelson's syndrome	1
Endocrinologically silent	2
FSH/LH-cell adenoma	10–15
TSH-cell adenoma	1
Null-cell adenoma	20
Nononcocytic	15
Oncocytic	5
Unclassified adenoma	1

GH, growth hormone; PRL, prolactin; FSH, follicle-stimulating hormone; LH, leuteinizing hormone; TSH, thyroid-stimulating hormone.

[a]Collectively, growth hormone producing tumors comprise 20–25% of all pituitary adenomas, plurihormonal adenomas being the principal subtype.

Used with permission from ref. *11a*.

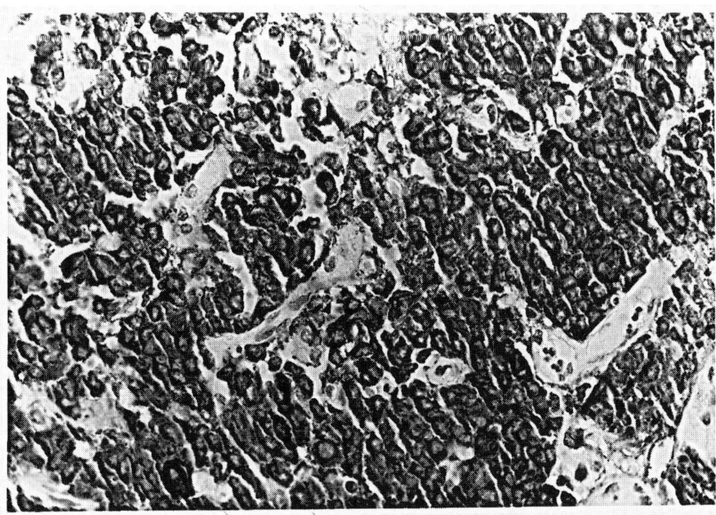

Fig. 8. Most prolactinomas are diffusely immunoreactive throughout the tumor for prolactin. Peroxidase-antiperoxidase technique for prolactin (original magnification × 350).

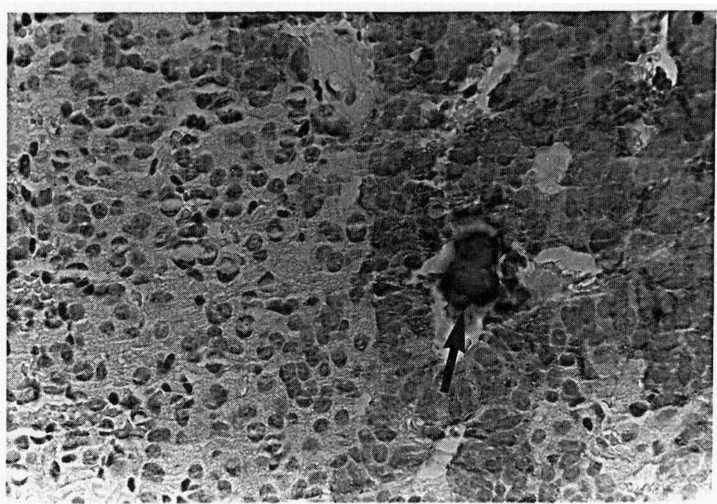

Fig. 9. Many pituitary adenomas display more patchy immunoreactivity for hormones; this chromophobic corticotrophic pituitary adenoma removed from a 48-yr-old man showed focal immunoreactivity for alpha-subunit (at right) in 10% of the adenoma tissue. The majority of the adenoma showed the sheet-like pattern seen at the left of the photograph, which was negative for alpha-subunit (as illustrated), but positive for ACTH (not shown). Also note the unusual feature of microcalcification in an adenoma (arrow). Peroxidase–antiperodixase technique for alpha-subunit (original magnification × 350).

ficult markers to utilize to screen for gonadotroph adenomas. Elevation of α-subunit in the serum is more commonly utilized as a marker for such tumors *(15)*. The TSH producing pituitary adenomas are the least common hypersecretory type. Coexistence of TSH-immunoreactive cells in GH-cell adenomas, null-cell adenomas, or plurihormonal adenomas is more frequent than pure TSH secreting adenomas.

Plurihormonal adenomas are being recognized more frequently than was once appreciated, owing to the increasing sensitivity of immunocytochemical methods. These generally have only one or two of the multiple hormones secreted in sufficient quantity to cause elevated serum hormone levels or clinical syndromes. Many in fact have a minimal hypersecretory state associated with them. The coexistent hormones are usually growth hormone, prolactin, α-subunit, FSH, and LH. Such a degree of plurihormonality is not seen with ACTH adenomas. This coexistence of the GH/prolactin and gonadotrophic line in the same adenoma raises interesting questions about the common origin or mode of differentiation in this group of anterior pituitary cells.

To summarize, IHC has greatly enhanced our understanding of the origin and diversity of pituitary adenomas. As more chemical agonists and antagonists become available, there may be even greater influence of this subclassification schema on medical therapy for pituitary adenomas, either primary or postoperative residual disease. Whereas subclassification by immunohistochemistry does not correlate well with adenoma invasiveness or metastatic potential (pituitary carcinoma), recognition that some subtypes of adenomas are particularly indolent or aggressive in their growth pattern *(16)* may more widely influence decisions in the future regarding external beam radiotherapy.

IMMUNOHISTOCHEMISTRY IN INVESTIGATIVE STUDIES

The development of IHC antibodies to various growth factors, transcription factors, and oncoproteins has led to a number of preliminary studies on the expression of these proteins in pituitary adenomas. Whereas this list will already be out of date by publication, many of the proteins important in systemic tumors have been investigated in pituitary adenomas, largely in an attempt to correlate biological behavior with some histochemical marker. As noted above, the microscopic appearance and hormonal content of pituitary adenomas correlates poorly with tumor invasiveness, growth rate, and/or metastatic potential. Hence it was hoped that other predictive markers could be found.

Raghavan et al. evaluated the oncoprotein products *fos*, *jun*, and *myc* of the c-*fos*, c-*jun*, and c-*myc* genes, and compared immunoreactivity in pituitary adenomas with an in vitro index of cell proliferation, Ki-67 *(17)*. Also used as indicators of biological aggressiveness were the radiographic appearances of the tumor, especially bony erosion. They found that oncoprotein immunoreactivity was present in 32 of 33 cases studied, but noted that it did not correspond to the type of hormone secreted, the degree of bony erosion, or the labeling index of the tumors *(17)*. Takino et al. looked at the purine binding factor nm23 gene expression in pituitary adenomas; previous work had shown reduced expression of the gene in highly metastatic melanoma cell lines. These investigators looked at both H1 and H2 isoform expression using a ribonuclease protection assay and immunohistochemistry. The nm23 H2 messenger RNA expression was significantly reduced in invasive tumors and correlated strongly with cavernous sinus invasion, but sequencing of the nm23 gene did not reveal a mutation. Immunohistochemical staining for nm23 H2 was very reduced in invasive tumors, whereas nm23 H2 was highly expressed in noninvasive ones; expression was thought to have a dampening effect on aggressive tumor behavior *(18)*. Pei et al. investigated 17 patients with pituitary tumors for a loss of heterozygosity of the retinoblastoma susceptibility gene. All 13 of the 17 malignant/highly invasive adenomas showed RB-allelic loss, although immunohistochemical staining revealed the presence of RB protein, suggesting that another tumor suppressor gene on chromosome 13q other than RB may be important for pituitary tumor progression in humans *(19)*. Investigation of neural-cell adhesion molecule expression (NCAM) in pituitary adenomas showed no correlation between immunostaining for NCAM and tumor aggressiveness *(20)*.

Other proteins investigated via immunohistochemical staining, albeit not specifically with intent to correlate with tumor aggressiveness, include transforming growth factor-α *(21)*, endothelin *(22)*, peptidylglycine α-amidating monooxygenase (PAM) *(23)*, epidermal growth factor *(24)*, epidermal growth factor receptor *(24)*, and oncoprotein erbB-2 *(24)*, fibronectin *(25)*, p53 protein *(26)*, and Pit-1 protein *(27)*.

REFERENCES

1. Miller DC. Histopathologic evaluation of pituitary tumors: Help for the clinician in diagnosis and management of pituitary adenomas. In: Cooper PR, ed. Contemporary Diagnosis and Management of Pituitary Adenomas. American Association of Neurological Surgeons Publication, Park Ridge, IL, 1991, pp. 37–52.

2. Burger PC, Scheithauer BW, Vogel FS. Region of the Sella Turcica. In: Surgical Pathology of the Nervous System and its Coverings. 3rd ed., Churchill Livingstone, New York, 1981, pp. 503–568.
3. Kovacs K, Horvath E. Tumors of the pituitary gland. Atlas of Tumor Pathology. Second Series, Armed Forces Institute of Pathology, Washington, DC, 1986, pp. 90, 128.
4. Rush S, Newall J. Concepts in integrating radiotherapy into pituitary tumor management. In: Cooper PR, ed. Contemporary Diagnosis and Management of Pituitary Adenomas. American Association of Neurological Surgeons, Park Ridge, IL, 1991, pp. 151–164.
5. Boenisch T. Bone Immunohistochemistry. In: Naish SJ, ed. Handbook of Immunohistochemical Staining Methods. Dako Corporation, Carpinteria, CA, 1989, pp. 7,8.
6. Shi S-R, Key ME, Kalra, KL. Antigen retrieval in formalin-fixed, paraffin-embedded tissues: an enhancement method for immunohistochemical staining based on microwave oven heating of tissue sections. J Histochem Cytochem 1991; 39:741–748.
7. Rosai J. Special techniques in surgical pathology. In: Rosai J, ed. Ackerman's Surgical Pathology. Mosby, St. Louis, MO, 1989, pp. 31–51.
8. Stefaneau L, Kovacs K. Light microscopic special stains and immunochemistry. In: Lloyd RV, ed. The Diagnostic of Pituitary Adenomas in Surgical Pathology of the Pituitary Gland. Saunders, Philadelphia, PA, 1993, pp. 34–51.
9. Pahlman S, Esscher T, Nitsson K. Expression of "subunit of enolase, neuron-specific enolase in human non-neuroendocrine tumors and derived cell lines. Lab Invest 1986; 54:554–560,
10. Juneau P, Schoene WC, Black P. Malignant tumors in the pituitary gland. Arch Neurol 1992; 49:555–558.
11. Kleinschmidt-DeMasters BK, Winston KR, Rubinstein D, Samuels MH. Ectopic pituitary adenoma of the third ventricle. Case report. J Neurosurg 1990; 72:139–142.

11a. Burger PC, Scheithauer BW, Vogel FS. Surgical Pathology of the Nervous System And Its Coverings. Churchill Livingstone, New York, 1991.

12. Asa SL, Gerrie SM, Singer W, Horvath E, Kovacs K, Smyth HS. Gonadotrophin secretion in vitro by human pituitary null cell adenomas and oncocytomas. J Clin Endocrinol Metab 1986; 62:1011–1019.
13. Furahata S, Kameya T, Tsuruta T, Naritaka TH, Toya S. Colocalization of growth hormone (GH) and glycoprotein subunit alpha in GH-producing pituitary adenomas in acromegalic patients. Acta Neuropathol 1994; 87:568–571.
14. Charpin C, Hassoun J, Oliver C, Jaquet P, Argemi B, Grisoli F, Toga M. Immunohistochemical and immunoelectron-microscopic study of pituitary adenomas associated with Cushing's disease. A report of 13 cases. Am J Pathol 1982; 109:1–7.
15. Demura R, Jibiki K, Kubo O, Odagiri E, Demura H, Kitamura K, Shizume K. The significance of alpha subunit as a tumor marker for gonadotropin producing pituitary adenomas. J Clin Endocrinol Metab 1986; 63:564–569.
16. Kovalic JJ, Mazoujian G, McKeel DW, Fineberg BB, Grigsby PW. Immunohistochemistry as a predictor of clinical outcome in patients given postoperative radiation for subtotally resected pituitary adenomas. J Neuro Oncol 1993; 16:227–232.
17. Raghavan R, Harrison D, Ince PG, James RA, Daniels M, Birch P, Caldwell GI, Kendall-Taylor P. Oncoprotein immunoreactivity in human pituitary tumours. Clin Endocrinol 1994; 40:117–126.
18. Takino H, Herman V, Weiss M, Melmed S. Purine-binding factor (nm23) gene expression in pituitary tumors: marker of adenoma invasiveness. J Clin Endocrinol Metab 1995; 80:1733–1738.
19. Pei L, Melmed S, Scheithauer B, Kovacs K, Benedict WF, Prager D. Frequent loss of heterozygosity at the retinoblastoma susceptibility gene (RB) locus in aggressive pituitary tumors: evidence for a chromosome 13 tumor suppressor gene other than RB. Cancer Res 1995; 55:1613–1616.
20. Kleinschmidt-DeMasters BK, Conway D, Franklin WA, Lillehei KO, Kruse C. Neural cell adhesion molecule expression in human pituitary adenomas. J Neuro Oncol 1995; 25:205–213.
21. Ezzat S, Walpola IA, Ramyar L, Smyth HS, and Asa SL. Membrane-anchored expression of transforming growth factor-alpha in human pituitary adenoma cells. J Clin Endocrinol Metab 1995; 80:534–539.
22. Lange M, Pagotto U, Hopfner U, Ehrenreich H, Oeckler R, Sinowatz F, Stalla GK. Endothelin expression in normal human anterior pituitaries and pituitary adenomas. J. Clin. Endocrind. Metab. 1994; 79:1864–1870.
23. Steel JH, Martinez A, Springall DR, Treston AM, Cuttitta F, Polak JM. Peptidylglycine α-amidating monooxygenase (PAM) immunoreactivity and messenger RNA in human pituitary and increased expression in pituitary tumors. Cell Tissue Res 1994; 276:197–207.
24. Chaidarun SS, Eggo MC, Sheppard MC, Stewart PM. Expression of epidermal growth factor (EGF), its receptor, and related oncoprotein *erbB-2* in human pituitary tumors and response to EGF *in vitro*. Endocrinology 1994; 135:2012–2021.

25. Farnoud MR, Farhadian F, Samuel JL, Derome P, Peillon F, and Li JY. Fibronectin isoforms are differentially expressed in normal and adenomatous human anterior pituitaries. Int J Cancer 1995; 61:27–34.
26. Levy A, Hall L, Yeudall WA, Lightman SL. p53 gene mutations in pituitary adenomas: rare events. Clin Endocrinol 1994; 41:809–814.
27. Asa SL, Puy LA, Lew AM, Sundmark VC, Elsholtz HP. Cell type-specific expression of the pituitary transcription activator Pit-1 in the human pituitary and pituitary adenomas. J Clin Endocrinol Metab 1993; 77:1275-1280.

Index

H

I

R

S

T

V

Z